HEALTH COMMUNICATION

FROM THEORY TO PRACTICE

Second Edition

Renata Schiavo

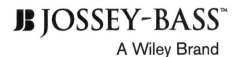

JOSSEY-BASS™

A Wiley Brand

Cover design: JPuda
Cover image : © Pixman/Imagezoo/Getty

Published by Jossey-Bass
A Wiley Brand
One Montgomery Street, Suite 1200, San Francisco, CA 94104-4594—www.josseybass.com

Limit of Liability/Disclaimer of Warranty: While the publisher and author have used their best
efforts in preparing this book, they make no representations or warranties with respect to the
accuracy or completeness of the contents of this book and specifically disclaim any implied
warranties of merchantability or fitness for a particular purpose. No warranty may be created or
extended by sales representatives or written sales materials. The advice and strategies contained
herein may not be suitable for your situation. You should consult with a professional where
appropriate. Neither the publisher nor author shall be liable for any loss of profit or any other
commercial damages, including but not limited to special, incidental, consequential, or other
damages. Readers should be aware that Internet websites offered as citations and/or sources for
further information may have changed or disappeared between the time this was written and
when it is read.

Jossey-Bass books and products are available through most bookstores. To contact Jossey-Bass
directly call our Customer Care Department within the U.S. at 800-956-7739, outside the U.S. at
317-572-3986, or fax 317-572-4002.

Wiley publishes in a variety of print and electronic formats and by print-on-demand. Some
material included with standard print versions of this book may not be included in e-books or in
print-on-demand. If this book refers to media such as a CD or DVD that is not included in the
version you purchased, you may download this material at http://booksupport.wiley.com. For
more information about Wiley products, visit www.wiley.com.

Library of Congress Cataloging-in-Publication Data
Schiavo, Renata, author.
   Health communication : from theory to practice / Renata Schiavo.—Second edition.
      pages cm.—(Jossey-Bass public health ; 217)
      Includes bibliographical references and index.
   ISBN 978-1-118-12219-8 (pbk.)—ISBN 978-1-118-41912-0 (pdf)—
ISBN 978-1-118-41639-6 (epub)
   1. Communication in medicine—United States. 2. Health promotion—United States. 3. Health
planning—United States. I. Title
   R118.S33 2014
   610.1′4—dc23
                                                                    2013025596

Printed in the United States of America
SECOND EDITION
HB Printing   10 9 8 7 6 5 4 3 2

CONTENTS

TABLES, FIGURES, EXHIBITS, AND NUMBERED BOXES

Tables

Figures

Exhibits

Numbered Boxes

For my wonderful daughters and husband,

Oriana, Talia, and Roger

Many colleagues and professionals from a variety of sectors have approached me since the first edition of *Health Communication: From Theory to Practice* was published in 2007. The book has often provided us with a framework and incentive to share information about our experiences and discuss many topics as they relate to society, health, and communication. Of great importance has also been the feedback of the many faculty members and students (including my own students) who have used the book as part of their courses in academic programs across the United States and around the world. I am thankful to all for contributing to my thinking and professional growth. Their input, suggestions, and our many conversations are among the main reasons for this second edition.

Other motivating factors for this second edition include health communication's own evolution, technological advances, and the need to capture recent experiences and theories that may have been less highlighted in the first edition. This second edition further emphasizes the importance of a people-centered and participatory approach to health communication interventions, which should take into account key social determinants of health and the interconnection among various health and social fields. While maintaining a strong focus on the importance of the behavioral, social, and organizational results of health communication interventions, this book also includes new or updated information, theoretical models, resources, and case studies on health equity, urban health, new media, emergency and risk communication, strategic partnerships in health communication, policy communication and public advocacy, cultural competence, health literacy, and the evaluation of health communication interventions as they relate to various health topics.

Finally, I myself have evolved as I am fortunate to continue to learn from my work and from the many people I have the pleasure to work with. My voice has become stronger in favor of health communication approaches that will encourage participation and community ownership of the overall communication process, yet will let people decide how much, when, and how to participate based on their cultural preferences. I also became increasingly connected to the reason I do this work: to make a difference in people's health and lives. My appreciation of the many challenges of disadvantaged groups has also grown along with my work, and has influenced my sense of urgency in encouraging people to switch from a disease-focused mind-set to a health communication approach that links health with related social, political, and environmental issues, while keeping a strong commitment to behavioral and social impact.

Put the public back in public health. Think globally, act locally. Tackle health disparities. These are not just catchy phrases. They are some of the principles that have been inspiring my work and this book.

ACKNOWLEDGMENTS

As for all projects that are in the making for a long time, this second edition is inspired by many people and is the fruit of years of thinking and work for which I am indebted to many colleagues. First and foremost, my heartfelt thanks go to my editors, Andy Pasternack and Seth Schwartz of Jossey-Bass, for their invaluable help and expert guidance with the many questions related to this project, as well as for their great support, cheers, and much-appreciated commitment to seeing things through. I could not have made it without them!

Thanks to Joshua Bernstein, Erin Driver, Rachel Gonzales, John Kowalczyk, Doris J. Laird, and C. J. Schumaker for their comments and feedback on the second edition revision plan and David Anderson, Ellen Bonaguro, Kathy Miller, and Mario Nacinovich for the invaluable suggestions that have considerably contributed to the significance of this second edition. Their helpful feedback was provided via Jossey-Bass's peer review process. My appreciation also goes to all professional friends and colleagues who provided suggestions on early drafts of the first and this second edition, or helped secure relevant case studies and interviews that are published here. Among them are Doug Arbesfeld, Susan Blake, Joe Casey, Lenore Cooney, Amanda Crowe, Gustavo Cruz, Chris Elias, Everold Hosein, Marina Komarecki, Destin Laine, Rafael Obregon, Sherry Michelstein, Elil Renganathan, and Lisa Weiss. Thank you also to the many authors of the case studies published in this book for their generosity, time, and willingness to contribute to this project. I am very grateful to Radhika Ramesh, a graduate of the New York University master's program in media, culture, and communication, as well as a former student and a colleague, who worked as a research and editorial assistant for this second edition, for her dedication and attention to detail. Also, my thanks go to Ohemaa Boahemaa who helped with the graphic design of many of the figures included in this book and managed to fit this in her busy schedule. Thanks to Prarthana Shukla who was a research assistant for the first edition and to other former public health students who have contributed feedback, most notably Lawrence Fung and Ellen Sowala, as well as other students and colleagues who used the book's first edition and provided suggestions for changes.

Thank you to colleagues from New York University and the CUNY School of Public Health at Hunter College, to whom I owe my academic and teaching experience: Marilyn Auerbach, Jo Ivey Boufford, Jessie Daniels, Nicholas Freudenberg, Sally Guttmacher, Susan Klitzman, James Macinko, and Kenneth Olden. Thanks also to the many other colleagues from either of these two institutions, with whom I have had many conversations on society, health, and communication or worked closely on different projects. Most noticeably, May May Leung, for her professionalism, graciousness, and sense of humor; Marcia Thomas and Lorna Thorpe, for our periodic lunch meetings and their professional friendship; and Jack Caravanos, Paula Gardner, Judith Gilbride, Barbara Glickstein, Lydia Isaac, Heidi Jones, Diana Mason, Khursheed Navder, Stacey Plitcha, Lynn Roberts, Diana Romero, Yumari Ruiz, Arlene Spark, and Christina Zarcadoolas. And a special thank-you to Sally Guttmacher, who encouraged me to write this book at the time of its first edition. I also want to acknowledge colleagues from Columbia University, James Colgrove, Leah Hopper, Lisa Melsch, and Marita Murrman, for the opportunity to start teaching in fall 2013 at the Mailman School of Public Health and their support as I get started. I look forward to our partnership.

There are many people to whom I owe my practical experience in health communication and related fields. These include the colleagues, partners, and clients with whom I have had the privilege to work over the years. I spent endless days (and nights) with many of them brainstorming and learned a great deal from all of them. The task of naming them all is quite daunting, so please forgive me if I do not mention someone who greatly contributed to my work or thinking over the years. A short list of colleagues with whom I have had the pleasure to work just in the last decade includes Upal Basu Roy, Ohemaa Bohaemaa, Patricia Buckley, Joe Casey, Paula Claycomb, Lenore Cooney, Samantha Cranko, Blake Crawford, Amanda Crowe, Gustavo Cruz, Isabel Estrada-Portales, Rina Gill, Matilde Gonzalez-Flores, Elena Hoeppner, Everold Hosein, Neha Kapil, Scott Kennedy, John London, Alka Mansukhani, LaJoy Mosby, Asiya Odugleh-Kolev, Lene Odum Jensen, Denisse Ormaza, Radhika Ramesh, Akiko Sakaedani Petrovic, Barbara Shapiro, Glenn Silver, Teresa (Tess) Stuart, Kate Tulenko, Marie-Noelle Vieu, Beth Waters, Jennifer Weiss, Lisa Weiss, and Sabriya Williams. And a special thank-you to past colleagues Daniel Berman and Frances Beves for their friendship of many years, and our many brainstorms.

I also want to acknowledge colleagues from *Cases in Public Health Communication and Marketing, Journal of Communication in Healthcare,* and *The Nation's Health*: Lorien Abroms, Samantha Ashton, Susan Blake,

Michelle Late, Craig Lefebvre, Esme Loukota, Ed Maibach, Kimberly Martin, Mario Nacinovich, Mark Simon, and Charlotte Tucker. Thank you all for the opportunity to help shape the content or direction of these publications that make such a great contribution to important health communication topics.

These acknowledgments wouldn't be complete without recognizing the role of the American Public Health Association (APHA) Health Communication Working Group (HCWG) of the Public Health Education and Health Promotion (PHEHP) section in my professional life. Not only has HCWG provided me with a home within the APHA but it has also given me the opportunity to enrich my experience and to network with many great colleagues, including those with whom I have had the pleasure of working closely on various HCWG activities: Gary Black, Marla Clayman, Rebecca (Becky) Cline, Carol Girard, Marian Hunman, Julia Kish Doto, Jennifer Manganello, Judith (Jude) McDivitt, John Ralls, Doug Rupert, J-J Sheu, Julie Tu Payiatas, Carin Upstill, and Meg Young. Thanks also to PHEHP colleagues Heather Brandt, Michelle Chuck, Regina Galer-Unti, Jeff Hallam, Stuart Usdan, and Katherine Wilson for their support on various projects in which I have been involved either with the HCWG or the PHEHP section.

My thanks to all people mentioned here—and to the ones whom I may have inadvertently omitted or with whom I worked prior to the last ten years, and I could not mention for space-related reasons—for contributing to my work and thinking. Also, thank you to all professionals in different parts of the world who have been championing and helping advance the field of health communication with their innovative and strategic thinking, creativity, and commitment.

Finally, many thanks to my husband, Roger Ullman, for his endless support and lifetime partnership, and to our daughters, Oriana and Talia, for inspiring my work ethics and life. And to my mother, Amalia Ronchi, who despite our differences, taught me perhaps the most important lesson in life: care about others and try to understand them. This lesson is also important in health communication.

In Memory of Andy Pasternack

"Hello from Jossey-Bass!" This is how I remember my first interaction with Andy. He had learned from one of Jossey-Bass' sales representatives that I was thinking to write a book on health communication and was emailing to talk and learn more about my idea. I didn't know at the time how much this was typical of Andy and his entrepreneurial spirit.

Andy was really passionate about providing new resources on what he believed to be important topics that may help advance people's work. He was proud of the fact that "authors preferred to work with Jossey-Bass" and was committed to creating a supportive environment that would be conducive to that. He cared about "his" authors and wanted to see them succeed in their professional endeavors. Always kind and cheerful, Andy loved to connect people, talked very fondly of his family and staff, and knew how to make things happen. His patience and encouragement were critical to my efforts to write this book . . . and I can't believe that he was corresponding with me about the back cover just a few weeks before his departure. Our professional community owes gratitude to Andy for his vision and professionalism. We will miss him.

THE AUTHOR

Renata Schiavo, PhD, MA, is a health and international communication, public health, and global health specialist with more than twenty years of experience in a variety of settings, including the United States and several countries in Europe, Latin America, and Africa. Currently, she is founding president and CEO of Health Equity Initiative, a nonprofit organization dedicated to building community, capacity, and strategic communication resources for health equity. Dr. Schiavo is also a senior lecturer, Columbia University Mailman School of Public Health, and has held academic appointments at the CUNY School of Public Health at Hunter College and New York University's MPH program.

Dr. Schiavo is a member of the board of directors, Public Health Foundation Enterprise (PHFE); a member of the Cultural Competence Interest Group of the New York Academy of Medicine (NYAM); and a member of the Steering Committee of the American Public Health Association (APHA) PHEPH Health Communication Working Group (HCWG), for which she also served as 2007–2008 chair. She serves on the advisory board of *The Nation's Health* (the APHA's official newspaper), as well as the editorial boards of *Cases in Public Health Communication and Marketing* and *Journal of Communication in Healthcare*. Among other international affiliations, Dr. Schiavo is a member of the UNICEF Communication for Development (C4D) Global Web Roster; the World Health Organization's Global Technical Network for Communication for Behavioral Impact (COMBI); and the Italian group Salute-Cura-Societa' (SaCS-Health-Cure-Society).

Dr. Schiavo is the author of dozens of publications in the health communication, public health, and global health fields. She has recognized international expertise in twenty-plus public health, global health, and social development areas, and has served on scientific, expert, and review panels for leading organizations, including the World Health Organization [WHO], the National Institutes of Health, and the American Public Health Association. Her work has been supported by the Office of Minority Health Resource Center, HHS Office of Minority Health; UNICEF; and WHO, among others.

Dr. Schiavo's professional interests lie at the intersection of strategic health communication for behavioral, social, and organizational change; multisectoral partnerships; health equity; community health; risk communication; and global health. Her recent work has focused on health equity–health disparities and social determinants of health, maternal and child health, public health and humanitarian emergencies, pandemic flu, global hand washing, childhood cancer, and malaria, among others. She has significant experience on strategy design; research design and implementation; program design, direction, and evaluation; and professional development, capacity building, and training.

Prior to founding Health Equity Initiative, Dr. Schiavo had the pleasure of serving as associate professor and director, Community Health/COMHE at the CUNY School of Public Health at Hunter College; founder and principal, Strategic Communication Resources; executive vice president, Cooney Waters Group; and head, corporate and marketing communications and social responsibility programs, Rhodia Farma-Brazil. Her recent consulting experience includes leading organizations such as the National Association of Pediatric Nurse Practitioners (NAPNAP); New York University College of Dentistry; the Office of Minority Health Resource Center, HHS Office of Minority Health; Solving Kids' Cancer; UNICEF; the World Bank; and the World Health Organization.

Renata has significant management experience, because in addition to current positions, she also served on the boards of directors of Solving Kids' Cancer and the Italian American Committee on Education, and was an elected voting member of the governing council of the American Public Health Association. Early in her career, Dr. Schiavo was a postdoctoral research scientist at Columbia University and New York University, where she worked on numerous molecular and cell biology projects. She holds a PhD in biological sciences from the University of Naples (Italy) and an MA in journalism and mass communication from New York University.

For additional information on Renata Schiavo's background and experience, visit www.renataschiavo.com.

Health communication operates within a very complex environment in which encouraging and supporting people to adopt and sustain healthy behaviors, or policymakers and professionals to introduce new policies and practices, or health care professionals to provide adequate and culturally competent care are never easy tasks. Moreover, most of these potential changes and behavioral and social results depend on various socially determined factors such as our living, working, and aging environments; access to health services and information; adequate transportation, nutritious food, parks and recreational facilities; socioeconomic opportunities; and social and peer support, among many others.

Childhood immunization, for example, is one of the greatest medical and scientific successes of recent times. Because of immunization, many diseases that were once a threat to the life and well-being of children have become rare or have been eradicated in many countries in the world. Yet as for most other health-related issues and interventions, changing public and professional minds and enabling parents to immunize their healthy children have required a worldwide multidisciplinary effort. Health communication has played a fundamental role in this success story since the introduction of the first childhood vaccine. Consider the case of Bonnie, the mother of a newborn child, who is offered a vaccine for her baby at birth or a few days after.

Bonnie, an American, is the twenty-five-year-old mother of a beautiful baby girl. She is thrilled about her child but quite fearful because parenting is new to her. She has read about the benefits of immunization but is too young to remember any of the diseases against which she should immunize her child. She does not know anyone who had polio or whooping cough or Hib (*Haemophilus influenzae* type B) disease. She has also heard conflicting information about the potential adverse events or risks that may be associated with immunization and is unsure about which of the available information is correct. She is confused and does not know whether she wants to immunize her child.

Bonnie's case is a typical example of issues that health communication interventions can successfully address:

- Engaging Bonnie, her peers, and her community in discussing their perceptions and opinions about the pros and cons of immunization as well as any barriers, social norms, or other socially determined factors that may influence their decisions

- Providing Bonnie with research-based and reliable information on immunization

- Encouraging participation of Bonnie, her peers, other community members, and professionals across sectors in developing a communication intervention that would address existing barriers to immunization, and effectively integrate the opinions, preferences, and needs of parents and other key groups and stakeholders

- Improving Bonnie's communication with her pediatrician or health care provider by empowering her with information and questions to ask at clinical encounters

- Raising awareness among health care providers of patients' needs and most frequent concerns, and equipping them with training and resources on cross-cultural health communication, health literacy, and health disparities

- Developing tools such as brochures, posters, web pages, and other informational vehicles from reputable sources that will reinforce the information Bonnie will hear from her health care provider

- Encouraging peer-to-peer support by establishing venues, events, and social media–based forums where new mothers can discuss immunization and be supported on their decisions

- Raising awareness of the impact of vaccine-preventable childhood diseases and benefits of immunization among the general public by targeting consumer media, parenting publications, social media sites, and other vehicles so that Bonnie and other parents can become familiar with the severity of vaccine-preventable diseases and the benefits of immunization

- Advocating for policies, mandates, and other regulations that would increase ease of access to timely immunization, convey the importance of immunization in child and community protection, and also be inclusive of vulnerable and underserved populations as it may relate to their specific needs and concerns

- Addressing socially determined factors (for example, access to or quality of health services and information, education, living and working conditions, and others) that may contribute to low immunization rates in specific segments of the general population

Health communication approaches will work only if they rely on an in-depth understanding of Bonnie's and other new mothers' lifestyles, concerns, beliefs, attitudes, social norms, barriers to change, and sources of information about newborns and immunization. It would also be important to research and understand the cultural, social, and political environment in which Bonnie lives. What kind of support does she get from family, friends, and her working environment? Who most influences her decisions on her child's well-being and upbringing? What does she fear about immunization? Is there any existing program in her community that focuses on childhood immunization? What are the lessons learned? Does she have access to timely immunization? Does she feel satisfied with the way her health care provider communicates on immunization (in other words, does she feel that she can understand and relate to the information her provider discusses)? These are just some of the many questions that need to be answered before developing a health communication program intended to promote behavioral and social change among Bonnie and her peers.

Most important, any kind of health communication intervention needs to be grounded in communication theory and lessons learned from past interventions as well as an in-depth understanding of the full potential of the field of health communication. Communication is considered an important discipline in the attainment of the Millennium Development Goals ("the eight MDGs—which range from halving extreme poverty rates to halting the spread of HIV/AIDS and providing universal primary education, all by the target date of 2015—form a blueprint agreed to by all the world's countries and all the world's leading development institutions" in 2000; United Nations, 2013) as well as the post-2015 global agenda. In fact, health communication can help integrate population, health, and environment-related issues to improve public health and social outcomes in different countries. For example, emerging best practices in health communication in Rwanda have led to the creation of a Population, Health, and Environment (PHE) Network. This newly established East Africa PHE Network is designed to "improve communication about PHE issues among policymakers, researchers, and practitioners within Rwanda and throughout eastern Africa. The PHE Network serves as a forum for information exchange about cross-cutting PHE issues, community networking, accessing resources" and also relies on various traditional communication channels (for example, community-level meetings, participatory planning) and mass and new media (for example, local radio, newspapers, and Internet).

In the United States, *Healthy People 2020*, the country's public health agenda for one decade, has defined several domains for health communication and health information technology, which are listed in the following.

Goal: Use health communication strategies and health information technology (IT) to improve population health outcomes and health care quality, and to achieve health equity.

The objectives in this topic area describe many ways health communication and health IT can have a positive impact on health, health care, and health equity:

- Supporting shared decision making between patients and providers
- Providing personalized self-management tools and resources
- Building social support networks
- Delivering accurate, accessible, and actionable health information that is targeted or tailored
- Facilitating the meaningful use of health IT and exchange of health information among health care and public health professionals
- Enabling quick and informed action to health risks and public health emergencies
- Increasing health literacy skills
- Providing new opportunities to connect with culturally diverse and hard-to-reach populations
- Providing sound principles in the design of programs and interventions that result in healthier behaviors
- Increasing Internet and mobile access

Source: US Department of Health and Human Services. Healthy People 2020. "Health Communication and Health Information Technology." http://healthypeople.gov/2020/topicsobjectives2020/overview.aspx?topicid=18. Retrieved July 2012b.

As you may realize yourself after reading this book, in many ways three of "these areas may encapsulate all others" (Schiavo, 2011b, p. 68): "Building social support networks . . . providing new opportunities to connect with culturally diverse and hard-to-reach populations . . . providing sound principles in the design of programs and interventions that result in healthier behaviors" (*Healthy People 2020*). These areas speak of innovation; the integration of different communication areas, strategies, and media, and health and social issues (after all, there is no magic fix in health communication); the need to include disadvantaged groups and effectively connect with them as part of the communication process; and the importance of making sure that communication is grounded in theoretical models, planning frameworks, and lessons learned from past experiences.

About This Book

Since its first edition in 2007, *Health Communication: From Theory to Practice* has provided students and professionals from the public health, health care, global health, community development, nonprofit, and public and private sectors with a comprehensive introduction to health communication as well as a strategic review of advanced topics and issues that affect the field's theory and practice, and a hands-on guide to planning, implementing, and evaluating health communication interventions. This second edition further emphasizes the importance of a people-centered and participatory approach to health communication interventions, which should take into account key social determinants of health and the interconnection among various health and social fields.

Although maintaining a strong focus on the importance of the behavioral, social, and organizational results of health communication interventions, the second edition also includes new or updated information, theoretical models, resources, and case studies on health equity, urban health, new media, emergency and risk communication, strategic partnerships in health communication, policy communication and public advocacy, cultural competence, health literacy, and the evaluation of health communication interventions as they relate to various health topics.

Who Should Read This Book

There are many people who I hope will read this book and, if willing, share their perspectives and feedback with me in the years to come. The following is only a short list of professionals and health and social change agents for which this book is designed with the intention to help in everyone's efforts to make a difference in people's health and lives.

Academics: If you are a faculty member in a school or program in public health, global health, health communication, community health, communication studies, health education, nursing, environmental health, nutrition, journalism, design for social innovation, medicine, health and life sciences, social work, public affairs, international affairs, or psychology, the multidisciplinary approach to health communication this book proposes will, I hope, complement other theoretical or practical approaches you may be using in your work, and provide you with a helpful didactic tool. I also hope that some of the theoretical concepts, lessons learned, and questions highlighted in this book will be further explored as part of your teaching and research efforts together with your colleagues, students, and relevant communities. The book is designed to fit most course schedules and to meet the needs of a variety of graduate and advanced undergraduate courses.

Students: Because health communication is an integral part of everyday life as well as various interventions for health and social change, I hope that this book will further motivate your interest in this field, and that some of its key concepts will stay with you throughout your career. The book is designed to provide you with some of the theoretical resources and practical skills to address the many challenges of any path you may decide to pursue. It also reflects my teaching philosophy, which is grounded in my commitment to help students develop essential strategic and critical skills, as well as my belief that all courses should be a forum for vibrant information exchange in which I learn from the students' perspectives while they learn from my experience. To this end, this second edition also incorporates the perspectives and suggestions of many of my students who used the first edition.

Health and social change agents: Regardless of whether you work in the public, nonprofit, academic, health care, or private sector, or a multilateral agency, I hope health communication, as described in this book, will complement your efforts to implement interventions that explore the connection between health and social issues, or support the creation of a movement for improved health outcomes and quality of life among different groups and populations, and ultimately promote behavioral, social, and organizational change. I hope that this book will help you achieve your vision.

Program managers: Because this book also includes many practical suggestions and a comprehensive hands-on guide, it is an easy-to-access resource for the development, implementation, and evaluation of health communication interventions, as well as for your training efforts of staff members and relevant partners.

Health care providers: Health communication is an increasingly important competency in provider-patient communication and professional medical communication settings because it is essential to improving patient outcomes and promoting widespread application of best clinical practices. This book covers both communication areas and also includes other relevant topics such as the role of health care providers in public health settings, using IT innovation to address emerging needs and global health workforce gaps, and prioritizing disparities in clinical education via increased training in cross-cultural health communication. These topics are designed to appeal to educators and health care providers in light of the expanded role of clinicians in patient, public health, and global health outcomes.

Community leaders: Although community leaders are by definition health and social change agents, I felt the need to include this specific category given the role communities in the United States and in international settings play or should play in the health communication process. I hope that community leaders from a variety of sectors read this and find it helpful in designing and implementing community-based interventions and forums to raise the influence of community voices on how we communicate about health and illness and the kinds of behavioral, social, and organizational results we seek to achieve.

Finally, one of the book's fundamental premises is the role good health (or lack thereof) plays either positively or negatively in influencing community development and people's ability to connect with socioeconomic opportunities. Because health communication can play a key role in raising awareness of the strong interconnection among these fields, or in advocating for policy and social change, and in promoting healthy behaviors, I certainly hope that colleagues from the community and social development fields will consider this book to be a useful resource on how to communicate about key social determinants of health as well as the influence health issues can have on their work and community and social outcomes.

Overview of the Contents

Two of the fundamental premises of this book are (1) the multidisciplinary and multifaceted nature of health communication and (2) the interdependence of the individual, social, political, and disease-related factors that influence health communication interventions, and, more in general, health and social outcomes. With these premises in mind, the division of topics in parts and chapters is only instrumental to the text's readability and clarity. Readers should always consider the connection among various theoretical and practical aspects of health communication as well as all external factors (political, social, cultural, economic, market, environment, and other influences that shape or contribute to a specific situation or health problem as well as affect key groups and stakeholders) that influence this field. This introduction is an essential part of the book and is instrumental to maximize use and understanding of the text.

This book is divided in four parts. Part One focuses on defining health communication—its theoretical basis as well as its contexts and key action areas. Part One also establishes the importance of considering cultural, geographical, socioeconomic, ethnic, age, and gender influences on people's concepts of health and illness, as well as their approach to health problems and their solutions. Finally, this part addresses the role of health communication in public health, health care, community development, as well as in the marketing or private sector contexts.

Part Two focuses on the different areas of health communication defined in Part One: interpersonal communication, mass media and new media communication; community mobilization and citizen engagement; professional medical communications; constituency relations and strategic partnership in health communication; policy communication, and public advocacy.

In all chapters in Part Two, key health communication issues are raised in the form of a question or brought to life in a case study. This is followed by a discussion of a specific communication approach or area. All chapters discuss specific communication areas in the context of the multidisciplinary nature of health communication and the need for an integrated approach. Special emphasis is placed on the importance of selecting and adapting health communication strategies, activities, materials, media, and channels to a fast-changing social, political, market, and public health environment. Case studies and testimonials from experts and practitioners in the field are included in many of the chapters in Part Two.

Part Three provides a step-by-step guide to the development, implementation, and evaluation of a health communication intervention. Each chapter covers specific steps of the health communication planning process or implementation and evaluation phases. Case studies, practical tips, and specific examples aim to facilitate readers' understanding of the planning process, as well as to build technical skills in health communication planning. Recent methodologies and trends in measuring and evaluating results of health communication programs are explored here, and so are specific strategies and tools to evaluate new media–based interventions.

Part Four examines select health communication case studies and related lessons. This last section of the book includes two chapters, respectively featuring case studies from the United States and global health communication. Yet, as discussed in Chapter Sixteen, and in light of the existing comprehensive definition of *global health*, key themes, emerging trends, and potential lessons that emerged from case studies in both chapters for the most part apply across geographical boundaries and health issues.

Appendix A contains resources and worksheets on health communication planning. Online resources listed in Appendix B point to job listings, conferences, journals, organizations, centers, and programs in the health communication field. The Glossary of key health communication planning terms at the end of the text should be used as a reference while reading this book, as well as a way to recap key definitions in health communication planning. Some of the key terms from the Glossary are highlighted in bold type and briefly defined the first time they are mentioned in the text so that readers can become familiar with them before approaching the chapters in Part Three that more specifically cover these topics. Other topic-specific definitions are included in all relevant chapters.

Many chapters start with a practical example or case study. This is often used to establish the need for communication approaches that should be based on an in-depth understanding of intended audiences' perceptions, beliefs, attitudes, behavior, and barriers to change, as well as the cultural, social, and ethnic context in which they live. Although referring to current theories and models, the book also reinforces the importance of the experience of health communication practitioners in developing theories, models, and approaches that should guide and inform health communication planning and management.

Each chapter ends with discussion questions for readers to reflect on, practice, and implement key concepts. Finally, all chapters are interconnected but are also designed to stand alone and provide a comprehensive overview on the topic they cover. An instructor's training supplement is available at www.josseybass.com/go/schiavo2e. Additional materials such as videos, podcasts, and readings can be found at www.josseybass publichealth.com. Comments about this book are invited and can be sent to publichealth@wiley.com, or via the contact form at www.renataschiavo.com.

Author's Note

As someone who has been spending a lot of time teaching, practicing, and thinking about health communication, I fully understand the complexity of communicating about health, behavior, and related social issues. Changing human and social behavior to attain better health outcomes and positively affect people's quality of life is often a lifetime endeavor, which is also intertwined with our own professional changes. We change, and our work and beliefs may change or evolve over time. In a way, I hope that we never stop questioning ourselves, and learning from professional and personal experiences, because this is the only way to stay true to what we should value the most: making a difference in people's health and lives.

My heartfelt appreciation and admiration go to all professionals, students, patients, policymakers, and ordinary people who every day dedicate their time to make a difference to their own health outcomes or those of their families, communities, special groups, or populations. These include all professionals and researchers in the public health, health care, community development, and urban planning fields; the students or young practitioners who have committed themselves to a rewarding but demanding career; the patients who strive to keep themselves informed and make the right health decisions; the health care providers who dedicate their lives to alleviate and manage human suffering; the urban planners and environmentalists who work to leave to our communities and children the kind of natural and built environments they need to stay healthy; the mass media, new media gurus, government officers, associations, advocacy groups, global health organizations from the public and private sectors, and everyone else who may have an impact on health and social change.

I believe that being aware of current health communication theories and experiences may ease the process of affecting health and social outcomes and make the task more approachable for all of these groups and individuals. I hope this book will help and will give you a glance into my world.

INTRODUCTION TO HEALTH COMMUNICATION

As readers approach Part One, I cannot help but wonder what they may already think or know about health communication. I wish this book had eyes and ears to listen to all of your discussions so I could learn about each one of you. I would love to know how health communication may help advance your professional goals and what you find helpful in achieving the kinds of behavioral, social, and organizational results that may support improved health outcomes in your neighborhoods, communities, and countries. After all, one of the main mantras of health communication is to get to know the groups we seek to engage and care about. This is why I hope that as for the first edition, many of you will write and share your experience with this book.

Part One is the backbone of the book. It focuses on defining health communication—its theoretical basis as well as its contexts and key action areas. It also establishes the importance of cultural, geographical, socioeconomic, ethnic, age, and gender influences on people's concepts of health and illness, as well as their approach to health problems and their solutions. Finally, this part addresses the role of health communication in public health, health care, community development, as well as in the marketing or private sector contexts.

This section is divided into three chapters, which are strictly interconnected in their scope and aim to provide a balanced theoretical and practical introduction to the field. Chapter One introduces readers to health communication, its key contexts and action areas, as well as its cyclical nature and the planning framework that we will discuss in detail in Part Three. Chapter Two provides an overview of key theoretical influences in health communication as well as contemporary health-related and public issues that influence or may influence its theory and practice. The chapter also includes a brief discussion of select planning frameworks and models used for the development of health communication interventions by a variety of US and international organizations. Chapter Three discusses the importance of cultural, ethnic, geographical, gender, age, and other factors in communicating about health and illness with a variety of groups and how communication is influenced by and influences all of these factors. It also provides examples of different concepts of health and illness and establishes cultural competence as a core competency for effective health communication.

Once again, welcome to my world!

CHAPTER 1

WHAT IS HEALTH COMMUNICATION?

Health communication is an evolving and increasingly prominent field in public health, health care, and the non-profit and private sectors. Therefore, many authors and organizations have been attempting to define or redefine it over time. Because of the multidisciplinary nature of health communication, many of the definitions may appear somewhat different from each other. Nevertheless, when they are analyzed, most point to the role that health communication can play in influencing, supporting, and empowering individuals, communities, health care professionals, policymakers, or special groups to adopt and sustain a behavior or a social, organizational, and policy change that will ultimately improve individual, community, and public health outcomes.

Understanding the true meaning of health communication and establishing the right context for its implementation may help communication managers and other public health, community development, and health care professionals identify early on the training needs of staff, the communities they serve, and others who are involved in the communication process. It will also help create the right organizational mind-set and capacity that should lead to a successful use of communication approaches to reach group-, stakeholder-, and community-specific goals.

CHAPTER OBJECTIVES

This chapter sets the stage to discuss current health communication contexts. It also positions the importance of health communication in public health, health care, and community development as well as the nonprofit and private sectors. Finally, it describes key elements, action areas, and limitations of health communication, and introduces readers to "the role societal, organizational, and individual factors" play in influencing and being influenced by public health communication (Association of Schools of Public Health, 2007, p. 5) and communication interventions in clinical (Hospitals and Health Networks, 2012) and other health-related settings.

Defining Health Communication

There are several definitions of health communication, which for the most part share common meanings and attributes. This section analyzes and aims to consolidate different definitions for health communication. This analysis starts from the literal and historical meaning of the word *communication*.

What Is Communication?

An understanding of health communication theory and practice requires reflection on the literal meaning of the word *communication. Communication* is defined in this way: "1. *Exchange of information,* between individuals, for example, by means of speaking, writing, or using a common system of signs and behaviors; 2. *Message*—a spoken or written message; 3. *Act of communicating;* 4. *Rapport*—a sense of mutual understanding and sympathy; 5. *Access*—a means of access or communication, for example, a connecting door" (*Encarta Dictionary*, January 2007).

In fact, all of these meanings can help define the modalities of well-designed health communication interventions. As with other forms of communication, health communication should be based on a two-way exchange of information that uses a "common system of signs and behaviors." It should be accessible and create "mutual feelings of understanding and sympathy" among members of the communication team and **intended audiences** or **key groups** (all groups the health communication program is seeking to engage in the communication process.) In this book, the terms *intended audience* and *key group* are used interchangeably. Yet, the term *key group* may be better suited to acknowledge the participatory nature of well-designed health communication interventions in which communities

intended audiences or key groups
All groups the health communication intervention is seeking to engage in the communication process

and other key groups are the lead architects of the change process communication can bring about. For those who always have worked within a participatory model of health communication interventions, this distinction is concerned primarily with terminology-related preferences in different models and organizational cultures. Yet, as *audience* may have a more passive connotation, using the term *key group* may indicate the importance of creating key groups' ownership of the communication process, and of truly understanding priorities, needs, and preferences as a key premise to all communication interventions.

Finally, going back to the literal meaning of the word *communication* as defined at the beginning of this section, **channels** or **communication channels** (the means or path, such as mass media or new media, used to reach out to and connect with key groups via health communication messages and materials) and messages are the "connecting doors" that allow health communication interventions to reach and engage intended groups.

Communication has its roots in people's need to share meanings and ideas. A review of the origin and interpretation of early forms of communication, such as writing, shows that many of the reasons for which people may have started developing graphic notations and other early forms of writing are similar to those we can list for health communication.

One of the most important questions about the origins of writing is, "Why did writing begin and for what specific reasons?" (Houston, 2004, p. 234). Although the answer is still being debated, many established theories suggest that writing developed because of state and ceremonial needs (Houston, 2004). More specifically, in ancient Mesoamerica, early forms of writing may have been introduced to help local rulers "control the underlings and impress rivals by means of propaganda" (Houston, 2004, p. 234; Marcus, 1992) or "capture the dominant and dominating message within self-interested declarations" (Houston, 2004, p. 234) with the intention of "advertising" (p. 235) such views. In other words, it is possible to speculate that the desire and need to influence and connect with others are among the most important reasons for the emergence of early forms of writing. This need is also evident in many other forms of communication that seek to create feelings of approval, recognition, empowerment, or friendliness, among others.

Health Communication Defined

One of the key objectives of **health communication** is to engage, empower, and influence individuals and communities. The goal is admirable because health communication aims to improve health outcomes by sharing

communication channels
The path selected by program planners to reach the intended audience with health communication messages and materials

health communication
A multifaceted and multidisciplinary field of research, theory, and practice concerned with reaching different populations and groups to exchange health-related information, ideas, and methods in order to influence, engage, empower, and support individuals, communities, health care professionals, patients, policymakers, organizations, special groups, and the public so that they will champion, introduce, adopt, or sustain a health or social behavior, practice, or policy that will ultimately improve individual, community, and public health outcomes

health-related information. In fact, the Centers for Disease Control and Prevention (CDC) define *health communication* as "the study and use of communication strategies to inform and influence individual and community decisions that enhance health" (CDC, 2001; US Department of Health and Human Services, 2012a). The word *influence* is also included in the *Healthy People 2010* definition of health communication as "the art and technique of informing, influencing, and motivating individual, institutional, and public audiences about important health issues" (US Department of Health and Human Services, 2005, pp. 11–12).

Yet, the broader mandate of health communication is intrinsically related to its potential impact on vulnerable and underserved populations. **Vulnerable populations** include groups who have a higher risk for poor physical, psychological, or social health in the absence of adequate conditions that are supportive of positive outcomes (for example, children, the elderly, people living with disability, migrant populations, and special groups affected by stigma and social discrimination). **Underserved populations** include geographical, ethnic, social, or community-specific groups who do not have adequate access to health or community services and infrastructure or information. "Use health communication strategies . . . to improve population health outcomes and health care quality, and to achieve health equity," reads *Healthy People 2020* (US Department of Health and Human Services, 2012b). **Health equity** is providing every person with the same opportunity to stay healthy or to effectively cope with disease and crisis, regardless of race, gender, age, economic conditions, social status, environment, and other socially determined factors. This can be achieved only by creating a receptive and favorable environment in which information can be adequately shared, understood, absorbed, and discussed by different communities and sectors in a way that is inclusive and representative of vulnerable and underserved groups. This requires an in-depth understanding of the needs, beliefs, taboos, attitudes, lifestyle, socioeconomics, environment, and social norms of all key groups and sectors that are involved—or should be involved—in the communication process. It also demands that communication is based on messages that are easily understood. This is well characterized in the definition of *communication* by Pearson and Nelson (1991), who view it as "the process of understanding and sharing meanings" (p. 6).

A practical example that illustrates this definition is the difference between making an innocent joke about a friend's personality trait and doing the same about a colleague or recent acquaintance. The friend would likely laugh at the joke, whereas the colleague or recent acquaintance might be offended. In communication, understanding the context

vulnerable populations

Includes groups who have a higher risk for poor physical, psychological, or social health in the absence of adequate conditions that are supportive of positive outcomes

underserved populations

Includes geographical, ethnic, social, or community-specific groups who do not have adequate access to health or community services and infrastructure or adequate information

health equity

Providing every person with the same opportunity to stay healthy or to effectively cope with disease and crisis, regardless of race, gender, age, economic conditions, social status, environment, and other socially determined factors of the communication effort is interdependent with becoming familiar with intended audiences. This increases the likelihood that all meanings are shared and understood in the way communicators intended them. Therefore, communication, especially about life-and-death matters such as in public health and health care, is a long-term strategic process. It requires a true understanding of the key groups and communities we seek to engage as well as our willingness and ability to adapt and redefine the goals, strategies, and activities of communication interventions on the basis of audience participation and feedback.

Health communication interventions have been successfully used for many years by public health and nonprofit organizations, the commercial sector, and others to advance public, corporate, clinical, or product-related goals in relation to health. As many authors have noted, health communication draws from numerous disciplines and theoretical fields, including health education, social and behavioral sciences, community development, mass and speech communication, marketing, social marketing, psychology, anthropology, and sociology (Bernhardt, 2004; Kreps, Query, and Bonaguro, 2007; Institute of Medicine, 2003b; World Health Organization [WHO], 2003). It relies on different communication activities or action areas, including interpersonal communication, mass media and new media communication, strategic policy communication and public advocacy, community mobilization and citizen engagement, professional medical communications, and constituency relations and strategic partnerships (Bernhardt, 2004; Schiavo, 2008, 2011b; WHO, 2003).

Table 1.1 provides some of the most recent definitions of health communication and is organized by key words most commonly used to characterize health communication and its role. It is evident that "sharing meanings or information," "influencing individuals or communities," "informing," "motivating individuals and key groups," "exchanging information," "changing behaviors," "engaging," "empowering," and "achieving behavioral and social results" are among the most common attributes of health communication.

Another important attribute of health communication should be "to support and sustain change." In fact, key elements of successful health communication interventions always include long-term program sustainability as well as the development of communication tools and steps that make it easy for individuals, communities, and other key groups to adopt or sustain a recommended behavior, practice, or policy change. If we integrate this practice-based perspective with many of the definitions in Table 1.1, the new definition on page 9 emerges.

Table 1.1 Health Communication Definitions

Key Words	Definitions
To inform and influence (individual and community) decisions	"Health communication is a key strategy to *inform* [emphasis added throughout table] the public about health concerns and to maintain important health issues on the public agenda" (New South Wales Department of Health, Australia, 2006).
	"The study or use of communication strategies *to inform and influence* individual and community decisions that enhance health" (CDC, 2001; US Department of Health and Human Services, 2005).
	Health communication is a "means to disease prevention through behavior modification" (Freimuth, Linnan, and Potter, 2000, p. 337). It has been defined as "the study and use of methods to *inform and influence* individual and community decisions that enhance health" (Freimuth, Linnan, and Potter, 2000, p. 338; Freimuth, Cole, and Kirby, 2000, p. 475).
	"Health communication is a process for the development and diffusion of messages to specific audiences in order to *influence* their knowledge, attitudes and beliefs in favor of healthy behavioral choices" (Exchange, 2006; Smith and Hornik, 1999).
	"Health communication is the use of communication techniques and technologies to (positively) *influence* individuals, populations, and organizations for the purpose of promoting conditions conducive to human and environmental health" (Maibach and Holtgrave, 1995, pp. 219–220; Health Communication Unit, 2006). "It may include diverse activities such as clinician-patient interactions, classes, self-help groups, mailings, hot lines, mass media campaigns, and events" (Health Communication Unit, 2006).
Motivating individuals and key groups	"The art and technique of informing, influencing and *motivating* individual, institutional, and public audiences about important health issues. Its scope includes disease prevention, health promotion, health care policy, and business, as well as enhancement of the quality of life and health of individuals within the community" (Ratzan and others, 1994, p. 361).
	"Effective health communication is the art and technique of *informing, influencing, and motivating* individuals, institutions, and large public audiences about important health issues based on sound scientific and ethical considerations" (Tufts University Student Services, 2006).
Change behavior, achieve social and behavioral results	"Health communication, like health education, is an approach which attempts to *change a set of behaviors* in a large-scale target audience regarding a specific problem in a predefined period of time" (Clift and Freimuth, 1995, p. 68).
	"There is good evidence that public health communication has affected health behavior . . . In addition, . . . many public agencies assume that public health communication is a powerful tool for *behavior change*" (Hornik, 2008a, pp. xi–xv).
	". . . *behavior change* is credibly associated with public health communication . . . " (Hornik, 2008b, p. 1).
	". . . health communication strategies that are collaboratively and strategically designed, implemented, and evaluated can help to improve health in a significant and lasting way. Positive results are achieved by empowering people *to change their behavior* and by facilitating *social change*" (Krenn and Limaye, 2009).
	Health communication and other disciplines "may have some differences, but they share a common goal: creating *social change* by changing people's attitudes, external structures, and/or *modify or eliminate certain behaviors*" (CDC, 2011a).
Increase knowledge and understanding of health-related issues	"The goal of health communication is to *increase knowledge and understanding* of health-related issues and to improve the health status of the intended audience" (Muturi, 2005, p. 78).
	"Communication means a process of *creating understanding* as the basis for development. It places emphasis on people interaction" (Agunga, 1997, p. 225).

Table 1.1   Health Communication Definitions *(continued)*

Key Words	Definitions
Empowers people	"Communication *empowers people* by providing them with knowledge and understanding about specific health problems and interventions" (Muturi, 2005, p. 81). ". . . transformative communication . . . seek[s] not only to educate people about health risks, but also to facilitate the types of social relationships most likely to *empower* them to resist the impacts of unhealthy social influences" (Campbell and Scott, 2012, pp. 179–180). "Communication processes are central to broader *empowerment* practices through which people are able to arrive at their own understanding of issues, to consider and discuss ideas, to negotiate, and to engage in public debates at community and national levels" (Food and Agriculture Organization of the United Nations and others, 2011, p. 1).
Exchange, interchange of information, two-way dialogue	"A process for partnership and participation that is based on *two-way dialogue*, where there is an interactive *interchange of information*, ideas, techniques and knowledge between senders and receivers of information on an equal footing, leading to improved understanding, shared knowledge, greater consensus, and identification of possible effective action" (Exchange, 2005). "Health communication is the scientific development, strategic dissemination, and critical evaluation of relevant, accurate, accessible, and understandable health *information communicated to and from intended audiences* to advance the health of the public" (Bernhardt, 2004, p. 2051).
Engaging	"One of the most important, and largely unrecognized, dimensions of effective health communication relates to how *engaging* the communication is" (Kreps, 2012a, p. 253). "To compete successfully for audience attention, health-related communications have to be polished and *engaging*" (Cassell, Jackson, and Cheuvront, 1998, p. 76).

Health communication is a multifaceted and multidisciplinary field of research, theory, and practice. It is concerned with reaching different populations and groups to exchange health-related information, ideas, and methods in order to influence, engage, empower, and support individuals, communities, health care professionals, patients, policymakers, organizations, special groups and the public, so that they will champion, introduce, adopt, or sustain a health or social behavior, practice, or policy that will ultimately improve individual, community, and public health outcomes.

Health Communication in the Twenty-First Century: Key Characteristics and Defining Features

Health communication is about improving health outcomes by encouraging behavior modification and social change. It is increasingly considered an integral part of most public health interventions (US Department of Health and Human Services, 2012a; Bernhardt, 2004). It is a comprehensive approach that relies on the full understanding and participation of its intended audiences.

Health communication theory draws on a number of additional disciplines and models. In fact, both the health communication field and its theoretical basis have evolved and changed in the past fifty years (Piotrow, Kincaid, Rimon, and Rinehart, 1997; Piotrow, Rimon, Payne Merritt, and Saffitz, 2003; Bernhardt, 2004). With increasing frequency, it is considered "the avant-garde in suggesting and integrating new theoretical approaches and practices" (Drum Beat, 2005).

Most important, communicators are no longer viewed as those who write press releases and other media-related communications, but as fundamental members of the public health, health care, nonprofit, or health industry teams. Communication is no longer considered a skill (Bernhardt, 2004) but a science-based discipline that requires training and passion, and relies on the use of different **communication vehicles** (materials, activities, events, and other tools used to deliver a message through communication channels; Health Communication Unit, 2003b) and channels. According to Saba (2006):

communication vehicles

A category that includes materials, events, activities, or other tools for delivering a message using communication channels

> In the past, and this is probably the most prevalent trend even today, health communication practitioners were trained "on-the-job." People from different fields (sociology, demography, public health, psychology, communication with all its different specialties, such as filmmaking, journalism and advertising) entered or were brought into health communication programs to meet the need for professional human resources in this field. By performing their job and working in teams, they learned how to adapt their skills to the new field and were taught by other practitioners about the common practices and basic "lingo" of health communication. In the mid-90s, and in response to the increasing demand for health communication professionals, several schools in the United States started their own curricular programs and/or "concentrations" in Health Communication. This helped bring more attention from the academic world to this emerging field. The number of peer-reviewed articles and several other types of health communication publications increased. The field moved from in-service training to pre-service education.

As a result, there is an increasing understanding that "the level of technical competence of communication practitioners can affect outcomes." A structured approach to health communications planning, a spotless program execution, and a rigorous evaluation process are the result of adequate competencies and relevant training, which are supported by leading organizations and agendas in different fields (Association of Schools of

Public Health, 2007; US Department of Health and Human Services, 2012b; American Medical Association, 2006; Hospitals and Health Network, 2012; National Board of Public Health Examiners, 2011). "In health communication, the learning process is a lifetime endeavor and should be facilitated by the continuous development of new training initiatives and tools" (Schiavo, 2006). Training may start in the academic setting but should always be influenced and complemented by practical experience and observations, and other learning opportunities, including in-service training, continuing professional education, and ongoing mentoring.

Health communication can reach its highest potential when it is discussed and applied within a team-oriented context that includes public health, health care, community development, and other professionals from different sectors and disciplines. Teamwork and mutual agreement, on both the intervention's ultimate objectives and expected results, are key to the successful design, implementation, and impact of any program.

Finally, it is important to remember that there is no magic fix that can address health issues. Health communication is an evolving discipline and should always incorporate lessons learned as well as use a multidisciplinary approach to all interventions. This is in line with one of the fundamental premises of this book that recognizes the experience of practitioners as a key factor in developing theories, models, and approaches that should guide and inform health communication planning, implementation, and assessment.

Table 1.2 lists the key elements of health communication, which are further analyzed in the following sections.

Table 1.2 Key Characteristics of Health Communication

- People-centered
- Evidence-based
- Multidisciplinary
- Strategic
- Process-oriented
- Cost-effective
- Creative in support of strategy
- Audience- and media-specific
- Relationship building
- Aimed at behavioral and social results
- Inclusive of vulnerable and underserved groups

People-Centered

Health communication is a long-term process that begins and ends with people's needs and preferences. In health communication, intended audiences should not be merely a *target* (even if this terminology is used by many practitioners from around the world primarily to indicate that a communication intervention will focus on, benefit, and engage a specific group of people that shares similar characteristics—such as age, socioeconomics, and ethnicity. It does not necessarily imply lack of audience participation) but an active participant in the process of analyzing and prioritizing the health issue, finding culturally appropriate and cost-effective solutions, and becoming effectively engaged as the lead change designer in the planning, implementation, and assessment of all interventions. This is why the term *key group* may better represent the role communities, teachers, parents, health care professionals, religious and community leaders, women, and many other key groups and stakeholders from a variety of segments of society and professional sectors should assume in the communication process. Yet, different organizations may have different cultural preferences for specific terminology even within the context of their participatory models and planning frameworks.

In implementing a people-centered approach to communication, researching communities and other key groups is a necessary but often not sufficient step because the effectiveness and sustainability of most interventions is often linked to the level of engagement of their key beneficiaries and those who influence them. Engaging communities and different sectors is often accomplished in health communication practice by working together with organizations and leaders who represent them or by directly involving members of a specific community at the outset of program design. For example, if a health communication intervention aims to reach and benefit breast cancer survivors, all strategies and key program elements should be designed, discussed, prioritized, tested, implemented, and evaluated together with membership organizations, patient groups, leaders, and patients who can speak for survivors and represent their needs and preferences. Most important, these groups need to feel invested and well represented. They should be the key protagonists of the action-oriented process that will lead to behavioral or social change.

Evidence-Based

Health communication is grounded in research. Successful health communication interventions are based on a true understanding not only of key groups but also of situations and sociopolitical environments. This includes existing programs and lessons learned, policies, social norms, key issues, work and living environments, and obstacles in addressing the specific health problem. The overall premise of health communication is that behavioral and social change is conditioned by the environment in which people live and work, as well as by those who influence them. Several socially determined factors (also referred to as **social determinants of health**)—including socioeconomic conditions, race, ethnicity, culture, as well as having access to health care services, a built environment that supports physical activity, neighborhoods with accessible and affordable nutritious food, health information that's culturally appropriate and accurately reflects literacy levels, and caring and friendly clinical settings—influence and are influenced by health communication (Association of Schools of Public Health, 2007). This requires a comprehensive research approach that relies on traditional, online, and new media-based research techniques for the formal development of a **situation analysis** (a planning term that describes the analysis of individual, social, political, environmental, community-specific, and behavior-related factors that can affect attitudes, behaviors, social norms, and policies about a health issue and its potential solutions) and **audience analysis** (a comprehensive, research-based, participatory, and strategic analysis of all key groups' characteristics, demographics, needs, preferences, values, social norms, attitudes, and behavior). The **audience profile**, a report on all findings, is the culminating step of a process of effective engagement and participation that involve all key groups and stakeholders in the overall analysis). Situation and audience analyses are fundamental and interrelated steps of health communication planning (the audience analysis is described in this book as a component of the situation analysis), which should be participatory and empowering in their nature, and are described in detail in Chapter Eleven.

Multidisciplinary

Health communication is "transdisciplinary in nature" (Bernhardt, 2004, p. 2051; Institute of Medicine, 2003b) and draws on multiple disciplines (Bernhardt, 2004; WHO, 2003). Health communication recognizes the complexity of attaining behavioral and social change and uses a multi-faceted approach that is grounded in the application of several theoretical frameworks and disciplines, including health education, social marketing, behavioral and social change theories, and medical and clinical models (see Chapter Two for a comprehensive discussion of key theories and models). It draws on principles successfully used in the nonprofit and corporate sectors and also on the people-centered approach of other disciplines, such as

social determinants of health
Different socially determined factors that affect health outcomes as well as influence and are influenced by health communication

situation analysis
A planning term that describes the analysis of individual, social, political, environmental, community-specific, and behavior-related factors that can affect attitudes, behaviors, social norms, and policies about a health issue and its potential solutions

audience analysis
A comprehensive, research-based, participatory, and strategic analysis of all key groups' characteristics, demographics, needs, preferences, values, social norms, attitudes, and behavior

audience profile
An analytical report on key findings from audience-related research (also called audience analysis) and one of the key sections of the situation analysis

psychology, sociology, and anthropology (WHO, 2003). It is not anchored to a single specific theory or model. With people always at the core of each intervention, it uses a case-by-case approach in selecting those models, theories, and strategies that are best suited to reach their hearts; secure their involvement in the health issue and, most important, its solutions; and support and facilitate their journey on a path to better health.

Piotrow, Rimon, Payne Merritt, and Saffitz (2003) identify four different "eras" of health communication:

> (1) The *clinic era*, based on a medical care model and the notion that if people knew where services were located they would find their way to the clinics; (2) the *field era*, a more proactive approach emphasizing outreach workers, community-based distribution, and a variety of information, education, and communication (IEC) products; (3) the *social marketing era*, developed from the commercial concepts that consumers will buy the products they want at subsidized prices; and, (4) . . . the era of *strategic behavior communications*, founded on behavioral science models that emphasize the need to influence social norms and policy environments to facilitate and empower the iterative and dynamic process of both individual and social change. (pp. 1–2)

More recently, health communication has evolved toward a fifth "era" of strategic communication for behavioral and social change that rightly emphasizes and combines behavioral and social science models and disciplines along with marketing, medical, and social norms–based models, and aims at achieving long-lasting behavioral and social results. However, even in the context of each different health communication era, many of the theoretical approaches of other periods still find use in program planning or execution. For example, the situation analysis of a health communication program still uses commercial and social marketing tools and models—even if combined with community dialogue and other participatory or new media–based methods (see Chapters Two and Ten for a detailed description)—to analyze the environment in which change should occur. Instead, in the early stages of approaching key opinion leaders and other key **stakeholders** (all individuals and groups who have an interest or share responsibilities in a given issue, such as policymakers, community leaders, and community members), keeping in mind McGuire's steps about communication for persuasion (1984; see Chapter Two), may help communicators gain stakeholder support for the importance or the urgency of adequately addressing a health issue. This theoretical flexibility should keep communicators focused on key groups and stakeholders and always on the lookout for the best approach and planning framework to achieve behavioral and

stakeholders
All individuals and groups who have an interest or share responsibilities in a given issue, such as policymakers, community leaders, and community members

social results by engaging and empowering people. In concert with the other features previously discussed, it also enables the overall communication process to be truly fluid and suited to respond to people's needs.

The importance of a somewhat flexible theoretical basis, which should be selected on a case-by-case basis (National Cancer Institute, 2005a), is already supported by reputable organizations and authors. For example, publications by the US Department of Health and Human Services (2002), and the National Cancer Institute at the National Institutes of Health (2002) points to the importance of selecting planning frameworks that "can help [communicators] identify the social science theories most appropriate for understanding the problem and the situation" (National Cancer Institute at the National Institutes of Health, 2002, p. 218). These theories, models, and constructs include several theoretical concepts and frameworks (see Chapter Two) that are also used in motivating change at individual and interpersonal levels or organizational, community, and societal levels (National Cancer Institute at the National Institutes of Health, 2002) by related or complementary disciplines.

The goal here is not to advocate for a lack of theoretical structure in communication planning and execution. On the contrary, planning frameworks, models, and theories should be consistent at least until preliminary steps of the evaluation phase of a program are completed. This allows communicators to take advantage of lessons learned and redefine theoretical constructs and **communication objectives** (the intermediate steps that need to be achieved in order to meet program goals and outcome objectives; National Cancer Institute, 2002) by comparing **program outcomes**, which measure changes in knowledge, attitudes, skills, behavior, and other parameters, with those that were anticipated in the planning phase. However, the ability to draw on multiple disciplines and theoretical constructs is a definitive advantage of the health communication field and one of the keys to the success of well-planned and well-executed communication programs.

communication objectives
The intermediate steps that need to be achieved in order to meet the overall program goals as complemented by specific behavioral, social, and organizational objectives

program outcomes
Changes in knowledge, attitudes, skills, behavior, social norms, policies, and other parameters measured against those anticipated in the planning phase

Strategic

Health communication programs need to display a sound strategy and plan of action. All activities need to be well planned and respond to a specific audience-related need. Consider the example of Bonnie, a twenty-five-year-old mother who is not sure about whether to immunize her newborn child. Activities in support of a strategy that focuses on facilitating communication between Bonnie and her health care provider make sense only if evidence shows all or any of the following points: (1) Bonnie is likely to be influenced primarily, or at least significantly, by her health care provider and not by family or other new mothers; (2) there are several gaps in the understanding of patients' needs that prevent health care providers from communicating effectively; (3) providers lack adequate tools to talk about this topic with patients in a time-effective and efficient manner; (4) research data have been validated by community dialogue and other participatory methods that are inclusive of Bonnie and her peers; and (5) Bonnie and her peers and organizations that represent them have participated in designing all interventions.

communication strategies
A statement describing the overall approach used to accomplish communication objectives

Communication strategies (the overall approach used to accomplish the communication objectives) need to be research-based, and all activities should serve such strategies. Therefore, we should not rely on any workshop, press release, brochure, video, or anything else to provide effective communication without making sure that its content and format reflect the selected approach (the strategy), and that this is a priority to reach people's hearts. For this purpose, health communication strategies need to respond to an actual need that has been identified by preliminary research and confirmed by the intended audience.

Process-Oriented

Communication is a long-term process. Influencing people and their behaviors requires an ongoing commitment to the health issue and its solutions. This is rooted in a deep understanding of key groups, communities, and their environments, and aims at building consensus among affected groups, community members, and key stakeholders about the potential plan of action.

Most, if not all, health communication programs change or evolve from what communication experts may have originally envisioned due to the input and participation of communities, key opinion leaders, patient groups, professional associations, policymakers, community members, and other key stakeholders.

In health communication, engaging key groups on relevant health issues as well as exploring suitable ways to address them is only the first step of a long-term, people-centered process. This process often requires theoretical flexibility to accommodate people's needs, preferences, and priorities.

While in the midst of many process-oriented projects, many practitioners may have noticed that health communication is often misunderstood. Health communication uses multiple channels and approaches, which, despite what some people may think, include but are not limited to the use of the mass media or new media. Moreover, health communication aims at improving health outcomes and in the process help advance public health and community development goals or create market share (depending on whether health communication strategies are used for nonprofit or for-profit goals) or encourages compliance to clinical recommendations and healthy lifestyles. Finally, health communication cannot focus only on channels, messages, and media. It also should attempt to involve and create consensus and feelings of ownership among intended audiences.

Exchange, a networking and learning program on health communication for development that is based in the United Kingdom and has multiple partners, views health communication as "a process for partnership and participation that is based on two-way dialogue, where there is an interactive interchange of information, ideas, techniques, and knowledge between senders and receivers of information on an equal footing, leading to improved understanding, shared knowledge, greater consensus, and identification of possible effective action" (2005). This definition makes sense in all settings and situations, but it assumes a greater relevance for health communication programs that aim to improve health outcomes in developing countries. Communication for development often needs to rely on creative solutions that compensate for the lack of local capabilities and infrastructure. These solutions usually emerge after months of discussion with local community leaders and organizations, government officials, and representatives of public and community groups. Word of mouth and the ability of community leaders to engage members of their own communities is often all that communicators have at hand.

Consider the case of Maria, a mother of four children who lives in a small village in sub-Saharan Africa together with her seventy-five-year-old father. Her village is almost completely isolated from major metropolitan areas, and very few people in town have a radio or know how to read. Maria is unaware that malaria, which is endemic in that region, poses a higher risk to children than to the elderly. Because elderly people benefit from a high hierarchical status in that region, if Maria is able to find money to purchase mosquito nets to protect someone in her family from mosquito bites and the consequent threat of malaria, she would probably choose that her father sleep under them, leaving her children unprotected. This is despite the high mortality rate from malaria among children in her village. If her village's community leaders told her to do otherwise, she would likely change her practice and protect her children. This may be the first building block toward the development and adoption of new social norms not only by Maria but also her peers and other community members.

Involving Maria's community leaders and peers in the communication process that would lead to a potential change in her habits requires long-term commitment. Such effort demands the involvement of local organizations and authorities who are respected and trusted by community leaders, as well as an open mind in listening to suggestions and seeking solutions with the help of all key stakeholders. Because of the lack of local capabilities and limited access to adequate communication channels, this process is likely to take longer than any similar initiative in the developed world. Therefore, communicators should view this as an ongoing process and applaud every small step forward.

Cost-Effective

Cost-effectiveness is a concept that health communication borrows from commercial and social marketing. It is particularly important in the competitive working environment of public health and nonprofit organizations, where the lack of sufficient funds or adequate economic planning can often undermine important initiatives. It implies the need to seek solutions that allow communicators to advance their goals with minimal use of human and economic resources. Yet, communicators should use their funds as long as they are well spent and advance their evidence-based strategy. They should also seek creative solutions that minimize the use of internal funds and human resources by seeking partnerships, using existing materials or programs as a starting point, and maximizing synergies with the work of other departments in their organization or external groups and stakeholders in the same field.

Creative in Support of Strategy

Creativity is a significant attribute of communicators because it allows them to consider multiple options, formats, and media channels to reach and engage different groups. It also helps them devise solutions that preserve the sustainability and cost-effectiveness of specific health communication interventions. However, even the greatest ideas or the best-designed and best-executed communication tools may fail to achieve behavioral or social results if they do not respond to a strategic need identified by research data and validated by key stakeholders from intended groups. Too often communication programs and resources fail to make an impact because of this common mistake.

For example, developing and distributing a brochure on how to use insecticide-treated nets (ITNs) makes sense only if the intended community is already aware of the cycle of malaria transmission as well as the need for protection from mosquito bites. If this is not the case and most community members still believe that malaria is contracted by bathing in the river or is a complication of some other fevers (Pinto, 1998; Schiavo, 1998, 2000), the first strategic imperative is disease awareness, with a specific focus on the cycle of transmission and subsequent protective measures. All communication materials and activities need to address this basic information need before talking about the use of ITNs and reasons to use them as an alternative to other potential protection methods. Creativity should come into play in devising culturally friendly tools to start sharing information about malaria and to engage community members in designing a community-specific communication intervention that would encourage protective behaviors and would benefit the overall community. In a nutshell, we should refrain from using creativity to develop and implement great, sensational, or innovative ideas when these do not respond to people's needs and key strategic priorities of the health communication intervention.

Audience- and Media-Specific

The importance of audience-specific messages and channels became one of the most important lessons learned after the anthrax-by-mail bioterrorist attacks that rocked the United States in October 2001. At the time, several letters containing the lethal agent *Bacillus anthracis* were mailed to senators and representatives of the media (Jernigan and others, 2002; Blanchard and others, 2005). The attack also exposed government staff workers, including US postal workers in the US Postal Service facility in Washington, DC, and other parts of the country, to anthrax. Two workers in the Washington facility died as a result of anthrax inhalation (Blanchard and others, 2005).

Communication during this emergency was perceived by several members of the medical, patient, and worker communities as well as public figures and the media to be often inconsistent and disorganized (Blanchard and others, 2005; Vanderford, 2003). Equally important, postal workers and US Senate staff have reported erosion of their trust in public health agencies (Blanchard and others, 2005). Several analyses point to the possibility that the *one message–one behavior approach* to communication (UCLA Department of Epidemiology, 2002)—in other words, using the same message and strategic approach for all audiences, which is likely to result in the same unspecific behavior that may not be relevant to specific communities or groups—led to feelings of being left out among postal workers, who in the Brentwood facility in Washington, DC, were primarily African Americans or individuals with a severe hearing impairment (Blanchard and others, 2005). They also point to the need for public health officials to develop the relationships that are needed to communicate with groups of different racial and socioeconomic backgrounds as well as "those with physical limitations that could hinder communication, such as those with hearing impairments" (Blanchard and others, 2005, p. 494; McEwen and Anton-Culver, 1988).

The lessons learned from the anthrax scare support some of the fundamental principles of good health communication practices. Messages need to be key group–specific and tailored to channels allowing the most effective reach, including among vulnerable and underserved groups. Because it is very likely that communication efforts may aim at producing multiple key group–appropriate behaviors, the one message–one behavior approach should be avoided (UCLA Department of Epidemiology, 2002) even when time and resources are lacking. As highlighted by the anthrax case study, in developing audience-specific messages and activities, the contribution of local advocates and community representatives is fundamental to increase the likelihood that messages will be heard, understood, and trusted by intended audiences.

Relationship Building

Communication is a relationship business. Establishing and preserving good relationships is critical to the success of health communication interventions, and, among other things, can help build long-term and successful partnerships and coalitions, secure credible stakeholder endorsement of the health issue, and expand the pool of ambassadors on behalf of the health cause.

Most important, good relationships help create the environment of "shared meanings and understanding" (Pearson and Nelson, 1991, p. 6) that is central to achieving social or behavioral results at the individual, community, and population levels. Good relationships should be established with key stakeholders and representatives of key groups, health organizations, community-based organizations, governments, and many other critical members of the extended health communication team. A detailed discussion of the dos and don'ts as well as the development of successful partnerships and relationship-building efforts is found in Chapters Eight and Thirteen.

Aimed at Behavioral and Social Results

Nowadays, we are transitioning from the "era of strategic behavior communications" (Piotrow, Rimon, Payne Merritt, and Saffitz, 2003, p. 2) to the *era of behavioral and social impact communication*. Several US and international models and agenda (for example, *Healthy People 2020*, COMBI, Communication for Development; see Chapter Two) support the importance of a behavioral and social change–driven mind-set in developing health communication interventions. Although the ultimate goal of health communication has always been influencing behaviors, social norms, and policies (with the latter often being instrumental in institutionalizing social change and norms), there is a renewed emphasis on the importance of establishing behavioral and social objectives early on in the design of health communication interventions.

"What do you want people to do?" is the first question that should be asked in communication planning meetings. Do you want them to immunize their children before age two? Become aware of their risk for heart disease and behave accordingly to prevent it? Ask their dentists about oral cancer screening? Do you want local legislators to support a stricter law on the use of infant car seats? Or communities and special groups to create an environment of peer-to-peer support designed to discourage adolescents from initiating smoking? Or encourage people from different sectors (for example, employers, clinicians, etc.) to provide social support and tools to members of underserved communities so they are more likely to adopt and sustain a healthy lifestyle? Answering these kinds of questions is the first step in identifying suitable and research-based objectives of a communication program.

Although different theories (see Chapter Two) may specifically support the importance of either behavioral or social results as key outcome indicators, these two parameters are actually interconnected. In fact, social change typically takes place as the result of a series of behavioral results at the individual, group, community, social, and political levels.

Inclusive of Vulnerable and Underserved Groups

With a precise mandate from *Healthy People 2020* and the fact that several international organizations, such as UNICEF, have been investing overtime in rolling out an equity-based approach to programming, health communication is increasingly considered a key field that can contribute to a reduction of **health disparities** ("diseases or health conditions that discriminate and tend to be more common and more severe among vulnerable and underserved populations" [Health Equity Initiative, 2012b]; or overall differences in health outcomes) and an advancement of health equity. Therefore, health communication programs need to be mindful and inclusive of vulnerable and underserved populations. Such inclusiveness is not only limited to making sure that programs intended for the general population or specific communities also have a measurable impact on disadvantaged groups but it also entails that such groups are involved in the planning, implementation, and evaluation of all interventions so that their voices are heard and considered as part of the overall communication process. This is also important to build leadership capacity among vulnerable and underserved groups

health disparities
Diseases or health conditions that discriminate and tend to be more common and more severe among vulnerable and underserved populations; or overall differences in health outcomes

so they can adequately address current and future health and community development topics and find their own solutions to pressing issues.

The Health Communication Environment

When looking at the health communication environment where change should occur and be sustained (Figure 1.1), it becomes clear that effective communication can be a powerful tool in seeking to influence all of the factors that are highlighted in the figure. It is also clear that regardless of whether these factors are related to the audience, health behavior, product, service, social, or political environment, all of them are interconnected and can mutually affect each other. At the same time, health communication interventions can tip the existing balance among these factors, and change the weight they may have in defining a specific health issue and its solutions as well as within the living, working, and aging environment of the people we seek to reach and engage in the health communication process.

Figure 1.1 also reflects some of the key principles of marketing models as well as the socioecological model (Morris, 1975), behavioral and social sciences constructs, and other theoretical models (VanLeeuwen,

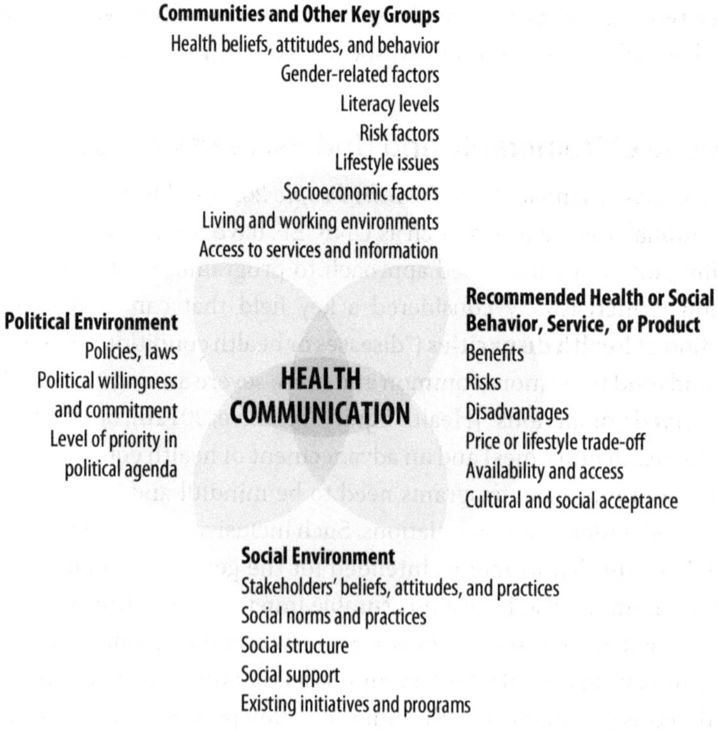

Communities and Other Key Groups
Health beliefs, attitudes, and behavior
Gender-related factors
Literacy levels
Risk factors
Lifestyle issues
Socioeconomic factors
Living and working environments
Access to services and information

Political Environment
Policies, laws
Political willingness
and commitment
Level of priority in
political agenda

HEALTH COMMUNICATION

Recommended Health or Social Behavior, Service, or Product
Benefits
Risks
Disadvantages
Price or lifestyle trade-off
Availability and access
Cultural and social acceptance

Social Environment
Stakeholders' beliefs, attitudes, and practices
Social norms and practices
Social structure
Social support
Existing initiatives and programs

Figure 1.1 The Health Communication Environment

Waltner-Toews, Abernathy, and Smit, 1999) that are used in public health, health care, global health, and other fields to show the connection and influence of different factors (individual, interpersonal, community, sociopolitical, organizational, and public policy) on individual, group, and community behavior as well as to understand the process that may lead to behavioral and social results. Health communication theoretical basis is discussed in detail in Chapter Two.

Health Communication in Public Health, Health Care, and Community Development

Prior to the recent call to action by many federal and multilateral organizations, which encouraged a strategic and more frequent use of communication, health communication was used only marginally in a variety of sectors. It was perceived more as a skill than a discipline and confined to the mere dissemination of scientific and medical findings by public health and other professionals (Bernhardt, 2004). This section reviews current thinking on the role of health communication in public health, health care settings, and community development, and also serves as a reminder of the need for increased collaboration among these important sectors.

Health Communication in Public Health

Health communication is a well-recognized discipline in public health. Many public health organizations and leaders (Bernhardt, 2004; Freimuth, Cole, and Kirby, 2000; Institute of Medicine, 2002, 2003b; National Cancer Institute at the National Institutes of Health, 2002; Piotrow, Kincaid, Rimon, and Rinehart, 1997; Rimal and Lapinski, 2009; US Department of Health and Human Services, 2005, 2012b) understand and recognize the role that health communication can play in advancing health outcomes and the general health status of interested populations and special groups. Most important, there is a new awareness of the reach of health communication as well as its many strategic action areas (for example, interpersonal communication, professional medical communications, community mobilization and citizen engagement, and mass media and new media communication).

As defined by *Healthy People 2010* (US Department of Health and Human Services, 2005), in the US public health agenda, the scope of health communication in public health "includes disease prevention, health promotion, health care policy, and the business of health care as well as enhancement of the quality of life and health of individuals within the community" (p. 11–20; Ratzan and others, 1994). Health communication "links the domains of communication and health" (p. 11–13) and is regarded as a science (Freimuth and Quinn, 2004; Bernhardt, 2004) of great importance in public health, especially in the era of epidemics and emerging diseases, the increasing toll of chronic diseases, the aging of large segments and percentages of the population of many countries, urbanization, increased disparities and socioeconomic divides, global threats, bioterrorism, and a new emphasis on a preventive and patient-centered approach to health. Finally, *Healthy People 2020* establishes health communication as a key discipline in contributing to advance health equity (US Department of Health and Human Resources, 2012b).

Health Communication in Health Care Settings

Health communication has an invaluable role within health care settings. Although provider-patient communications—which is perhaps the best known and most important use of communication within health care settings—is discussed in detail within Chapter Four, it is worth mentioning here that communication is also used to coordinate the activities of interdependent health care providers, encourage the widespread use of best clinical practices, promote the application of scientific advancements, and overall to administer complex and multisectoral health care delivery systems (see Chapter Seven and other relevant sections throughout this book).

As *Healthy People 2020* suggests, by combining effective health communication processes and integrating them with new technology and tools, there is the potential to

- Improve health care quality and safety.
- Increase the efficiency of health care and public health service delivery.
- Improve the public health information infrastructure.
- Support care in the community and at home.
- Facilitate clinical and consumer decision-making.
- Build health skills and knowledge (US Department of Health and Human Services, 2012b).

Among other things, *Healthy People 2020*'s recommendations reflect the support many reputable voices and organizations—in the United States and globally—have lent to the need for effective integration of the work and strategies from our public health and health care systems.

Health Communication in Community Development

As previously mentioned, health is influenced by many different factors and is not only the mere absence of illness. Health is a state of well-being that includes the physical, psychological, and social aspects of life, which in turn are influenced by the environment in which we live, work, grow, and age.

Community development refers to a field of research and practice that involves community members, average citizens, professionals, grant-makers, and others in improving various aspects of local communities. More traditionally, community development interventions have been dealing with providing and increasing access to adequate transportation, jobs, and other socioeconomic opportunities, education, and different kinds of infrastructure (for example, parks, community centers, etc.) within a given community or population. Yet, because all of these interventions or factors are greatly connected to people's ability to stay healthy or effectively cope with disease and emergency, many organizations have been calling for increased collaboration among the community development, health care, and public health fields (Braunstein and Lavizzo-Mourey, 2011).

community development
A field of research and practice that involves community members, average citizens, professionals, grant-makers, and others in improving various aspects of local communities

Health communication can play a key role in moving forward such a collaborative agenda. It can help bridge organizational cultures and showcase relevant synergies among the works of public health, health care, and community development organizations and professionals; increase awareness on how key social determinants of health influence health outcomes; establish "good health," and more in general health equity, as key determinants of socioeconomic development; and engage and mobilize professionals from different sectors to take action. Health communication can be instrumental in empowering community members and professionals from different sectors to implement such cross-sectoral collaborative agenda, which would benefit different communities and populations in the United States and globally. We will continue to explore this important theme throughout the book.

The Role of Health Communication in the Marketing Mix

As mentioned, health communication strategies are integral to a variety of interventions in different contexts. In the private sector, health communication strategies are primarily used in a marketing context. Still, many of the other behavioral and social constructs of health communication—and definitely the models that position people at the center of any communication intervention—are considered and used at least at an empirical level. As in other settings (for example, public health), health communication functions tend to be similar to those described in the "What Health Communication Can and Cannot Do" section of this chapter.

Many in the private sector regard health communication as a critical component of the marketing mix, which is traditionally defined by the key four Ps of social marketing (see Chapter Two for a more detailed description): product, price, place, and promotion—in other words, "developing, delivering, and promoting a superior offer" (Maibach, 2003). Chapter Two includes a more detailed discussion of marketing models as one of the key theoretical and practical influences of health communication.

Overview of Key Communication Areas

Global health communication is a term increasingly used to include different communication approaches and action areas, such as interpersonal communication, social and community mobilization, and advocacy (Haider, 2005; Waisbord and Larson, 2005). Well-planned health communication programs rely on an integrated blend of different action areas that should be selected in consideration of expected behavioral and social outcomes (WHO, 2003; O'Sullivan, Yonkler, Morgan, and Merritt, 2003; Health Communication Partnership, 2005a). Long-term results can be achieved only through an engagement process that involves key groups and stakeholders, implements participatory approaches to research, and uses culturally appropriate action areas and communication channels. Remember that there is no magic fix in health communication.

Message repetitiveness and frequency are also important factors in health communication. Often the resonance effect, which can be defined as the ability to create a snowball effect for message delivery by using multiple vehicles, sources, and messengers, can help motivate people to change by reminding them of the desired behavior (for example, complying with childhood immunization requirements, using mosquito nets for protection against malaria, attempting to quit smoking) and its benefits. To this end, several action areas are usually used in health communication and are described in detail in the topic-specific chapters in Part Two:

Interpersonal communication, which uses interpersonal channels (for example, one-on-one or group meetings), and is based on active listening, social and behavioral theories, as well as the ability to relate to, and identify with, the audience's needs and cultural preferences and efficiently address them. This includes "personal selling and counseling" (WHO, 2003, p. 2), which takes place during one-on-one encounters with members of key groups and other key stakeholders, as well as during group events and in locations where materials and services are available. It also includes provider-patient communications—which has been identified as one of the most important areas of health communication (US Department of Health and Human Services, 2005) and should aim at improving health outcomes by optimizing the relationships between providers and their patients, and community dialogue, which is an example of interpersonal communication at scale and is used in research and practice to solicit community input and engage and empower participants throughout the communication process.

(•) *Mass media and new media communication,* which relies on the skillful use of culturally competent and audience-appropriate mass media, new media, and social media, as well as other communication channels to place a health issue on the public agenda, raise awareness of its root causes and risk factors, advocate for its solutions, or highlight its importance so that key stakeholders, groups, communities, or the public at large take action.

(•) *Community mobilization and citizen engagement,* a bottom-up and participatory process that at times more formally includes methods for public consultations and citizen engagement. By using multiple communication channels, community mobilization seeks to involve community leaders and the community at large in addressing a health issue, participating in determining key steps to behavioral or social change, or practicing a desired behavior.

(•) *Professional medical communications,* a peer-to-peer approach intended to reach and engage health care professionals that aims to (1) promote the adoption of best medical and health practices; (2) establish new concepts and standards of care; (3) publicize recent medical discoveries, beliefs, parameters, and policies; (4) change or establish new medical priorities; and (5) advance health policy changes, among other goals.

(•) *Constituency relations and strategic partnerships in health communication,* a critical component of all other areas of health communication as well as a communication area of its own. Constituency relations refers to the process of (1) creating consensus among key stakeholders about health issues and their potential solutions, (2) expanding program reach by involving key constituencies, (3) developing alliances, (4) managing and anticipating criticisms and opponents, and (5) maintaining key relationships with other health organizations or stakeholders. Effective constituency relations often lead to strategic and multisectoral partnerships.

Policy communication and public advocacy, which include government relations, policy briefing and communication, public advocacy, and media advocacy, and use multiple communication channels, venues, and media to influence the beliefs, attitudes, and behavior of policymakers, and consequently the adoption, implementation, and sustainability of different policies and funding streams for specific issues.

The Health Communication Cycle

The importance of a rigorous, theory-driven, and systematic approach to the design, implementation, and evaluation of health communication interventions has been established by several reputable organizations in the United States and globally (Association of Schools of Public Health, 2007; US Department of Health and Human Services, 2012b; WHO, 2003). Chapter Two includes examples of theory-driven planning frameworks used by different types of organizations in a variety of professional settings.

As previously mentioned in the book's introduction, Part Three provides detailed step-by-step guidance on health communication planning, implementation, and evaluation and at the same time also highlights the cyclical and interdependent nature of different phases of health communication interventions. Although a comprehensive overview of the health communication cycle and strategic planning process can be found in Chapter Ten, Figure 1.2 briefly describes key phases of health communication planning and introduces the basic planning framework

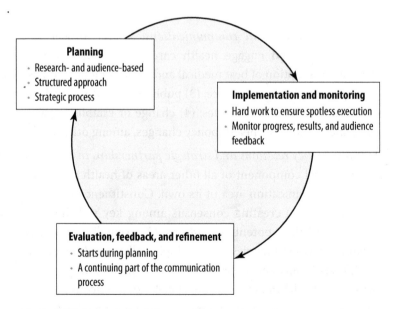

Figure 1.2   The Health Communication Cycle

that is discussed in detail in Part Three. Figure 1.2 also shows how strategic planning is directly connected to the other two stages of the health communication cycle (program implementation and monitoring, and evaluation, feedback, and refinement).

What Health Communication Can and Cannot Do

Health communication cannot work in a vacuum and is usually a critical component of larger public health or community development interventions or corporate efforts. Because of the complexity of health issues, it may "not be equally effective in addressing all issues or relaying all messages" (National Cancer Institute at the National Institutes of Health, 2002, p. 3), at least in a given time frame.

Health communication cannot replace the lack of local infrastructure (such as the absence of appropriate health services or hospitals or other essential services that would provide communities with enhanced opportunities to stay healthy, as, for example, parks, adequate transportation systems, recreational facilities, bike-sharing programs, and stores that sell nutritious food) or capability (such as an inadequate number of health care providers in relation to the size of the population being attended). It cannot compensate for inadequate medical solutions to treat, diagnose, or prevent any disease. But it can help advocate for change and create a receptive environment to support the development of new health services or the allocation of additional funds for medical and scientific discovery, or access to existing treatments or community services, or the recruitment of health care professionals in new medical fields or underserved geographical areas. In doing so, it helps secure political commitment, stakeholder endorsement, and community involvement to encourage change, devise community-specific solutions, and improve health outcomes.

Because of the evolving role of health communication, other authors and organizations have been defining the potential contribution of health communication to the health care and public health fields. For example, the US National Cancer Institute at the National Institutes of Health (2002) has a homonymous section, which partly inspired the need for this section, in one of its publications on the topic.

Understanding the role and the potential impact of health communication is important to take full advantage of the contribution of this field to health and related social outcomes as well as to set realistic expectations on what can be accomplished among team members, program partners, key groups, and stakeholders. Table 1.3 provides examples of what health communication can and cannot do.

Table 1.3   What Health Communication Can and Cannot Do

Health Communication Can Help . . .	Health Communication Cannot . . .
Raise awareness of health issues and their root causes to drive policy or practice changes	Work in a vacuum, independent from other public health, health care, marketing, and community development interventions
Engage and empower communities and key groups	Replace the lack of local infrastructure, services, or capability
Influence research agendas and priorities and support the need for additional funds for medical and scientific discovery	Compensate for the absence of adequate treatment or diagnostic or preventive options and services
Increase understanding of the many socially determined factors that influence health and illness so they can be adequately addressed at the population and community levels	"Be equally effective in addressing all issues or relaying all messages," at least in the same time frame (National Cancer Institute at the National Institutes of Health, 2002, p. 3)
Encourage collaboration among different sectors, such as public health, community development, and health care	
Secure stakeholder endorsement of health and related social issues	
"Influence perceptions, beliefs and attitudes that may change social norms" (National Cancer Institute at the National Institutes of Health, 2002, p. 3)	
Promote data and emerging issues to establish new standards of care	
"Increase demand for health services" (National Cancer Institute at the National Institutes of Health, 2002, p. 3) and products	
Show benefits of and encourage behavior change	
"Demonstrate healthy skills" (National Cancer Institute at the National Institutes of Health, 2002, p. 3)	
Provoke public discussion to drive disease diagnosis, treatment, or prevention	
Suggest and "prompt action" (National Cancer Institute at the National Institutes of Health, 2002, p. 3)	
Build constituencies to support health and social change across different sectors and communities	
Advocate for equal access to existing health products and services	
Strengthen third-party relationships	
Improve patient compliance and outcomes	

Key Concepts

- Health communication is a multifaceted and multidisciplinary field of research, theory, and practice. It is concerned with reaching different populations and groups to exchange health-related information, ideas, and methods in order to influence, engage, empower, and support different groups so that they will champion, introduce, adopt, or sustain a health or social behavior, practice, or policy that will ultimately improve individual, community, and public health outcomes.

- Health communication should be inclusive and representative also of vulnerable and underserved groups.

- Health communication is an increasingly prominent field in public health, health care, community development, and the private sector (both nonprofit and corporate).

- Health communication can play a key role in advancing health equity.

- Several socially determined factors (also referred to as *social determinants of health*) influence and are influenced by health communication.

- One of the key characteristics of health communication is its multidisciplinary nature, which allows the theoretical flexibility that is needed to consider and approach each situation and key group for their unique characteristics and needs.

- We are now in the era of behavioral and social impact communication. In fact, several US and international models and agendas support the importance of a behavioral and social change–driven mind-set in developing health communication interventions.

- Health communication is an evolving discipline that should always incorporate lessons learned and practical experiences. Practitioners should take an important role in defining theories and models to inform new directions in health communication.

- It is important to be aware of key features and limitations of health communication (and more specifically what communication can and cannot do).

- Health communication relies on several action areas.

- Well-designed programs are the result of an integrated blend of different areas that should be selected in light of expected behavioral and social outcomes.

FOR DISCUSSION AND PRACTICE

1. Did you have any preliminary idea about the definition and role of health communication prior to reading this chapter? If yes, how does it compare to what you have learned in this chapter?

2. In your opinion, what are the two most important defining features of health communication and why? How do they relate to the other key characteristics of health communication that are discussed in this chapter?

3. Can you recall a personal experience in which a health communication program, message, or health-related encounter (for example, a physician visit) has influenced your decisions or perceptions about a specific health issue? Describe the experience and emphasize key factors that affected your decision and health behavior.

4. Did you ever participate in the development or implementation of a health communication intervention? If yes, what were some of the key learnings and how do they relate to the attributes of health communication as described in this chapter?

5. Can you think of examples of health communication interventions that seek to benefit and address the needs of vulnerable and underserved groups in your neighborhood, community, city, and country? If yes, did you observe any results or impact among these groups?

KEY TERMS

audience analysis

audience profile

channels

communication channels

communication objectives

communication strategies

communication vehicles

community development

health communication

health disparities

health equity

intended audiences

key groups

program outcomes

situation analysis

social determinants of health

stakeholders

underserved populations

vulnerable populations

CHAPTER 2

CURRENT HEALTH COMMUNICATION THEORIES AND ISSUES

Over several decades, the field of health communication has experienced a dramatic growth and evolution, which is still continuing. The multidisciplinary nature of health communication, one of its most important characteristics, has been recognized by several organizations and leaders (Institute of Medicine, 2003b; Bernhardt, 2004; World Health Organization [WHO], 2003; Kreps, 2012b; Rimal and Lapinski, 2009).

Although several authors and organizations have been defining the theoretical basis of health communication, the intersection among many different disciplines (for example, behavioral and social sciences, social marketing, development theories, and health education) as well as between social sciences and the humanities is still a growing field of research and practical application (Health Communication Partnership, 2005b). Some authors have been referring to a "family tree" (Waisbord, 2001, p. 1) of communication theories and models; others do not emphasize the chronological sequence and interdependence of communication theories, but focus primarily on the impact theories may have on program design and outcomes (Institute of Medicine, 2002). At the same time, current health-related issues and topics influence the theory and practice of health communication so that communication interventions can effectively address the health and social challenges of the twenty-first century.

CHAPTER OBJECTIVES

This chapter provides readers with (1) a brief overview of major theories and planning frameworks and their implications in health communication; (2) a basic foundation to apply theory and strategy-based communication principles across different settings and key groups (Association of Schools of Public Health, 2007); and (3) a review of key current issues that influence the theory and practice of health communication.

Use of Communication Models and Theories: A Premise

Theories and planning models are particularly important for students and young practitioners in this field. Theories help clarify how to approach a health issue and plan to address it through a health communication intervention. They also have a significant weight at all levels in communication research, donor-sponsored programs, retrospective analyses, outcome and impact evaluation, and all other circumstances that demand a rigorous program design. Theories can also provide a powerful tool to organize one's thoughts and to design interventions that clearly have in mind specific behavioral and social outcomes. Communication theories and frameworks are used in a less rigorous way in the commercial, nonprofit, and private sectors in the interest of time. The downside to this approach is that it may be more difficult to link any specific behavioral or social outcome to the actual health communication program, which is already a notably complex task in health communication (see Chapter Fourteen).

Overall, communication models and theoretical constructs are often used to

- Provide a basis for communication planning, monitoring, and evaluation.
- Inspire specific communication approaches.
- Help implement a specific phase of a health communication program.
- Support a true understanding of key groups as well as the health communication environment as part of the planning, implementation, and evaluation processes.

When reviewing these theories and models, junior health communication practitioners and students should remember that these are just selected references, which ideally should prompt further inquiries and readings on the theory of health communication. They should also keep in mind that theories, models, and planning frameworks should (1) be considered part of a tool kit and selected on a case-by-case basis, (2) respond to an audience's needs, (3) address the specific health situation and all factors that play a role in determining it, (4) inform and guide message development as well as the identification of appropriate communication channels, and (5) be revisited in light of emerging factors and needs. This selection process should take into account expected program outcomes and the behavioral or social impact the communication program seeks to achieve. For all other readers (including current health communication practitioners, researchers, health care providers, and other professionals), the following overview should provide an updated summary of selected theories and models that currently inspire our field, as well as key issues and topics that influence its theory and practice.

Key Theoretical Influences in Health Communication

Health communication is influenced by different disciplines and theoretical approaches (see Figure 2.1). Some of the most important theories can be divided into the following categories: behavioral and social science theories, mass communications theories, new media influence theories,

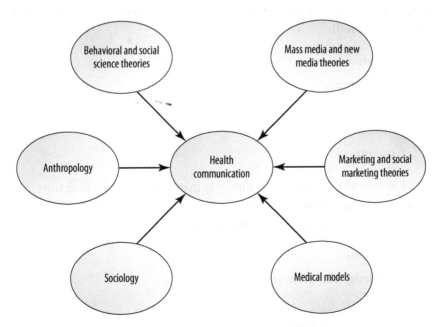

Figure 2.1 Health Communication Theory Is Influenced by Different Fields and Families of Theories

marketing and social marketing, and other theoretical influences, including medical models, sociology, and anthropology. In addition, several planning frameworks and models have been developed to reflect or incorporate key principles from some or all of these categories. The overview that follows focuses on select theories and models as well as their potential or actual impact on health communication practice.

Selected Behavioral and Social Sciences Theories

Behavioral and social sciences theories seek to analyze and explain how change occurs at the individual, community, and social levels. Some of these theories focus primarily on the key steps that may lead to behavioral or social change and others look at communication processes and group dynamics. Most of them also emphasize the interconnection and mutual dependence of individual and external factors. As previously mentioned, this connection is of great importance in health communication.

Diffusion of Innovation Theory

Initially developed by Everett Rogers (1962, 1983, 1995), the diffusion of innovation theory addresses how new ideas, concepts, or practices can spread within a community or "society, or from one society to another" (National Cancer Institute at the National Institutes of Health, 2002, p. 226). The theory identifies and defines five subgroups on the basis of their characteristics and propensity to accept and adopt innovation (Beal and Rogers, 1960):

- Innovators
- Early adopters
- Early majority
- Late majority
- Laggards

The overall premise of this theory is that change occurs over time and is dependent on the following stages (Rogers, 1962, 1983, 1995; Waisbord, 2001; Health Communication Partnership, 2005c):

- Awareness
- Knowledge and interest
- Decision
- Trial or implementation
- Confirmation or rejection of the behavior

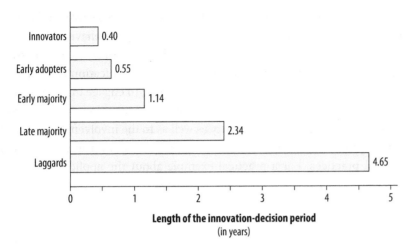

Figure 2.2 Attributes of the Audience

Source: Beal, G. M., and Rogers, E. M. *The adoption of two farm practices in a central Iowa community.* Special report no. 26, p. 14.
Ames, Iowa: Agricultural and Home Economics Experiment Station, Iowa State University, 1960. Used by permission.

It also observes that innovators usually decide much faster than any other subgroup on whether to adopt new ideas, concepts, or practices (Beal and Rogers, 1960; see Figure 2.2). Therefore, innovators can act as role models and persuade other subgroups (including laggards) to accept and adopt new behaviors and social practices.

Similar to many other theories in any field, diffusion of innovation has been misused and misinterpreted at times (Health Communication Partnership, 2005c). Some critics have observed that the trickle-down approach, from the innovators to the laggards, may not work in all situations (Waisbord, 2001). Rogers himself modified the theory to change the focus from "a persuasion approach (transmission of information between individuals and groups)" to "a process by which participants create and share information with one another in order to reach a mutual understanding" (Waisbord, 2001, p. 5; Rogers, 1976).

Nevertheless, diffusion of innovation still plays a key role in health communication research, evaluation, and planning. The major contribution of the theory is its early audience segmentation model, which supports the importance of looking at intended audiences as a complex puzzle of different subgroups, stages, needs, and priorities that should be considered in developing communication messages and activities. The theory can also provide a valid framework for "innovator studies" that seek to assess program impact within an initial group of adopters (Schiavo, Gonzalez-Flores, Ramesh, and Estrada-Portales, 2011).

Finally, the individuals' stage model provides a perspective on the time and the external conditions that are needed to achieve behavioral or social change. It is a useful tool in thinking about the levels of awareness, knowledge, and interest among key groups (Health Communication Partnership, 2005c). It is also a valid reminder that continuing to engage innovators and early adopters, or their representatives, in program planning and evaluation is essential to program sustainability as well as to the involvement of larger segments of the intended population in promoting innovative behaviors or social practices. For a practical example about the application of this theory, see Box 2.1.

BOX 2.1. DIFFUSION OF INNOVATION THEORY: A PRACTICAL EXAMPLE

Luciana, a nineteen-year-old college student, lives in a coastal town in southern Italy and loves going to the beach. During her summer vacation and many of the late spring weekends, she spends four to six hours each day basking in the sun while talking with her friends or playing beach volleyball or swimming. She uses sunscreen lotion with a low sunscreen protection factor (SPF), and only at the beginning of the season, to avoid sunburn. Once she is tanned, she may not use it at all. Most of her friends rarely use any sunscreen protection and, if they do, use the same kind with a low SPF. During the winter, Luciana keeps her tan by using artificial ultraviolet sunlamps.

In the summer, getting a nice *tintarella*, the Italian word for *suntan*, is one of Italians' favorite pastimes and is considered very attractive. People compliment each other on their tintarella. Although Luciana and some of her friends may be somewhat aware that prolonged and continual sun exposure is a risk factor for skin cancer, the aesthetic appeal and social approval of a tanned skin allay their doubts about sun exposure. Luciana also feels she is too young to worry about skin cancer, does not know enough about it, and therefore does not feel the need to use much stronger sunscreen protection.

A review of the literature on the subject (for example, Monfrecola, Fabbrocini, Posteraro, and Pini, 2000) shows that Luciana's fictional profile is somewhat representative of frequent beliefs and behavior among a percentage of Italian young people who live on the Mediterranean coast.

According to the diffusion of innovations theory, Luciana could be considered an innovator or early adopter in her peer group if she starts using higher sunscreen protection and limiting her use of sunlamps. Ideally, she could talk with her peers and circle of friends about following her example. In fact, most of them do not use any sunscreen and may be slower to change than Luciana.

There are a few facts that are good indicators that she could become an innovator or early adopter: her education level (she is a college student), socioeconomic background (both of her parents hold advanced degrees and professional jobs and have raised Luciana to question existing behaviors in light of new information), personality (she is rational, resourceful, and charming, and often perceived as a leader in her peer group), exposure to media (she is well read and relies on a variety of media for information and entertainment), attitude toward change (she is willing to experiment with new things and behaviors if she understands them and perceives their benefits), and social involvement (she is an active member of several student organizations and other social and political groups).

If we look at the different stages of the diffusion of innovation theory (awareness, knowledge and interest, decision, trial or implementation, confirmation or rejection of the behavior), the first step is to make Luciana aware of skin cancer's severity, recent increase, and strong link to sun exposure and sunlamp use. Recent facts and incidence data should be used to reinforce her awareness and to point to the need for sunscreen use.

If research shows that Luciana is already aware of the disease severity and related risk factors, communication messages and interactions should focus on making skin cancer relevant to her and her peers (the second stage of the diffusion theory). Knowledge that skin cancer can also occur among young people, and that the sun's damaging effects begin at an early age (National Cancer Institute, 2005b) may help increase Luciana's concern about sun exposure. Still, her perception that a tanned body is more attractive than an untanned one may prevent her from taking action and should be addressed early as part of the overall intervention. Focusing on the damaging effects of sun exposure on the skin's appearance and overall aging process may appeal to Luciana's aesthetic values.

Social support as well as the ability to sustain the recommended behavior should be encouraged by using adequate communication tools and activities while Luciana goes through the three remaining stages of the diffusion of innovation theory as she decides, tries, and, ideally, continues to use sunscreen and limit her use of sunlamps. In these stages, Luciana will need to perceive the advantages of behavioral change, find it acceptable for her lifestyle, and find it easy to implement and sustain. Sunscreen samples and detailed instructions on when to apply the sunscreen (not only to prevent skin burning) can facilitate early use, but social support and peer validation is critical to sustainability.

The program should also address her other concerns: the appeal of an untanned or lightly tanned body (Broadstock, Borland, and Gason, 1992; Monfrecola, Fabbrocini, Posteraro, and Pini, 2000), which could be reinforced by celebrities, institutions, older family members, or others who could act as role models; and the reduced risk for a potentially life-threatening disease. Change would occur only if all tools and activities are designed to take into account Luciana's needs and rely on her input as a key actor in the overall change process. If these needs are adequately met, Luciana may become an ambassador (innovator) for the importance of sunscreen use among her circle of friends, peers, and social groups. (An example on the topic of skin cancer is given in Weinreich [1999].)

In approaching the rest of this chapter, readers may find it helpful to apply Luciana's fictional example or other examples to all theories and models that are discussed in it. At a minimum, this would prompt awareness of different ways of organizing one's thoughts when dealing with the same health issue using different theoretical frameworks. It will also provide a tool to organize audience-related research.

Health Belief Model

The health belief model (HBM) (Becker, Haefner, and Maiman, 1977; Janz and Becker, 1984; Strecher and Rosenstock, 1997) was originally intended to explain why people did not participate in programs that could help them diagnose or prevent diseases (National Cancer Institute at the National Institutes of Health, 2002). The major assumption of this model is that in order to engage in healthy behaviors, key groups need to be aware of their risk for severe or life-threatening diseases and perceive that the benefits of behavior change outweigh potential barriers or other negative aspects of recommended actions. HBM is one of the first theories developed to explain the process of change in relation to health behavior. It has also inspired—among many other models—the field of health education. Health education is defined in *Healthy People 2010* as "any planned combination of learning experiences designed to predispose, enable, and reinforce voluntary behavior conducive to health in individuals, groups, or communities" (US Department of Health and Human Services, 2005, p. 11–20; Green and Kreuter, 1999).

HBM has the following key components:

- *Perceived susceptibility:* The individual's perception of whether he or she is at risk for contracting a specific illness or health problem
- *Perceived severity:* The subjective feeling on whether the specific illness or health problem can be severe (for example, permanently impair physical or mental functions) or is life threatening, and therefore worthy of one's attention
- *Perceived benefits:* The individual's perceptions of the advantages of adopting recommended actions that would eventually reduce the risk for disease severity, morbidity, and mortality
- *Perceived barriers:* The individual's perceptions of the costs of and obstacles to adopting recommended actions (includes economic costs as well as other kinds of lifestyle sacrifices)

* *Cues to action:* Public or social events that can signal the importance of taking action (for example, a neighbor who is diagnosed with the same disease or a mass media campaign)

* *Self-efficacy:* The individual's confidence in his or her ability to perform and sustain the recommended behavior with little or no help from others

In describing the HBM, Pechmann (2001) referred to it as a "risk learning model because the goal is to teach new information about health risks and the behaviors that minimize those risks" (p. 189). The overall premise of the HBM is that knowledge will bring change. Knowledge is brought to intended groups through an educational approach that primarily focuses on messages, channels, and spokespeople (Andreasen, 1995).

"Some authors caution that the HBM does not pre-suppose or imply a strategy for change" (Rosenstock and Kirscht, 1974, p. 472; Andreasen, 1995, p. 10). Nevertheless, the major contribution of the HBM to the health communication field is its emphasis on the importance of knowledge, a necessary but not sufficient step to change. HBM can also be used for audience-related research because it provides a useful framework to organize one's thoughts in developing an audience profile and refining health communication programs as part of research and evaluation. Box 2.2 provides a case study on how the health belief model was used to evaluate a mass media campaign for HIV prevention.

BOX 2.2. THE ADDED-VALUE OF THEORETICAL MODELS IN EVALUATING MASS MEDIA CAMPAIGNS

Situation and Program Description

In 1988, the National AIDS Program (NAP) of the Ministry of Health of Peru conducted a household survey on knowledge, attitudes, and practices related to sexual behavior and HIV transmission with technical and financial support from Johns Hopkins University, Population Communication Services, and the Population Council. The results showed high levels of misconceptions about HIV transmission routes and a low percentage of respondents (13 percent) reporting condom use in the last month before the survey (Saba and others, 1992). In order to educate the public on HIV transmission and prevention, the NAP and its partners agreed to conduct a six-week mass media campaign using TV spots, radio spots, and movie theater advertisements.

Theory-Based Evaluation

The impact of the campaign was evaluated by comparing the baseline with a follow-up survey.[1] The evaluation team created a rating scale (health belief model [HBM] index) and related evaluation parameters based on the constructs of the HBM (Jette and others, 1981). The rating scale ranged from 0 to 3 depending on the individual's perception of none, one, two, or three of the following variables: (1) susceptibility to HIV infection, (2) severity of the disease, and (3) perceived benefits of condoms as effective protection against HIV. Thus, respondents who consider themselves as susceptible to HIV infection, consider AIDS as a severe disease, and perceived condoms effective for prevention got a score of 3. Those who did not have any of these three beliefs were given a score of 0. There were values of 1 and 2 in between.

The evaluation showed an increase in perceived susceptibility, perceived severity, and perceived benefits of condom use after exposure to the mass media campaign. Self-reported condom use increased from 13 to 16 percent (a difference of 3 percentage points). To better understand the profile of the respondents who changed their behavior, the HBM index was correlated with self-reported condom use. It was observed that for individuals exposed to the campaign, the proportion of high scorers on the HBM index who used condoms was significantly greater than low scorers on the HBM index. In fact, 20 percent of the respondents who scored high in the HBM index used condoms after exposure to the campaign, compared with only 9 percent of the individuals who scored low in the HBM index[2] (a difference of 11 percentage points). High scorers were clearly the most susceptible to change.

Conclusions

As for this case study, the use of a theoretical model guides and organizes data interpretation when evaluating the mass media campaign. Theory guides assumptions about the profile of the population who are more susceptible to change if exposed to a "cue to action" such as an educational campaign. The "predictability" offered by the theoretical model can be very valuable for audience segmentation, message design, and campaign evaluation so that program efforts can be tailored to address existing perceptions, attitudes, needs, and behaviors among key audiences.

Notes

[1]The pre- and postcampaign survey consisted of structured questionnaires applied to two samples of 1,913 and 2,443 men and women aged fifteen to forty-four from middle, lower middle, and lower socioeconomic strata before and after the six-week campaign.

[2]Scores of 2 or 3 in the HBM index were considered high whereas scores of 0 or 1 were considered low.

References

Jette, A. M., and others. "The Structure and Reliability of Health Belief Indices." *Health Services Research*, 1981, *16*(1), 81–98.

Saba, W., and others. "The Mass Media and Health Beliefs: Using Media Campaigns to Promote Preventive Behavior." Unpublished case study, 1992, 1–25.

Source: Saba, W. "The Added-Value of Theoretical Models in Evaluating Mass Media Campaigns." Unpublished case study, 2012a. Used by permission.

Social Cognitive Theory

Also known as social learning theory, social cognitive theory (SCT; Bandura, 1977, 1986, 1997) explains behavior as the result of three reciprocal factors: behavior, personal factors, and outside events. Any change in any of these three factors is expected to determine changes in the remaining ones (National Cancer Institute at the National Institutes of Health, 2002). Behavior is viewed as influenced by a combination of personal and outside factors and events.

One of SCT's key premises is its emphasis on the outside environment, which becomes a source of observational learning. According to SCT, the environment is a place where individuals can observe an action, understand its consequences, and, as a result of personal and interpersonal influences, become motivated to repeat and adopt it. SCT has these key components (Bandura, 1977, 1986, 1997; National Cancer Institute at the National Institutes of Health, 2002; Health Communication Partnership, 2005d):

- *Attention:* People's awareness of the action being modeled and observed.

- *Retention:* People's ability to remember the action being modeled and observed.

- *Reproduction (trial):* People's ability to reproduce the action being modeled and observed.

- *Motivation:* People's internal impulse and intention to perform the action. Motivation depends on a number of social, affective, and physiological influences (for example, the support of peers and family members to perform the action, the knowledge that the action will improve physical performance), as well as the perception of self-efficacy.

• *Performance:* The individual's ability to perform the action on a regular basis.

• *Self-efficacy:* The individual's confidence in his or her ability to perform and sustain the action with little or no help from others, which plays a major role in actual performance.

SCT can provide a framework to approach several different questions in program research and planning, but its major contribution to health communications is to understand the mechanisms and factors that can influence retention, reproduction, and motivation (Health Communication Partnership, 2005d) on a given behavior.

Theory of Reasoned Action

The theory of reasoned action (TRA; Ajzen and Fishbein, 1980) suggests that behavioral performance is primarily determined by the strength of the person's intention to perform a specific behavior. It identifies two major factors that contribute to such intentions (Ajzen and Fishbein, 1980; Health Communication Partnership, 2005e; Coffman, 2002):

• A person's attitude toward the behavior. In general, attitudes can be defined as positive or negative emotions or feelings toward a behavior, a person, a concept, or an idea (for example: "I ___ eating fruit and vegetables"; "I ___ my friend's boyfriend").

behavioral beliefs
A term used within the theory of reasoned action that refers to a person's own beliefs about the consequences of a given behavior

• A person's subjective norms about the behavior. In the TRA, subjective norms are defined as the opinion or judgment, positive or negative, that loved ones, friends, family, colleagues, professional organizations, or others may have about a potential behavior (for example, "My friends do not approve that I smoke marijuana"; "My doctor recommends that I exercise at least twice per week").

normative beliefs
A term used within the theory of reasoned action that refers to whether a person may believe significant others will approve or not of his or her behavior

Under the TRA, attitudes toward a specific behavior are a function of the person's own beliefs about the consequences of such behavior (for example, "smoking marijuana may have a negative impact on my concentration and work performance"). These are called **behavioral beliefs**.

Subjective norms are influenced by **normative beliefs**, which refer to whether a person may think significant others will approve or not of his or her behavior (for example, "I think that if I start to smoke marijuana, some of my friends may not approve of it"). Another component of normative beliefs is the person's motivation to comply with other people's ideas and potential approval (Coffman, 2002). For example, if one's normative belief is, "I think that if I start to smoke marijuana, some of my friends may not approve it," the person's motivation to comply can be assessed by asking the following question: "Do I care enough about these specific friends to avoid smoking marijuana?" In other words, "Do I care about what people may expect of me?"

TRA is an influential theory in health communication and is frequently used also in program evaluation (Coffman, 2002). However, it is important to be cautious about concluding that the intention of adopting a certain behavior may always translate in actual behavior adoption. Communication can play an important role in supporting behavioral intentions and increasing the likelihood that they would become actual behaviors. This requires the development of interventions and tools that would increase social support and community engagement as well as make it easy for people to try, adopt, and integrate new health behaviors in their lifestyle.

TRA is particularly useful in analyzing and identifying reasons for action and what may change people's attitudes toward a health or social behavior. It is also a good tool in profiling **primary audiences** (people whom the program seeks to engage more directly and would most benefit from change) and **secondary audiences** (individuals and groups who may have an influence on the primary audience) (Health Communication Partnership, 2005e).

primary audiences
The people whom the program seeks to engage more directly and would most benefit from change

secondary audiences
All individuals, groups, communities, and organizations that may influence the decisions and behaviors of the primary audiences

Social Norms Theory

Several theories address the influence of **social norms** (group-held beliefs on how people should behave in a social situation or group setting) on behaviors. This is of particular importance for health communication interventions because understanding and influencing such norms via a community- or population-centered process is often critical to attaining behavioral and social results. Social norms–centric theories predicate that most people may be willing to adopt or sustain a specific behavior not only if they are able to see a definite benefit in that change but also if they are convinced that other people will do the same.

Several authors have developed social norms theories. Among them, Bicchieri's (2006) new theory of social norms challenges key assumptions from the field of social sciences by arguing that people conform to social norms as an automatic response to cues they receive in a specific social situation. According to this theory, too much emphasis is placed on the rational

social norms
Group-held beliefs on how people should behave in a social situation or group setting

process of decision making because decisions are often made without much deliberation, (1) as a result of people's understanding of social expectations or (2)—in the case of "moral norms"—as an unconditional response to emotional reactions to a situation (Bicchieri, 2006).

That is why, in order to achieve almost any kind of behavioral or social result in health or community development settings, it is necessary to consider, understand, and influence existing social norms. For example, we have case study–based evidence that in pandemic flu or other emergency settings, social norms may prevent the implementation of recommended emergency response measures, such as social distancing, avoiding crowded places, safely caring for loved ones, or handling dead bodies (Schiavo, 2009b).

Yet, in applying social norms theories it may be equally important to research and develop a **key influentials roadmap** (identifying and mapping groups and stakeholders whose opinions, moral values, and expectations actually matter in the eyes of specific groups or populations) for each intended group. Although social norms theories rightly assume a horizontal and participatory process to addressing and influencing current norms, the moral and social authority of specific gatekeepers (for example, elderly, community, or religious leaders, etc.) or other stakeholders should not be underestimated. Social cues and emotional reactions to situations are dependent on cultural values and the specific peer groups with whom people interact. Therefore, it's important that gatekeepers and other relevant groups are engaged in the process of influencing social norms.

key influentials roadmap

Identifying and mapping groups and stakeholders whose opinions, moral values, and expectations actually matter in the eyes of specific groups or populations

Ideation

The ideation theory (Kincaid, Figueroa, Storey, and Underwood, 2001; Rimon, 2002; Cleland and Wilson, 1987) refers to "new ways of thinking and diffusion of those ways of thinking by means of social interaction in local, culturally homogenous communities" (O'Sullivan, Yonkler, Morgan, and Merritt, 2003, pp. 1–3; Bongaarts and Watkins, 1996). This theory is used in strategic behavior communications to identify and influence ideational elements (Rimon, 2002; Kincaid, Figueroa, Storey, and Underwood, 2001), such as attitudes, knowledge, self-efficacy, social and peer approval, and other factors that can affect and determine health behavior (see Figure 2.3).

One of the key premises of the ideation theory is "that the more ideational elements that apply to someone, the greater the probability that they will adopt a healthy behavior" (Kincaid and Figueroa, 2004). In other words, individual and community behaviors are influenced by the social contexts in which people live and work.

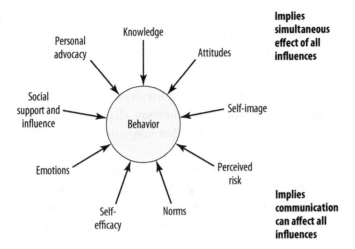

Figure 2.3 Ideation Theory

Sources: Kincaid, D. L., and Figueroa, M. E. *Ideation and Communication for Social Change.* Health Communication Partnership Seminar, April 23, 2004. Used by permission. Rimon, J. G. *Behaviour Change Communication in Public Health. Beyond Dialogue: Moving Toward Convergence.* The Communication Initiative, 2002. www.comminit.com/strategicthinking/stnicroundtable/sld-1744.html. Retrieved Nov. 2005. Used by permission.

Convergence Theory

Similar to other theories in the social process category (O'Sullivan, Yonkler, Morgan, and Merritt, 2003), the convergence theory (Kincaid, 1979; Rogers and Kincaid, 1981) emphasizes the importance "of information sharing, mutual understanding and mutual agreement" on any collective or group action that would bring social change (Figueroa, Kincaid, Rani, and Lewis, 2002, p. 4). It is based on the perspective that individual perceptions and behavior are influenced by the perceptions and behaviors of members of the same group, such as members of professional associations, colleagues, and family members, and by people "in one's personal networks," such as peers, friends, or personal or professional acquaintances (O'Sullivan, Yonkler, Morgan, and Merritt, 2003, p. 1-4).

This theory is characterized by three distinctive features (Kincaid, 1979; Rogers and Kincaid, 1981; Figueroa, Kincaid, Rani, and Lewis, 2002):

* Information is shared using a participatory process in which there is no sender or receiver but everyone creates and shares information. Participants in this process include individuals, community groups and organizations, and different kinds of institutions, such as professional associations, churches, and schools.

* Communication emphasizes individual perceptions and interpretations of the information being shared, encourages an ongoing dialogue, and fosters mutual understanding and agreement on common meanings.

* Communication is horizontal and involves two or more participants. In a horizontal model of communication, all participants are equal and aim to reach mutual agreement that may stimulate a group action.

This theory has contributed to redefining communication as a process in which all participants need to respect and take into account other people's feelings, emotions, and beliefs. It has also highlighted the importance of social networks and key influentials in defining the path to social change.

Stages of Behavior Change Model

The stages of behavior change model, also known as the *transtheoretical model* (Prochaska and DiClemente, 1983; Grimley, Gabrielle, Bellis, and Prochaska, 1993; Prochaska and Vellicer, 1997), defines behavioral change as a process that goes through different stages or steps. Each stage describes different "levels of motivation or readiness to change" (National Cancer Institute at the National Institutes of Health, 2002, p. 221; Prochaska and Vellicer, 1997). The model identifies five stages of change (Prochaska and Vellicer, 1997; Weinreich, 2011):

1. *Precontemplation*, in which individuals have no intention of adopting a recommended health behavior but are learning about it

2. *Contemplation*, in which individuals are considering adopting the recommended behavior

3. *Decision*, in which people decide to adopt the recommended health behavior

4. *Action*, in which people try to adopt the recommended behavior for a short period of time

5. *Maintenance*, in which people continue to perform the recommended health behavior for a long period of time (at least over six months) and, ideally, incorporate it in their routine and lifestyle

In health communication, these stages of change can be used in the phase in which intended audiences are segmented (see Chapter Ten) to identify key groups that, among other related characteristics, will also have similar levels of motivation and readiness for behavioral change (Weinreich, 1999). Therefore, this theory can be instrumental in designing communication objectives, messages, and strategies for each of these groups (National Cancer Institute at the National Institutes of Health, 2002).

Communication for Persuasion Theory

This theory was developed by social psychologist William McGuire and focuses on how people process information. McGuire (1984) highlighted twelve interdependent steps in the process of persuasive communication (McGuire, 1984; National Cancer Institute at the National Institutes of Health, 2002; Alcalay and Bell, 2000). He suggested that in order to assimilate and perform a new behavior, a person should do the following (McGuire, 1984; National Cancer Institute at the National Institutes of Health, 2002):

1. Be exposed to the message.
2. Pay attention to it.
3. Find it interesting or personally relevant.
4. Understand it.
5. Figure out how the new behavior could fit in his or her life.
6. Accept the change that is being proposed.
7. Remember and validate the message.
8. Be able to think of the message in relevant contexts or situations.
9. Make decisions on the basis of the retrieved information or message.
10. Behave in line with that decision.
11. Receive positive reinforcement for that behavior.
12. Integrate the new behavior into his or her life.

This model also suggests that these twelve steps are interdependent. Achieving any of them is strictly contingent on success at all prior steps. Message design, messenger credibility, communication channels, and the characteristics of both the intended audiences and the recommended behavior, which should be intended to fit easily in people's lives, all influence behavioral outcomes.

Although the current focus of health communication is more on engaging intended groups than persuading them, keeping in mind McGuire's steps for persuasion can provide a valid framework for approaching key groups and stakeholders to secure their initial involvement and input in the health issue. In doing so, it is also important to remember that key values and needs may change over time. This should prompt communicators to incorporate these changes in communication planning and evaluation as well as redefine recommended behaviors depending on people's lifestyles, preferences, and needs.

Intergroup Theories

Intergroup theories seek to explain intergroup behavior within the context of communication and decision-making settings and may provide useful constructs for the development of intercultural communication interventions and message design strategies. A comprehensive discussion of all theories in this group goes beyond the scope of this book. Yet, sample contemporary intergroup theories that continue to influence the field of health communication include the *anxiety and uncertainty management (AUM) theory* and the *problematic integration theory.*

Developed by William B. Gudykunst, AUM theory assumes that at least one person in an intercultural or group encounter is a stranger. The theory explains how intergroup communication's effectiveness may be enhanced by "the mindful management of anxiety and uncertainty levels of interaction" (Littlejohn and Foss, 2009a). AUM explores the roles of motivation, knowledge, skills, and cultural differences in effective communication as well as people's ability to manage anxiety and uncertainty (Gudykunst, 1993). The theory also has implications for risk communication in epidemics and emergency settings where managing people's psychological reaction to crisis is strictly dependent on the ability of key professional and community groups and leaders to adequately manage the anxiety and uncertainties that accompany the process of communicating about risk.

Similarly, problematic integration theory (PI) (Babrow, 1992, 2007) also examines "the role of communication in producing and copying with subjective uncertainty" (Bradac, 2011, p. 456). PI theory analyzes the process through which people receive, process, and react to communication and life's experiences. "Although PI theory is a general perspective on communication in difficult situations, many applications have been made in the area of health communication" (Littlejohn and Foss, 2009b). Some of the main premises of PI theory is that communication processing and integration is related to social and cultural beliefs and constructs, which determine people's ability to integrate new information and experiences within their existing beliefs and cultural identity, either in harmony with them or in a problematic way. Babrow (1992) identified several different manifestations of problematic integration, which may be symptomatic of cognitive, emotional, communicative, or motivational discomfort. PI theory has great implications for cross-cultural health communication interventions because it points to the importance of identifying and adequately addressing cultural and social constructs among groups and stakeholders we seek to engage in the health communication process.

Mass and New Media Communication Theories

This section includes sample mass media and new media theories that influence the practice of health communication and provides useful guidance on communication principles as they relate to media use and influence within the context of health communication interventions. Many of these principles transcend mass media and new media and also apply to other action areas of health communication.

Mass Media

No one can dispute the ability of the mass media to reach significant percentages of interested groups and audiences. If adequately used and selected in response to audience's needs and preferences, radio, television, printed media, and the Internet are powerful connectors between communicators and their audiences.

Mass communication theories include research and studies that focus on the impact of the mass media on intended populations. However, many of their key principles and observations can apply in general to the overall field of global health communication. The following definitions are important when looking at this family of theories:

- *Media effects* are simply the consequences [on the groups they reach] of what the mass media do, whether intended or not.
- *Media power*, on the other hand, refers to a general potential on the part of the media to have effects, especially of a planned kind.
- *Media effectiveness* is a statement about the efficiency of media in achieving a given aim and always implies intention or some planned communication goal. (McQuail, 1994, p. 333)

Although several authors divide mass communication theories into different eras and subgroups (McQuail, 1994; Health Communication Partnership, 2005b), a comprehensive discussion of all of them is beyond the scope of this book. Therefore, the theory presented next represents only an example of models and studies in this category.

Cultivation Theory of Mass Media   Developed by George Gerbner, the cultivation theory "specifies that repeated, intense exposure to deviant definitions of 'reality' in the mass media leads to perceptions of the 'reality' as normal" (Communication Initiative, 2003a; Gerbner, 1969; Gerbner, Gross, Morgan, and Signorielle, 1980). "The result is a social legitimization of the reality depicted in the mass media, which can influence behavior" (Communication Initiative, 2003a; Gerbner, Gross, Morgan, and Signorielle, 1980). In other words, the media have the power to portray a behavior to make it socially acceptable by shaping public perceptions and feelings toward that behavior. Cultivation refers to the ability of the mass media to produce long-term effects on intended audiences by nurturing their feelings through continual message exposure. This process also relies on the ability of the mass media to "transcend traditional barriers of time, space and social grouping" (Communication Initiative, 2003a; Gerbner, 1969).

Cultivation is a concept that transcends the mass media and applies to the overall field of health communication. In fact, nurturing the feelings of key stakeholders and groups through continual message exposure, using all kinds of communication channels including the mass media, is a practice that frequently helps secure their involvement in the health issue and its solutions.

New Media Theories

new media
"Those media that are based on the use of digital technologies, such as the Internet, computer games, digital television, and mobile devices, as well as the remaking of more traditional media forms to adopt and adapt to new media technologies" (Williams and others, 2008; Flew, 2002)

There is a lot of excitement about the widespread use of **new media** ("those media that are based on the use of digital technologies, such as the Internet, computer games, digital television, and mobile devices, as well as 'the remaking of more traditional media forms to adopt and adapt to new media technologies,'" Williams, Zraik, Schiavo, and Hatz, 2008, p. 161; Flew, 2002, p. 11) and their ever increasing potential in health communication. Emerging new media theories have been focusing primarily on attempting to explain the process through which new media may help build community around a health or social issue, influence people's participation, share knowledge, expand one's social networks, test messages and strategies, and ultimately influence behavior and social change (Dholakia, Bagozzi, and Pearo, 2004; Hsu, Ju, Yen, and Chang, 2007).

Of interest, Dholakia, Bagozzi, and Pearo (2004) developed a social influence model to connect and identify personal and social motives for people's participation in virtual communities. According to this model, many of the motivating factors (for example, social enhancement, entertainment value, and self-discovery) for participation in virtual communities mirror those that play a key role in motivating people to participate in real-world communities.

Yet, the lack of visual cues and the overall anonymity that new media and **social media** (a subgroup of new media and social sites that aim primarily to create community and connect people, such as Facebook [Stelzner, 2009]) provide users, may change group dynamics and, depending on the health or social topic, may also shift perceptions of others "from being primarily interpersonal to being group-based perceptions (stereotyping)" (Lea, Spears, and de Groot, 2001, p. 527). In health communication, the appeal of the anonymous connotation of new media may vary depending on cultural values of specific groups and health and social issues.

Although a comprehensive discussion on the use of new media among different groups and kinds of organizations, as well as planning and evaluation methodologies for new media–based interventions is included in Chapters Five and Fourteen, it is worth mentioning here that—as with other communication channels—new media–based approaches should be integrated with the many other forms of communication we discuss in this book (and others) in order to maximize behavioral and social impact of all programs.

social media
A subgroup of new media and social sites that aim primarily to create community and connect people. Social media (for example, YouTube) are tools for sharing and discussing information (Stelzner, 2009)

Marketing-Based Models

In the private (commercial and nonprofit) sector, the field of marketing refers to strategic activities that encourage the use of products or services by consumers or special groups. Over time, marketing-based models have also inspired public health, health care, and community development interventions that encourage the adoption of new or existing health products, services, or behaviors. The two models that are presented next have many similar features and contribute to the theoretical basis of health communication.

Social Marketing

Social marketing has been defined as "the application of commercial marketing technologies to the analysis, planning, execution, and evaluation of programs designed to influence the voluntary behavior of intended audiences in order to improve their personal welfare and that of their society" (Andreasen, 1995, p. 7). Similar to commercial marketing, behavior change is the ultimate goal of social marketing. However, in commercial marketing, behavior change is sought primarily to benefit the sponsoring organizations (Andreasen, 1995), even if, in some cases, marketing activities also encourage the adoption of healthy behaviors, such as immunization or compliance to medication, which can improve the health conditions of intended populations.

Social marketing practices are consumer centered (Andreasen, 1995; Kotler and Roberto, 1989; Lefebvre, 2007) and stress the importance of four elements, referred to as the four Ps of social marketing:

- *Product:* The behavior, service, product, or policy that the organization or program seeks to see adopted by intended audiences. In social marketing, products can be tangible (for example, condoms or mosquito nets being sold and distributed as part of a social marketing campaign) or intangible (for example, the behavior being recommended and adopted by intended audiences).

- *Price:* The price of the product that is being promoted or the emotional, physical, community, or social cost of adopting the new behavior, policy, or practice.

- *Place:* The product distribution channels (for example, point-of-service locations, wholesale distributors) or the place where it is most likely to reach intended audiences with communication messages and tools to facilitate the adoption of the new behavior.

- *Promotion:* How a message is conveyed. It thus refers to how to motivate intended audiences so they try and perform the recommended behavior or adopt a new policy or practice.

Social marketing is also considered a planning framework to be used with other theories and models in health communication planning (National Cancer Institute at the National Institutes of Health, 2002). Additional theoretical constructs should closely fit the specific health issue and its potential solutions and, most important, sustain community participation and involvement (Waisbord, 2001).

Critics of social marketing view this approach as a top-down model that does not allow the level of community participation required for effective change, especially in the case of developing countries: "For them, social marketing is a non-participatory strategy because it treats most people as consumers rather than protagonists" (Waisbord, 2001, p. 9). Yet, social marketing models and interventions over the years have been incorporating community engagement and mobilization and other participatory strategies. In several of its applications, social marketing has evolved into a theoretical and practice-based model that may also apply to social change (Lefebvre, 2013). Moreover, *Healthy People 2020* includes social marketing–specific objectives as part of the health communication and health information technology topic area (US Department of Health and Human Resources, 2012b).

One of social marketing's key contributions to the health communication field is a systematic people-centered and market-driven approach to program research. Social marketing techniques and tools are particularly helpful in developing key group profiles, situation and marketing analyses, and defining the health problem and potential solutions. Although these analyses occur in a participatory context, which involves members of key groups and should be always encouraged, many research tools and techniques are imported from social marketing and marketing practices (see Chapter Eleven).

Another contribution is related to the importance of cost-effectiveness and competitive analyses. The social marketing approach to competition encourages the analysis and understanding of all alternatives, such as alternative behaviors or programs or products that people may have (Andreasen, 1995). This helps develop a desirable "product" that is likely to be adopted and to fit people's lifestyle, beliefs, and needs. However, in health communication, "products" are always intangible and should coincide with behavioral or social outcomes (for example, changes in immunization or AIDS prevention practices or policies).

Finally, social marketing strategies have been shown to be helpful in raising disease and risk awareness (see the example in Box 2.3) as well as contributing to achieving behavioral and social results among different groups and populations. In public health, other models and techniques complement and integrate social marketing theory and practice in order to further encourage program sustainability as well as a long-lasting community involvement (Waisbord, 2001) and the building of local capacity to address health and development issues.

BOX 2.3. RAISING AWARENESS OF INFANT MORTALITY DISPARITIES IN SAN FRANCISCO

In San Francisco, African American infants suffer a mortality rate two to three times higher than white infants. In an attempt to address this disparity, the San Francisco Public Health Department (SFDPH) partnered with community-based organizations and the Family Health Outcomes Project at the University of California, San Francisco, and with funding from the Centers for Disease Control (CDC) REACH 2010 initiative, created the Seven Principles Project. The project included a social marketing campaign aimed at (1) raising awareness of the gap in infant mortality rates among African Americans who live in San Francisco, (2) increasing knowledge of specific practices and risk factors that have been associated with higher incidence of sudden infant death syndrome (SIDS), and (3) encouraging families to take action.

Methods

Working together with African American residents and using focus groups to secure program feedback, the Seven Principles Project developed three multimedia campaigns. The three campaigns all used the same media to disseminate information. These included advertorials on buses and at bus stops in the neighborhoods where the majority of African Americans reside, as well as posters, cards, brochures, handouts, church fans, and radio public service announcements on radio stations that are popular with the African American community. Main messages included the information that (1) black babies die at twice the rate of all babies in San Francisco; (2) to reduce the chance of SIDS, babies sleep best on their backs; and (3) stop black babies from dying—take action. The campaign also provided a telephone number that people could call to get involved with the project.

The campaign's main concepts and activities were based on research findings on knowledge, attitudes, and beliefs about infant mortality and SIDS among African Americans. Prior to the design of the Seven Principles Project, the SFDPH conducted several focus groups to assess existing awareness levels and to help develop effective intervention strategies. Focus groups included 250 African American community members. Focus group findings revealed that prior to the campaign, over half of the participants did not know about any disparity in infant mortality in San Francisco. In addition, a baseline telephone survey of 804 African Americans ages eighteen to sixty-four showed that only 39.6 percent knew about the disparity. Moreover, 28.5 percent of survey respondents were not aware that placing an infant on his or her back to sleep may reduce the risk of SIDS. Because the disparity in infant mortality rates has persisted for years, clearly this message had not been effectively communicated to the African American community. The Seven Principles Project aimed to address this information gap.

Results

A follow-up telephone survey conducted with 654 African Americans indicated substantial community exposure to the awareness campaign. It also revealed a statistically significant increase in awareness about the existing disparity in infant mortality when compared to the data collected prior to the campaign (62.7 percent of respondents who participated in the postsurvey were aware of the disparity versus only 39.6 percent of respondents in the precampaign survey). Although there was no overall significant increase (70.4 percent versus 71.7 percent) in knowledge about proper sleep positions to prevent SIDS, respondents who reported any exposure to this campaign were more likely to know about proper sleep positions (79.7 percent versus 64.3 percent).

Source: Rienks, J., and others. "Evidence That Social Marketing Campaigns Can Effectively Increase Awareness of Infant Mortality Disparities." Paper presented at the Annual Meeting of the American Public Health Association, Philadelphia, Dec. 13, 2005. Used by permission.

Integrated Marketing Communications

Integrated marketing communications (IMC), a planning concept "that recognizes the added value of a comprehensive plan that evaluates the strategic roles of a variety of communication disciplines and combines these disciplines to provide clarity, consistency, and maximum communication impact" (Belch and Belch, 2004), is a strategic approach used in the private sector to develop, implement, and evaluate brand communication programs. It takes into account and addresses the consumer's perspective, needs, beliefs, and perceptions and relies on the strategic integration of measurable objectives and approaches (Schultz and Schultz, 2003; Nowak and others, 1998). It is considered an avant-garde marketing approach, has been incorporated in several academic programs, and forms part of the curricula of many departments (New York University, 2013; University of Utah, 2013; Emerson College, 2013). IMC principles are also reflected in some models for strategic behavior communications.

IMC recognizes that the flow and volume of information is constantly increasing for most audiences around the world (Schultz, Tannerbaum, and Lauterborn, 1994; Renganathan and others, 2005). Therefore, message clarity and consistency as well as "an integrated and coordinated approach with credibility is vital" (Renganathan and others, 2005, p. 310). The most important contribution of IMC to health communication is its emphasis on the significance of a multifaceted and strategic approach, which is based on people's point of view, and address their key needs.

Select Models for Strategic Behavior and Social Change Communication

Several models incorporate or combine behavioral, social, mass media, new media, or marketing theories described in this chapter. Select examples of these models and planning frameworks are described next.

Communication for Development (C4D)

The concept of development communication (DW communication) was born over half a century ago to address key issues and lessons learned from the developing world. The field of DW communication has been evolving since the 1970s and strongly emphasizes community ownership and participation. It has been defined as "the art and science of human communication linked to a society's planned transformation from a state of poverty to one of dynamic socio-economic growth that makes for greater equity and the larger unfolding of individual potential" (Quebral, 1971, 1972, 2001).

Inspired by DW theories and lessons learned, communication for development (C4D) is a broad term that refers to all kinds of communications that need to take place in society—and within different levels of society—if sustainable democratic development and behavioral and social change are to occur.

Several international and multilateral organizations have been using C4D as a planning framework for communication interventions aiming to achieve behavioral and social change. At UNICEF, for example, "C4D is defined as a systematic, planned and evidence-based strategic process to promote positive and measurable individual behavior and social change that is an integral part of development programs, policy advocacy and humanitarian work. C4D ensures dialogue and consultation with, and participation of children, their families and communities. In other words, C4D privileges local contexts and relies on a mix of communication tools, channels and approaches" (UNICEF, 2012, 2013a).

Although some of these concepts (for example, focus on participation, horizontal communication, and collective action) have been already incorporated by a variety of other communication models and planning frameworks, C4D further embraces them via its human rights–based approach to programming and by ultimately seeking to create equality of distribution of social benefits, which in turn may help sustain long-term behavioral and social changes. At UNICEF, C4D has been used to improve "health, nutrition, and other key social outcomes for children, their families" and their communities (UNICEF, 2012). Several academic programs in the United States and internationally (Ohio University, 2013; Malmo University, 2013 [Sweden]) specifically focus on the theory and practice of communication for development.

Communication for Behavioral Impact

Communication for behavioral impact (COMBI) is an integrated model and planning framework for social mobilization and strategic behavior communication interventions (Parks and Lloyd, 2004; Renganathan et al., 2005; Schiavo, 2007b; Hosein, Parks, and Schiavo, 2009). COMBI's theoretical foundation and "ten-step planning methodology have progressively matured from work started in 1994 at New York University on integrated marketing communication applied to social development challenges, with the input also of UNICEF and UNFPA" (Hosein, 2008; Hosein, Parks, and Schiavo, 2009). It was later absorbed by WHO in its social mobilization work in Geneva in 2000. "To date, WHO and its partners have trained public health professionals and government agencies in COMBI from more than fifty countries in Africa, Asia, Eastern Europe, Latin America, the Caribbean, and North America. This training has increased local strategic communication capacity and resulted in the development and implementation of more than sixty COMBI programs worldwide" (Hosein, 2008).

Although COMBI has been applied primarily in the health care field, its key principles and methodologies may be relevant to other areas. For example, COMBI has been used as part of UNICEF's programs on child protection and juvenile justice in Moldova (E. Hosein, personal communication, 2005, 2006). Similar efforts were undertaken with UNICEF in Albania and Jordan. A very successful program also using COMBI for antenatal care was carried out by UNICEF in Cambodia in 2009 (E. Hosein, personal communication, 2012, 2013). "Moreover, COMBI has been used and has the potential to be used in combination with other strategic communication models . . . of other U.S. and international organizations for the development of tools and planning resources" (Hosein, Parks, & Schiavo, 2009, p. 547; Johns Hopkins University, 2005; UNICEF, 2006c).

With its emphasis on behavioral impact, COMBI uses a research-based, participatory approach to identify and address behavioral issues that may have an impact on health outcomes (Renganathan and others, 2005; E. Hosein, personal communication, 2005, 2006). COMBI is based on two fundamental principles. "First: Do nothing—produce no T-shirt, no posters, no leaflets, no videos, until you have set out clear, precise, specific behavioral objectives (SBOs). Second: Do nothing—produce no T-shirts, no posters, no leaflets, no videos, until you have successfully undertaken a situational 'market' analysis in relation to preliminary behavioral objectives" (Schiavo, 2007b, p. 51; Renganathan and others, 2005). The situational market analysis calls for taking the recommended behavior back into the community and listening to its members to identify the "communication keys" to help secure their involvement (E. Hosein, personal communication, 2005, 2006). The key marketing principle here is to listen to the consumer. According to COMBI principles, an example of behavioral objectives is to prompt X number of people to swallow four to six tablets a day at home in the presence of filaria prevention assistant (or go to the distribution point) on filaria day (Renganathan and others, 2005). Evaluation of COMBI programs is specific to the achievement of the behavioral objectives specified early in program planning.

COMBI focuses on addressing specific diseases and related health behaviors, but it may also have an impact on social change. For example, the initial focus of COMBI primarily has been on communicable diseases that have been jeopardizing the socioeconomic development of entire communities and countries, especially in the developing world (WHO, 2003; Renganathan and others, 2005). With this in mind, COMBI's contribution to development and social change is its potential to "remove a significant obstacle that keeps people in poverty" (Renganathan and others, 2005, p. 318), as well as to reduce the mortality rates of diseases that affect entire families and communities. It also contributes to strengthen people's health literacy and disease-related self-reliance.

As with most other kinds of interventions and models, COMBI alone is not sufficient to address development issues (Renganathan and others, 2005) and public health deficiencies. Yet, it can help make a difference. Addressing broader social issues such as health disparities, poverty, and injustice, all factors contributing to poor health, requires many different kinds of public health strategies and interventions, which should all rely on long-term commitment, a step-by-step approach, people's participation, and a series of behavioral changes at the policymaker, stakeholder, funding agency, population, community, and individual levels. COMBI operates within this larger context as an approach to minimize the burden of disease and strengthen health services. In doing so, it supports one of the fundamental goals of public health.

COMBI integrates principles and methodologies from multiple disciplines, including marketing, mass communications, information education communication, social mobilization, anthropology, and sociology. It models its integrated approach on recent developments and lessons learned from IMC, which is widely used in the private and commercial sectors. As in IMC, COMBI uses a strategic blend of activities, channels, and audience-specific messages to address people's perceptions, attitudes, and behaviors (WHO, 2003; Renganathan and others, 2005; Hosein, Parks, and Schiavo, 2009).

COMBI takes into account key IMC learnings, including what the influence of people's perceptions—in other words, what people "believe to be important or true" (Renganathan and others, 2005, p. 309)—have on attitudes and behaviors. It also stresses the importance of clear, credible, and consistent communication messages in relation to the healthy behaviors, products, or services that people are asked to endorse and use (WHO, 2003; Renganathan and others, 2005).

Precede-Proceed Model

Designed by Lawrence Green and Marshall Kreuter (Green and Kreuter, 1991, 1999; Green and Ottoson, 1999), the precede-proceed model "is an approach to planning that analyzes the factors contributing to behavior change" (National Cancer Institute at the National Institutes of Health, 2002, p. 219). The model assumes that long-lasting change always occurs voluntarily (Communication Initiative, 2003b; National Cancer Institute, 2005a) and is determined by the individual motivation to become directly involved with the process of change. Individuals need to feel empowered to change their quality of life (National Cancer Institute, 2005a), and in doing so are influenced by their community and social structure.

The key factors influencing behavior change are divided in three categories (National Cancer Institute at the National Institutes of Health, 2002, p. 219):

⬧   Predisposing factors—the individual's knowledge, attitudes, behavior, beliefs, and values before intervention that affect willingness to change

⬧   Enabling factors—factors in the environment or community of an individual that facilitate or present obstacles to change

⬧   Reinforcing factors—the positive or negative effects of adopting the behavior (including social support) that influence continuing the behavior

This model reinforces the importance of considering the individual as part of the social environment. It also supports the notion of individual empowerment and capacity building at both the individual and community levels, one of the most important components of sustainable behavior and social change. In some ways, this model is in contrast with social norms theories previously discussed in this chapter, which assume that people usually take decisions without too much deliberation in response to social expectations. In real life, a combination of both processes is likely to occur depending on the specific group and issue.

Communication for Social Change

Communication for social change (CFSC) is a participatory model for communication planning, implementation, and evaluation. It was developed with the original input and sponsorship of the Rockefeller Foundation, which in 1997 convened a conference to explore the connection between communication and social change. The actual model was developed on the basis of the recommendations from all participants at this initial conference as well as follow-up meetings (Figueroa, Kincaid, Rani, and Lewis, 2002).

CFSC is defined as "a process of public and private dialogue through which people define who they are, what they want and how they can get it" (Gray-Felder and Dean, 1999, p. 15). It is an integrated model that describes an "iterative process" to community dialogue that "starts with a catalyst/stimulus that can be external or internal to the community," and "when effective, leads to collective action and the resolution of a common problem" (Figueroa, Kincaid, Rani, and Lewis, 2002, p. iii).

In this model, outcome indicators of social change include "leadership, degree and equity of participation, information equity, collective self-efficacy, sense of ownership, and social cohesion" (Figueroa, Kincaid, Rani, and Lewis, 2002, p. iv). In applying this model, it is important to recognize that social change (for example, less poverty, less HIV/AIDS) can take a long time and demands intermediate evaluation parameters to assess progress (Rockefeller Foundation Communication and Social Change Network, 2001). Social change is always the result of a series of gradual behavioral changes at the individual, group, and community levels. Therefore, behavioral outcomes should remain an important evaluation parameter in health communication even in the context of social change models.

Other Theoretical Influences and Planning Frameworks

Several other models and planning frameworks influence the theory and practice of health communication. A few examples, including medical models and logic models, are discussed next.

Medical Models

Communication is also influenced by general beliefs about the intrinsic causes of health and illness. Over time, two *medical models* have been influencing communication in the provider-patient setting as well as how health organizations and professionals perceive what kinds of topics and factors should be addressed as part of a public health intervention.

The first of the two models, the biomedical model, has been around for many centuries and is based on the assumption that poor health is a physical phenomenon that "can be explained, identified, and treated with physical means" (du Pré, 2000, p. 8; Twaddle and Hessler, 1987). Therefore, the biomedical model does not take into account the person's psychological conditions, individual and social beliefs, attitudes and norms, or other factors that can affect health and illness. As a result, communication efforts that are based on this model tend to be informative, strictly scientific, doctrinarian, authoritarian, "efficient," and "focused" (du Pré, 2000, p. 9). Communication relies on a top-down approach in which medical providers or health organizations limit their efforts to transferring their knowledge on the medical and scientific causes of an illness and to prescribing a solution.

This approach lacks empathy with the patient or intended group's feelings and social experiences (Friedman and DiMatteo, 1979; Laine and Davidoff, 1996; du Pré, 2000). Moreover, it does not take into account current knowledge that most diseases and their prognoses are heavily influenced by social and cultural habits, as well as the individual's psychological status. For example, health conditions such as obesity, diabetes, and depression are clearly influenced by external factors, which can include lifestyle issues, emotional stress, and cultural beliefs and preferences. Finally, disease prevention is not considered under this model because its practice is closely related to the ability of health professionals and organizations to engage interested individuals and communities in the act of prioritizing a recommended behavior by reaching out to their core beliefs, feelings, and needs.

The second model, the biopsychosocial model, is based on the premise that poor health is not only a physical phenomenon but "is also influenced by people's feelings, their ideas about health, and the events of their lives" (du Pré, 2000, p. 9; Engel, 1977). Given current emphasis on a patient-centered approach to health, the biopsychosocial model has been gradually substituting the biomedical model in most settings, also thanks to the work of many professional societies (for example, the American Medical Association and the American Academy of Family Physicians) and several hospitals and universities, which have guidelines and courses on provider-patient communications and highlight the importance of relating to patients' feelings, culture, literacy levels, needs, and other key factors that may help improve patient compliance and outcomes. More broadly, the model also fits well with many of the current practices and theories in health communication. Under this model, communication tends to be empathetic, sensible to people's needs and feelings, motivational, truly interdependent, and also aims to generate understanding of scientific and medical issues.

Logic Modeling

Logic modeling is a flexible framework that has been used for program planning and evaluation in the fields of education (Harvard Family Research Project, 2002), public-private partnerships (Watson, 2000), health education (University of Wisconsin, Extension Program Development, 2005), and many other programmatic areas. In general, it is a one-page summary of

logic modeling
A flexible framework that has been used for program planning and evaluation in the fields of education, public-private partnerships, health education, and many other programmatic areas

key factors that contribute to a specific health or social issue, the program's key components, the rationale used in defining program strategies, objectives, and key activities, and expected program outcomes and measurement parameters that will be used in evaluating them. In sum, logic models are used to explain the relationship among key factors contributing to a health or social issue, program components, and related outcomes.

Logic models are considered helpful tools in the planning and evaluation of public communication campaigns (Coffman, 2002) and other health communication interventions. They are tools for organizing one's thoughts in considering all program-related options as well as to provide key stakeholders, partners, and team members with a quick snapshot of a specific program and its rationale. Logic models can be constructed using different theories and assumptions so they fit the health issues and the needs of the audiences under consideration. Yet, the first step in logic modeling is always analyzing the situation, its contributing factors, and the environment we seek to influence (Morzinski and Montagnini, 2002) in order to develop adequate strategies and activities and establish realistic outcome objectives.

Appendix A provides a list of online resources for the development of logic models for health communication planning. See Figure 2.4 for an example of a logic model we developed to evaluate the impact of a national infant mortality prevention program (Schiavo and others, 2011). This program was developed and implemented by the Office of Minority Health Resource Center (OMHRC), Department of Health and Human Services (DHHS) Office of Minority Health (OMH).

Current Issues and Topics in Public Health and Health Care: Implications for Health Communication

In addition to theories and models, a number of issues influence the theory and practice of health communication. Many of them are specific to a certain country, environment, political situation, health issue, or population, among other factors. Because of the large variety and number of such issues, a comprehensive discussion of all of them is beyond the reach of this book. Therefore, the topics explored next are just examples of some of the issues that are currently influencing the field of health communication.

Project name: *A Healthy Baby Begins with You*

Long-term health issue and problem: High rate of preventable infant mortality (defined as death of an infant before age one) among African Americans

Long-term goal: Reduced incidence of infant mortality in the United States and more specifically among African Americans

Contributing Factors	⇒⇒⇒	Strategies and Tactics	⇒⇒⇒	Outcomes and Impact

⇓ ⇓ ⇓   ⇓ ⇓ ⇓   ⇓ ⇓ ⇓

Contributing Factors	Strategies and Tactics	Outcomes and Impact

• Lack of awareness of disproportionate infant mortality rates among African Americans
• Poor understanding of link between infant mortality prevention and preconception care
• Lack of understanding of timing, importance, and definition of preconception care as well as related behaviors
• Impact of chronic stress re: history of discrimination on health outcomes among African Americans, including infant mortality rates
• Limited community engagement and social support especially in most affected cities and neighborhoods
• Limited support and involvement of men and other family members
• Lack of focus on preconception health within provider-patient settings
• Conflicting priorities, access to care, and other obstacles to healthy lifestyle and preconception health
	• Engagement of college-age African-American population via
	  ○ Tailored health messages
	  ○ Development of pool of health ambassadors and peer educators via preconception peer education training
	  ○ Increased OMH involvement with (minority-serving) colleges and institutions
	• Establishment of partnerships with health departments and programs and other local and state health organizations
	• Faith-based community outreach
	• High school outreach
	• Community canvassing and health fairs
	• Mass media communications
	• Education of health care providers
		Short-term/<u>intermediate</u> process-related parameters
		• Message retention at key events re: core program information
		• Increased awareness of high burden of infant mortality among African Americans and related risk factors and causes
		• Increased awareness of link between infant mortality prevention and preconception care
		• Increased awareness of key behaviors that are part of preconception care
		• Increased number of people reporting having the intention of adopting and sustaining preconception health behaviors
		• Increased community engagement and number of community-based outreach efforts on this topic
		• Increased focus and support on preconception care within the provider-patient setting
		• Increased number of local and statewide partnerships on this topic
		Summative evaluation outcomes
		• Increased number of women and men who adopt and sustain at least three to four recommended behaviors that are part of preconception health and care
		• Increased number of health care providers who discuss preconception care at routine visits
		• Increased number of community-based and other health organizations that would develop programs to address infant mortality prevention and preconception care and regard them as a key organizational priority

Figure 2.4 Logic Model and Evaluation Design for a National Program for Infant Mortality Prevention by the Office of Minority Health, Department of Health and Human Services

Source: Schiavo, R., Gonzalez-Flores, M., Ramesh, R., and Estrada-Portales, I. "Taking the Pulse of Progress Toward Preconception Health: Preliminary Assessment of a National OMH Program for Infant Mortality Prevention." *Journal of Communication in Healthcare,* 2011, *4*(2), 106, Figure 1. © W. S. Maney & Son Ltd. 2011. Used by permission.

Health Disparities

As previously discussed, the concept of health equity has rightly emerged worldwide as one of the guiding principles for the work of many organizations in the public health, health care, and community development fields. Health equity addresses the importance of eliminating health disparities (see Chapter One for definitions of *health equity* and *health disparities*) by minimizing or removing differences in the well-being and health status of diverse populations and groups. As Dr. Martin Luther King Jr. is often quoted to have said, "Of all forms of inequality, injustice in health is the most shocking and the most inhuman" (Randall, 2002).

"The United States National Institutes of Health (NIH) defines health disparities as the 'differences in the incidence, prevalence, mortality, and burden of diseases and other adverse health conditions that exist among specific population groups in the United States'" (Center for Health Equity Research and Promotion, 2005). Unfortunately, "health disparities continue to undermine opportunities for economic and social development of too many communities in the United States and globally" (Health Equity Initiative, 2012b). They are "linked to diverse factors that are likely to be community-specific, including socio-economic conditions, race, ethnicity and culture, as well as having access to health care services, a built environment that supports physical activity, neighborhoods with accessible and affordable nutritious food, well-designed housing that is sited to minimize community exposure to environmental and other health hazards, efficient transportation that enable vulnerable groups to connect with services and support systems, culturally appropriate health information that accurately reflects literacy levels, and caring and friendly clinical settings" (Health Equity Initiative, 2012b). Some health disparities are also related to "genetic and biological differences among ethnic groups or between men and women" (Center for Health Equity Research and Promotion, 2005).

Although "health is the foundation for civil society, for social and cultural growth, for political stability, and for economic sustainability" (Families USA, 2012), only 59 percent of US adults are aware of health disparities, and this includes the ethnic and social groups that are most affected by such differences in health status and outcomes (Benz, Espinosa, Welsh, and Fontes, 2011). Over one decade, awareness of health disparities has increased only a mere 5 percent (Benz, Espinosa, Welsh, and Fontes, 2011), whereas disparities have increased or stayed the same among many disadvantaged groups. Health communication can contribute to reducing or eliminating health disparities by doing the following, for example:

- Raising awareness of health disparities and their root causes (for example, social determinants of health)

- Encouraging community action and multisectoral partnerships to identify, design, and implement community-specific solutions

- Reaching disadvantaged groups across cultures, socioeconomic conditions, geographic boundaries, and other factors that may influence health outcomes

- Developing programs, tools, and resources that would result in behavioral, social, and organizational results in support of health equity

- Creating a professional and social movement in support of health equity

- Ultimately, facilitating the long-term social change process that is needed to achieve health equity

Patient and Community Empowerment

Patient empowerment is an important concept in modern medicine and one of the central pillars of health communication strategies within health care settings. However, definitions and expectations generated by this term vary by health settings, contexts, and environments. For example, the term can refer to patient awareness about a disease and its treatment, which allows patients to engage in informed discussions with their health care providers, and therefore participate in treatment and prevention decisions. It can imply the patient's ability to feel competent to adhere to recommended treatment or prevention measures, or to engage in behaviors that may improve health outcomes. And it can include the patient's involvement in the public debate about policies, health care regulations, medical practices, research funding, and social change.

Partnering for Patient Empowerment Through Community Awareness (2005) and the Standing Committee of European Doctors (2004) are two organizations that focus on expanding consumer awareness about diseases and health resources or improving patient-provider communications. Others have effectively mobilized and engaged patient groups in the process of policy and social change. AIDS and other life-threatening conditions have taught important lessons to patients around the world. Over time, AIDS activists have had a tremendous impact on drug approval regulations, research funding, policies, and access to AIDS drugs, as well as public perception of AIDS, just to name a few topics.

Because of the different levels of patient involvement, it is important to refrain from using the term *patient empowerment* in a general way.

When a planned health communication intervention is seeking to engage patients or the general public, consideration should be given to what patients ideally should be able to do and what kind of empowerment may help advance patient outcomes. This should inform all capacity building and outreach efforts.

Similarly, community engagement, participation, and empowerment form a central mantra of effective health communication interventions. It is only when communities get together and understand the connection among health, community development and the availability of a variety of services (within and outside of health care) as it relates to improving community health and well-being that communication interventions have an actual opportunity to generate sustainable results and to mediate the kind of social support that is needed to implement and maintain complex health and social behaviors. Community mobilization and engagement are further discussed in Chapter Six.

The Rise of Chronic Diseases

Over the past few decades, the burden of chronic diseases (for example, obesity, diabetes, cardiovascular disease, etc.) has exponentially increased. In many settings, chronic diseases have now replaced infectious diseases as the predominant cause of death. In New York City, for example, chronic diseases account for 75 percent of all deaths versus the 9 percent of deaths that can be attributed to infectious diseases (Lee, 2012). The trend has been growing since the 1940s and sharply differs from data from the year 1880 in which only 13 percent of all deaths occurring in New York City could be attributed to chronic diseases and 57 percent to infectious diseases (Lee, 2012). Worldwide, chronic diseases are the largest cause of death (WHO, 2005c).

Because chronic diseases are influenced by multiple factors and shaped by the environment in which people live, work, and play, a social determinants of health-based perspective needs to be incorporated in all interventions. Health behaviors to prevent and manage chronic diseases need to be implemented during a person's lifetime, which also adds to the complexity of communication interventions that seek to address them. Health communication interventions can help prevent and manage chronic diseases at different levels (Halpin, Morales-Suárez-Varela, and Martin-Moreno, 2010):

- *Social level:* By advocating for policies, bans, adequate urban planning, access to services and information (including, but not limited to, health care services) that would help create a healthy social context and environment

- *Community level:* By encouraging community action and multisectoral partnerships to promote social support for healthy behaviors, identify solutions to community-specific needs and issues, and mobilize communities around this issue

- *Health care level:* By encouraging widespread use of best clinical practices, building capacity for **cultural competence** (defined as the ability to relate to other people's values, feelings, and beliefs across different cultures, and effectively address such differences as part of all interactions) among health care providers, addressing health literacy issues, promoting community and patient participation in clinical care, and continuing to build awareness of the importance of preventive care

cultural competence
The ability to relate to other people's values, feelings, and beliefs across different cultures, and effectively address such differences as part of all interactions

- *Individual level:* By promoting healthy behaviors and routine medical checkups among different populations and groups

Given the complexity and multifactoral nature of chronic diseases, only sustainable and multilevel communication interventions are likely to produce long-term results.

Limits of Preventive Medicine and Behaviors

Despite the medical and scientific advances of the past few centuries, preventive medicine cannot eliminate disease. However, preventive medicine and behaviors have contributed to extending life expectancy and improving the overall quality of life for many populations.

Still, preventive medicine does not work all the time. This concept may be troublesome for some people and therefore should be considered in designing health communication interventions. Consider the example of Eduardo, a fifty-year-old low- to middle-class Puerto Rican man who smokes and is being pressured by his family to quit because of the risk of oral cancer. They also want him to have regular checkups with his doctor and break his habit of seeking medical help only when he is seriously ill. The family has been alarmed by the recent death of a close cousin who was a heavy smoker and developed oral cancer. However, Eduardo has a very good friend who never smoked in his life and still developed oral cancer. He makes several arguments against his family's request to change his health-related habits:

- Quitting smoking will not guarantee that he will not get cancer.

- He enjoys smoking and drinking alcohol.

- Why is his family worried about oral cancer? What happened to their cousin is a rare event.

- He is too busy for regular checkups with his doctor.

Eduardo is right about the limits of preventive medicine and habits. However, there are a few facts that may help him see his family's point of view if discussed as part of a comprehensive and culturally competent health communication intervention:

- Oral cancer incidence is two times higher among men in Puerto Rico than among mainland US Hispanics (Hayes and others, 1999) and higher than that observed in white males living on the mainland United States (Ho and others, 2009; Parkin and others, 1997; Suarez and others, 2009).

- Together with alcohol consumption, tobacco use is a primary risk factor for oral cancer (Blot and others, 1988; Mashberg and others, 2006). Actually, their joint effect appears to be more than additive, if not multiplicative. The risk for oral and pharyngeal cancers is between six and fifteen times greater for smokers who are also heavy drinkers compared to individuals who neither smoke nor drink (Mashberg and Samit, 1995).

- Smoking cessation is a standard preventive measure against the risk for oral cancer (Lewin and others, 2000; Matiella, Middleton, and Thaker 1991; US Department of Health and Human Services, 1986, 1994).

- Social support (for example, from friends, peers, and others) help people quit smoking (Mermelstein and others, 1986), so talking with family and friends about one's intention and the benefits of quitting smoking, and seeking their support and involvement, may help people succeed in adopting new behaviors.

Of course, many other issues need to be considered and addressed in order to motivate Eduardo to quit smoking—for example, his social context, the potential difficulty of succeeding in quitting smoking, the priority assigned by his health care provider to oral cancer screening, and the friendliness and support of clinical settings and peers. Still, it is important to remember that most people are not aware of disease risk factors and other relevant information. Incorporating disease statistics and information in health communication interventions legitimizes the quest for behavior and social change. It also helps attract people's attention by positioning the health issue in a larger context than the family and circle of friends in which they live. Finally, it may help people accept the limits of preventive medicine and behavior by showcasing whenever possible the high percentage of cases in which disease can be prevented. Prevention does not work in all cases, but it still works in most cases.

A Mobile, On-Demand, and Audience-Driven Communication Environment

The Internet, mobile technology, and other advances have significantly extended "the scope of health care beyond its traditional boundaries" (Eysenbach, 2001, p. e20) and consequently have changed the practice of health communication. Increasingly, patients, health care professionals, the general public, and the overall health care community rely on the Internet and mobile technology for a variety of services and communications, which include advice on health issues, virtual pharmacies, distance learning for practitioners, medical or public health information systems (for example, disease surveillance systems), patient support groups, and health records, to name a few applications (Gantenbein, 2001; Eysenbach, 2001).

E-health has emerged as "a field in the intersection of medical informatics, public health and business, referring to health services and information delivered or enhanced through the Internet and related technologies" (Eysenbach, 2001, p. e20). In health communication, the increasing reliance on the Internet and mobile technology by consumers and professionals has opened the way to the use of interactive health communication tools (for example, websites, Internet-based games, mobile applications, online press rooms, disease symptoms simulations, opinion polls, seminars), which are often designed as part of larger health communication interventions. It has also prompted several initiatives and research studies that attempt to analyze the impact of the Internet and mobile technology on health beliefs, behaviors, outcomes, and policies, as well as health-related encounters and communications such as provider-patient interactions. Finally, it has raised questions about the accuracy of sources of information on all kinds of new media as well as the importance of understanding the implications of Internet and mobile technology use in relation to issues of patient privacy and equal access to information by those who may not have the resources or skills to take advantage of new technologies, especially in relation to health matters (Eysenbach, 2001; Cline and Haynes, 2001). Most important, the advent of new technology has created a mobile, on-demand, and audience-driven communication environment, which in integration with other communication areas and channels is quick to create community around health issues, and has also been used to validate ideas and new interventions, secure audience feedback on variety of issues, support people who want to quit smoking, and remind pregnant women to see their health care providers, among other initiatives (Abroms, Padmanabhan, Thaweethai, and Phillips, 2011; Evans and others, 2012). These topics as well as the use of the Internet, mobile technology, and new media and their implications in health communication are discussed in detail in Chapter Five.

Interactive health communication has been defined as the "interaction of an individual—consumer, patient, caregiver or professional—with or through an electronic device or communication technology to access or transmit health information or to receive guidance and support on a health-related issue" (Robinson, Patrick, Eng, and Gustafson, 1998, p. 1264). Several other disciplines influence or contribute to interactive health communication (Gantenbein, 2001). These include areas of public health informatics, defined as "the systematic application of information and computer science and technology to public health practice, research and learning" (US Department of Health and Human Services, 2005, p. 23); medical informatics, "the field that concerns itself with the cognitive, information processing, and communication tasks of medical practice, education and research" (Greenes and Shortliffe, 1990, p. 1114); and consumer health informatics, "the branch of medical informatics that analyzes consumers' needs for information; studies and implements methods of making information accessible to consumers; and models and integrates consumers' preferences into medical information systems" (Eysenbach, 2000, p. 1713).

In addition to extending the outreach of health communication programs, the use of the Internet, mobile technology, and other new platforms provides health communication practitioners with an opportunity to advocate for policy efforts on expanding access and new media literacy among disadvantaged communities both in the United States and globally, as well as helping people evaluate the accuracy, credibility, and relevance of the information found on different kinds of new media. As "health communication and health information technology (IT) are central to health care, public health, and the way our society views health" (US Department of Health and Human Services, 2012b), health communication research and practice can prove instrumental in promoting understanding, and expanded and effective use of, technological advances.

Low Health Literacy

Low health literacy is the inability to read, understand, and act on health information, options, and services (Zagaria, 2004; Zarcadoolas, Pleasant, and Greer, 2006). Health literacy is a significant prerequisite to the effectiveness of how people make health-related decisions in a variety of contexts and communication settings (Schiavo, 2009d) and one of the most important issues in health communication. No matter how accurate, compelling, or graphically appealing information appears to be, the purpose of any material or verbal communication is defeated if people cannot understand it. Health literacy levels affect how we communicate about health and illness in a variety of settings and countries, and also have a well-documented impact on several health issues (Schiavo, 2009d).

Low health literacy affects all different age groups and ethnic backgrounds. "Nearly half of all American adults—90 million people—have difficulty understanding and acting upon health information" (Institute of Medicine, 2004, p. 1). In Canada, a significant percentage of the population lacks basic literacy skills (for example, the ability to work well with words and numbers or read and understand printed materials) that are needed to process complex information, including health information (Gillis, 2005).

In addition to inadequate reading, writing, or math skills, other factors may contribute to low health literacy (Institute of Medicine, 2004; Zorn, Allen, and Horowitz, 2004; Schiavo, 2009d):

- Poor or insufficient speaking, listening, or comprehension ability

- Language barriers and skills

- Low ability to advocate for oneself and navigate the health care system

- Inadequate background information

- Low socioeconomic status

- Lack of Internet access, computer skills, and new media literacy

- Gender and cultural roles

- Overall level of engagement in health decisions

Healthy People 2010 describes **health literacy** as "the degree to which individuals have the capacity to obtain, process, and understand basic health information and services needed to make appropriate health decisions" (US Department of Health and Human Services, 2005, p. 11–20; Selden and others, 2000). Health communication can help improve this capacity by taking into account health literacy levels in all phases of strategic planning and program implementation. Health communication interventions should be designed to address different areas, including culture and society, health care and public health systems, and education (Institute of Medicine, 2004). Health communication can also contribute to breaking down barriers by relying on culturally relevant messages, materials, and activities that reflect the language ability and preferences of intended groups. Specific health

health literacy
"The degree to which individuals have the capacity to obtain, process, and understand basic health information and services needed to make appropriate health decisions" (US Department of Health and Human Services, 2005, p. 11–20; Selden and others, 2000)

literacy objectives included as part of *Healthy People 2020* "to improve the health literacy of the population" include the following (US Department of Health and Human Services, 2012b):

- Increase the proportion of persons who report their health care provider always gave them easy-to-understand instructions about what to do to take care of their illness or health condition

- Increase the proportion of persons who report their health care provider always ask them to describe how they will follow the instructions

- Increase the proportion of persons who report their health care providers' office always offered help in filling out a form

Because health literacy has implications for different kinds of communication areas within and outside clinical settings (including provider-patient communication, community engagement and mobilization, and mass media and new media communication), a strong focus should be placed on people's needs and preferences, as well as on the **health literacy–health communication continuum** (health literacy improves communication and at the same time communication improves health literacy levels) (Schiavo, 2009d).

health literacy–health communication continuum

Health literacy improves communication and at the same time communication improves health literacy levels (Schiavo, 2009d)

Health communication interventions can also play a key role in building the skills needed to improve overall health literacy levels. They can help sensitize health care providers, public health officers, community leaders, industry representatives, and others in the health care field about the need to reach out to patients and the general public in these groups' own terms. Sample online resources on health literacy are included in Appendix A. Health literacy is considered and mentioned throughout this book.

Impact of Managed Care and Other Cost-Cutting Interventions on Health

The advent of managed care in the United States has had an overall impact on provider-patient relationships as well as the way health care may be perceived by the media, the general public, and health care providers. This is not only a US-based phenomenon. Cost-cutting interventions are being implemented in many places around the world. For example, several countries in Asia are increasingly adopting managed care plans (Gross, 2001), and the UK health care reform has been gradually opening doors for the managed care industry (Royce, 2012).

Managed care organizations essentially manage the costs and the delivery of health services to patients. Many aspects of health care (for example, the choice of a primary care physician, the eligibility for medical tests and other procedures) that traditionally were decided only by the health care provider or the patient are now scrutinized and influenced by managed care. Other worldwide cost-cutting interventions are part of the same trend that over the past few decades has been shifting responsibilities for health care from the government to companies (such as managed care organizations) or individuals.

The time that providers can dedicate to an individual patient has been reduced by the need to see an increasing number of patients each workday. From the patient's perspective, the quality of care may seem inferior and lacking the human touch that much longer conversations with physicians and indiscriminate access to tests and other medical procedures may provide.

Although the debate on the pros and cons of cost-cutting interventions is beyond the scope of this book, it may be worth considering the implications of the current health care environment for health communication interventions:

• Health communication planning should take into account both the provider's and patient's opinion on cost-saving interventions and their perceived impact on their professional and personal lives.

• Health communication activities can help health care providers improve their communication skills and optimize their time with patients by managing expectations, addressing questions in a brief but efficient manner, and showing empathy with patients' needs and worries.

• Through advocacy, mass media campaigns, professional and government relations, and other strategic activities, health communication can help create a climate in which managed care organizations, legislators, and other key groups would feel compelled to preserve the right balance between quality of care and cost-saving measures.

These are just a few examples of the kinds of considerations that should be given to the current cost-saving environment and how this could be incorporated in strategic health communication planning.

Reemergence of Communicable Diseases

The reemergence of many infectious diseases that had started to decline or disappear has influenced health communication in two different but related ways. First, it is one of the reasons for the health communication renaissance. Because of the rising incidence of several reemerging diseases such as tuberculosis (CDC, 1994a), many authors and organizations have pointed to the need to raise awareness of the ongoing risk for communicable diseases by using the health communication approach (Freimuth, Cole, and Kirby, 2000).

In fact, many infectious diseases may again become a public threat in the absence of effective prevention and communication strategies. For example, pediatricians in the United States and many other countries have been witnessing increasing parental complacency about the need for childhood vaccines (Macartney and Durrheim, 2011). Vaccines have become victims of their own success because many parents and young health care providers may have never seen the devastating effects of diseases (National Foundation for Infectious Diseases, 1997; Vernon, 2003), such as polio or *Haemophilus influenzae* type B, the leading cause of bacterial meningitis and acquired mental retardation in US children before the vaccine was introduced (National Association of Pediatric Nurse Practitioners, 2005).

Still, five cases of polio among children in an Amish dairy farm community in Minnesota in 2005 (Harris, 2005) are a powerful reminder that even vaccine-preventable infectious diseases remain a threat everywhere, including in the developed world. In most cases, they are just a train ride or flight away. Communicating about the ongoing risk for infectious diseases has become a strategic imperative.

The second implication of this topic in health communication is related to the attempt by the health care community to redefine risk communication, which is assuming greater prominence, and also incorporating principles and strategies from crisis and emergency communication. Risk communication has been identified by *Healthy People 2010* as one of the relevant contexts of health communication. It is defined as "the dissemination of individual and population health risk information" (US Department of Health and Human Services, 2005, p. 11-13). *Health People 2020* also includes a specific objective on risk communication: "Increase the proportion of crisis and emergency risk messages intended to protect the public's health that demonstrate the use of best practices" (US Department of Health and Human Services, 2012b).

Health communication has traditionally used strategies that raise awareness of disease severity and risk among interested groups and populations so that people can relate to this risk and learn how to minimize it. Now, a more systematic approach to risk communications has been dictated by new attitudes toward disease prevention (or the lack of) that have led to the reemergence of many infectious diseases, as well as the need to engage relevant communities in all steps related to the preparedness and response phases of public health and humanitarian emergencies. To this end, several related fields have been converging to harness best practices and models. These include risk communication (which traditionally has been long-term, frequent, behavior-centered, expert-led, and focused on "hazards, consequences and cultural beliefs and attitudes" [Schiavo, 2009c] among other distinguishing features); and crisis communication (which traditionally has been reactive, nonroutine, focused on crisis update and status, led by authority figures, and short term) (Schiavo, 2009c; Reynolds and Seeger, 2005). **Crisis and emergency risk communication** integrates approaches from both fields (risk and crisis communication) in preparing for, responding to, and recovering from epidemics, emerging disease outbreaks, and other hazards (CDC, 2013b).

A definition of risk communication that attempts to represent the complexity of the process related to communicating and managing risk during public health emergencies is the one offered by the US Department of Health and Human Services (2002, p. 4), which defines **risk communication** as "an interactive process of exchange of information and opinion among individuals, groups, and institutions." The definition also includes a discussion and related actions about risk types and levels as well as methods, strategies, and activities for managing risks in a variety of settings. Given the complexity of risk communication in public health emergency (also called **emergency risk communication**) and other settings, this process is or should be characterized by the participation of different key groups, communities, stakeholders, and segments of society so that risk—and its social determinants—can be adequately addressed by effective, multisectoral, and integrated communication interventions, which rely on multiple action areas (for example, mass media and new media communication, community mobilization and citizen engagement, policy communication and public advocacy) and strategies.

Worldwide Urbanization

Cities and urban living have assumed greater relevance in relation to overall public health outcomes. "In 2008, for the first time in history, more than half of the world's population will be living in towns and cities. By 2030 this number will swell to almost 5 billion, with urban growth concentrated in Africa and Asia" (UNFPA, 2012). Strategic health communication interventions in urban settings present many similarities with health communication planning, implementation, and evaluation in other settings. However, a specific set of issues, trends, and challenges may

crisis and emergency risk communication
Integrates risk and crisis communication in preparing for, responding to, and recovering from epidemics, emerging disease outbreaks, and other hazards

risk communication
"An interactive process of exchange of information and opinion among individuals, groups, and institutions" (US Department of Health and Human Services, 2002). "The dissemination of individual and population health risk information" (US Department of Health and Human Services, 2005, pp. 11–13)

emergency risk communication
Risk communication as applied to public health and humanitarian emergency settings

influence interventions in urban settings and should be addressed as part of training modules and sessions intended for public health, health care, and community development professionals, nonprofit organizations, and government agencies.

For example, a 2009–2010 exploratory survey revealed several areas of need for capacity-building efforts on strategic communication in urban health settings (Schiavo and Ramesh, 2010; Communication Initiative, 2010; Schiavo, 2010b). Key findings from this survey emphasize the need for "training modules and sessions that address the issues of diversity and health disparities, which are very prominent in urban settings. Respondents pointed to the need for tools and strategies that would help them tailor communication interventions to different populations (both in relation to different racial and ethnic groups as well as various socioeconomic levels) within highly diverse contexts and given potential limitation of resources. Specific training needs were primarily related to the following topics: health disparities, diversity, communication framing and tailoring, and communication planning and evaluation methods" (Schiavo and Ramesh, 2010). As urban areas continue to grow—and to pose new challenges and opportunities regarding the way we communicate on health and illness—research and capacity-building efforts on strategic health communication in urban settings will intensify to address the needs and preferences of urban communities. This theme will be further explored throughout relevant sections of this book.

The Threat of Bioterrorism

The threat of bioterrorism has forced public health officials, governments, and key community leaders and organizations to revisit their communication strategy in light of the possibility of an emergency situation. A few general principles about the key characteristics of communications efforts aimed at averting a potential public health disaster have emerged from the lessons learned from the 2001 anthrax-by-mail bioterrorist attacks in the United States (see Chapter One):

- Clear, timely, accurate, and audience-specific messages
- Credible spokespeople
- Strategic planning
- Coordinated efforts
- Adequate channels
- Culturally competent attitude to communication

Although all of these elements are standard attributes of well-designed and well-implemented health communication programs, the issue of preparedness assumes a greater importance in emergencies. In health communication, preparedness relates to the following (Schiavo, 2009b, 2010a):

- Clarity of behavioral results

- A standard protocol that different organizations and multilateral agencies can use in a coordinated effort within countries and globally

- Risk assessment and related preparedness measures that are specific for each at-risk group

- Community dialogue and consultations to secure community buy-in on emergency mitigation measures and assess existing obstacles, community-specific preferences, and needs that may jeopardize their implementation

- Involvement and training of social mobilization partners (for example, teachers, religious leaders, community leaders, health care providers, etc.)

- Early selection and training of key spokespeople who can address intended groups

- Advance preparation to address potential questions from different groups or from the mass media

- Other group- and issue-specific tools and activities

International Access to Essential Drugs

The HIV/AIDS crisis in Africa and other developing regions, where the high incidence of AIDS has been threatening not only lives but also the regions' economic and social development, dramatically pointed to the importance of equal access to life-saving medications (Ruxin and others, 2005). It would certainly be a failure of modern medicine if treatment could not be delivered to those most in need of it.

In developing countries, access to medications is primarily influenced by cost, capacity for storage and drug delivery, adequate medical training, local infrastructure for drug distribution, hospital and treatment center conditions, and political willingness (Ruxin and others, 2005). All of these factors are equally important in ensuring that medications are available to people and can be effectively used to treat them.

Different efforts and campaigns have been developed and implemented by several organizations in the AIDS and public health fields (for example,

Doctors Without Borders, Medicus Mundi, World Health Organization). Yet, multisectoral partnerships are emerging as suitable models to work in multiple countries and bring together local governments, companies, local nongovernmental organizations, and other key stakeholders in sharing responsibility for guaranteeing access. This is a complex issue that deserves a book of its own and has been shaping interactions among different key players in the health care, public health, and community development fields as well as government or organizational policies. The overall point is that health communication, together with other kinds of interventions, can help advance this debate by creating consensus and raising awareness about adequate strategies, lessons learned from previous experiences, as well as the importance of a cohesive approach in which different stakeholders would assume their share of responsibility. It is a topic that those who enter the health care field cannot ignore, and one that is being greatly emphasized by global health interventions. It is also strictly interconnected to access to health services and adequately trained health workers, which is discussed in the next section.

Global Health Workers Brain Drain and Other Capacity-Building Needs in Developing Countries

Health communication cannot replace the lack of adequate local capacity, training, or infrastructure. When health services are unavailable or too distant from specific groups, health communication interventions should help create the political and social willingness that is needed to build hospitals, recruit and train local health care providers, and make health products available.

This is a major issue in developing countries. Nevertheless, lack of capability or training often affects health care in developed countries, too. For example, underserved populations around the world are faced with a shortage of medical supplies in local hospitals or inadequate numbers of nurses or physicians per number of patients (Physicians for Human Rights, 2004; Colwill and Cultice, 2003). Among others, health communication can play a role in the process of expanding local capacity and infrastructure in these ways:

- Increasing understanding of the key factors contributing to brain drain
- Advocating for increased funds for health care provider training and retention strategies, patient clinical care, and task-shifting interventions that incorporate community engagement and peer-to-peer communication strategies into clinical care

- Engaging local leaders and government officers in the process of assessing local needs and subsequently creating or updating health services

- Raising awareness among local health care providers of standard medical practices they may not use routinely

- Training patients and family caregivers so they can ask the right questions in physicians' offices, local meetings, and all other venues where health care–related decisions are made

- Increasing the visibility of leaders and organizations that focus on a specific health issue, disease, or local need

- Creating local awareness of disease severity and risk so that the issue can be prioritized and addressed in the community through adequate services and training

Lack of local capacity and training should force communicators to reflect on the limits of communication interventions. It should make them prioritize those strategies that together with other public health interventions would help develop critical masses, political willingness, and innovative processes to address existing deficiencies.

Key Concepts

- The theoretical basis of health communication is influenced by the behavioral and social sciences, health education, social marketing, mass and speech communication, new media theory, medical models, anthropology, and sociology.

- In this chapter, the most prominent theories and models are divided into the following categories: behavioral and social science theories, mass and new media communication theories, marketing-based models, and other theoretical influences and planning frameworks, including medical models and logic modeling.

- There is recognition of the multidisciplinary nature of health communication.

- Theories, models, and planning frameworks can influence different aspects and phases of health communication planning, evaluation, and management. They should all be considered as part of a comprehensive tool kit and selected in response to situational and group-related issues and needs.

- A number of issues and topics influence the practice of health communication and need to be considered in the analysis of the current health care environment.

FOR DISCUSSION AND PRACTICE

1. Select a theory addressed in this chapter and use a practical example on a health issue of your choice to illustrate how changes in health behaviors may occur according to the steps highlighted by the theory you selected. Box 2.1 provides a practical example on the diffusion of innovation theory. This example can be used as a model for this exercise.

2. In your opinion, what is the main benefit of using theoretical frameworks and planning models in health communication? Do you have experience with any theory-based health communication interventions? If yes, identify your key learnings.

3. Which of the current issues highlighted in this chapter do you think most affect health communication practice, and why? Do you have any experience in addressing these issues or participating in health-related programs that focus on them? What, if anything, have you recently heard in the news about these topics? Is there any other issue that you think may shape the practice of health communication in the near future?

4. Using the logic model featured in this chapter (see Figure 2.4), research and discuss with your fellow students key contributing factors to a health issue or condition you are aware of either professionally or personally.

5. Analyze and present on common elements of different theories within the same category or compare key elements of theories in two different categories (or family of theories) as described in this chapter.

KEY TERMS

behavioral beliefs

crisis and emergency risk
   communication

cultural competence

emergency risk communication

health literacy

health literacy–health
   communication continuum

key influentials roadmap

logic modeling

new media

normative beliefs

primary audiences

risk communication

secondary audiences

social media

social norms

CHAPTER 3

CULTURE AND OTHER INFLUENCES ON CONCEPTIONS OF HEALTH AND ILLNESS

In 1976, as the United States celebrated its Bicentennial, the US Congress passed the American Folklife Preservation Act (Public Law 94–201) [1976]. In writing the legislation, Congress had to define folklife. Here is what the law says: "American folklife" means the traditional expressive culture shared within the various groups in the United States: familial, ethnic, occupational, religious, regional; expressive culture includes a wide range of creative and symbolic forms such as custom, belief, technical skill, language, literature, art, architecture, music, play, dance, drama, ritual, pageantry, handicraft; these expressions are mainly learned orally, by imitation, or in performance, and are generally maintained without benefit of formal instruction or institutional direction. (Hufford, 1991)

Traditional expressions of any culture influence everyday decisions, both big and small. They are reflected in the choice of the cake people have for their children's birthday, and also in major decisions related to child rearing. They influence the slang children and doctors or handymen use to address their peers or others (Hufford, 1991). They are recalled when grandparents come to visit through tales and stories they transmit to the next generation. They are verbal and nonverbal cues that affect how information on any topic is received, accepted, and elaborated.

These traditions, habits, and beliefs also influence ideas of health and illness among different groups. The reality is that conceptions of health and illness are related to people's upbringing as well as their cultural, religious, ethnic, and gender-related values and beliefs, to name just a few components. In health communication, these values and beliefs assume a critical importance in the design and implementation of programs that can reach across cultural boundaries and produce behavioral and social results.

CHAPTER OBJECTIVES

Through a comparative review of examples of different religious, ethnic, cultural, age, and gender-related influences on the concepts of health and illness, this chapter (1) establishes the need for research-based communication interventions that always take into account audience-specific beliefs, behaviors, and characteristics and (2) provides information and reflections that would help readers "assess cultural, environmental, and social justice influences on the health of communities" (Association of Schools of Public Health, ASPH Education Committee, 2009, p. 11) and "engage communities in creating evidence-based, culturally competent programs" (p. 11).

What Is Culture?

Culture has been rightly compared to an iceberg (Peace Corps, 2011). "Just as an iceberg has a smaller visible section above the waterline and a larger, invisible section, below the waterline" (Peace Corps, 2011, p. 10), so culture has some observable aspects (observable behaviors) and others that can only be intuited, imagined, and ultimately researched (see Figure 3.1). Culture is both influencing and influenced by **universal values** (emotions and feelings that people may share across different groups within the same

universal values
Emotions and feelings that people may share across different groups within the same culture or in some cases across cultures

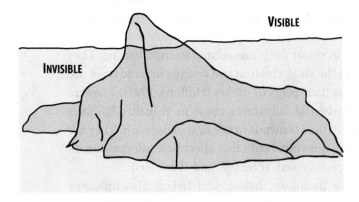

Figure 3.1 Comparing *Culture* to an Iceberg

culture or in some cases across cultures) and **personal values** (emotions and feelings that derive from personal, group, or community past experiences) (Peace Corps, 2011). As previously mentioned, culture is one important dimension of human behavior and, along with other factors (for example, age, religious beliefs, geographic location) influences people's concepts of health and illness.

personal values
Emotions and feelings that derive from personal, group, or community past experiences

Approaches in Defining Health and Illness

Defining the meanings of health and illness may appear to be an easy task. After all, in Western countries, people seem to know when they are sick with a cold or other illness. Why should it be so complicated? Yet, in reality, health and illness have been defined in different ways across cultures around the world. Most authors agree that individual ideas on health and illness have a tremendous impact on people's attitudes toward healthy behaviors as well as disease prevention and treatment.

Following are two of the many models that over time have been used to define health. Although the models need to be considered in the context of the cultural and geographical attributes of key groups and stakeholders, they can still help us comprehend the evolution of the definitions of health and illness over time.

Medical Concept of Health

Under the medical concept of health, health is strictly defined as the lack of disease (Balog, 1978; Boruchovitch and Mednick, 2002) and, more specifically, the absence of physical symptoms and signs associated with illness. This concept mirrors the biomedical model discussed in Chapter Two and takes into account only the physiological nature of health and illness. It was particularly popular among physicians and other health care professionals in the first half of the twentieth century (Boruchovitch and Mednick, 2002).

However, as with the biomedical model, the medical concept of health neglects to consider the influence that other factors, such as psychological or lifestyle issues, have on many diseases. Moreover, it defines health by highlighting illness (Boruchovitch and Mednick, 2002) and therefore does not take into account that often a healthy status is more of a general condition of well-being.

Several studies have shown that people tend to feel "healthy" when they are happy, energetic, and feel invulnerable to disease (Andersen and

Lobel, 1995; Campbell, 1975; Pew Research Center, 2006; Veenhoven, 2008). At times, this applies also to cases in which they are "concurrently ill" (Andersen and Lobel, 1995, p. 132). Healthy people tend to bounce back from illness faster and with better outcomes than unhealthy ones (for example, people who are under a lot of physical or emotional stress) (Dougall and Baum, 2012; Gouin and Kiecolt-Glaser, 2011; Godbout and Glaser, 2006), so there is something more to a healthy status than just being disease free. For example, chronic stress associated with low socioeconomics or a history of social discrimination may be linked to higher incidence of preterm births and higher infant mortality rates among African Americans (*California Newsreel*, 2008; Lu and Lu, 2007).

World Health Organization Concept of Health and Its Connection to the Social Determinants of Health

One of the key principles of the World Health Organization (WHO) Constitution (1946) is a definition of health, which in the past few decades has changed the perspective of many health care and public health professionals on the concepts of health and illness. "Health is a state of complete physical, mental and social well-being and not merely the absence of disease and infirmity" (p. 2). This concept of health refers to the need for a balanced interaction among different physical, medical, psychological, social, and lifestyle-related factors. Balance, and the need for a balanced life that may help achieve good health, becomes a key principle in this definition, which also somewhat reflects the biopsychosocial model discussed in Chapter Two.

In fact several factors—or determinants of health—affect health outcomes. Such factors (see Figure 3.2) pertain to different categories: the living, working, and aging environment; community-, population-, or group-specific factors, such as culture, gender, race, and other social influences, including the kind of social support people are used to giving and receiving as it relates to health and social behaviors they currently practice or plan to change; socioeconomic opportunities and related policies; access to services and information as they relate not only to health care but also to other essential services such as transportation, recreational facilities and parks, community centers, and others.

The concept of balance is also echoed in the definition of health in many populations and cultures. For example, health beliefs of traditional Southeast Asians, such as most Chinese people, revolve around the concept of balance between yin and yang, the two life forces (Matsunaga, Yamada, and Macabeo, 1998). Yin is the female force and is described as dark,

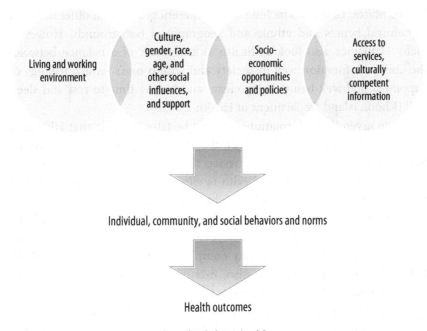

Figure 3.2   Health Outcomes as a Complex and Multidimensional Construct

Source: Adapted from Schiavo, R., Boahemaa, O., Watts, B., and Hoeppner, E. "Raising the Influence of Community Voices on Health Equity: Introducing Health Equity Exchange." *Journal of Communication in Healthcare*, Aug. 2012a. http://maneypublishing.com/images/pdf_site/Health_Equity_Exchange_-_Renata_Schiavo.pdf.

cold, and wet. Yin illnesses need to be treated with yang (hot) to restore health and the right balance. Hot foods such as chicken or herbal mixtures may be recommended to treat yin illnesses (Rhode Island Department of Health, 2005d; Raven, Chen, Tolhurst, and Garner, 2007). Yang is the male force and is considered "light, hot and dry" (Matsunaga, Yamada, and Macabeo, 1998, p. 49). Yang diseases may be treated with cold foods, such as vegetables (Rhode Island Department of Health, 2005d) or herbs. In traditional Chinese culture, hot and cold do not refer to actual temperature but are used to define and characterize opposite forces (Matsunaga, Yamada, and Macabeo, 1998). Cancer is an example of a yin disease, whereas an ear infection is considered a yang disease (Rhode Island Department of Health, 2005d).

As another example, drinking a lot of cold fluids, such as water or orange juice, to nurture a bad cold may appear strange in some traditional Hispanic cultures, because illness, treatment, and foods are also viewed in terms of seeking a balance between hot and cold (Rhode Island Department of Health, 2005b), this time referring to actual temperature. Among Hispanics, hot soups or teas may be viewed as an option to becoming healthy. In the

United States, Hispanics include many different groups that differ in terms of cultural beliefs and ethnic and geographical backgrounds. However, many Hispanics also look at health as the result of a balance between the ability to function well in society and within one's family, feelings of happiness and well-being, being clean, and having time to rest and sleep well (Rhode Island Department of Health, 2005b).

Even given this information, it would be false to imply that Hispanics or Chinese are unaware of the medical basis of diseases and the role germs may play at the onset of many illnesses; they are actually aware. However, as with many other cultures, health is viewed as the result of a sense of well-being with oneself and others, which goes beyond being disease free.

One of the potential limitations of the WHO model of health is its lack of specificity (Lewis, 1953; Boruchovitch and Mednick, 2002) and measurable parameters. This may complicate the evaluation of medical, behavioral, and social results. Also, it is important to take into account that although conditions such as obesity, diabetes, and depression are more heavily influenced by a number of social and individual factors, a sudden stroke or a head trauma needs immediate and urgent medical intervention that at least initially is limited to addressing medical causes and symptoms. This intervention focuses on restoring health by addressing only physical symptoms, which is the key assumption of the medical model.

Understanding Health in Different Contexts: A Comparative Overview

The definition of *healthy* varies from culture to culture and region to region. Ethnic, religious, socioeconomic, and age-related factors influence perceptions about health and healthy behaviors. For example, in some countries where malnutrition and poverty may be predominant, a large body size is considered a sign of a healthy lifestyle because it is associated with wealth and enough food (Mokhtar and others, 2001). In many Western countries, however, people often regard heavy weight as a sign of an unhealthy lifestyle (for example, lack of exercise or poor eating habits).

Religious and spiritual factors are also relevant in medicine because they influence beliefs about the nature of illness as well as the ability to cope with disease or adhere to recommended treatments. Several questionnaires and standard models, such as the Royal Free Interview for Religious and Spiritual Beliefs, have been developed and translated in many languages to assess religious and spiritual ideas and their potential influence on patients' behaviors and outcomes. Among other things, the Royal Free Interview is designed to investigate the extent to which people attribute sickness to

God's will or rely on religious beliefs and practices to cope with the stress of an illness (Pernice and others, 2005).

In assessing the impact of religion and spirituality on ideas of health and illness, it is important to distinguish between the two terms because they refer to different levels of involvement in organized religious practices. *Religion* is usually defined as a series of spiritual practices and behaviors within an organized religious structure (for example, the Catholic church), which in some cases may also recommend or inspire specific health behaviors; *spirituality* is a larger concept that includes people's values, questions about the meaning of life, and, potentially, some level of involvement in organized religious activities (Emblen, 1992; Mueller, Plevak, and Rummans, 2001; Hill and Pargament, 2003; Pernice and others, 2005). "Spirituality is expressed through art, poetry and myth, as well as religious practice. Both religion and spirituality typically emphasize the depth of meaning and purpose in life. One does not, of course, have to be religious for life to be deeply meaningful, as atheists will avow. Yet, although some atheists might not consider themselves spiritual, many do. Spirituality is thus a more inclusive concept than religion" (Dein, Cook, Powell, and Eagger, 2010, p. 63). Both can play a key role in the way disease is perceived and addressed in different cultures. In fact, religion and spirituality include traditions and values that may affect people's understanding of the causes of illness, compliance to treatment and physician recommendations, or feelings of optimism or fatalism about disease outcomes, to name just a few examples. Religious beliefs have been reported to overrule clinical recommendations in influencing patients' decisions (Coward and Sidhu, 2000). This points to the need for a culturally competent approach to disease prevention and management in which intended groups' religious or spiritual assumptions should be respected and understood.

Age is another contributing factor in defining health and healthy behaviors. For example, in Canada, awareness of the importance of adequate nutritional habits in relation to health tends to increase with age. When choosing food to eat, older Canadians "place more emphasis on nutrition" than younger Canadians (Health Canada, 2002). As another example, some authors have shown that even within a sample representing different ethnic backgrounds, a significant number of older people in the United States are fatalistic about the cause of many diseases, feel powerless about treatment, and tend to consider disease "a normal part of aging" (Goodwin, Black, and Satish, 1999). In general, concepts of health and illness change over time and often become increasingly more complex with older age.

Finally, access to recent advances in technology has also contributed to defining what people think it means to be healthy. For those who have regular access to it, the Internet and mobile technology have contributed to the merging of cultural perspectives and the understanding of many diseases. Similarly, radio and television have brought into many homes across the world images of models and lifestyles from different countries and cultures that over time can be assimilated or emulated by a given culture. However, it would be naive to expect that people will not incorporate their traditional beliefs and social values in redefining health as a result of new information and models. For any given culture, new ideas of health and illness tend to be the result of a carefully balanced combination of preexisting and new concepts.

Health communicators should be aware that programs designed to achieve awareness of a specific health issue and its solutions may also have an impact on existing concepts of health and illness because of people's exposure to new models and beliefs. This potential impact should be considered early in program design as well as monitored and evaluated over time. Cross-cultural communication efforts should always be envisioned as an opportunity to integrate cultures and not to convince people of the rightness of a single culture. Adequate resources and tools should be developed to support people who initially adhere to new concepts and behaviors so they can be encouraged in their new beliefs by their social and family circles. Consider the following story that exemplifies how miscommunication about the ideas of health and illness, and the consequential clash of two different cultures, may produce disastrous results (Fadiman, 1997):

> Lia Lee was a three-month-old Hmong child with epilepsy. Her doctors prescribed a complex regimen of medication designed to control her seizures. However, her parents felt that the epilepsy was a result of Lia "losing her soul" and did not give her medication as indicated because of the complexity of the drug therapy and the adverse side effects. Instead, they did everything logical in terms of their Hmong beliefs to help her. They took her to a clan leader and shaman, sacrificed animals and bought expensive amulets to guide her soul's return. Lia's doctors felt her parents were endangering her life by not giving her the medication so they called Child Protective Services and Lia was placed in foster care. Lia was a victim of a misunderstanding between these two cultures that were both intent on saving her. The results were disastrous: a close family was separated and Hmong community faith in Western doctors was shaken. (American Medical Student Association, 2005)

Table 3.1 provides a comparative overview of ideas of health and illness among different populations and groups. This table offers a useful perspective on the many variations of these two fundamental concepts that need to be considered in researching and approaching any key group or community. The information in the table includes only sample facts, which come from published data and reviews in this field and may not apply to all people in the groups being featured. In fact, people in these groups may have individual conceptions that are shaped not only by sociocultural factors but also by their family upbringing, gender, educational level, life experiences, and living environment. Moreover, many other audience- or issue-specific factors that are not highlighted here may influence conceptions of health and illness and should be analyzed on a case-by-case basis.

Gender Influences on Health Behaviors and Conceptions of Health and Illness

Gender refers to the role and responsibilities that men and women respectively assume in their society and family. It is distinguished from *sex*, which is a biological trait (Zaman and Underwood, 2003). Although these two terms are often used interchangeably, only *gender* refers to cultural values that are associated with a given sex. Communication, culture, and gender are interconnected, and communication needs to take into account what gender means and how meanings of gender change in relation to cultural values, organizations, and activities through which such meanings are expressed (Wood, 2009).

In many cultures, gender roles and responsibilities tend to be different. Conceptions of health and illness often reflect this diversity. However, in approaching gender communication, it is important to refrain from applying gender-related stereotypes. The right approach is to research how gender attributes have evolved over time in a given culture and have influenced health care–related decisions and definitions.

In many settings, women's ideas of health and illness have been influenced by their role as wives and mothers in providing health care for the rest of the family. This role has also traditionally influenced the epidemiology and control of many diseases (Vlassoff and Manderson, 1998). For example, Finerman (1989) reports that in rural Ecuador, women may be reluctant to defer medical care to professionals or other people outside their home. They are motivated by their need to protect their privileged and well-respected role as the family's caretaker, which could be questioned by

Table 3.1   A Comparative Overview of Ideas of Health and Illness

Population or ethnic group	Good health is	Illness is
African Americans (United States)	The result of "keeping spiritual harmony [among] mind, body and soul" (University of Michigan Health System, 2005) "Feelings of well-being" and the capacity "to fulfill one's role" in society without excessive pain or stress (Rhode Island Department of Health, 2005a)	The consequence of natural causes, inadequate diet, too much wind or cold (University of Michigan Health System, 2005) God's punishment for bad conduct (University of Michigan Health System, 2005)
Vietnamese (country of origin and United States)	The proper balance between *am* and *duong* opposing forces, which are the same as yin and yang in Chinese culture (Matsunaga, Yamada, and Macabeo, 1998; Rhode Island Department of Health, 2005d)	An indication that "the body is out of balance" (Rhode Island Department of Health, 2005d)
Koreans (country of origin and United States)	A balance between organic and inorganic elements, mind and body (Matsunaga, Yamada, and Macabeo, 1998; Pang, 1980)	Imbalance among the many elements that make a person (Matsunaga, Yamada, and Macabeo, 1998)
Hispanics (United States)	A feeling of *bienestar* (well-being), which is related to achieving balance in the emotional, physical, and social spheres; a balance between hot and cold body humors (Rhode Island Department of Health, 2005b)	An imbalance among emotional, physical, and social factors; an unevenness between hot and cold in the body (Rhode Island Department of Health, 2005b)
Native Americans (United States)	A cycle that symbolizes perfection and equality; a balancing act among mind, body, spirit, and nature (Rhode Island Department of Health, 2005c)	
Chinese (country of origin and United States)	Balance among body, mind, and spirit, commonly expressed as yin and yang (Centers for Disease Control [CDC], 2008a)	Imbalance of yin and yang, unbalanced qi (life energy), lack of emotional harmony, or because of fate, interference from ancestors and others in the spirit world who seek revenge (CDC, 2008a)
Somali (country of origin and United States)		"Caused by angry spirits or 'evil eye,' which can stem from excessive praise of someone (i.e., flattery about a person's beauty can curse the person receiving the compliment)" (CDC, 2008b)
Religious groups		
Catholics		A reflection of fallen nature and something evil; a result of the sin of Adam (Ukrainian Catholic Church in Australia, New Zealand, and Oceania, 2006)
Muslims	A state of dynamic equilibrium (Al-Khayat, 1997)	A punishment; a way of washing sins away (CancerBACKUP, 2006)

Table 3.1   A Comparative Overview of Ideas of Health and Illness (*Continued*)

Population or ethnic group	Good health is	Illness is
Hindus and Sikhs	The result of good karma ("the cyclical process of life and rebirth," Sheikh, 1999, p. 600), which is the total effect of a person's actions and determines the person's destiny (Sheikh, 1999; CancerBACKUP, 2006)	A punishment for wrongdoings in the current and previous lives (CancerBACKUP, 2006)
Age groups		
Children (Brazil)	"Positive feelings" (Boruchovitch and Mednick, 1997)	"Negative feelings associated with being ill"; "not being healthy" (Boruchovitch and Mednick, 1997)
Elderly (Mexico)	Something to be grateful to God for; dependent on the situations one lives in (Zunker, Rutt, and Meza, 2005)	Normal at their age; because of lack of knowledge about how to keep healthy during youth (Zunker, Rutt, and Meza, 2005)
Elderly (United States)		A normal part of aging (Goodwin, Black, and Satish, 1999)

outside interventions. The desire to preserve a woman's role as a primary caretaker has an important impact on the way diseases are managed, controlled, and prevented.

Gender also affects women's access to health information, financial resources for treatment interventions, and ways to respond to disease in comparison with men (Vlassoff and Manderson, 1998). Moreover, in the case of diseases that are highly stigmatized, such as AIDS or tuberculosis, women tend to be marginalized more than men by family and social circles.

In addition, in many cultures, the imbalance of power between men and women has created the need for developing different role models and recommended behaviors that are specific to each gender (Zaman and Underwood, 2003). For example, there are gender-related differences in talking with adolescents about sex and risky behaviors. Teaching girls about being assertive and demanding that their partners use condoms to prevent sexually transmitted diseases (STDs) is an additional but fundamental gender-specific element of most STD awareness efforts intended for adolescent girls.

More recently, the advent of the Internet and other technologies has left women behind and created a large gender divide in many countries or communities across the world. For example, Obayelu and Ogunlade (2006) report that in Nigeria some women are influenced by local culture and other kinds of social pressures to believe that "working with *ICTs (Information-Communication-Technologies)* would drive women mad."

Others "considered the word 'technology' to have male connotations, even though 'information' seemed more feminine" (Obayelu and Ogunlade, 2006, p. 55). In developing countries, access to ICT training and literacy is connected to economic and social opportunities, as well as the ability to network across regions and genders. "ICTs also provide options for women, including overcoming illiteracy, creating opportunities for entrepreneurship, allowing women to work from home and care for their families, accessing ICTs from rural locations, and enhancing and enriching their quality of life" (Obayelu and Ogunlade, 2006, p. 55). Therefore, one of the priorities for health communication in the twenty-first century is to close the gender divide as it relates to the understanding and use of technological advances and to create the cultural change that is needed to empower women and include them.

As for concepts of health and illness, changes in gender-related roles and responsibilities may be one of the effects of a health communication program on a particular health issue (Zaman and Underwood, 2003). Therefore, gender attributes in the health care setting need to be understood, monitored, and evaluated over time in relation to the influence that health communication programs may have on them. These changes could potentially influence gender-related concepts of health and illness and become one of the many examples of how different elements of the health communication environment are interconnected.

Health Beliefs Versus Desires: Implications for Health Communication

Meeting and managing expectations is a critical attribute of most professional and personal interactions in result-oriented societies such as Western cultures. However, achieving what has been promised to others is important in all cultures.

In the public health and health care fields, when one asks others to change behaviors, it is usually for better health. But the concept of health and illness varies across cultures and groups, and so are culturally related and group-specific health beliefs. Health beliefs influence how people estimate the likelihood that different outcomes may be linked to the recommended behavior. If people feel competent about managing their health, they are more likely to feel optimistic about their ability to reverse negative patterns and become healthier. If instead they feel that illness is God's punishment for some past wrongdoing (as in the case of a few cultural or religious groups), they may be more pessimistic about their ability to change what they view as their fate, or they may rely on prayer to seek help. Table 3.2

Table 3.2   Examples of Disease-Specific Ideas of Illness

Epilepsy is a "loss of soul" (American Medical Student Association, 2005; Fadiman, 1997)—Hmong

Tuberculosis is due to God's curse, evil spirits, or sin (Kapoor, 1996)—Indians

Mental retardation is due to the "spirit of dead horse" (Chan, 1986; Erickson, Devlieger, and Sung, 1999)—Koreans

"Malaria is caused by mosquito bite and when the child walks or spends too much time in the hot sun, his blood becomes hot and this causes malaria" (Ahorlu and others, 1997, p. 492)—Igbo in Nigeria

"Diabetes is permanent in the body leading to [a] terrible, pessimistic and hard future resulting in loss of independence" (Meeto and Meeto, 2005)—Asians

"Schizophrenia is split personality or multiple personality. People with schizophrenia are violent and dangerous" (Health Canada and Schizophrenia Society of Canada, 1991)—North America

Some types of TB are caused by hard work, too much worrying, or passed down from older generations to younger (Le and Nguyen, 2013)—Vietnamese

". . . people get the 'shaking illness [Parkinson's disease] through witchcraft after taking forcefully something belonging to other people . . . " (Mshana, Dotchin, and Walker, 2011, p. 5)—rural northern Tanzania

HIV is a punishment from God and condoms cannot be trusted; HIV/AIDS can be caused by sorcery; . . . HIV is added to the lubricant in condoms (Bogart and others, 2011)—South Africa

provides a few examples of disease-specific definitions of illness that may affect how people from different cultures view specific diseases. These ideas have been reported in existing literature on the topic and may evolve over time.

Beliefs also affect how people rate the desirability of a certain outcome. In evaluating potential outcomes and their individual, social, and cultural appeals, people are influenced by logical and emotional arguments. It is important to understand and rate the level of priority and appeal placed on potential consequences of recommended behaviors.

Take the example of Julie, a fifty-two-year-old woman who is severely overweight. At her annual checkup, her physician finds out that she has type 2 diabetes, which is frequently associated with obesity and characterized by high blood sugar (glucose) levels. So far, Julie does not have any of the major symptoms of diabetes, with the exception of feeling tired and having a few episodes of blurred vision. She has attributed these symptoms to the long hours she spends working in a local manufacturing company and to recent personal events that "make her feel she wants to sleep more." Therefore, when her physician recommends that she lose weight because of the potential long-term effects of diabetes, which include eye complications, kidney disease, and an increased risk for heart attack, stroke, and poor circulation problems (American Diabetes Association, 2005), she does not see the need to follow these instructions. She has no interest in minimizing the potential impact of her diabetes because she does not have any obvious symptoms.

Diabetes prevention and control is only one of the many benefits of weight loss in obese or severely overweight patients. Others are the potential reduction of the psychological effects of obesity, which is a highly stigmatized condition and often limits opportunities in education, employment, personal relationships, and other areas (Wang, Brownell, and Wadden, 2004), and a lower risk for many other conditions associated with obesity, including some forms of cancer, alterations in pulmonary function, hypertension, and cardiovascular disease (Bray, 2004).

Well-planned health communication programs should consider all of these potential outcomes and evaluate their level of importance to key groups. In order to convince people to prioritize weight loss (as in Julie's case), communicators and health care providers should identify the most desirable outcomes to the patient. This should become the entry message of all interactions and communication efforts, which creates a receptive environment to introduce and discuss the benefits of other potential outcomes and relate to and address patients' needs and preferences.

Regardless of the context in which they take place (for example, the physician's office or a public forum), communication interactions and related health practices should be effective and efficient. *Effective* refers to the ability to achieve desired outcomes (for example, in Julie's case, diabetes control or reduction of psychological effect). *Efficient* refers to the ability of achieving these outcomes with minimal time and cost (both economic and emotional).

Of equal importance are people's expectations about the overall quality of the experience. Factors that may influence the quality of the experience are the level of difficulty in complying with recommended activities (for example, limiting consumption of sweets), the kind of support received by friends and family, access to healthy food in one's neighborhood, and many others that are social, community, or individual-specific. Potentially negative consequences of weight loss should also be considered in order to assess the overall appeal of the recommended behavior and its outcomes.

Many experiences have emphasized the importance of understanding and managing health beliefs and desires. As Babrow (1991) reports on the topic of smoking cessation, the probability of achieving expected outcomes, as well as the value placed on positive (for example, "improve health, quit successfully, save money") and negative (for example, potential "weight gain, stress, loss of time") consequences of smoking cessation strongly relate to the intention of smokers to participate in programs that would help them quit (Babrow, 1991, p. 102).

Health communication programs can highlight the cause-and-effect relationship between desirable outcomes and recommended behaviors. They can also contribute to the development of tools and resources that will recommend easy-to-achieve steps for recommended behaviors and set realistic expectations. Finally, as Babrow (1991, p. 96) suggests, communication messages "might inculcate optimism, hope or faith," depending on people's health beliefs and related cultural values.

Cultural Competence and Implications for Health Communication

Cultural competence has been defined as "the capacity to function effectively as an individual and an organization within the context of the cultural beliefs, behaviors and needs presented by consumers and their communities" (US Department of Health and Human Services, 2006b). In simpler terms, cultural competence is the ability to relate to the unique characteristics and values of each population, community, or ethnic group and address them in an efficient way that would create bridges across cultures and different opinions. Culturally appropriate care, defined as the ability of health care professionals to provide medical care within a socially and culturally acceptable framework that may vary from patient to patient, can actually lead to enhanced patient outcomes (Frable, Wallace, and Ellison, 2004) and can also help reduce health disparities. In health communication and, more broadly, public health and health care, cultural competence is increasingly important, given the diversity of most urban and other settings.

cultural competence
The ability to relate to other people's values, feelings, and beliefs across different cultures, and effectively address such differences as part of all interactions

Recent consensus among public health and health communication experts and organizations has highlighted the role culture plays in health outcomes and behaviors, as well as in increasing the effectiveness of health communication interventions (Kreuter and McClure, 2004; Institute of Medicine, 2002, 2003b; Liu and Chen, 2010). Well-designed and well-executed health communication programs should rely on an in-depth understanding of intended groups and be tailored to their needs and beliefs. This implies a true knowledge of cultural values that inspire the people with whom we interact.

In fact, although shared values and other cultural expressions are often related to age, race, religion, gender, and geographical boundaries, it is likely that even within the same racial or age group, there may be different subgroups with specific cultural connotations or different stages in terms of their understanding and involvement in a certain health issue. For example, it would be naive to believe that a single smoking cessation program could be designed for teenagers who live in the inner city and affluent neighborhoods of a metropolitan area and have different smoking-related habits and beliefs. Some of the program's key elements may be the same, but others should address the unique characteristics and preferences of these different groups.

audience segmentation
The practice of understanding large groups and populations as part of smaller groups (segments) that have similar characteristics, preferences, and needs; one of the key steps of the situation and audience analysis and completes the audience profile

Audience segmentation, which is defined as the practice of understanding large groups and populations as part of smaller groups (segments) that have similar characteristics, preferences, and needs (Boslaugh, Kreuter, Nicholson, and Naleid, 2005; Moss, Kirby, and Donodeo, 2009), is a well-established process in health communication as well as in related disciplines. Although a detailed discussion of audience segmentation is included in Chapter Eleven, readers should start thinking about the potential uniqueness of the cultural, behavioral, psychological, demographic, socioeconomic, and geographical characteristics and risk factors of different audience segments and try to apply them to a recent health situation they encountered. For example, would you use just one approach to help your friends quit smoking, regardless of whether they are aware of the potential risk for smoking-related complications and diseases? What about the approach you would take to help a friend who is surrounded by peers who regard smoking as cool versus someone who feels guilty about not being able to quit and lives with people who disapprove of smoking? There are many variables in approaching audience segmentation, and culture is one of them (Kreuter and McClure, 2004).

Although audience segmentation is a term that health communication borrows from marketing disciplines, our emphasis on a participatory approach to communication planning, implementation, and evaluation demand innovative methods, including community consultation and dialogue and community-driven assessments to understand the uniqueness of each group with whom we interact.

The concept of cultural competence establishes the need for tailored communication interventions, which usually use a multifaceted approach to address the concerns, preferences, and needs of a specific group (Kreuter and Skinner, 2000; Slater, 1996; Kreuter and McClure, 2004). Cultural competence is key to a program's success and is strictly related to how information is exchanged, processed, and evaluated by intended groups. It also points to the importance of tailoring language and cultural references to the specific audience, customizing message delivery to different learning styles, and using credible messengers. (For additional discussion on the role that culture and cultural competence should play in message development and delivery, as well as in the selection of appropriate communication channels and spokespeople, see Chapter Thirteen.)

Key Concepts

- Culture has been rightly compared to an iceberg (Peace Corps, 2011). Just as an iceberg has some visible sections and others are below the waterline, culture has some observable aspects (observable behaviors) and others that can only be intuited, imagined, and ultimately researched.

- Conceptions of health and illness are influenced by culture, race, ethnicity, age, gender, socioeconomic conditions, and geographical boundaries, among other factors.

- Gender influences not only ideas of health and illness but also access to health information, financial resources for treatment interventions, and ways to respond to disease. In many cultures, it may also determine differences in the level of social marginalization experienced by those who suffer from highly stigmatized diseases, such as AIDS or tuberculosis.

- Health communication interventions should analyze and take into account different ideas of health and illness in order to be effective in reaching out to intended groups.

- Tensions between health beliefs and desires influence people's willingness to adopt and sustain health behaviors and are influenced by culture. Health communication can highlight the cause-and-effect relationship between recommended behaviors and desirable outcomes.

- Cultural competence is critical in health communication.

- Major implications of cultural competence in health communication include the need for audience segmentation and capacity building in a variety of professional and community settings, as well as the development of group-specific messages, channels, and messengers.

FOR DISCUSSION AND PRACTICE

1. While reflecting on the chapter's definitions, list some universal values and personal values that influence your culture. Please provide examples of how such values may have influenced your own health-related decisions.

2. What is your reaction to the section in this chapter about Lia Lee, a Hmong child? What (if anything) do you think should have happened differently?

3. When can you say that you feel in good health? Do any family or cultural beliefs affect your ideas of health and illness? Does your family or ethnic group have any special way to deal with illness? Can you think of an experience in which your health was affected by physical as well as mental and social factors?

4. Describe a personal experience with cross-cultural communication—for example, a health-related encounter with a health care provider from a different cultural or ethnic background or participation in research studies or programs that involved different groups or populations.

5. In health communication, what are the major implications of the potential tension between patients' health beliefs and desires? Can you provide a practical example or personal experience that illustrates how culturally competent communications can help address such issues?

KEY TERMS

audience segmentation   personal values

cultural competence   universal values

PART TWO

HEALTH COMMUNICATION APPROACHES AND ACTION AREAS

By the time readers approach Part Two, they have probably already had an opportunity to discuss different topics in health communication with peers, colleagues, and others. In most cases readers have had a chance to practice or reflect on how some of the concepts and theories we discussed in Part One may apply to their current or future endeavors. Because Part Two focuses on the different areas of health communication defined in Part One, some of you may come directly to this section of the book for special topics on a specific communication area.

Part Two focuses on the different action areas of health communication, related theoretical and practical approaches, and case studies. Key areas in this section include interpersonal communication (Chapter Four), mass media and new media communication and public relations (Chapter Five), community mobilization and citizen engagement (Chapter Six), professional medical communications (Chapter Seven), constituency relations and strategic partnerships in health communication (Chapter Eight), and policy communication and public advocacy (Chapter Nine). Although each chapter focuses on a specific action area, all six chapters in this section also reinforce the importance of an integrated approach to health communication interventions, which relies on a strategic blend of communication areas (and related media channels) to mirror how people talk about health and illness—in public forums, and with family members, at the doctor's office and over the Internet, via new media and in community settings, just to cite a few examples—and to encourage behavioral and social change in support of improved patient, community, and public health outcomes.

CHAPTER 4

INTERPERSONAL COMMUNICATION

In 1999, Harry Depew, the 2000 Family Physician of the Year of the American Academy of Family Physicians (AAFP), began his comments to the AAFP Congress of Delegates by first addressing the audience in sign language: "If you were a hearing person in a deaf world, where you could not understand sign language, how would you feel communicating with your doctor?" Then he asked out loud (AAFP, 1999). His question refers to a specific communication need and area of interpersonal communication (provider-patient communication). Still, the feelings of isolation and frustration that may be elicited by the situation Depew describes are likely quite similar to those we may feel in all instances in which health information, or another kind of information, is misunderstood or blocked out because we cannot relate to the person who is speaking.

Interpersonal communication is an important action area of health communication programs aimed at behavioral (World Health Organization [WHO], 2003) or social change. It includes provider-patient communications as well as community dialogue (interpersonal communication at scale) and counseling and personal selling (the one-on-one engagement of key groups in their own homes, offices, or places of work and leisure), which are activities that find applicability in many different phases and aspects of the communication process.

CHAPTER OBJECTIVES

This chapter reviews some of the key factors in the dynamics of interpersonal behavior and communication. It also focuses on practical aspects of community dialogue, counseling, personal selling, and provider-patient communications, which are all key areas of interpersonal communication. In doing so, it highlights the importance of considering all encounters as an opportunity for a two-way exchange of information and ideas, as well as the potential beginning of a long-lasting partnership.

The Dynamics of Interpersonal Behavior

Interpersonal behavior is influenced by several cultural factors. Although each individual has his or her own style of interacting with others, social conventions or norms, as well as traditions and values in a given group or community, play an important role in how behavior and communication take place and are interpreted and perceived.

All interactions comprise both verbal and nonverbal signs and symbols that contribute to the meanings of behavior and communication actions. Social psychologists tend to consider *signs* to be involuntary behaviors. *Symbols* are defined as voluntary acts, such as using verbal expressions to describe one's feelings (Krauss and Fussell, 1996). According to these definitions, saying "I am embarrassed" is a symbol, whereas blushing in response to feelings of embarrassment is a sign.

Symbols are the result of social conventions and agreement (Sebeok, 2001; Lim, Liu, and Lee, 2011). For example, the significance of the word *embarrassed* is well known and shared by all English-language users (Krauss and Fussell, 1996). Therefore, using it in this context is supported by social norms and conventions.

A number of so-called signs may be controlled and therefore assume a symbolic value (Krauss and Fussell, 1996). For example, facial expressions can be controlled and modified to induce others to believe what we want them to believe and disguise what we are really feeling (Kraut, 1979; Porter and ten Brinke, 2008). Most people can recall situations in which they met a colleague or attended a business party immediately after a painful disagreement with a loved one. Chances are that facial expressions were controlled to disguise all feelings related to the recent disagreement. As this example demonstrates, it is difficult to strictly apply the theoretical distinction between signs and symbols (Krauss and Fussell, 1996). Still, this distinction can provide a useful framework to explain some of the components of interpersonal behavior and communication.

It is also critical to take into account the impact of culture on the interpretation of signs and symbols. Culture starts influencing meanings quite early in life. In fact, the process of socialization that begins within the family, and aims at preparing children for their adult role, is influenced by social norms and cultural factors of a given population or group (Moment and Zaleznik, 1964; Grusec, 2011; Berns, 2013). How a child will address teachers and elderly members of his or her family and community depends on the educational level, cultural values, age, and traditions of the parents, as well as their social environment.

Differences in power and social status also affect the dynamics of interpersonal behavior and the potential intimacy or level of formality of relationships (Hwa-Froelich and Vigil, 2004; Hofstede, 1984, 2001). In some cultures, people are assigned a higher social status in relation to their age, economic wealth, education, profession, or birth order (Hwa-Froelich and Vigil, 2004). For example, in the Chinese language, the eldest sister is addressed with a special word that conveys respect (Hwa-Froelich and Vigil, 2004).

Signs and symbols often assume different meanings in different cultures. Posture, social cues, and facial and idiomatic expressions all influence interpersonal relationships. In interpreting people's behavior, it is important to be aware of cultural differences that may have a powerful effect on the dynamics of interpersonal behavior. Lack of understanding of these differences often undermines the impact of well-meant communication efforts.

In the public health and health care fields, understanding how cultural variables and interpretations affect interpersonal behavior has a positive influence on communication that may lead to better patient outcomes, increased patient compliance to treatment, or a better chance for disease control in a given group or population, to name just a few potential positive effects. Table 4.1 compares examples of different aspects of culture that may influence interpersonal relationships and communication during a health care–related encounter. Because these are just sample cultural norms and values, they may not apply to all situations or may evolve over time. As previously mentioned in Chapters Two and Three, cultural competence is essential to effective health communication within the context of interpersonal behavior and interactions as well as in a variety of organizational and professional settings. Table 4.1 provides useful insights to manage diversity in the interpersonal setting but also applies to other communication areas and settings.

Table 4.1   Comparing Cultural Norms and Values

Aspects of culture	US health care culture	Other cultures
Sense of self and space	Informal Handshake	Formal Hugs, bows, handshakes
Communication and language	Explicit, direct communication Emphasis on content; meaning found in words	Implicit, indirect communication Emphasis on context; meaning found around words
Dress and appearance	"Dress for success" ideal Wide range in accepted dress More casual	Dress seen as a sign of position, wealth, and prestige Religious rules More formal
Food and eating habits	Eating as a necessity; fast food	Dining as a social experience Religious rules
Time and time consciousness	Linear and exact time consciousness Value on promptness Time equals money	Elastic and relative time consciousness Time spent on enjoyment of relationships
Relationship, family, friends	Focus on nuclear family Responsibility for self Value on youth; age seen as handicap	Focus on extended family Loyalty and responsibility to family Age given status and respect
Values and norms	Individual orientation Independence Preference for direct confrontation of conflict Emphasis on task	Group orientation Conformity Preference for harmony Emphasis on relationships
Beliefs and attitudes	Egalitarian Challenging of authority Gender equity Behavior and action affect and determine the future	Hierarchical Respect for authority and social order Different roles for men and women Fate controls and predetermines the future
Mental processes and learning style	Linear, logical Problem-solving focus Internal locus of control Individuals control their destiny	Lateral, holistic, simultaneous Accepting of life's difficulties External locus of control Individuals accept their destiny
Work habits and practices	Reward based on individual achievement Work has intrinsic value	Rewards based on seniority, relationships Work is a necessity of life

Source: Gardenswartz, L., and Rowe, A. *Managing Diversity: A Complete Desk Reference and Planning Guide.* New York: McGraw-Hill, 1993, p. 57. © The McGraw-Hill Companies, Inc. Reprinted with permission.

Social and Cognitive Processes of Interpersonal Communication

Interpersonal behavior is usually affected by social cues, preferences, needs, and factors as well as cognitive processes that may vary at the individual level. Social and cognitive factors play a key role in how information is shared, evaluated, processed, and absorbed.

Social Cues, Needs, and Factors

Change occurs when people are able to share common meanings and understand each other. In health communication, messages affect attitudes only when people understand, process, and remember them (Krauss and Fussell, 1996) and feel motivated to apply them in their everyday life.

In order to be effective, communication needs to respond to specific social cues and needs. This general principle also applies to different types of interpersonal communication, such as one-on-one teaching, counseling, personal selling, and provider-patient communications.

Several authors explain people's behavior in the interpersonal communication context in terms of the desire to satisfy a specific need (Step and Finucane, 2002; Kellerman and Reynolds, 1990; Roloff, 1987; Schutz, 1966; Frisby and Martin, 2010). Rubin, Perse, and Barbato (1988) developed the Interpersonal Communication Motives scale to explain the dynamics and motivation of interpersonal communication. Based on this model, people interact and speak with each other to satisfy specific needs:

- Being part of a social group or including others in one's group
- Appreciating others
- Controlling other people's actions and increasing behavioral compliance
- Being amused and entertained
- Escaping and being distracted from routine activities
- Relaxing and relieving stress

In their analysis, Rubin, Perse, and Barbato (1988) also showed that people tend to be less anxious when their motivation to communicate is to include others or to feel included. Having a good life, which entails overall satisfaction, good health, economic security, and social gratification, among other factors, also influences the reasons for which people communicate (Barbato and Perse, 1992; Step and Finucane, 2002).

Age and gender also influence motives for interpersonal communication. For example, young people between eighteen and twenty-five years old often use communication as a means for having fun, relaxing, feeling part of a social group, or escaping from routine activities (Javidi and others, 1990; Step and Finucane, 2002; Barbato, Graham, and Perse, 2003). Alternatively, middle-aged or older adults tend to communicate more to express appreciation or feel appreciated (Javidi and others, 1990; Step and Finucane, 2002). Barbato and Perse (1992) found that elders with greater life satisfaction and higher levels of social activity reported pleasure and affection as motives for communication, whereas those who were less healthy, mobile, and socially active communicated for control or comfort. There are gender differences in interpersonal communication as well: women seem to communicate more "to express emotions" or appreciation, whereas men's motivation is primarily control (Step and Finucane, 2002, p. 95; Barbato and Perse, 1992). To this effect, for example, gender communication interventions need to rely on an in-depth understanding of the communication styles and attitudes different genders bring to all interactions. These may include differences in the way of processing information, attitudes toward tasks and relationships, gender-specific values, leadership styles, and motivational factors. Yet, this kind of analysis is needed not only for different genders but also should expand to all groups and stakeholders we seek to reach and engage in the communication process.

Many other elements contribute to the quality and tone of interpersonal interactions. Some obvious factors are common cultural references: similar upbringing, level of intimacy and mutual trust, level of competence about the topic being discussed, openness to new ideas, and individual states of mind.

Most people can relate to the feeling of recognizing themselves in the values and expressions of those who were born in the same part of the world. This is a good predictor of potentially good interpersonal interactions but needs to be complemented by feelings of trust and respect about the other person's competence or level of empathy on the subject being addressed.

Personal experiences can also affect interpersonal communication and influence relationships with those who previously shared one's cultural values and beliefs. For example, a couple from a conservative country where women are not allowed to participate with men in any kind of social event may reevaluate their beliefs and interact differently with their fellow citizens after living in a country where the concept of equality between men and women is widely accepted. When travelers return from such a trip, their interpersonal relationships may be affected by the urge to change beliefs, whereas before such beliefs were based on shared values and the need to conform to them.

This example points to the importance of cultural and social factors in interpersonal interactions and communication. It also suggests that interactions and communication may change over time according to people's beliefs and values. Therefore, communication needs to be sensitive to belief and attitude changes and recognize that these changes are often the result of other interpersonal relationships and communications. It is important to acknowledge the cause-and-effect impact of interpersonal communication and promptly adapt to change.

Cognitive Processes

The process of acquiring knowledge by the use of reasoning, intuition, or perception is strictly related to communication and its modalities. Every time people interact with others, they share information. How new or existing information is acknowledged and processed depends on the approach one takes to communication.

For example, psychologists have long pointed out that people's performance in trying to solve a problem is influenced by the way the problem is presented (Glucksberg and Weisberg, 1963; Chiu, Krauss, and Lau, 1998). In the United States, an "I-can-do" attitude toward professional tasks is considered a major asset. Can-do people feel that all tasks are within their reach and competence, and there is no such thing to them as an insurmountable problem. They also tend to transmit their enthusiasm and confidence to subordinates and colleagues. They present problems and situations with an optimistic flair. This is likely to make people feel competent and able to solve problems and may enhance their performance. By contrast, if a problem is presented by highlighting all the worst scenarios and expressing doubts about the possibility of addressing it, chances are that people may feel that whatever they do may not work.

Knowledge and attitude change are also influenced by the way information is presented. Establishing open and trusting communication is often the first step in creating a receptive environment in which information can be perceived as reliable and worthy of consideration. All successful communications and interactions usually require a reasonably good understanding of the other person's point of view (Brown, 1965; Park and Raile, 2010). Openness and trust are usually contagious. People can induce the same kind of open and trusting communications in others just by beginning first. Cooperation creates and is created by, among other things, openness in communication and trusting and friendly attitudes (Deutsch, 2012). Figure 4.1 shows two different scenarios and their potential impact on knowledge, attitude, and behavior after a mother's conversation with her infant daughter's pediatrician.

Still, it is important to remember that the sole or singular use of verbal expressions has been shown to have only a temporary impact on attitude change (Chiu, Krauss, and Lau, 1998). Eiser and Pancer (1979) studied the

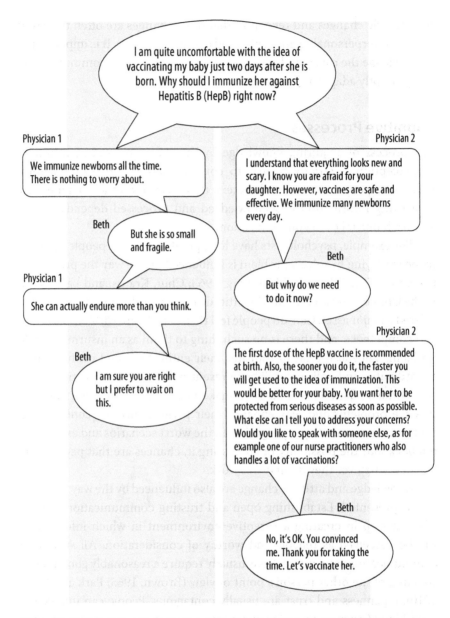

Figure 4.1 The Potential Impact of Interpersonal Communication on Behavior: A Practical Example

effect of biased language on attitudinal changes by asking study participants to write their views on capital punishment. Some of the subjects
were directed to use words in their essays that were pro–capital punishment. Others were told to use words that were anti–capital punishment.
Although the attitude of study participants toward capital punishment
initially changed to reflect the words they had used in their essays, they

had reverted to their original perspectives within six days from when they wrote their papers (Eiser and Pancer, 1979; Chiu, Krauss, and Lau, 1998).

In health communication, it is not enough to define a recommended behavior as "healthy" or "life-saving." In order to determine a more permanent attitude change, all statements need to reflect local cultural values, be supported by evidence (Chiu, Krauss, and Lau, 1998), and translated into tools to facilitate their practical application. This is an important concept in message development in both interpersonal communication and other action areas of health communication. Facts and tools are critical to lend credibility to verbal expressions and motivate people to change.

Community Dialogue as an Example of Interpersonal Communication at Scale

Listening to communities and their members and responding to their needs by encouraging action and partnerships across sectors are or should be key cornerstones of any kind of health communication intervention. **Community dialogue** is a process that seeks to create a favorable environment in which communities feel comfortable putting forward their ideas and interests and providing input and opinions on specific matters on which they are consulted. "Unlike debate, dialogue emphasizes listening to deepen understanding. It develops common perspectives and goals, and allows participants to express their own interests" (Agriculture and Agri-Food Canada, 2012). Dialogue is a conversation that takes place at the community level and can take many forms: from a small group of people around a kitchen table, to a large consensus process in a community center, to dialogues over the Internet and other kinds of new media, and workshops or polling. In this way, community dialogue is a form of interpersonal communication at scale to which all of the principles of interpersonal communication as well as the dynamics of interpersonal behavior rightly apply. As some other authors have also suggested community dialogue processes "are based on the belief that such inclusion is a citizen's right, may improve the accuracy of decision making and may assist in the community's acceptance of decisions" (Duignan and Parker, 2005, p. 2).

Community dialogue methods and tools have been incorporated in a variety of communication planning frameworks (including communication for development, communication for behavioral impact, and others; see Chapter Two), and have been used by different kinds of community organizations, citizens, and institutions. Because community dialogue is an integral component of community mobilization and citizen engagement,

community dialogue
A process that seeks to create a favorable environment in which communities feel comfortable putting forward their ideas and interests and providing input and opinions on specific matters on which they are consulted

further discussion of this topic and its practical applications is included in Chapter Six.

The Power of Personal Selling and Counseling

personal selling
Refers to (1) one-on-one engagement of different groups in their own homes, offices, or places of work and leisure and (2) the ability to sell one's image and expertise, an important skill in most counseling activities

Personal selling is a well-established practice in the commercial sector that also has many applications in public health, health care, and health communication. In the commercial sector, it refers to the one-on-one, "door-to-door engagement" (WHO, 2005b, p. 27) of potential customers or special groups in their own homes, offices, or places of work and leisure. In the health care industry, the figure that comes to mind is the pharmaceutical sales representative who goes to physicians' offices to present a product.

Personal selling is also widely used for nonprofit causes and to spread the word about recommended new health behaviors and practices. In public health and health communication, personal sellers are usually volunteers, social workers, trainers, health professionals, or representatives of community development organizations who go door-to-door or attend events where health services are provided. Their role is to engage key groups in interpersonal interactions to explain, recommend, and show benefits of a specific health behavior or practice. Often this role is coupled with actual service delivery. It also serves the purpose of answering questions and addressing fears and concerns about recommended health services and practices.

Door-to-door immunization is considered a core strategy of the worldwide polio eradication campaign, for example (Joyner, 2001; WHO, 2012b). House-to-house "mop-up" campaigns were part of a four-pronged strategy employed to eliminate polio in the Americas (Aylward and Heymann, 2005). WHO, UNICEF, and their partners in the polio-eradication effort organize national immunization days in which thousands of volunteers and health professionals travel to remote villages and poor areas in the developing world to set up one-day clinics in schools, markets, and other places where they can reach a large number of people and persuade them to vaccinate their children. In India alone, during National Immunization Day in 1999, "2.5 million volunteers and health professionals traveled by any available means, including by camel and on foot following dry riverbed[s], carrying the vaccine on ice to their immunization posts" (Joyner, 2001). Another door-to-door campaign aiming to immunize seventy-seven million African children against polio in one year was launched by UNICEF and its partners in 2005 (Li, 2005). Polio immunization campaigns in South Sudan targeted 3.2 million children under the age of five and conducted door-to-door national immunization days in all ten states of South Sudan in February and March 2012 (WHO, 2013b).

Personal selling does not work in a vacuum. In most cases, personal selling efforts need to be complemented by other communication interventions, such as new media and mass media outreach, community mobilization, and other communication approaches discussed later in this book (see the example in Box 4.1). All of these other activities help create social consensus and support about the importance of responding to the call for action of volunteers, health workers, or school children who would knock on people's doors. Without creating a supportive environment in which people feel motivated to listen to the recommendations of the so-called agents of change, most personal selling efforts may fail or produce only minimal results. Still, in the case of polio, door-to-door immunization enables the vaccination of millions of children in areas where war, lack of infrastructures, and poverty would otherwise make vaccine access and delivery impossible (Joyner, 2001). Similarly, personal selling was one of the key success factors in a WHO effort to prevent lymphatic filariasis in several endemic countries (see Box 4.1).

BOX 4.1. PERSONAL SELLING AND COUNSELING CASE STUDY

Lymphatic Filariasis

India, Kenya, Nepal, Philippines, Sri Lanka, and Zanzibar

Lymphatic filariasis (LF) is a painful and disfiguring disease caused by threadlike worms that live in the human lymphatic system. LF is transmitted from person to person by mosquitoes. Around 120 million are affected by LF, with more than one billion people at risk of infection.

LF is one of seven diseases targeted for elimination by WHO. The strategy adopted for elimination in 1997 at the World Health Assembly is to treat entire endemic communities once a year, for five to six years, with two coadministered antiparasitic drugs. For the strategy of mass drug administrations to be successful over 70 percent of the total population should take the prescribed number of LF prevention pills. The other fundamental aspect of the program is to provide support for those already suffering from LF-related disabilities.

Impact

Country	Total population targeted	Coverage rate achieved (% of total population)
India: Tamil Nadu	28 million	74
Kenya	1.2 million	81
Philippines	4.5 million	87
Sri Lanka	9.5 million	86
Zanzibar	1 million	83

The behavioral objective: Take your LF pills from your filaria prevention assistants on filaria day.

COMBI plans were designed for India (the state of Tamil Nadu), Kenya, Nepal, Philippines, Sri Lanka, and Zanzibar. The campaigns had a sharp, singular focus on the behavioral result expected: the ready acceptance and swallowing of the tablets on a chosen day.

The heart of the entire effort were a group of dedicated individuals (health workers, teachers, and volunteers) called *filaria prevention assistants*, going door-to-door hand-delivering a set of tablets to all eligible individuals. They also carried out two preparatory visits to households explaining the elimination program, showing the tablets, describing what was expected, and answering any queries or concerns. The filaria prevention assistants were supported by intense community mobilization, massive advertising, high media coverage, and political and religious leadership backing.

Source: World Health Organization. Mediterranean Center for Vulnerability Reduction. "COMBI in Action: Country Highlights." 2004a. http://wmc.who.int/pdf/COMBI_in_Action_04.pdf. Used by permission.

Still, the practice of personal selling is an acquired communication skill that relies on many of the principles of interpersonal communication discussed so far in this chapter, as well as on individual characteristics and strengths. It requires training, awareness of people's needs, strong listening skills, and the ability to engage others, as well as to counter objections by acknowledging the other person's perspective and empathizing with it. It involves the ability to resolve conflicts by brainstorming and finding common ground. In the case of a specific health communication campaign or public health intervention, it requires a level of competence and knowledge on the subject matter that, at a minimum, should be sufficient to elicit trust among the groups and communities we may reach.

Furthermore, the term *personal selling* can refer to the ability to sell one's image and expertise, a helpful skill in most kinds of consulting activities. This second definition refers primarily to a communication skill, whereas the first definition is related to a key area of interpersonal communication. These two meanings are strongly connected and interdependent in their practical application.

Personal selling (the ability to sell one's image and expertise but also a skill that is needed in the one-on-one engagement of key groups and stakeholders) is dependent on a number of verbal and nonverbal signals that should be recognizable by such groups. Among others, these include posture, overall confidence, speech and expressions, dress code (casual versus formal), and the ability to relate to others and express genuine concern. However, signs and symbols are not the same across differing populations and cultures. As previously discussed (see Table 4.1), several cultural and social factors may influence people's ability to sell their image, competence, and expertise among members of different key groups and populations.

In **counseling**, which could be defined as the help provided by a professional on personal, psychological, health, or professional matters, personal selling skills are a powerful determinant of one's ability to have an impact on the beliefs, attitudes, and behavior of the person who is seeking counsel. In fact, personal selling skills may affect the ability of health communication practitioners to counsel others on communication strategies or engage opinion leaders in prioritizing a given health issue. Personal selling also influences patient-provider relationships and treatment compliance.

counseling
The help provided by a professional on personal, psychological, health, or professional matters, including via one-on-one interactions, personal selling, and other interpersonal communication approaches

Because of their special role in giving advice and shaping other people's professional or personal lives, counselors, whether they are physicians, nurses, psychologists, lawyers, health communication practitioners, community organizers, health science librarians, or other public health, community development, or health care professionals, need to be trusted and respected by the people they seek to reach. The audiences (whether they are patients or nonprofit organizations or others) need to have faith in the counselors' commitment to a common cause (for example, a patient's well-being or the success of a communication intervention) in order to relate to them and follow their advice.

Most important, people need to feel a sense of ownership of the issue on which they are being advised. And how could it be otherwise? Even if health professionals are knowledgeable about a given disease or health problem, it is the patient's life that is directly affected by its symptoms and potential consequences. And what about key stakeholders, such as professional organizations, senior government officials, community development organization, foundations, or top physicians who decide to endorse a health issue after being solicited by health communication practitioners or other public health professionals? Given their busy schedule and conflicting priorities, they are likely to dedicate significant portions of their time to addressing a specific issue only if they feel needed and can make a significant contribution to the problem's solution.

Several cultural nuances may affect these general concepts. In some cultures, patients tend to defer more to their physicians or do not participate as much in treatment and prevention decisions because of their views of illness as God's will or punishment or other cultural beliefs. Nevertheless, in all situations, the role of counselors, including health care providers, is to reach out, bridge cultural differences, and try to transform each encounter into a productive partnership.

Because of the documented impact of provider-patient communications on patient outcomes and overall satisfaction, the rest of this chapter focuses primarily on this important form of interpersonal communication in health care. In doing so, it provides a practical and research-based perspective on how to transform ordinary relationships into successful partnerships that may lead to improved disease outcomes.

Communication as a Core Clinical Competency

Being sick is among one of the most vulnerable times in people's lives, especially in the case of severe, chronic, or life-threatening diseases. It is also a time in which patients need to understand and feel comfortable with the information their provider shares with them. From a patient's perspective, it is important to feel that their case is a key priority for the health care provider they have selected. From a provider's perspective, conflicting priorities, managed care requirements (see Chapter Two), time barriers, or insufficient communication training may limit the ability to establish trusting and open relationships with patients.

Still, effective communication has been shown to have a positive impact on patient compliance to health recommendations, patient satisfaction, patient retention rates, overall health outcomes, and even a reduced number of malpractice suits (DiMatteo and others, 1993; Garrity, Haynes, Mattson, and Engebretson, 1998; Lipkin, 1996; Lukoschek, Fazzari, and Marantz, 2003; Belzer, 1999; Zolnierek and DiMatteo, 2009). As Lukoschek, Fazzari, and Marantz (2003) highlighted, the patient-provider encounter offers one of the most important opportunities "to have a major impact on reducing morbidity and mortality of chronic diseases, through personalized information exchange" (p. 209). Box 4.2 provides a health care provider's perspective on the impact of effective communication on patient outcomes and well-being, as well as on key social determinants of health (for example, the level of social support and the kind of interactions with peers and others that people experience in their living and working environment).

BOX 4.2. THE IMPACT OF EFFECTIVE PROVIDER-PATIENT COMMUNICATION ON PATIENT OUTCOMES: A PEDIATRIC NURSE PRACTITIONER'S PERSPECTIVE

Mary Beth Koslap Petraco, CPNP, is the coordinator for child health in the Suffolk County Department of Health Services, New York; chair of the Immunization Special Interest Group of the National Association of Pediatric Nurse Practitioners; and a clinical assistant professor at the State University of New York at Stony Brook. Her thoughts on the importance of provider-patient communications (interview and other personal communications with the author, 2006) reflect her extensive patient-related experience.

Cultural competence is very important in nursing. US nurses are specifically educated to put aside their cultural bias and work with the patient's cultural beliefs. This is a unique attribute of US-educated nurses and helps establish effective relationships with patients.

Good provider-patient communications are very important in changing patients' attitudes toward disease, helping them use their culture in a positive way, and empowering them to make the changes in their lives that are associated with better health outcomes.

I learned a long time ago that the parents of the children I see know more than I do. When I acknowledge this fact, it's much easier to guide parents to make the changes that are needed for their children as well as to reinforce the positive things they are already doing.

There are a number of key factors that help establish a good provider-patient relationship. First, give patients respect. Introduce yourself and explain the role you will play in their care. Don't talk down to them. Use language the patient understands. Acknowledge positive points and accomplishments. Always think of them as people with their unique needs and beliefs.

Nurses are well positioned to establish good provider-patient relationships because of their education and training. Nursing is at the same time an art and a science and is based on the same key steps (assessment, implementation, and evaluation) of effective communication.

Patient-provider encounters should be used not only to determine the physical fitness of the patient and treat potential illnesses but also to assess the patient's overall well-being. For example, when a twelve-year-old Hispanic girl presented with vague stomach complaints that were preventing her from attending school, we discovered that physical symptoms and causes had nothing to do with her condition. The girl was happy at home and loved her mother, who was a domestic worker and spoke only Spanish. She was also a very good student. Yet, recently she had refused to go to school. By talking with her and her mother, we discovered that she had been bullied and threatened with physical assault by a group of children in the school.

We taught both her and her mother to talk to the school counselor, request a Spanish translator, and speak with the families of the other children. We did a role-play with the mother so she would feel comfortable once at school. We also recommended she mention that the police would get involved if this would not stop.

It was priceless to see the smile on the mother's face when she came back to our office a few weeks later for a follow-up visit. It is also priceless to know that the girl is now happy in school and doing very well academically.

Nurses can make a difference in their patients' lives. This is why I think nurses should always advocate for their patients' rights, especially in the case of underserved populations.

In all disease areas, effective communication is part of the cure. So, what is the best way to make it happen and overcome existing barriers to good patient-provider relationships?

One important step is to recognize that communication is a core clinical competence that can help improve effective use of time and help patients comply with recommended treatment and healthy behaviors, as well as optimize overall patient satisfaction and outcomes. As with other kinds of interpersonal interactions, understanding the patient's cultural values, language preferences, differences in style, living and working environments, life stressors, and specific meanings attributed to verbal and nonverbal expressions (see Table 4.1) are fundamental in establishing a satisfactory relationship.

It all starts with training. Some studies have shown that a patient's comprehension of health information is highly influenced by physicians' attitudes toward the importance of sharing information with their patients, which is shaped by their experience during medical training (Lukoschek, Fazzari, and Marantz, 2003; Eisenberg, Kitz, and Webber, 1983). For example, after three years of training, most medical residents tend to maintain a participatory attitude toward the decision-making process related to treatment and other recommendations. But after the same time period, surgical residents have switched to a more authoritarian attitude, even if they started with similar views as those of medical residents. This may reflect the hierarchical status and the task-oriented characteristics of surgeons' medical training (Eisenberg, Kitz, and Webber, 1983). Still, it would be unfair to generalize these findings without taking into account personal and cultural factors and experiences.

The example in Box 4.3 shows how different physician attitudes toward communication may result in different outcomes. It also points to the importance of an empathetic and participatory approach to provider-patient communications, which may be better suited to motivate patient compliance and establish true partnerships.

BOX 4.3. IMPACT OF PHYSICIAN ATTITUDES ON PATIENT BEHAVIOR: A TRUE STORY

Carmen was a sixty-one-year-old Spanish woman visiting her relatives in the United States. (The name of the patient and some other facts have been changed to protect the patient's and physicians' privacy.) During her trip, she was hospitalized for emergency spine surgery. She had been suffering from excruciating back pain that her physicians in Spain had misdiagnosed. While in the United States, her pain had worsened, and it turned out that a major infection had almost destroyed two of her vertebrae and was threatening her ability to walk.

The surgery was successful. However, Carmen felt isolated in a foreign hospital where she could not communicate with physicians and nurses. She spoke no English. Her relatives visited her as often as they could, but they also needed to deal with work and family obligations. They hired an interpreter for a few hours each day so Carmen could communicate with the hospital staff and perhaps feel a little less lonely.

Approximately fifteen days after the surgery, one of Carmen's physicians recommended that she try to stand up and sit on a chair. When he went to visit Carmen, he did not speak to her through the interpreter. He just instructed the nurse to help her and did not show much empathy for Carmen's pain. Carmen tried to get out of bed, but her pain was really bothering her. After the first attempt, she asked her interpreter to tell the physician that she was tired; she needed to rest and might try later.

A few hours later, her internal medicine specialist came by. She had been alerted about the earlier events and had called Carmen's relatives to discuss how to approach this issue. She greeted Carmen warmly and started to speak with her through her interpreter. Carmen talked about her attempt to stand up. She was still in a lot of pain. Despite the words of reassurance by her relatives who had just telephoned her, she was not sure she wanted to try again. After all, in most countries, patients who have this kind of surgery, or even less invasive surgery, are confined to bed rest for much longer. Carmen found the request unreasonable.

The internist explained to Carmen that this was a common procedure in the United States and helped improve and accelerate a patient's rehabilitation. She highlighted the benefits of early ambulation. She also showed empathy for Carmen's pain. She mentioned that she would consult pain specialists to see whether they could do something to reduce her pain while she tried to regain mobility. Through the interpreter, she made sure that Carmen understood all the information and also asked if she had additional questions.

Carmen decided to try again with the help of the nurse and her interpreter. After a few attempts, she stood up and managed to sit on a chair. The entire team—the physician, the nurse, and the interpreter—encouraged and congratulated her for trying. She was still in a lot of pain, but she was happy about having succeeded. After all, this was a sign that things might go back to normal soon.

The physicians' recommendations proved to be effective. Less than a month after her surgery, Carmen was able to walk with the aid of a cane. Without the skillful communication intervention of the internal medicine specialist, this story might have had a different outcome. Carmen might have taken longer to stand up and perhaps suffered some of the medical consequences of prolonged immobility.

Finally, it is also important to remember that most health care providers care about communicating well with their patients. For most physicians, nurses, and other care providers, helping others is one of the primary reasons they chose their professions. However, lack of communication training or other patient- or physician-related barriers may prevent some of them from being effective in establishing productive partnerships with their patients.

Prioritizing Health Disparities in Clinical Education

Health and health care disparities continue to exist and, in some cases to increase, for many populations in the United States and globally. For example, "recent studies have shown that despite the steady improvements in the overall health of the United States, racial and ethnic minorities experience a lower quality of health services and are less likely to receive routine medical procedures and have higher rates of morbidity and mortality than non-minorities. Disparities in health care exist even when controlling for gender, condition, age and socio-economic status" (American Medical Association, 2013).

The issue of quality and equality of care has assumed greater prominence in the era of urbanization and increasing diversity, both at the general population and patient levels. At the same time, diversity and inclusion have been recognized as core elements to the pursuit of excellence in clinical care, and ultimately, to addressing institutional and community priorities (Nivet, 2012). Several prominent organizations and authors (New York Academy of Sciences, 2012; Lunn and Sanchez, 2011; American Medical Association, 2013) have been encouraging physicians and other health care providers to look at their own practices to eliminate inequalities in clinical care, and medical schools to prioritize health disparities in clinical education.

Among others, **cross-cultural health communication** (which refers to a systematic approach to health communication programming and interpersonal communication that emphasizes one key aspect of the health communication process: the ability to communicate across cultures, be culturally competent, be inclusive and mindful of diversity, and to bridge cultural differences so that community and patient voices are heard and properly addressed) has emerged as a prominent field also in clinical education on health disparities. In clinical settings, the importance of cross-cultural health communication strategies and skills continues to grow since the Institute of Medicine report *Unequal Treatment* (2003a) recommended cultural competence training for health care professionals as one of the key activities toward attaining health care equality.

Of great importance in the development of cultural competence and cross-cultural communication training curricula is the inclusion of information, resources, and easy-to-implement tools for physicians, nurses, and other health care providers to assess the socioeconomic and living environment of patients so that barriers to patient compliance can be readily identified and addressed. Health care providers as well as the institutions they serve can play a key role in developing and implementing new community-driven models for the provisions of health care services so that peer-to-peer communication and community engagement strategies can help reinforce clinical recommendations, increase cultural competence in clinical settings, and address key social determinants of health that affect patient outcomes. As the journey toward quality and equality of care progresses, it is important to make sure that clinical education also addresses key barriers to effective provider-patient communications that are discussed in the following section.

cross-cultural health communication
A systematic approach to health communication programming and interpersonal communication that emphasizes one key aspect of the health communication process: the ability to communicate across cultures, be culturally competent, be inclusive and mindful of diversity, as well as to bridge cultural differences so that community and patient voices are heard and properly addressed

Barriers to Effective Provider-Patient Communication

Although many health care providers and public health professionals believe in the importance of optimal provider-patient communications, data suggest that many interactions could be improved. For example, in the United States, studies have shown that the average patient speaks for eighteen to twenty-two seconds before the physician interrupts (Belzer, 1999; American Medical Association, 2005c). Additional research shows that "if allowed to speak freely, the average patient would initially speak for less than 2 minutes" (American Medical Association, 2005a). Most important, in this short period of time, the patient would be able to

Table 4.2 Barriers to Effective Provider-Patient Communication: Patient Factors

Education level

Health literacy level

Language barriers

Cultural or ethnic differences

Age

Cognitive limitations

Lack of understanding of medical jargon and scientific terms

Disease-related stress

Power imbalance compared to health care providers

Socioeconomic conditions (including living and working environment)

express most of his or her concerns and symptoms (Belzer, 1999). This is likely to translate to a better provider-patient relationship as well as to "less follow-up visits, and shorter, more focused, interactions" (American Medical Association, 2005c).

Time is not the only barrier that could be addressed by effective communication. Most of the patient-related barriers in Table 4.2 could be removed by improved interactions and simplified information. For example, research shows that education level and language barriers may lead to low comprehension of medical information among patients (Lukoschek, Fazzari, and Marantz, 2003), so the use of jargon and complex medical terms negatively affects patients' comprehension. As the American Medical Association (2005d) suggests, most patients, regardless of their education level, prefer health information that is simple and easy to understand. In fact, most people can relate to the feelings of vulnerability and stress associated with the diagnosis of a chronic or life-threatening disease or the fear that a temporary medical condition may jeopardize imminent events in their life. In these situations, even well-educated patients may prefer not having to deal with the additional burden of making an effort to understand their provider's suggestions.

As previously discussed in Chapter Two, health literacy is another key issue that affects quality and equality of care and should be prioritized in addressing barriers to provider-patient communication. Providers who are aware of, and able to address, different health literacy levels, and at the same time be culturally competent, are more likely to do the following (Schiavo, 2009b):

- Contribute to building and maintaining a caring, engaging, and friendly clinical environment

- Use simple and direct language
- Listen to patient's concerns
- Have a proactive attitude toward asking questions
- Have the ability to recognize nonverbal clues
- Use repetition, feedback, and follow-up mechanisms to increase patient recollection of medical information, assess patient comprehension levels, and motivate patient compliance

Similarly, language and cultural barriers can be addressed by the use of interpreters as well as an increased emphasis on cultural sensitivity and competence during medical training and cross-cultural communication training sessions (both before and after graduation), which should engage and provide physicians and other health care providers with essential concepts and skills in this area. Research shows that patients may attribute different connotations to words that are used interchangeably by health professionals (Lukoschek, Fazzari, and Marantz, 2003; Heurtin-Roberts and Reisin, 1992). For example, African Americans attribute a different meaning to the words *hypertension* and *high blood pressure* (Lukoschek, Fazzari, and Marantz, 2003; Heurtin-Roberts, 1993), and this may affect their compliance to providers' suggestions (Heurtin-Roberts and Reisin, 1992).

As Heurtin-Roberts (1993) reports, the term *hypertension* is often replaced by "*high-pertension*, a chronic folk illness related to the biomedical hypertension and involving blood and nerves" (p. 285). A percentage of African Americans consider hyper-tension (or high-pertension) different from high blood pressure. High-pertension is regarded as a chronic condition that may become worse with older age and may be related to being "high tempered" (p. 290). Because it is considered a chronic illness, high-pertension is often a way to cope with difficult living conditions and is "one of the few means of controlling the behavioral environment available to the individual" (p. 285).

Some health care providers are quite savvy about cultural differences and other kinds of barriers, whereas others may not have had an opportunity to focus on them throughout their careers. From the provider's perspective, the demands and long hours of most health care professions are often too burdensome to leave time for pleasantry and more effective communication. Physicians in the primary care or pediatric environment are being required to see an increasing number of patients to satisfy managed care policies and other cost-cutting interventions (see Chapter Two).

In the United States, the number of office visits per year has increased by more than 40 percent, rising from 581 million in 1980 to approximately

838 million in 2003 (Robert Graham Center, 2005). Pediatricians, for example, see an average of 93.6 patients per week (American Academy of Pediatrics, 2005a). In addition, only 30 percent of them feel they have received adequate training in counseling and behavior modification techniques. Most are fulfilled by many elements of their professional life, but more than half feel "stressed trying to balance work and personal responsibilities" (American Academy of Pediatrics, 2005b).

Still, when most health care providers are given an opportunity to attend a communication training session, a most common reaction is pleasant surprise about skills, methods, and facts they may not have considered but that may help save time, improve overall patient satisfaction, and avoid conflicting or stressful patient-related situations. After some initial reluctance and skepticism, most providers enjoy testing their knowledge about communication methodologies as well as their skills as effective communicators. For many of them, hearing that most physicians do not let their patients speak for more than eighteen to twenty-two seconds without interrupting is often a surprise.

Trends in Provider-Patient Communication

For several decades, people in Western countries have witnessed an ongoing shift in provider-patient relationships. Patients have become more involved with their own care and are more educated about health issues. Several patient organizations have worked to reinforce patients' rights and to create networks and tools that contribute to patient education and empowerment. Patient activism and lessons learned from the AIDS crisis, which have shown the importance of patient and public participation in health care decisions and policies, have contributed a new perspective on more traditional provider-patient communications. At least among the most affluent segments of society, the Internet and other new media have also contributed to a variety of new forums where medical information is discussed, questioned, and analyzed with peers, experts, and others.

Physicians, nurses, and other health care providers have been adapting to, and in many cases encouraging, a new kind of relationship in which the power balance weighs less heavily on the physician's side. Although many providers have been enjoying and adapting to this new trend, others have been struggling to find the time to accommodate patients' increasing requests and demands. Providers who have made successful transitions have thriving practices (patients like physicians who are good communicators and personable) and have relied on a number of tools developed by their professional associations.

Recent initiatives by the American Medical Association (2005a), the American Academy of Family Physicians (1999), and the Association of American Medical Colleges (AAMC) (1999) highlight the importance of provider-patient communications and aim to equip physicians with skills and tools to communicate effectively with patients and incorporate communication as a core competency at all levels of medical education.

Among them, the AAMC (1999), which represents all 141 accredited medical schools in the United States, 17 medical schools in Canada, and more than 400 teaching hospitals, has identified several communication-related goals for medical students. Also, the AMA Foundation (2005b) has become a member of the Partnership for Clear Health Communication, which includes several organizations and industry leaders, in an attempt to address the problem of low health literacy. In 2007, the Partnership for Clear Health Communication joined forces with the National Patient Safety Foundation (2007).

Health care providers are increasingly learning communication skills that may help them break bad news. For example, special communication courses teach oncologists how to talk with cancer patients about their diagnosis, life expectancy, treatment, and other sensitive issues in an empathetic and effective way. Some of these courses use standard communication techniques, such as role-playing, to help providers practice their communication approach with actors who pose as patients (Zuger, 2006).

Moreover, some professional organizations have been focusing on equipping practitioners and patients with communication skills and tips. Ask Me 3, an initiative of the Partnership for Clear Health Communication, teaches patients to ask their providers three questions that will help them understand their problem and recommended solutions (American Medical Association, 2005d). This approach may help patients stay focused, ask the right questions, and minimize miscommunication with their providers if integrated with broader health literacy interventions. At the same time, it is a service to health care providers because it may lead to shorter and more focused conversations.

Although there is still a lot to do in the area of provider-patient communication, new trends and initiatives in Western countries have established a path for a more participatory attitude to health care. The hope is that this will teach patients to make the best use of encounters with providers and help providers to be more effective at conveying information. In most developing countries, as well as in many traditional cultures where the power balance has not shifted yet, health communication training and other kinds of interventions can help encourage people to become more responsible for health care decisions by communicating better with their physicians. In doing so, it is important to remember that models that have worked in Western countries may not work in other regions of the world or among members of different ethnic groups. For example, "many Asian Indians (especially older patients) prefer their doctors to make health-related decisions on their behalf, as opposed to a more participatory style of decision making where the doctor presents them with options to be discussed. They often consider doctors to be authority figures and are more accustomed to answering questions than asking them. Asian Indian patients may thus be more inclined to play a passive role and may hesitate to express their concerns" (Health Equity Initiative, 2011). These kinds of examples further support the need for understanding patients' preferences and culture as well as the importance of cross-cultural communication training in clinical education.

Transforming Provider-Patient Relationships into Partnerships

By definition, partnerships require that all partners are equally committed to pursuing a common cause and are aware of their role. In the provider-patient relationship, the common cause is the patient's health.

Health communication can help improve provider-patient relationships by raising awareness of common communication issues as well as roles and responsibilities in achieving good health outcomes. Training in communication methodology and message development may help health care providers sharpen their communication skills and address patients' questions and concerns in a more effective way. It may also help physicians conduct conversations in a way so that patients will stay on topic and feel that their provider is truly concerned about their health.

In summarizing many of the ideas discussed in this chapter, ideally, communication training for health care providers should focus on these topics:

- A brief overview on communication methodologies and how to affect behavioral change
- How communication skills can help make effective use of time
- Benefits of effective communication
- Common barriers and how to address them
- Differences in cultural and ethnic factors, age, and gender as they relate to health beliefs and attitudes

- Impact of the social determinants of health on patient outcomes (including practical tips on how to discuss with patients how their living and working environment may affect their health)

- Practical tips and examples on all topics

- Interactive session in which health care providers practice and test their communication skills in different potential scenarios

Some practical tips that may help providers establish good and trusting relationships with their patients are common to all human interactions:

- Greet patients properly and according to their cultural and ethnic preferences. For example, calling patients by their first name is appropriate in many Western countries and can help break down barriers but is not advisable when addressing Korean patients, who prefer to be called by their full name (Matsunaga, Yamada, and Macabeo, 1998).

- Put patients at ease by smiling, asking about the patient's family, and establishing good eye contact (if culturally appropriate).

- Do not make patients feel that the next patient may be more important by looking at the watch or at the door (Belzer, 1999).

- Show empathy about patients' concerns and needs.

- Listen and avoid interrupting.

- Help patients stay focused on their medical issues.

- Recognize nonverbal clues.

- Reinforce key messages and recommendations by providing written materials and scheduling follow-up visits or contacts.

Focusing on only the communication skills of health care providers may not be sufficient to achieve an effective provider-patient partnership. As patients' participation in health decisions increases, communication tools and events intended for patients may help them do their share in establishing a true partnership with their providers. Primarily, training can help patients in several ways:

- Asking the right questions

- Staying focused

- Becoming familiar with common medical terms

- Understanding how to differentiate between credible and noncredible informational sources (on the Internet as well as in other settings)

- Dealing with conflicts or other kinds of impediments that may prevent them from following or trusting a provider's recommendations
- Showing respect for the provider's time and experience
- Identifying and discussing key factors in their living and working environments that may affect their health or ability to comply with clinician recommendations

Communication specialists can help address issues in provider-patient relationships by helping professional associations, patient groups, and individual health care providers understand the issues at stake as well as improve overall communication skills. They can also help influence policies and medical curricula to recognize the central role that effective communication can have on health outcomes.

Implications of Interpersonal Communication for Technology-Mediated Communications

A discussion about interpersonal communication would not be complete without acknowledging the impact that the advent of the Internet, video technology, telephone, mobile technology, and other media has had on interpersonal relationships over several decades. Increasingly, many interactions are mediated by technology and take place using e-mail, voice mail, videoconferencing, texting, or other media channels. This may shape the quality and implications of communication by depriving it of nonverbal expressions (for example, facial expressions, gestures) and other influences (for example, the potential impact of different venues—formal versus informal venues—on health care or business conversations) that are usually common in face-to-face encounters.

Still, as several authors report, even when people rely on electronic media, they continue to engage in the process of *grounding*, which refers to the ability to find, understand, and share common meanings (Brennan and Lockridge, 2006; Brennan, 1990, 2004; Clark and Brennan, 1991; Clark and Schaefer, 1989; Clark and Wilkes-Gibbs, 1986; Schober and Clark, 1989). Take the example of an e-mail in which a mother asks a close friend to pick her child up from school. If the e-mail states only, "Could you please pick my child up from school?" the request may not be clear unless the recipient already knows the school's address, the dismissal time, the names of the child and the teacher, as well as where he or she should bring the child. These additional facts will allow the recipient to evaluate and eventually rule out the existence of potential conflicts (for example, previous work commitments) or other impediments. Still, the mother would have to wait for her friend's reply. This dynamic is quite similar to what occurs in face-to-face encounters. As other authors highlight, the interpersonal exchange in both cases has two phases: the presentation phase, when the mother asks her friend for help and describes the task's requirements, and the acceptance phase, which implies the need for the friend's reply to confirm that he or she understood and accepted the task (Brennan and Lockridge, 2006; Clark and Schaefer, 1989).

As it related to health, technology-mediated communications have provided a private forum to discuss sensitive matters, connect with others who may have experienced similar health issues, network, and learn about new medical solutions, among other actions. They have also affected provider-patient relationships. For example, some physicians may complain about the number of unnecessary questions and concerns that patients raise because of noncredible medical facts found on the Internet. Yet the Internet and other technology advances have improved the ability of patients and the general public to participate in personal and public health decisions.

In the case of life-threatening conditions such as HIV/AIDS, the use of the Internet has increased people's ability to deal with their illness. For example, the use of the Internet has influenced the coping skills of people living with HIV by promoting individual empowerment, increasing social support, and helping them help others (Reeves, 2000; Coursaris and Liu, 2009).

The influence of media technology on interpersonal communication and other aspects of health communication varies from population to population and group to group. It is related to media access, socioeconomic conditions, media literacy levels, as well as specific media uses and preferences that may vary from group to group. A more comprehensive discussion on new media communication is included in Chapter Five.

Still, when using any form of technology to communicate about health matters, it is important to remember and apply all general principles and values that pertain to interpersonal communication. Gender, age, and cultural, ethnic, and geographical factors as well as literacy levels still influence technology-mediated communications and should be considered. This is about using one of the many kinds of media to have a heart-to-heart discussion about health and health behaviors.

Key Concepts

- Interpersonal communication is an important action area of health communication.

- Interpersonal behavior and communication are highly influenced by cultural-, social-, age-, and gender-related aspects, as well as literacy and health literacy levels and individual factors and attitudes.

- The dynamics of interpersonal communication are determined by signs (for example, involuntary acts) and symbols (for example, use of verbal expressions) that may differ among cultures and groups.

- Examples of interpersonal communication are community dialogue, personal selling, counseling, and provider-patient communication.

- Community dialogue is an example of interpersonal communication at scale. It is a process that seeks to create a favorable environment in which communities feel comfortable putting forward their ideas and interests and providing input and opinions on specific matters on which they are consulted.

- Personal selling refers to (1) one-on-one engagement of different groups in their own homes, offices, or places of work and leisure and (2) the ability to sell one's image and expertise, an important skill in most counseling activities. It is an acquired communication skill that requires training but is also dependent on individual, social, and cultural factors. The two definitions are strongly connected and interdependent in their practical application.

- Personal selling interventions may not be very effective in the absence of other communication activities (for example, public relations, community mobilization) that would help create a receptive environment for door-to-door interventions.

- In counseling, which could be defined as the help provided by a professional on personal, psychological, health, or professional matters, personal selling is a powerful determinant of one's ability to have an impact on the beliefs, attitudes, and behavior of the person who is seeking counsel.

- Provider-patient communications is an important area of interpersonal communication and has been shown to affect patient satisfaction, retention, and overall health outcomes.

- Further emphasis should be placed on prioritizing health disparities in clinical education—including training in cross-cultural health communication—to address differences in quality and equality of care.

- Effective communication in the provider-patient setting depends on several patient- and physician-related factors as well as external factors (for example, time constraints and managed care requirements).

- Communication specialists can help improve provider-patient communications. They can help health care providers and patients understand the issues at stake and improve their communication skills. They can also work with professional associations, patient groups, and individual health care providers to help them influence policies and university curricula, including communication as a core clinical competency.

- Technology advances have had a tremendous impact on interpersonal communication. Many types of interpersonal communication are now mediated by technology and take place using e-mail, videoconferencing, telephone, texting, and other media.

- Technology-mediated communications are influenced by many of the same factors that rule other types of interpersonal communication, such as literacy and health literacy levels and age, gender, cultural, ethnic, and individual factors.

FOR DISCUSSION AND PRACTICE

1. Describe the most common verbal and nonverbal clues that, according to your culture, age group, gender, family values, personal preferences, or other factors, may affect your level of satisfaction with health-related encounters and communications and prompt you or your peers to comply with the health care provider's recommendations. For example, how do you like to be greeted by your physician? Is there any specific personal or cultural value or belief that you need to have acknowledged in order to trust and comply with the health information being presented to you? Is there any nonverbal clue that you may find confusing or offensive?

2. Maria is a forty-one-year-old Caucasian woman who is expecting her first baby. Eight weeks into the pregnancy, it becomes clear that she is likely to have a miscarriage. She really wants the baby and may be very upset at the idea of a miscarriage, especially because she fears she may not become pregnant again. Think of how her physician should break the bad news in a way that would acknowledge Maria's feelings and set realistic expectations. Use role-playing to simulate the actual discussion, and try to envision some of Maria's potential questions. Evaluate the pros and cons of potential physician approaches and attitudes toward communication on this matter.

3. Have you ever participated in any kind of community dialogue or read about it in the media? Use your own experience or research an example of community dialogue to discuss how this process helped a community identify key priorities and next steps on a health issue.

4. In this chapter, personal selling is defined as (1) one-on-one, door-to-door engagement of key groups and stakeholders and (2) the ability to sell one's image and expertise. Discuss practical examples from your professional or personal experience or recent readings that illustrate these two definitions.

5. Review Figure 4.1 and use five to ten adjectives to describe the style and communication approaches of physicians 1 and 2. Then discuss key factors that in your opinion influenced the mother's decision in both scenarios.

6. Reflect on and discuss when the use of technology (e-mail, texting, etc.) is appropriate within clinical settings. Provide examples of when, in your opinion, health care providers should or should not communicate with their patients via e-mail.

KEY TERMS

community dialogue   cross-cultural health communication

counseling   personal selling

CHAPTER 5

MASS MEDIA AND NEW MEDIA COMMUNICATION, AND PUBLIC RELATIONS

"Years ago, Americans grabbed toast and coffee for breakfast. Public relations pioneer Edward Bernays changed that" (Spiegel, 2005). Bernays, whom many regard as the historical father of public relations, referred to many theories of his uncle, Sigmund Freud, in developing a public relations campaign to help convince Americans that "bacon and eggs was the true all American breakfast" (Spiegel, 2005; Museum of Public Relations, 2005) and that it was ultimately healthier. Bernays's campaign in the mid-1920s was successful at changing the public's mind (Museum of Public Relations, 2005). Although bacon and eggs have been somewhat eclipsed by new habits, such as eating cold cereals or not eating breakfast at all (ABC News, 2005), they remain a very popular breakfast: only one in ten Americans usually eats toast or some other kind of bread or pastry (ABC News, 2005).

Outside the breakfast setting, public relations strategies and activities are usually used for mass communication or to create interest among multiple publics about an idea, a new policy, a product or service, a recommended behavior, a professional field, a company, an institution, or a nonprofit organization. Ethical public relations relies on reputable facts and figures, and has found many applications as part of health communication interventions in the commercial, nonprofit, health care, and public health sectors. Yet, in the new media age, public relations theory and practice has evolved to develop new models and strategies for the use of new and social media as part of health communication programs.

CHAPTER OBJECTIVES

This chapter reviews the relationships among mass communication, public relations, mass media, and new media, and discusses them within the context of health communication in the new media age, establishes public relations as a key action area in mass communication and other health communication interventions, and provides an overview of mass media and new media use and strategies. Finally, it also provides practical suggestions on key success factors of mass media and new media communication programs, and discusses select mass media- and new media–specific evaluation parameters.

Health Communication in the New Media Age: What Has Changed and What Should Not Change

We live in an exciting time for health communication. Communication-related technologies (Internet, mobile, etc.) have been fast advancing at an unprecedented pace, and have been adopted by different groups and populations across the world. Technology provides communicators with myriad new channels and strategic options, which can no longer be ignored and need to be efficiently integrated as part of comprehensive multimedia health communication interventions. Through a variety of media (for example, professional and personal blogs, social media sites, podcasts, chat rooms, and mobile applications, among others), e-health (see definition in Chapter Two and the Glossary) and **mHealth** (the use of mobile and wireless technology devices for health-related interventions that seek to improve patient and public health outcomes) have been rising to provide innovative ways to communicate about health and community development issues with many different groups.

mHealth
The use of mobile and wireless technology devices for health-related interventions that seek to improve patient and public health outcomes

In this multimedia environment the distinction between **mass media** (means of communication reaching large audiences or percentages of a given population; what can act as mass media may vary in different countries or groups) and new media is always evolving and being debated. For example, for some of its information-related applications (for example, websites, online journals, and libraries) and related functions (for example, health information seeking and retrieving), the Internet acts—and in many cases substitutes—more traditional mass media, such as print and broadcast media and books (Flanagin and Metzger, 2001; Schiavo, 2008, 2009a). Yet, this is primarily true in North America, Europe, and several Asian countries. In fact, several developing countries and underserved and vulnerable groups in developed countries continue to lag behind in

mass media
Means of communication to reach large audiences or percentages of a given population; what can act as mass media may vary in different countries or groups

this technological revolution despite several initiatives that are underway to bridge the digital divide. Depending on the country and the specific group or population, such a digital divide occurs because of a combination of technology access and quality, costs of Internet connectivity—which in some African countries may be hundreds of times higher than in the United States or most European countries (World Health Organization [WHO], 2007)—and most important, media and health literacy.

In several African countries, for example, "even where institutions and individuals have Internet access, the connection often has little practical value for more than a few elite users" and "tests of actual Internet speeds indicate that, while users at large European or American universities enjoy Internet connections which deliver 17 million bits per second, users at African institutions operate at speeds that are 500 to 600 times slower" (WHO, 2007). In the United States, many groups may still lack the capacity to retrieve, assess, and understand health information. About one-third of Americans lack health literacy (National Opinion Research Center, 2010). Lack of health and media literacy as well as cultural preferences in relation to the use of online tools or limited access to computer skills and technology may negatively affect the use of online media among underserved groups and communities with significant health disparities. For all of these groups, it may be a bit of stretch to say that the information-related features of the Internet can be considered to act in the same way as mass media, at least for the time being.

New media (see Chapter Two and the Glossary for a relevant definition) and social media penetration has been exponentially increasing (see Table 5.1), and is projected to continue to increase, and helps people connect on many different issues, create online communities, and work together across geographic boundaries. Yet, the use of interactive functions of the Internet and mobile technology—such as social media, texting, and online forums—cannot yet be considered the same as mass media in their application to health issues, at least not across different socioeconomic, age, and ethnic groups. In fact, "Web 2.0 is not familiar ground for the majority of the US population . . . When you hear the phrase '2.0' you are hearing about an online world that is familiar to what we call the 'Elite Tech Users,' who make up one-third of all adults" (Fox, 2008). Similarly, although "social network sites are popular, they are used only sparingly for health updates and queries" (Pew Internet & American Life Project, 2011e). Although these trends will continue to evolve, technology-mediated messages tend to reach those segments of the population that are already highly motivated about their health, therefore leading to "increasing gaps between the health haves and the have-nots" (Dutta, 2009, p. 71) and to the need for

Table 5.1   Internet and New Media Penetration

United States	International
Eighty-one percent of US adults use the Internet.	Thirty-two and one-half percent of the world uses the Internet.
• Seventy-one percent visit video-sharing sites (YouTube/ Vimeo).	North America, Oceania, and Europe have the highest Internet penetration.
• One in three read blogs.	Asia is the leading world region for Internet use.
• Sixty-nine percent use social networking sites (Facebook, Twitter, LinkedIn, Instagram, Pinterest).	Ninety-six percent of Canadian households own a computer.
	Africa is becoming a fast-growing mobile market:
Ninety-five percent of US teenagers use the Internet.	• Mobile phone penetration rate of 62 percent in 2011.
Fifty-three percent of US adults sixty-five and older use the Internet and e-mail.	• Penetration expected to grow to 84 percent by 2015.
Seventy-two percent of Internet users admitted looking for health information online.	• Nigeria, Egypt, and South Africa are the fastest-growing markets.
Eighty-seven percent of US adults have cell phones.	
• Fifty-five percent use the Internet on their mobile phones.	

Source: GSMA (2011); International Telecommunication Union (2012); *Internet World Stats* (2012); Pew Internet & American Life Project (2011b, 2011c, 2012a, 2012b, 2013a, 2013b, 2013c, 2013d).

developing adequate strategies to bridge the digital divide, increase overall media literacy, and continue to integrate the use of new media with other health communication areas and channels.

Yet, new media are increasingly used in mass communication and community-based communication. In approaching health communication planning, implementation, and evaluation, it is important to take into account what has changed and what should not change in this new media age so that we continue to stay focused on achieving behavioral, social, and organizational results that ultimately help improve population and community health outcomes.

This chapter focuses on mass media and new media communication as they relate to practical applications for **mass communication** (a field of research and practice that is concerned with communication with large segments of the population and the general public, which is also a key action area in health communication) as well as other kinds of interventions intended for specific communities, populations, and groups. Given the prominence of new media in the twenty-first century, this brief overview identifies key elements of what has changed and what should not change in the new media age (see Table 5.2), and serves as a premise for discussing the relationship among mass communication, multiple kinds of media, and public relations.

mass communication
A field of research and practice that is concerned with communication with large segments of the population and the general public, which is also a key action area in health communication

Table 5.2 Health Communication in the Media Age: What Has Changed and What Should Not Change

What has changed . . .	What should not change . . .
It is an exciting time for new media and health communication. Communication environment has become mobile, searchable, customizable, and on-demand.	New media–based interventions "need to be part of an integrated approach with other health communication areas" (Schiavo, 2008).
Now is a horizontal media environment in which every reader is a publisher; every click contributes to whether a new idea, product, or service will make or break it.	● Integration supports effectiveness, expanded reach, and mirrors how people communicate every day.
● There is increased participation and real-time feedback from different groups. ● Online communities provide opportunity for feeling part of a group and help people cope with disease and crisis.	"A technology-based revolution more than a health communications revolution" (Schiavo, 2008)
Convergence of computer, Internet, telecommunications, televisual technologies presents users with myriad choices.	● Interventions should still be designed to achieve group-specific behavioral and social objectives. ● Theory- and strategy-driven communication principles should continue to inform new media–based interventions.
● Information overload: There is more total media time but less information time.	
Digital divide and computer skills are key factors in health literacy and the ability to navigate health systems.	Each key group and stakeholder have specificity, needs, and preferences that are central to intervention design.
● Vulnerable populations are still excluded from new media revolution. ● New media is English-dominated; non-English speakers also largely excluded.	● As with other communication areas, evaluation also essential to new media–based interventions. ● Need to go beyond counting and tracking and assess real-life effectiveness.
News spreads fast, so do communication hoaxes and cyberbullying.	
There are new challenges and opportunities for a variety of key groups and stakeholders.	

References: Schiavo, R. "The Rise of E-Health: Current Topics and Trends on Online Health Communications." *Journal of Medical Marketing*, 2008, *8*, 9–18. Schiavo, R. "E-Health: Current Trends, Strategies, and Tools for Online Health Communications." Presented at the Office of Minority Health Resource Center, Rockville, MD, Mar. 24–25, 2009a. Schiavo, R. "Health Communication in the New Media Age: What Has Changed and What Should Not Change." Workshop presented at Health Equity Initiative, 2012b.

Although many of the topics listed in Table 5.2 are discussed in further detail in the "New Media and Health" section of this chapter and other relevant sections of the book, the table seeks to establish the need to use this exciting new channel strategically and in integration with other kinds of health communication interventions and areas. New media–based interventions should continue to be grounded in communication theory and rigorous planning frameworks, and, most important, be people-centered. After all, these same mantras apply to all other communication areas, media, and channels, because there is no magic way to promote health and social change. This is also relevant for mass communication, a key area of health communication, which relies on public relations strategies and multimedia platforms to communicate with large segments of the US and global populations about health and social matters of public interest.

The Media of Mass Communication and Public Relations

In general terms, the basic function of mass communication is to inform, educate, entertain, motivate action, and build community on issues of public interest. As it relates to health and social development, purposeful mass communication is instrumental to creating a favorable environment on new or recurring health issues or social determinants of health, policies, products, and services, which may support and open the way to other kinds of communication areas and activities. In turn, this may motivate people to participate in community events or new social movements, and to adopt new health and social behaviors.

Creating the feeling of "I heard this from many places" among intended groups and populations is strictly related to the main challenge of mass communication, which is to reach as many people as possible. To do so, communication should rely on common meanings and styles to which large segments of the population may relate. Yet, mass communication is increasingly multicultural and no longer knows geographic boundaries. As mass communication at the global scale has become a recent cultural phenomenon (ISeek Education, 2013), the challenges of finding common meanings have increased and evolved, and so has the demand for a stronger understanding of the theory and practice of mass communication and the specific characteristics and current or potential use of different kinds of media among students and practitioners.

Within and outside health communication, the media of mass communication are composed of a strategic blend of what some people may define as "old" media (print, radio, broadcast, entertainment and motion media, which have been evolving over the years and look nothing like "old") and new media, which include blogs, wikis, videocasts, podcasts, social networking sites, mobile technology, and texting, just to name a few examples. These media are being used in innovative ways across issues and sectors. In this scenario, media literacy—both as consumers and purveyors of media—is an increasingly important skill within most health-related and professional sectors.

Public relations (PR), which is defined as "the art and science of establishing and promoting a favorable relationship with the public" (*American Heritage Dictionary of the English Language*, 2011) has been the backbone of mass communication for several decades. Yet, the conceptualization and models of public relations have evolved over time to mirror not only new communication theories and trends but also the characteristics of available media and the evolution of journalism's standards and practice (Duhe, 2007).

Without any doubt, the advent of new media has also been changing the practice of public relations. If nothing else, as "large, hierarchical entities, tend to lag behind smaller, more nimble organizations in the adoption and applications of new media technologies . . . dominant voices are now accompanied, challenged, and sometimes overshadowed by voices previously marginalized" (Duhe, 2007, p. x). The new media have created an interactive environment in which organizations and their public can tell and compare their stories from beginning to end. Whether relying on mass media, new media, or other communication channels, public relationships continue to be part of the communication process, because there is no way to replace the human factor.

public relations
"The art and science of establishing and promoting a favorable relationship with the public" (*American Heritage Dictionary of the English Language*, 2011)

Public Relations Defined: Theory and Practice

The word *relationship* is fundamental to all definitions of PR as well as their practical applications. As with other action areas of health communication, PR is a relationship-based discipline. Similarly, health care or public health PR is based on an in-depth understanding of its publics as well as their needs, wants, and desires. This overall concept applies to all functions of PR listed and defined in Table 5.3: public affairs, community relations, issues or crisis management, media relations, and marketing PR.

Public Relations Theory

Historically, the theoretical basis of PR has been influenced not only by Bernays's relationship with Sigmund Freud, the father of psychoanalysis, but also by many other observations and models. Nevertheless, some of Bernays's theoretical assumptions still apply to the modern practice of PR. If you want people to do what you want, "you don't hook into what they say. You try to find out what they really want" (National Public Radio, 2005), according to Bernays. This concept recognizes the importance of psychological, emotional, and subconscious factors in human behavior, one

Table 5.3 Public Relations Functions in Public Health and Health Care

Public affairs	A strategic approach to promote public discussion and, eventually, agreement on health policies or administrative procedures that may be practiced by a given organization or its key stakeholders and intended audiences.
Community relations	An area of PR practice through which practitioners and organizations establish, cultivate, and strive to maintain mutually beneficial relationships with the **communities** (defined as groups with common values, causes, needs, and sharing the same geographic location) that can affect or are affected by their actions. Community relations is one of the many aspects of constituency relations and building (see Chapter Eight) and a component of all other health communication areas.
Issues management	A multifaceted and "formal management process to anticipate and take appropriate action on emerging trends, concerns, or issues likely to affect an organization and its stakeholders" (Issue Management Council, 2005).
Crisis management	A proactive approach based on the advance development of contingency plans and activities to anticipate, avert, and deal with potential crises. It often includes a strong focus on the use of mass media to help organizations ensure their publics that a solution is being implemented and a specific concern or issue is being addressed.
Media relations	A proactive and reactive approach that aims at interacting with key health journalists, bloggers, and offline and online pundits, and makes "use of the media in a planned way" (Economic and Social Research Council, 2005a). This includes print, broadcast, entertainment, and online journalists, bloggers, and writers.
Marketing public relations	An area of PR that focuses on developing strategic programs and relationships that would support endorsement and use of the organization's health products and services among its key stakeholders and publics.

communities

A variety of social, ethnic, cultural, or geographical associations, for example, a school, workplace, city, neighborhood, organized patient or professional group, or association of peer leaders; groups with common values, causes, and needs

of the main ideas Freud developed (National Public Radio, 2005; Museum of Public Relations, 2005), which is also more recently supported by social norms theory (see Chapter Two).

Some of the theories in PR also highlighted the relevance of psychological aspects of human personality in moving intended groups through the three desirable effects of PR interventions: "attention, acceptance and action" (Smith, 1993, p. 193). For example, some authors advocate the use of the psychological type theory in public relations practice (Smith, 1993). This theory has been primarily used in education, religion, and business to understand and predict "patterns of human interaction" (p. 177). According to Smith, if applied in PR, it could help practitioners tailor their messages to key groups and stakeholders by taking into account their personal psychological type and learning preferences. As Table 5.4 shows, Smith (1993) identified four primary types:

ST: Sensitive/thinking

SF: Sensitive/feeling

NT: Intuitive/thinking

NF: Intuitive/feeling

Table 5.4   Characteristics of Psychological Types Relevant to Public Relations

	ST	SF	NT	NF
People who prefer . . .	Sensing and thinking	Sensing and feeling	Intuition and thinking	Intuition and feeling
Focus on . . .	Facts: What is . . .	Facts: What is . . .	Possibility: What could be	Possibility: What could be
Make decisions based on . . .	Impersonal analysis; reason	Personal warmth; emotion	Personal warmth; reason	Impersonal analysis; emotion
Tend toward . . .	Practical and pragmatic	Sympathetic and friendly	Logical and ingenious	Enthusiastic and insightful
Adept at . . .	Applying facts and experience	Meeting daily needs of people	Developing theoretical concepts	Recognizing aspirations of people
Sensitive to . . .	Cause and effect	Feelings of others	Technique and theory	Possibility for people

Note: ST: Sensitive thinking; SF: Sensitive feeling; NT: Intuitive thinking; NF: Intuitive feeling.
Source: Smith, R. D. "Psychological Type and Public Relations: Theory, Research, and Applications." *Journal of Public Relations Research,* 1993, *5*(3), 177–199.
© Lawrence Erlbaum Associates. Used by permission.

Each of these types has distinct characteristics and learning habits (listed in Table 5.4) that influence their decision-making process, as well as the way they may react to different ways that information is presented (for example, factual information versus information that appeals primarily to emotions).

Although the psychological type theory may be difficult to apply rigorously to actual PR practice (in fact, data on psychological types exist for only select audiences and may be too expensive to collect in a timely and statistically significant manner), keeping in mind the influence of both "reason and sentiment" (Smith, 1993, p. 195) on people's beliefs and behavior is quite common among PR practitioners. Understanding people's learning styles and other preferences is part of the process of preparing for the development of a PR program. This is equally important in new media communication in which people's action (both in sharing information via social networking sites and other media and actually acting on the information being shared) is immediate and messages need to have an emotional and graphic appeal to resonate with the groups we intend to engage and ultimately to be shared on others' social networks and media.

Similarly, the notion of multiple publics and the need to address them differently in response to their characteristics, needs, desires, and issue-specific beliefs has been historically addressed by PR theory and practice. It is also one of the main assumptions of field dynamics models and methods, which, in their application to PR, attempt to explain the relationship between an organization and its different publics, as well as the mutual interaction among such publics. For example, one method describes and compares this interaction in terms of "dominance-submissiveness, friendly-unfriendly, and group versus personal orientation" (Springston, Keyton, Leichty, and Metzger, 1992, p. 81). In practice, when there is public debate about an organization, an idea, a product, or a behavior, it is quite common to find a variety of opinions, levels of involvement (for example, leaders versus followers), and interest and attitudes among multiple audiences. PR interventions often tip the preexisting balance and prompt a shift in the attitudes and opinions of multiple key groups. As a result, they may also change the dynamics of the relationship among such groups.

Within this perspective, PR is considered "the management function that establishes and maintains mutually beneficial relationships between an organization and the publics on whom its success or failure depends" (Cutlip, Center, and Broom, 1994, p. 2). The concept of PR as a relationship management discipline has emerged as a fundamental part of its theoretical basis (Ledingham, 2003) and finds application in actual PR practice. As Center and Jackson (1995) observe, "the proper term for the desired outcomes of public relations practice is public relationships. An organization with effective public relations will attain positive public relationships" (p. 2).

In the new media era, not much has changed in relation to PR's emphasis on relationships. "Public relations specialists were some of the first people to embrace the power of social media, and as a result are often the ones leading the way in the social space, whether they are consulting with clients from an agency point of view or strategizing on an in-house PR team" (Swallow, 2010). No matter which tools PR professionals use to connect with media members, most agree and emphasize "the fact that personal relationships will continue to propel the bond between social media and PR," and also report spending "80% of their time talking with journalists, bloggers and other influencers about issues and macro topics" (Swallow, 2010). In other words, "the critical step has historically been, and will remain, the human element" (Swallow, 2010). Online relationship and reputation management is only one of the many areas in which PR has been reinventing itself and applying the field's relationship-based theory and practice.

The value of PR practitioners to the general public and the organizations they serve is often determined by the extent and closeness of their contacts with the media and community representatives, as well as other key stakeholders. In this way, PR strategies and activities become a fundamental tool of larger health communication, health care, and public health interventions by expanding the reach of health messages as well as using the power of mutually beneficial relationships to advance the discussion and solution of a given health issue. In order to be effective, PR practitioners ought to read, understand, and follow their audiences (whether online or offline), and then use the power of mass and new media as well as community relations to talk to and with them. Several other authors or organizations also include PR among communication's key action areas (WHO, 2003) or recognize, among other fields, the role or influence of PR in health communication and mass communication (Springston and Lariscy, 2001).

Public Relations Practice

Although the practice of public relations is less than a hundred years old, PR is now employed by a broad variety of organizations beyond companies that sell products, including universities, foundations, nonprofit organizations, schools, hospitals, and associations. In fact, the official definition of PR by the Public Relations Society of America (PRSA) highlights the widespread use of PR by different types of organizations and the existence of multiple publics from which these organizations "must earn consent and support" (PRSA, 2005b). PRSA (2005b) also notes that "public relations helps an organization and its publics adapt mutually to each other." In most cases, PR also helps organizations and their publics discuss and eventually come to an agreement on ideas, recommended behaviors, products, or services—a process increasingly common in the new media era. In this way, it becomes an essential area of mass and health communication.

Over the past few decades, PR growth has been related to the diversification of mass media and its increasing influence on society, with the Internet having a huge impact on the work of PR professionals in the last decade. More recently, social media have pretty much changed the face of PR in relation to some of the tools being used as well as the constant evolution of social platforms and need for connectivity among all of them. New media and social media have kept PR professionals on their toes and fostered an evolution that the PR world seems to have enjoyed (see later sections of this chapter for a discussion of tools and specific media).

Yet, PR strategies have, for the most part, remained unchanged. In the commercial world, PR helps create market share and secure product endorsement and use. In the public health world, it helps create a receptive public environment that can motivate people to change their health or social behavior and act on community needs. In doing so, it provides the public with widespread access to information and helps build support for behavioral, social, and policy changes.

Nonprofit and commercial efforts to feature a specific disease area or health issue sometimes complement each other. For example, in promoting a product through the mass media, companies often discuss other important facts, such as awareness about a disease, disease incidence, or risk factors. If the information is based on reputable sources and scientifically relevant data, these efforts may contribute to the disease awareness endeavors of many nonprofit and government organizations in the same field. In some cases (see Box 5.1), corporations have helped tackle a general public health or health care–related problem by providing resources, funds, and programs to elicit interest in the subject.

BOX 5.1. JOHNSON & JOHNSON'S CAMPAIGN FOR NURSING'S FUTURE INITIATIVE

Recognizing that the United States was experiencing the most severe nursing shortage in history, Johnson & Johnson, a multinational health care company, launched the Johnson & Johnson Campaign for Nursing's Future in 2002. This is a multiyear, nationwide effort to enhance the image of the nursing profession, recruit new nurses, and retain nurses currently in the system.

Campaign elements have included a national television, print, and interactive advertising campaign in English and Spanish celebrating nursing professionals and their contributions to health care; a multifaceted and highly visible public relations campaign with press releases, video news releases, and satellite radio tours available to hundreds of media outlets across the country; recruitment materials including brochures, pins, posters, and videos in English and Spanish distributed free of charge to hospitals, high schools, nursing schools, and nursing organizations; fundraising efforts for student scholarships, faculty fellowships, and grants to nursing schools to expand their program capacity; celebrations at regional nursing events to create enthusiasm and feelings of empowerment among local nursing communities; a website (www.discovernursing.com) about the benefits of a nursing career featuring searchable links to hundreds of nursing scholarships and more than one thousand accredited nursing educational programs; and activities to create and fund retention programs designed to improve the nursing work environment. Numerous organizations, including the White House, with the Ron Brown Award for Corporate Leadership, the American Hospital Association, the American Organization of Nurse Executives, the National Student Nurses Association, the American Nurses Association, and *NurseWeek*, have honored Johnson & Johnson for this campaign and their overall contribution to addressing the current nursing shortage.

Key Outcomes[*]

- Forty-six percent of eighteen- to twenty-four-year-olds who participated in a 2002 Harris Poll survey recalled the campaign.
- Sixty-two percent had discussed a nursing career for themselves or a friend.
- Twenty-four percent of the respondents in this group said the campaign was a factor in their consideration.

- The discovernursing.com website traffic has tallied over three million unique visitors, spending an average of twelve to fifteen minutes exploring the site.

- Surveys show that recruitment materials are being used by 97 percent of high schools and 73 percent of nursing schools.

- Eighty-four percent of nursing schools that received the materials reported an increase in applications and enrollment for the fall 2004 semester.

- The campaign has raised over $8 million [up to the date of this case study] at regional fundraising events. These funds have been used to provide scholarships to thousands of nursing students and nurse educators and have been complemented by more than one hundred Johnson & Johnson grants to area nursing schools to help them expand their program capacity and, therefore, accept more students.

- The American Association of Colleges of Nursing reported that baccalaureate nursing school enrollments have seen double-digit increases every year since the launch of the campaign in 2002.

Key Success Factors

- Relevance of the issue to Johnson & Johnson's key publics as well as the community at large and organizational competence to address it

- Strong relationship-building effort in support of the campaign with organizations including health care systems, nursing schools, and professional associations around the country

- Multimedia strategy with consistent messages in broadcast, print, publicity, special events, printed materials, videos, and the Internet

*Outcomes include only results that had been analyzed at the time this case study was developed.

Source: Johnson & Johnson. "Campaign for Nursing's Future Initiative." Unpublished case study, 2005b. Used by permission.

Although the issue of partnerships with commercial entities will be discussed in Chapters Eight and Thirteen as part of the broader subject of partnerships in health communication, it is worth mentioning here that many reputable nonprofit and government organizations, including the US National Cancer Institute (National Cancer Institute at the National Institutes of Health, 2002), consider collaborations or partnerships with for-profit entities. In doing so, many of them have developed strict guidelines and criteria that help them protect the public interest and avoid endorsing specific products or services (see Chapter Eight).

PR practice must be held to high ethical standards. The ongoing debate on PR ethics and related dos and don'ts is legitimate and should never be abandoned. However, although it is fair to assume that the main motivation of any industry is profit, it would be unfair to think that all companies would go to any length to sell their products.

Media power, on which PR relies, can be abused if facts are misrepresented or inflated. However, in the battle for free media coverage and the high number of social media followers, this is a risk that the general public may encounter with a variety of organizations (even those with the best intentions) if they become too enamored with an idea or the opportunity to raise their own profile and visibility. Because of the nature of their profession, PR practitioners need to meet the challenges of serving their client's interests (whether their client is a business, a nonprofit, or a government organization) while preserving an honest and ethical relationship with the publics they cultivate and address. Most professional societies in this field, including the PRSA (2005a), have a comprehensive code of ethics for their members.

Table 5.5 lists some of the key characteristics of ethical PR programs. Many of them are common sense but should always be considered in designing and implementing a multimedia PR campaign.

In addition to promoting public discussion of ideas, policies, services, or behaviors, PR also contributes to increasing the visibility of nonprofit organizations, commercial entities, and other kinds of institutions, as well as their mission, activities, and spokespeople. This is a fundamental function of PR that helps establish organizations and their experts as leaders in a field. Together with other kinds of activities, PR helps them gain the favorable reputation and the public respect that are needed to have an impact on behavioral and social change, as well as to encourage others to join the debate on a health issue and its potential solutions.

As an example of PR activities reaching out to multiple publics, Box 5.2 shows the media and public relations page of the website of the Schepens Eye Research Institute, an affiliate of Harvard Medical School.

Table 5.5   Key Characteristics of Ethical Public Relations Programs

Based on research
Feature reputable and scientifically relevant facts and figures
Strive to maintain an honest and direct relationship with the publics they address
Adhere to general ethical principles such as identifying sources, conflicts of interest, and grant disclosures
Seek to establish trusting and long-term relationships between organizations and their publics and therefore discourage unethical approaches that may harm relationships
Include standard procedures to promptly correct potential mistakes and misinformation
Encourage free information exchange and seek to engage different publics
Preserve the public interest

The page includes information that helps position the institute as a resource for the media about eye diseases and related research and treatment news. By providing resources on the institute's history, mission, and activities, as well as the background and expertise of its faculty and spokespeople, the page appeals to journalists and bloggers in search of story ideas and resources on the subject, and experts interested in authoring guest editorials and blogs, and also provides news to feature on social media. In addition, it appeals to many different key groups and stakeholders (for example, health care providers, professional organizations, patient groups) that may have an interest in this field and may want to engage in collaborations or just participate in the public debate on eye disease research and treatment. Recently, this page, located at www.schepens.harvard.edu/news room/newsroom/newsroom.html, has evolved to include a much more comprehensive news section with posts that can be easily shared on different media, versus the traditional press releases that were more often featured until 2011.

BOX 5.2. USING THE INTERNET AS A KEY PUBLIC RELATIONS CHANNEL: THE SCHEPENS EYE RESEARCH INSTITUTE

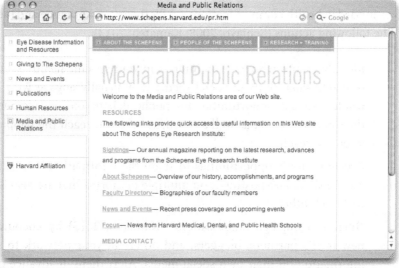

Source: Schepens Eye Research Institute. "Media and Public Relations." 2003. www.schepens.harvard.edu/news room/newsroom/newsroom.html. Used by permission.

PR Versus Advertising: The Differences

Media coverage as well as the virality level and the number of social kudos of a post stemming from PR campaigns is free of charge, but placing a story requires an in-depth understanding of the media, journalists, bloggers, influentials, and audiences among PR practitioners and the organizations they represent. For example, faced with countless choices for story ideas, journalists select what they cover primarily on the basis of newsworthiness, which is what they think their audiences may find interesting (Fog, 1999; De Nies and others, 2012). Other parameters include level of comfort or knowledge about the topic, the way the information is framed and presented to them, and the relationship they have with their sources, such as PR practitioners, organizations, and politicians. In this highly competitive environment, achieving national media coverage is a major endeavor.

In the new media era, PR practitioners can borrow from advertising its experience in creating visual opportunities for complex concepts. Although PR practitioners already work in multidisciplinary teams including graphic designers and web and new media developers, further emphasis on advertising techniques may help increase people's ability to connect and identify with new media sites and information via the power of imagery and evocative taglines.

Yet, the success of new media–based communication interventions is linked to several research- and relationship-centered factors, which are grounded in health communication and PR theory and practice and include the following actions (Schiavo, 2008; Kamateh, 2013):

- Identify groups who have an interest in your specific health issue and research what kinds of social media they usually engage with. This would increase opportunities for public debate and engagement on the topic of interest as well as to make sure you reach the people you intend to reach.

- Create multiple opportunities to share the information by making it easy to share and posting it on multiple platforms that are also linked with each other.

- "Identify campaign ambassadors" (Kamateh, 2013) by encouraging new media partners, bloggers, and others in your network to share information on their own social media. Alert them in advance of the campaign and send them relevant links at launch and throughout the campaign.

- "Encourage message co-creation" by identifying opportunities for the groups you seek to engage "not only to repost your materials but convey the message in their unique and perhaps more relatable way" (Kamateh, 2013). Take into account that this is not very different from the other communication areas discussed in this book in which the role of influencers and community leaders has a major impact on the trust, significance, and transparency of all communications.

- Use an integrated approach that relies on a variety of media and communication settings and areas to maximize impact.
- Go beyond tracking and counting in evaluating results. Create measurable behavioral, social, and organizational objectives for all interventions.
- Update your media frequently to continue to engage online communities.

Whether offline or online, PR is a less controlled but more credible way to approach the media than advertising. In advertising, organizations pay for the print, online, or broadcast space to place their ads, so the media have no editorial power on the ad content. The ad content is immediately recognized and identified with a specific health organization by the media's audiences. In PR, the media placement is free of charge, but its final tone and content are determined by the journalist or the new media publics who author or contribute to the story. In the absence of breakthrough news, achieving media coverage using PR strategies is not easy and requires strategic efforts and tools, long-term relationships with the media, and a true understanding of the concept of newsworthiness and community engagement, as well as the ability to track online communities and listen to their needs, concerns, and preferences. Most important, it requires patience and perseverance.

Mass Media, Health-Related Decisions, and Public Health

No one can dispute the power of mass media. Part of this power stems from the media's influence on public opinion and everyday decisions. Often the general public views the mass media as an objective source of information. Another important factor is related to the media's relationships with important decision makers and stakeholders around the world, including governments and multilateral organizations as well as the nonprofit and business sectors. In addition to the entertainment appeal of the media, both of these factors have contributed to the increasing power of the mass media.

In the Internet era—and more specifically in the United States, Canada, and several countries in Europe—mass media also include websites, blogs, online libraries, magazines, and journals, prerecorded webcasts and podcasts, and all other information-related functions of the Internet. In these contexts, health information–seeking behavior has dramatically changed since the advent of the Internet, which is functioning as other established mass media. For example, in the United States, eight out of ten (80 percent) of Internet users look online for medical or health information (Pew Internet & American Life Project, 2011c). Similarly, more than one-third of Canadian adults searched for health information online (Underhill and Mckeown, 2008), with these numbers continuing to increase. As previously discussed, this does not apply to many disadvantaged and low health literacy groups in both developed and developing countries, and therefore supports the need for a research-based approach to health communication planning, which includes the selection of adequate group-specific media and channels.

Yet, because mass media are the main channels of mass communication, competition for media coverage and to stand out in the online space is quite fierce. People rely on mass media as their main source of news and information, and their health, political, and life choices are increasingly conditioned by what they hear or read. For example, a well-documented impact of the Internet is on the quality and nature of patient-provider communications, because the Internet has enabled additional patient participation in clinical settings and decisions (Pew Internet & American Life Project, 2007). Similarly, mass media campaigns that use other kinds of mass media, more specifically television, radio, and newspapers, have been shown to produce positive changes or to prevent negative changes within the context of health-risk behaviors (for example, "use of tobacco, alcohol, and other drugs, heart disease risk factors, sex-related behaviors, road safety, cancer screening and prevention, child survival, and organ or blood donation") across large populations (Wakefield, Loken, and Hornik, 2010, p. 1261).

One of the major accomplishments of many successful organizations from a variety of sectors, other than the programs, services, or goods they manufacture and provide, is the success of their advertising and media coverage efforts as well as their online reputation and reach, which helps strengthen their credibility and stake on key issues and increase their visibility. In public health, the media can influence people's perception of disease severity, their views about the potential risk of contracting the disease, or their feelings about the need for prevention or treatment. Media coverage can also affect what people eat or do in their leisure time. It can help reduce the stigma associated with many diseases or break the cycle of misinformation and silence about health conditions that are underdiagnosed, undertreated, or underreported. It can help convince policymakers to develop new prevention or treatment policies or address specific social determinants of health to benefit large segments of the population.

In summary, especially in the United States and most of Europe, where there is a widespread media culture, mass media can have an enormous impact on people's health behaviors. The typical American watches over thirty-five hours of TV every week (Nielsen, 2010). Also, Americans spend an average of thirty-two hours a month online versus sixteen hours a month globally (GoGulf, 2012). People do not see their best friends that often, so the media may become more influential than actual people.

Mass media campaigns have proven to be effective in helping to increase immunization rates (Porter and others, 2000; Paunio and others, 1991), vaccination knowledge (McDivitt, Zimicki, and Hornik, 1997), cervical cancer screening among Hispanic women (Ramirez and others, 1999), people's ability to cope with disease (Pew Internet & American Life Project, 2007), and dieting and fitness regimens (Pew Internet & American Life Project, 2007). The list of media influences (positive or negative) on health beliefs and behaviors is enormous. Most important, mass media have been defining the concept of health and fitness by bringing into everyone's homes seductive images of men and women, such as healthy and fit celebrities with whom average people would like to identify. Sometimes these images are used for the right purpose (for example, encouraging people to exercise or remember their annual medical checkup), but at other times they promote unhealthy behaviors such as smoking. The power of mass media is such that not everyone can understand what is really behind a seductive image and make the right health decision.

Vulnerability to the power of the mass media and some of the unhealthy behaviors the media may consciously or subconsciously promote is related to many factors, including educational level, prior knowledge, or experience on the subject, age, socioeconomic conditions, personal experience, psychological status, and health and media literacy. For example, in 1998, recognizing the vulnerability of young adults and adolescents to media messages that encourage smoking, the US government limited forms of advertisement or PR activities that would directly target this age group with positive messages on smoking (Centers for Disease Control [CDC], 1999; Advertising Law Resource Center, 2006). Similarly, in many countries, direct-to-consumer advertising is prohibited for prescription drugs and other kinds of products that are used for the treatment or prevention of serious diseases (DES Action Canada and Working Group on Women and Health Protection, 2006; Mintzes and Baraldi, 2006; Ventola, 2011).

This brings us back to the discussion on the ethics of PR as well as the importance of following the code of ethics highlighted by many professional societies, keeping in mind the suggestions in Table 5.5.

Fortunately, most PR practitioners think that preserving the ethics of their actions is in the best interest of their own practice as well as the publics and organizations they serve.

Dos and Don'ts of Media Relations

Interacting with the media is an acquired skill. Because of limited time and conflicting priorities, journalists do not like to be approached by people who sound incompetent about the story they are trying to place or show little awareness of the media industry and its rules. This also applies to news websites and popular blogs in search of guest bloggers or information on an issue of interest. It is not very different (other than the format of the tools being used) to pitch the *Huffington Post* (www.huffingtonpost.com), a very popular US news website, content aggregator, and blog, which covers US politics, entertainment, style, world news, and comedy, than pitching a popular newspaper or television station. It requires the same understanding of what they may be interested in covering, the right contact person at the selected media outlet, and ultimately a great and newsworthy story.

In an attempt to help junior PR practitioners approach the media in the way the media want to be approached, several professional societies, including the Public Relations Society of America, organize workshops and lunch meetings in which journalists speak about their daily routine, their preferred communication channels (for example, e-mail, telephone, social media), and the kind of health issues and stories they may be interested in covering. More recently, such events also include popular bloggers and journalists from online news websites so that PR practitioners can develop relevant skills. Because PR is increasingly recognized as an important skill in public health as well as a key area of health communication, one of the sessions of the 2005 annual meeting of the American Public Health Association focused on media advocacy and featured journalists from broadcast and print media who discussed the dos and don'ts of media and press relations with public health professionals.

In approaching the media, it is essential to remember that they are just another audience, so it is important to know them well. Because of their influence on many of the publics of PR and larger health communication interventions, knowing them and understanding how to spur their interest in a story and its core messages is even more critical than with many other audiences.

The average US reporter now receives approximately two hundred e-mails each day, and some receive as many as five hundred per day (101PublicRelations, 2005). "Their Twitter networks churn out an endless stream of updates, links, and photos. Their RSS (really simple syndication) feeds offer innumerable stories from their favorite blogs and websites" (Phillips, 2012). Also, given recent changes in the media industry, some journalists who work in some kinds of media outlets (for example, print media) are gradually being replaced by online reporters and therefore work within limited human resources settings. They have time to read only a small portion of their e-mails, and usually it is the first few lines. The **media pitch**—defined as a brief summary statement or e-mail message that explains why the information is new, relevant to the journalist's intended audience, and worth covering—should be the focus of these first few lines. Only stories that stand out for their newsworthiness and relevance to the publication's audience are actually published; each reporter files no more than one to three stories on any given day.

media pitch
A brief summary statement, letter, or e-mail message that explains why a piece of information is new, relevant to a journalist's intended audience, and worth covering

Using the mass media to publicize the core messages and activities of a larger health communication or public health intervention can help expand the reach of the program to different key groups and publics. It can also help create a critical mass in support of the recommended health behavior or social change. However, getting there, and seeing a story published, is a process in itself. Once the first stories are published, it is still important to secure ongoing attention from multiple media to reach new audiences or reinforce the message over time. Table 5.6 highlights some of the dos and don'ts of media relations as they apply to more traditional mass media (print, broadcast, and radio) and online media sites and outlets. All of them are based on PR practice. Others may apply to specific situations, countries, reporters, or media channels.

What Makes a Story Newsworthy

The concept of newsworthiness is strictly related to the preferences, needs, and interests of the intended audience of a given publication or media outlet. For example, it is not a surprise that most parenting magazines in the United States and Europe dedicate a lot of space to stories on babies or toddlers and their sleeping habits. Sleep deprivation is a common problem among new parents as well as parents of toddlers who struggle to teach their children how to go to sleep on their own and stay asleep for the entire night. Parenting magazines and other consumer publications perceive the topic as something that sells the magazine to their audience. In fact, in 2005 alone, there were at least seventy-four articles on "getting your baby to sleep" or related topics in different kinds of consumer publications (LexisNexis, 2006). Over time, "babies and sleep" continues to be a popular topic with at least seventy-eight articles in US magazines and newspapers from January 2012 to April 2013 (ProQuest, 2013).

Table 5.6   Dos and Don'ts of Media Relations

DO	DON'T
Identify the names and interests of journalists, bloggers, or online reporters who usually cover health generally or specific health topics	Waste reporters' or bloggers' time by pitching them randomly regardless of their specific interests
Establish long-term relationships or cultivate media interest in a specific topic by posting frequently on media they may follow	Use jargon or technical terms in writing news pieces and speaking with reporters (Economic and Social Research Council, 2005a)
Be aware of reporters' and bloggers' deadlines and respond in a timely fashion	Agree to disclose information off the record unless you have a special relationship with a reporter; you are always at risk of seeing that information in print
Be polite, accurate, and helpful, and most important, responsive; for example, prime time on television fills up quickly, so reply as fast as you can	Call repeatedly or leave multiple voice messages or send multiple e-mails on the same topic
Understand why reporters are calling; determine whether they are seeking to quote you, do they want only a background briefing (Economic and Social Research Council, 2005a), or do they want to ask you to author a guest blog or a piece for a news site	
Make yourself available for a few days after issuing any kind of news	
Make sure all partners in your program are aware of their media-related roles and responsibilities (Economic and Social Research Council, 2005a)	
Media train key spokespeople	
Use media tools that are specific to the kind of media and can be easily shared offline and online	
Learn when reporters are on deadline and don't call at that time	
Read the news (online and offline) and relevant blogs; it is the best way to understand the media and what they may cover	

Sometimes newsworthy topics for specific publications can be found in the publication name. For example, the *Chapel Hill News* (both online and print versions) looks primarily for stories that appeal to the residents of Chapel Hill, North Carolina. *Infectious Diseases News* includes breaking news, editorials, and feature articles that appeal primarily to infectious disease specialists, and also to other health care providers (for example, family physicians, pediatricians, and internal medicine specialists) who are involved in preventing and managing infectious diseases among their patients. The type of media (print, radio, television, or online publications) influences the concept of newsworthiness as well.

Understanding the relevance of a story to the media's intended audiences is only the first step in defining whether the story may be newsworthy. Many other criteria need to be met to maximize the chances for media coverage of an organization's data, information, and messages:

* The story's time line: it just happened or is about to happen

- The existence of new data or information from clinical trials, opinion surveys, and other kinds of studies and their potential impact on the media's intended publics

- The presentation of these new data or information at a major professional, community, or interdisciplinary meeting or their publication in a prestigious peer-reviewed journal, which would legitimize the public impact and relevance of the information

- Reputable spokespeople, such as opinion leaders (for example, top physicians, researchers, and community leaders), top executives, athletes, or other celebrities who appeal to the media's intended audiences

- A new angle to a story of current interest or to an issue that has not been covered for a while; reading the news is the best way to find new media hooks

- Human interest stories, such as the testimonial of a mother who decided not to immunize her child who then died or almost died of a vaccine-preventable disease or the personal story that is behind a celebrity's endorsement of a specific cause

- The announcement of a new large program or event for the media's intended audiences and either providing a unique health-related service or social benefit or conveying big names in the field

- The use of appropriate media tools, which are developed to create connections and to reach and engage intended groups, whether virtually or offline

The following PR tools are the ones most commonly used for mass media communication.

- *Press release:* A written announcement of an event, program, or other newsworthy items for distribution to the media. It includes information on the details of the event, program, or news item and the organization that issues the press release; facts and data on the topic being featured; telephone and e-mail of a media contact person; and the name and credentials of an expert or celebrity spokesperson to interview. In the new media era, press releases are often substituted by **virtual newsrooms** (see, for example, Cooney Waters Group, 2013), dedicated webpages where the announcement is linked to videos and other resources that can help reporters, online newsletter editors, and bloggers write the story or just link to it. In some other cases the announcement is featured in the news or media section of the organization's website. Yet, copies of press releases and other

virtual newsrooms
Dedicated webpages where the event announcements or other newsworthy items are linked to videos and other resources that can help reporters, online newsletter editors, and bloggers write the story or just link to it

information are still being sent as PDF files to some reporters. Although in the United States and many other countries the emphasis is on making sure that the news release is sharable on a variety of social media, standard techniques to approach reporters and online gurus to secure media coverage are often country- and media-specific.

- *Media alert:* A one-page announcement including information on the what, when, where, and who of a specific event and the telephone number and e-mail address of a media contact. It is used for media distribution to announce press conferences, speakers' availability for telephone interviews, and program kick-off events, for example. This is often included as part of the virtual newsroom in the new media era.

- *Op-ed article:* A signed article expressing a personal opinion and the viewpoint of a specific group or organization. It is usually published on the page opposite the editorial page of a newspaper and is targeted to one publication and not sent to multiple publications simultaneously. In the online space, the equivalent of an op-ed article is often a guest blog or an opinion piece submitted to a news website.

- *Public service announcement:* Noncommercial advertising for distribution to radio, broadcast, or print media that includes information and a call to action for the public good. The format varies to accommodate the characteristics of print, radio, online, and broadcast media. It can also be sent to multiple media outlets for free and unrestricted use.

- *Radio news release:* The radio version of the press release, sent to radio stations for free use, and lasting forty-five to sixty seconds. It includes a sound bite from one of the PR program's spokespeople. In developing countries, where community and national radios are still one of the most valuable communication channels in terms of audience reach and influence, radio news releases are still widely used for a variety of health communication programs. Their use is now less frequent in the United States and other Western countries.

- *Radio actuality:* A recorded segment of a speech, statement, or other speaking engagement. It can be posted online or distributed as a media file to relevant radio stations. "Usually, the biggest news stations will not use actualities, as they consider them spoon-fed news. Some of the smallest stations do not have the equipment necessary to record actualities over the phone. This leaves a large number of mid-sized stations to target for actuality distribution" (Families USA, 2013).

- *Video news release:* A video segment designed in the style of a news report and distributed to local and national television and cable networks for free and unrestricted use. It is rarely used in the United States but remains somewhat common in some European countries. Media outlets often use only portions of the release.

- *B-roll:* A series of video shots on a specific topic, packaged in the format of unedited material (footage) and distributed to local and national televisions and cable networks. It is sometimes used in the United States to pitch a story to local TV news shows.

- *Mat release:* A ready-to-use feature story, usually including a photograph or some artwork, for distribution to community newspapers and other local and smaller publications. Digital mat releases are designed for online outlets and include backlinks to additional information and the source's website. Mat releases are designed to be easily incorporated in print or online news outlets.

Selecting the right tools for target media is not an optional step. Because all of these tools are designed to facilitate the reporter's or blogger's job and make it easy to cover the story, using the wrong tool sends a negative message to the media about the source's knowledge of the media industry and, potentially, his or her level of competence in the issue at hand. Table 5.7 identifies the mass media channels and most common PR tools used to address each of them specifically.

New Media and Health

Young professionals just completing their studies or entering the workforce have never known a world without the Internet and, in most cases, new media. This is an important point to reflect on when we think about whether or not to include new media as part of health communication interventions in the public health, health care, or community development fields. The answer is an unmistakable yes!

New media have changed the way we think about connecting with each other and are increasingly playing an important role in public health, health care, and community development interventions. They have broadened the traditional and more elitist notion of expert knowledge, connected people across disciplines and created collaborations beyond traditional geographic boundaries, enabled the development of strong online communities that help people cope with specific situations or just do their job better and more effectively, and, depending on the issue and specific groups, also contributed to raising awareness of health and community development issues.

The opportunity new media provides to create groups and communities that share the same interest in health or social topics has been

Table 5.7   Mass Media Channels and Related Public Relations Tools

Media	Tools
Print media (for example, national newspapers, magazines)	Press releases, op-ed articles, letters-to-editor, print public service announcement, media alerts
Radio (local and national radio stations)	Radio news release, radio public service announcement, radio actuality, media alerts, live interview with expert (by telephone or in a studio)
Broadcast (national and local TV stations)	Press release, video news release, B-roll, public service announcement, media alerts, and videos—often packaged as part of virtual newsroom on a dedicated page
Local publications and community newspapers	Mat release
Online news websites	Virtual newsrooms (including press releases or news announcements, media alerts, video or audio files, and other relevant documents), opinion pieces (guest blogs, opinion pieces on news website), public service announcements, digitized mat releases, audio and video files (including podcasts, webcasts, and so on)

influencing not only information-seeking behavior but also treatment and research efforts in many areas. For example, "online patient groups have become an increasingly powerful voice . . . raising funds for research, and offering patient information and support. As the cumulative power of the membership grows, these groups are becoming invaluable partners to researchers and physicians searching for a cure" (*Wall Street Journal*, 2007). New media use is growing among a variety of different professional, patient, voluntary, and advocacy organizations, as illustrated in Table 5.8, which includes sample—and ever evolving—uses of the Internet and new media by health organizations.

Yet, are the new media the new magic tools? In this case, the answer is an unmistakable no! Although new media (and generally, the Internet) have created great opportunities for an increased democratization of the knowledge-sharing process and have changed power levels in many contexts, both online and offline (including the patient-provider setting), they have also presented professional and lay communities with a variety of serious challenges and, too often, hidden roadblocks and pitfalls. Think about the many people who, because of their lack of methodological training or low health literacy status, may not know how to discern between real and misleading or fake data; or struggle to decide whether they should follow dieting and fitness advice from the American Dietetic Association—which bases

Table 5.8 Most Common Uses of the Internet and New Media by Health Organizations

Professional health organizations	Voluntary, patient, and advocacy organizations
Continuing medical education (CME)	Virtual support groups for patients and family caregivers
Professional networking	Community building and organizing
Dissemination of new health policies and standards of care	Volunteer recruitment
Online publications and reports	Disease profiling and risk assessment tools
Publicity of ongoing activities, programs, events (online and offline)	
Disease-specific resources	
Organizational visibility	
Media and press relations	
Advocacy	
Fundraising	

Source: Adapted from Schiavo, R. "The Rise of E-Health: Current Topics and Trends on Online Health Communications." *Journal of Medical Marketing,* 2008, *8*, 15, Table 2. © Palgrave Macmillan, LTD. Used by permission.

its recommendations on lessons learned from research and clinical results among many people—or the Amazing Adventures of Dietgirl, which is a valuable one-person anecdotal experience that may not work for all, given the complexity of people's body build, health status, or concurrent health conditions, social support levels, just to name a few reasons. Think about the opportunities new media have created for hoaxes, self-publicity, and instant celebrity, even when information or celebrity status may not be deserving attention and aims to trick people into buying harmful products or services.

Most important, think about the digital divide among the haves and have-nots because of differences in computer skills, access to new technology, and health and new media literacy. Technological advances may help reduce health disparities through the potential to make information available to all, advocate for access to important services (within and outside health care), and support partnership building and management. However,

> when new information is delivered indiscriminately via the mass media, it is acquired at a faster rate among those of higher socioeconomic status. . . . Given that the wealth gap between white and non-white is widening, with the median wealth of white households now twenty times that of non-Hispanic black households and eighteen times that of Hispanic households, research is needed to examine the processes which give rise to communication equalities. . . . Given the constant evolution of the media landscape, comprehensive efforts will

be needed to ensure that all groups are benefiting equally from health messages on the internet. If not, the rise of new media may serve only to exacerbate already apparent disparities in health. (Richardson, 2012)

Although an important function of health communication interventions is, or should be, to address and enhance health literacy and new media skills among underserved and vulnerable populations, the tension between the pace of capacity-building efforts on health and new media literacy and the advent of new technology will continue to exist for the foreseeable time. In other words, many disadvantaged groups may not be able to keep up with the pace of technological progress at all times. These are just some of the arguments in favor of continuing to use new media in integration with other communication areas, strategies, and activities so that our efforts will not only be more inclusive of cultural preferences and group-specific needs but will also mirror the way communication about health and illness actually happens: via myriad interpersonal, community, professional, mass media, and new media channels in a variety of settings.

Other authors have pointed to many of the lessons learned from Barack Obama's campaign to become the forty-fourth president of the United States of America, and how these lessons may be relevant to public health or health care communication theory and practice. Obama's campaign strategy, which relied heavily on new media, was able to rally an unprecedented level of public engagement that translated to donations, volunteers, and the kind of excitement in intensity and numbers not seen too often in US politics. In analyzing the campaign, although recognizing that very few public health campaigns may be funded at the same level as Obama's presidential campaign, Abroms and Lefebvre (2009, p. 420) highlighted the following take-away messages for public health interventions that use new media:

- Consider new media—social network sites, uploaded videos, mobile text messages, and blogs—as part of a comprehensive media mix.

- Encourage horizontal (i.e., peer-to-peer and social network) communications of campaign messages as social influence and modeling are important drivers of behavior.

- Embrace user-generated messages and content, especially in the case where top-down campaign messages are straightforward and translatable by the public.

- Use new media to encourage small acts of engagement. Small acts of engagement are important for relationship building and can lead to larger acts of engagement in the future. Additionally, small acts of engagement can have effects that ripple throughout a social network.

- Use social media to facilitate in-person grassroots activities, not to substitute for them.

Perhaps the most important lesson learned from the Obama campaign was the campaign's ability to translate online engagement into offline action. This leads to another take-away message:

Make sure that the online and offline worlds actually support each other's efforts via integrated and synergic activities and strategies that maximize their combined or individual impact.

So, we are back to the importance of integrating different action areas, strategies, activities, and channels of health communication. In doing so, it's important to stay abreast of new media current use and future potential as well as factors that contribute to use and perceptions of new media tools among different groups, because these influence or should influence the selection of new media channels for specific health communication interventions (see Table 5.9 for sample factors in the public's perception and use of new media–specific tools). As an example, Box. 5.3 includes information on a program that integrates different kinds of media and action areas.

Table 5.9   Sample Factors in Public Perception and Use of New Media–Specific Tools

Task appropriateness
Organizing strategies; ease of navigation
Message content and complexity
Adequate health literacy levels and cultural competence of all information
User attitudes toward technology and new media literacy
Frequency of use of specific new media among key groups
Format, presentation style, visual appeal
Stage of illness
Size and composition of network and online community
Visibility of information, specific topic, organization
Level of comfort of your organization and partners with specific new media tool
Feasibility for integration with other communication areas and services
Can this be tailored to meet the needs of the end user?

References: Schiavo, R. "The Rise of E-Health: Current Topics and Trends on Online Health Communications." *Journal of Medical Marketing*, 2008, *8*, 9–18; George Mason University. "Review of Literature: Impact of Interactive Health Communications." F. Alemi (ed.). 1999. http://gunston.gmu.edu/healthscience/722/Review.htm.

BOX 5.3. SPORTS FOR HEALTH EQUITY: A MULTIFACETED NATIONAL PROGRAM

Health disparities continue to compromise the ability of vulnerable and underserved communities across the United States to thrive. These disparities are linked to diverse factors, including socioeconomic conditions, race, ethnicity, and culture, as well as access to health care services, affordable and nutritious food, culturally appropriate health information, caring and friendly clinical settings, and a built environment that supports physical activity. Communities with greater disparities experience higher rates of infant mortality, higher incidence of several diseases and health conditions, and lower life expectancy.

Any progress toward health equity is predicated on raising awareness that these inequities exist. Studies have shown that there are low levels of awareness among racial and ethnic minority groups regarding disparities that disproportionately affect their own communities (Benz, Espinosa, Welsh, and Fontes, 2011), and that there have only been very modest gains in awareness in the last decade among all Americans, despite the national goal to reduce health disparities introduced by *Healthy People 2000* and reemphasized by *Healthy People 2010* and *Healthy People 2020*. There is an urgent need for innovative approaches to educate people about health disparities and encourage them to talk about health equity in their communities with the goal of assessing their own health-related needs and working together across sectors to achieve key changes.

Goals and Objectives

Sports for Health Equity is a national program launched in late 2012 by Health Equity Initiative (HEI), a nonprofit organization, to raise awareness and promote community action about health equity. The program uses sports as its central theme to engage young people and members of their communities. The campaign has featured Essence Carson, WNBA All Star, NY Liberty player, recording artist, writer, and producer as its Sports for Health Equity ambassador. The program's goal is to increase the awareness and understanding of health equity, including social determinants of health and how health disparities can negatively affect socioeconomic status and opportunity, among teens, their families, their communities, and the general public. Other key objectives include encouraging healthy behaviors and lifestyles and promoting youth as key agents of change. The project aims to create increased community action on health equity and to enable multiple sectors to join forces to develop long-term sustainable solutions to reduce health disparities.

Communication Strategies and Activities

The campaign employs a multifaceted approach to enlist students, their families, teachers, coaches, communities, community-based businesses, and organizations and professionals from multiple sectors in the health equity movement. Current and future activities have included or may include in the future a national media campaign to help create a receptive environment for community-based dialogue on health equity, awareness-raising basketball shoot-a-thons at middle schools and high schools, virtual and community town hall meetings on health equity and neighborhood involvement, a turnkey kit on how to organize a community town hall, a pledge campaign that will encourage families to talk about health equity issues around the kitchen table, a public information campaign of fact sheets, PowerPoint presentations that can be used by teachers and coaches within middle and high school settings, and other sample educational materials examining health equity and social determinants of health that can be integrated into middle and high school social studies and health studies courses.

The campaign capitalizes on elements vital to sports and to achieving health equity, such as teamwork, collaboration, focus, unity, and a sense of community, and emphasizes how sports and the movement for health equity can bring together people from all different backgrounds, ethnicities, and socioeconomic categories to work for the common goal of finding community-specific solutions. Health Equity Initiative also conducted a new and social media outreach campaign that included a video featuring Essence Carson, which was publicized on various social media outlets and websites.

Program Launch Results

As a testimonial to the power of mass media and new media, in less than six months since its launch, the program already reached over 1.24 million people via mass media, new and social media, event-based outreach, and presentations of the video at national conferences and film festivals. Celebrity endorsement and participation were key to media and event placement. Other key elements in securing media coverage included the personal story appeal of the program's video, and preexisting experience with key media that cover this kind of topic. Future evaluation efforts will focus on assessing results vis-à-vis the program's key elements and objectives.

Source: Health Equity Initiative. "Sports for Health Equity: A Multi-faceted National Program." Unpublished Case Study, 2013b. Used by permission.

New Media Use: Blogs, Podcasts, Social Networks, and More

A comprehensive discussion of the use of different new media goes beyond the scope of this book. Yet, this section highlights how different groups are using select new media such as blogs, podcasts, and social networks. By the time this book is published, the new media discussed here as well as others that are still in their infancy may have further evolved. The main purpose of this section is primarily to make sure that practitioners and students approach the use of new media as part of health communication interventions with the same research- and evidence-based attitudes that we use or should use for all other communication channels and provide examples of current uses and facts that should be researched and understood in the planning phase. In considering any kind of existing or emerging new media, the key to integrating them strategically within health communication interventions is to understand how they are used and perceived by different groups.

Blogs

blog
An abbreviation of the term *web log* and a discussion or an online informational site consisting of brief and conversational entries called *posts*

Blogs (an abbreviation of the term *web log* and a discussion or an online informational site consisting of brief and conversational entries called *posts*) are often used to make public hallway conversations on health and illness and to publicize and discuss health-related experiences, news, studies, opinions, and statistics. Many blogs act as online journals or diaries, whereas others function as online branding forums for an organization, an individual, a service, or a product. Well-established blogs such as the *Huffington Post* (www.huffingtonpost.com) act primarily as news websites where readers go periodically to stay informed on a variety of news topics. Although their interactivity distinguishes them from other media, these kinds of blogs act as mass media because of their wide reach.

For the most part, blogs continue to focus on sharing personal experiences or practical knowledge or keeping in touch with friends and family (Pew Internet & American Life Project, 2006). Fewer blogs focus on larger themes or have reached the kind of popularity that is typical of more-established mass media. Yet, blogs, as a kind of media, have reached mainstream popularity and have accounted for some of the decline of print media, as well as for influencing political agendas and conveying different viewpoints, including, sometimes, opinions that do not have factual validation (one of the main pitfalls of blogs and more, in general, of new media).

"Overall, bloggers are a highly educated and affluent group. Nearly half of all bloggers earned a graduate degree, and the majority have a household income of $75,000 per year or higher (Sussman, 2009). When considering influence, mommy bloggers are very powerful. Close to 71% of US female Internet users turned to them for useful information and 52% read them for product recommendations (*eMarketer Digital Intelligence*, 2010)" (CDC, 2011b, pp. 32–33). Bloggers are now 7 percent of US social media users (Knowledge Networks and MediaPost Communications, 2011) and more recently tend to team up to contribute to a specific multiauthor blog (MAB). MABs from universities, think tanks, popular newspapers, interest groups, and other organizations account for an increasing quantity of blog traffic (*Wikipedia*, 2013). Many bloggers have moved over to other media, whether they have appeared on popular television and radio programs, published a book on the content of their blog, or converted their blog into an online magazine. See, for example, the case of *Street Fighters of Public Health* in Box 5.4.

BOX 5.4. *STREET FIGHTERS OF PUBLIC HEALTH:* USING ONLINE TOOLS TO CREATE NETWORKING OPPORTUNITIES IN PUBLIC HEALTH

At a recent American Public Health Association annual meeting, public health professionals wore bright orange badges on which they had written their strengths, or "super powers," in the field of public health. Produced and distributed by the blog *Street Fighters of Public Health (SFoPH)*, www.streetfightersofpublichealth.com, these badges became known as "sticky ice breakers." Designed to decrease barriers to networking among public health professionals, the stickers showed off the wearer's areas of interest and qualifications, thereby facilitating an ice-breaking conversation with conference attendees and potential employers.

The blog *Street Fighters of Public Health* was founded in 2009 by Kate Swartz while pursuing her master's in public health degree in health communication at the Keck School of Medicine of the University of Southern California. The blog started as a practice in simplifying public health issues for the public with an approachable voice. However, while mentoring and attending public health meetings, Swartz found that public health professionals were spending enormous amounts of money attending conferences, only to leave with unpaid internships and few valuable contacts. She found that these individuals in the field wanted to learn more about career development, networking, and solutions in the public health workplace.

The innovative nature of *Street Fighters of Public Health* is twofold in both authorship and content that diverts from conventional online publishing and academia. Authorship changed when *SFoPH* transitioned from a blog to an online magazine in which professionals were given the opportunity to self-promote by contributing and publishing articles on public health topics online. In a formative evaluation of the contribution network, the first candidate contributor was given the opportunity to research content and write material and successfully published an average of two articles every week. Unlike the traditionally objective and technical descriptions of public health issues found in academic journals, the network of contributors at *SFoPH* are encouraged to engage a public audience with stories about public health that relate to current events or personal experience in addition to research citations.

"Public health professionals focus on improving the well-being of the community. I wanted to form the community that improves the well-being of the public health professional," says Swartz. In order to develop an "army of street fighters" the blog employs social media mechanisms such as Twitter, Facebook, and Blogger to attract public health professionals who are new to the field. In order to help professionals better advocate for themselves, the staff began hosting social hours and providing networking advice and mentoring services for individuals in the field. "It is important to polish new talent, and make young professionals feel welcome in public health; they'll be running the show soon," says Swartz. The site accepts blog entries on public health topics from interested parties willing to subscribe.

Source: Swartz, K. "Street Fighters of Public Health: Using Online Tools to Create Networking Opportunities in Public Health." Interview and other personal communications with author, 2012 and 2013.

One of the most important features of blogs is their interactivity, which allows readers to leave comments and start new conversations. Yet, "in most online communities [including blogs], 90% of users are lurkers who never contribute, 9% of users contribute a little, and 1% of users account for almost all the action" (Nielsen Norman Group, 2006). Also, in the United States, only one in three Internet users (Pew Internet & American Life Project, 2013a) and 12 percent of social media users age thirteen to eighty (Knowledge Networks and MediaPost Communications, 2011) read blogs, with Internet users under age thirty-four significantly more likely to read blogs.

So, what do the statistics we discussed so far tell us? That blogs may be best suited (at the least at the moment) to build awareness of health issues than engaging communities; that blogs still do not reach a significant segment of the US population so they should be used in combination with other culturally competent and audience-specific media; and that perhaps they may be best suited to reach mothers, affluent groups, online teens, and adults age eighteen to thirty-three when compared to other age or social groups. These and many other facts are the kinds of information that need to be researched and analyzed in considering and integrating blogs as a communication channel for any health communication intervention in the public health, community development, or health care fields.

podcasts
Multimedia digital files made available on the Internet for downloading to a portable media player or computer

Podcasts

Podcasts (digital or audio files that can be downloaded from a website to a media player or a computer) are increasingly used by a variety of organizations and publications in the health field. For example, podcasts are commonly used to do the following:

- Provide a valuable and user-friendly continuing medical education or continuing education "to-go" (Korioth, 2007) option, which can be usually downloaded from a members-only webpage.

- Bring to life complex issues, such as the role of scientists in health communication (*Biotechnology Journal*, 2007).

- Stir debate on recent medical advances and fuel innovation, as, for example, the podcast series by Solving Kids' Cancer (2012), an organization dedicated to find, fund, and manage therapeutic development for life-threatening kinds of pediatric cancer.

- Discuss health news and topics of public interest via a themed series or special podcasts.

- Be a part of new media and mass media news releases.

Podcasts are a cost-effective option to expand the reach of expert panels, conferences, and other professional and community-based events. Currently, they are an extremely common audio file on a variety of online resources in the Unites States and other Western countries. As technology evolves, the use of podcasts is expected to expand and change to include new applications and options.

Social Media and Social Networking

It is difficult to think of a starting point to describe the use of social media and social networking in health communication. Although the two terms are often lumped together, "**social media** [emphasis added] (for example, YouTube) are tools for sharing and discussing information. **Social networking** [emphasis added] is the use of communities of interest to connect to others" (Stelzner, 2009). Some media (for example, Facebook and Twitter) combine both functions (Stelzner, 2009).

Perhaps, the most common uses of these media by different organizations, professionals, and lay people are to build community and raise awareness on specific health issues (for example, via Facebook or Twitter); validate ideas and organizational strategies via the number of social kudos or "likes" one may receive on Facebook, or the number of followers on Twitter; expand event and meeting outreach; solicit opinions and ideas across geographic boundaries; mobilize communities in support of addressing specific health issues; build professional connections and relationships (for example, via LinkedIn); create virtual identities for oneself or test messages and strategies of health communication programs on virtual world networks such as Whyville and Second Life; share photos (Flickr); or fundraise

social media
A subgroup of new media. "Social media (for example, YouTube) are tools for sharing and discussing information" (Stelzner, 2009)

social networking
A type of new media that uses "communities of interest to connect to others" (Stelzner, 2009)

for organizational causes and special projects not only via social media and fundraising sites (for example, JustGive.org) but also via crowd-funding sites such as rockethub.com.

Social media are constantly evolving and being used in new ways. As the evaluation of social media impact is a relatively new and evolving practice, we can expect the next decade to add clarity on what social media actually can and cannot do within a variety of settings, groups, and health issues. Given the high number and variety of social media, a detailed description of the use of specific media is beyond the scope of this book. Therefore, this section is indicative only of the current and potential uses of social media. For additional case studies on social media and their use, see Chapters Fifteen and Sixteen.

mHealth

Mobile health (mHealth) technologies have rapidly advanced and hold the promise to provide health information and services on the go. mHealth is the delivery of select public health and clinical information and services via mobile technologies (including texting, apps, and others). It is one of the many approaches that could help personalize and revolutionize health and medicine.

Several authors (Nilsen and others, 2012, p. 5) refer to mHealth's "potential to greatly impact health research, health care, and health outcomes." Recent experiences have already demonstrated the promise of mHealth within interventions on different but interconnected areas such as maternal and child health, chronic diseases, smoking cessation, and skilled delivery attendance (Evans and others, 2012; Abroms and others, 2012; Katz, Mesfin, and Barr, 2012; Lund and others, 2012). In Zanzibar, for example, a mobile phone intervention in twenty-four facilities (Lund and others, 2012) was associated with an increase in the number of women of urban residence who delivered their babies with skilled attendance (in other words with the help of a midwife, nurse, or physician or other health professional who had been educated and trained to proficiency to manage childbirth).

Yet, as technology progresses, so should be the science behind mHealth applications and evaluation. "mHealth requires a solid, interdisciplinary scientific approach that pairs the rapid change associated with technological progress with a rigorous evaluation approach" (Nilsen and others, 2012, p. 5). Several tools, trainings, and resources to strengthen research and evaluation capacity in this field as well as to encourage multidisciplinary collaborations are already underway and include work by the National Institutes of Health (Office of Behavioral and Social Sciences Research,

2013) and the United Nations Foundation (2013). A proposed logic model for the evaluation of new media-based interventions, including mHealth, is featured in Chapter Fourteen.

As with other health communication areas and interventions, a list of the top ideal features of an mHealth intervention include the following:

- Integration within the socioeconomic and political contexts in which health communication operates, as well as other synergic communication areas

- Clarity of expected behavioral and social results at the outset of the intervention

- Interdisciplinary collaborations and partnerships to maximize impact

- Robust planning, research, and evaluation processes and efforts

The mHealth system is at the intersection of three different fields: health, technology, and grant-making philanthropy (with the last fueling innovation and providing adequate resources for scaling up and replication in a variety of settings). It is also influenced by local, national, and international policies and regulations. There are a large number of groups and stakeholders involved in the mHealth system who are invested in realizing the promise of new technology. Research and evaluation are core functions of this system as well as critical to guaranteeing a sound review of lessons learned and their applicability in a variety of real-life settings.

Therefore, as mHealth evolves, of equal importance is the continual monitoring of actual and perceived uses of mobile technology as a channel for health information and services among different groups, as well as in relation to their culture, gender, and age-related preferences, health and media literacy levels, and access to technology, among others. For example, although mobile application popularity continues to increase in the United States and many other countries, smartphones—which are essential to applications functioning—are only owned by 35 percent of the US adult population (Pew Internet & American Life Project, 2011d) and about one in four American teens (Pew Internet & American Life Project, 2012c), with the majority of users under the age of forty-five (Pew Internet & American Life Project, 2011d). This kind of analysis is needed every time that we approach a new mHealth intervention to ensure maximum reach and impact in integration with other mHealth interventions, such as texting, and communication areas.

Reaching the Underserved with Integrated New Media Communication

As previously noted, underserved and vulnerable populations are essential beneficiaries of the new media and other technological revolutions to address health disparities. As with all technological advances (including new treatment and prevention options), new media have the potential to help mitigate gaps in services and information that may lead to better health outcomes among disadvantaged groups. It definitely would be a failure of public health, health care, and, more in general, of community development, if those groups most in need of progress won't benefit from it.

As with all other group-specific communication, reaching the underserved with integrated new media communication starts with listening, building trust, and understanding current needs, preferences, and priorities of specific groups. Whether the new media intervention is engaging mothers from ethnic minorities, the elderly, or communities from low-income countries or affected by social discrimination and stigma, or other vulnerable groups, all interventions should be grounded in a rigorous communication process and inspired by models for behavioral and social change. Formative research is crucial and should also include a comprehensive health literacy assessment and health issue–specific risk mapping, as well as rely on a combination of quantitative and qualitative methods (see Chapter Fourteen for more details) to uncover unknown insights into health and community development issues. Most important, no intervention should be designed without the participation and active engagement of representatives from vulnerable and underserved populations.

In order to help bridge the digital divide and effectively reach the underserved, new media communication interventions need to focus on the following key factors and features, among others:

- Integration of community voices in all phases of program planning, implementation, and evaluation as well as relevant and culture-friendly visual pieces, including the use of online and offline videos to motivate change and mobilize communities. For example, *The Waiting Room*, a documentary and social media project, features the stories of patients and their families and friends who attend an overcrowded emergency room in Oakland, California. People in the waiting room speak about community, language barriers, family violence, chronic diseases, poverty, access to care, taking action, and many other relevant subjects in addressing health disparities (*The Waiting Room*, 2012). The film has won several awards and is the central piece of screenings and community outreach efforts throughout the United States (*The Waiting Room*, 2012).

* Community-specific role models and champions who are recognized by underserved communities.

* Culture- and user-friendly selection of new media channels. For example, mobile technology is by far more common than Web. 2.0 in underserved and minority communities in the United States. Adults from underserved communities "use a much wider range of their cell phones' capabilities," with text messaging, for example, being used by "70% of *all* African-Americans and English-speaking Latinos vs. just over half of whites" (Smith, 2010).

* Tailored risk-assessment tools and messages for change, which seek to showcase risk and health outcomes as they relate to family, generational, and group-specific facts and time periods.

* Focus on increasing new media literacy via a variety of programs that use public libraries and other "usual suspect" kinds of contexts (for example, clinical settings) as key venues for training sessions and programs, and show, instead of telling, how to use new media.

* Integration of new media activities with community-based and other offline interventions. For example, in the research and issue assessment phase, focus groups including low literate and underserved groups could be turned into long-term support groups for interested participants, which could also include a social media component to spread their impact. Similarly, online communities can be connected to resources and local groups in relevant cities and neighborhoods.

These and other key features of new media interventions may help expand new media reach to include vulnerable and underserved populations and realize the promise of this technological revolution as it relates to improved access to care, health outcomes, patient engagement, and management of chronic diseases, among many other actions, also within low-income and other disadvantaged settings.

Mass Media- and New Media–Specific Evaluation Parameters

Although the results of mass media and new media–based interventions should be evaluated as part of the larger behavioral and social outcomes of the health communication program for which the strategies and activities are designed, a few specific parameters are commonly used to measure quantitative and qualitative results of mass media campaigns that rely on traditional mass media such as print, radio, and broadcast. Similarly, specific parameters apply to the counting and tracking of new media campaign results. (A complete discussion of evaluation parameters and methodologies of health communication interventions is included in Chapters Twelve, Thirteen, and Fourteen. The methodologies discussed here apply more specifically only to mass media and new media and reflect current practice.)

As with all other areas of health communication, evaluation and measurement of the mass media component of a program should be related to the specific and measurable goals and objectives defined at the outset of the program. Some of these measures are defined by PR theory and practice, especially in the context of mass media campaigns (Institute for Public Relations, 1997, 2003; Yaxley, 2013). In other words, what was the mass media component of the program trying to accomplish? What are or were the specific objectives of each strategy or activity? Which of them were accomplished?

The Institute for Public Relations (1997, 2003) and Yaxley (2013) define three categories to measure PR-driven mass media programs:

- *PR outputs:* Short-term and process-oriented measurements, such as the number of stories published by the media, the number of times a specific spokesperson is quoted, the tone and content of the media coverage, and the number of Internet **hits**, likes, or shares received by an online article

hits
Total number of downloads (photos, text, HTML, etc.) on all the pages, including all times users came in contact with any of the different elements and components on all pages of a given site

- *PR outtakes:* The way the PR program is received by the media and other target key groups and stakeholders as well as overall message recall and retention. For example, did the media find the design and content of press materials or the virtual newsroom appealing and easy to use? Was the language used in press releases, virtual newsrooms, and other materials received favorably, or did the media have problems understanding and using it? Did the actual message recipients (for example, the media's intended audiences such as consumers or professionals) respond positively to the message? Did the recipients ask for more information by, for example, going to a recommended website? Did they write any letters to the editor or commentaries in response to media coverage, or did they comment on a specific blog post that was part of the mass media outreach?

- *PR outcomes:* The evaluation and measurement of changes in the opinions, attitudes, behaviors, or levels of engagement in the media's audiences regarding a given issue

Similar to some new media-specific measurements, PR outputs can be measured simply by "counting, tracking and observing" (Institute for Public Relations, 1997, 2003, p. 7). In media and press relations efforts, a common parameter to measure PR outputs is the number of media impressions, defined as "the number of people who might have had the opportunity to be exposed to a story that has appeared in the media" (Institute for Public Relations, 2006, p. 9). It is related to the total circulation (for example, number of copies sold by a newspaper or number of viewers of a TV news program) of a given publication or broadcast media outlet (Institute for Public Relations, 2002). For example, in 2010, the *New York Times* had an audited circulation of approximately 900,000 (daily issues) to 1.3 million (Sunday issue) readers (New York Times Company, 2013). Therefore, a story in the *Times* will generate 900,000 to 1.3 million media impressions, depending on whether it is published on a weekday or on a Sunday.

PR outcomes and to some extent PR outtakes (for example, for the part concerning the evaluation of message recall and retention by key groups and stakeholders) can be measured only through extensive pre- and postintervention studies (Institute for Public Relations, 1997, 2003; Macnamara, 2006; Futerra Sustainability Communications, 2010) and are difficult and expensive to assess. "Measurement of any process requires pre-activity measurement, followed by post-activity measurement . . . For instance how can you show you have increased employee understanding of company policies if you have not measured what they were before you implemented your communication?" (Macnamara, 2006, p. 14). Common methodologies for evaluating PR outcomes as well as some types of PR outtakes are similar to those generally used in health communication. (These are discussed in Chapters Twelve, Thirteen, and Fourteen.)

Similarly, new media–specific measurements often focus on the following measurements (Williams, Zraik, Schiavo, and Hatz, 2008; Abroms, Schiavo, and Lefebvre, 2008):

- **Unique visitors:** The total count of how many different people accessed a specific website or media
- **Visits:** Total number of visits (including returning visitors and users who are no longer unique)
- **Page views:** Total number of times users viewed each unique page on

unique visitors
The total count of how many different people accessed a specific website or media

visits
Total number of visits (including returning visitors and users who are no longer unique)

page views
Total number of times users viewed each unique page on a given site, meaning the total number of pages users viewed when they visited a specific site

a given site, meaning the total number of pages users viewed when they visited a specific site

- **Hits:** Total number of downloads (photos, text, HTML, etc.) on all the pages, including all times users came in contact with any of the different elements and components on all pages of a given site

keyword mentions
Total count of mentions of the program's name or issue on the web (on websites, blogs, social media, and others)

- **Keyword mentions:** Total count of mentions of the program's name or issue on the web (on websites, blogs, social media, and others)

responses to text messages
Total number of mobile users who reply to program texts or number of total responses per user received in reply to a text messaging program

- **Responses to text messages:** Total number of mobile users who reply to program texts or number of total responses per user received in reply to a text messaging program

- **Text messaging readership:** Total number of mobile users who report reading messages from a text messaging program

text messaging readership
Total number of mobile users who report reading messages from a text messaging program

- **Use of mobile interactive features:** Total number of mobile users who use interactive features associated with the mHealth program (for example, apps, links to websites, and digital resources, etc.)

use of mobile interactive features
Total number of mobile users who use interactive features associated with the mHealth program

Ultimately, the contribution of the mass media and new media components of a health communication intervention should be measured as part of the overall evaluation of such interventions in relation to the impact on social and behavioral results of the overall program, and the attainment of its public health, patient-related, community development, or organizational goal. For a discussion of specific tools and models that apply to new media, see the section in Chapter Fourteen called "Evaluating New Media–Based Interventions: Emerging Trends and Models."

Key Concepts

- Mass media and new media communications are important components of health communication interventions.

- We live in an exciting time for health communication. Communication-related technologies (Internet, mobile, etc.) have been fast advancing at an unprecedented pace, and have been adopted by different groups and populations across the world.

- In approaching health communication planning in the new media age, special attention should be given to what has changed and what should not change as well as to analyzing specific opportunities and challenges.

- The media of mass communication include print, broadcast, radio, entertainment, and motion media, and information-related features of the Internet (for example, news websites, blogs, online journals, and libraries). Yet, the definition of mass media may be group-specific because it depends on several factors, including access to technology, cultural preferences, and health and new media literacy.

- The use of interactive functions of the Internet and mobile technology—such as social media, texting, and online forums—cannot yet be considered the same as mass media in their application to health issues, at least not across different socioeconomic, age, ethnic groups, and country settings. This will evolve over time and will continue to be group-specific.

- Public relations (PR), which is defined as "the art and science of establishing and promoting a favorable relationship with the public" (*American Heritage Dictionary of the English Language*, 2011), has been the backbone of mass communication for several decades.

- Whether relying on mass media, new media, or other communication channels, public relationships continue to be part of the communication process, because there is no way to replace the human factor.

- Key theoretical constructs of PR recognize the importance of psychological, emotional, and subconscious factors in human behavior; understanding and addressing multiple publics in light of their unique characteristics as well as their mutual relationships and interaction; and understanding its role in relationship management. PR theory and practice has significantly evolved and adapted in the new media age.

- Because of the significant power of the mass media on public opinion and the potential risk for manipulation and misrepresentation, PR ethics should be always held to the highest standards. Professional codes of ethics as well as key characteristics of ethical PR programs should be considered in developing mass media and new media communication programs.

- The success of media-based campaigns depends on the story's newsworthiness, ability to listen to and engage relevant groups, as well as the effectiveness of media relations and media-specific tools.

- Mass media and new media communications alone are not as effective in affecting and engaging the public, and encouraging behavioral and social change as larger and multifaceted interventions that rely on other action areas of health communication; use community-based strategies and activities; and complement existing or future public health, health care, and community development programs.

- Underserved and vulnerable populations need to be included as essential beneficiaries of the new media and other technological revolutions to address health disparities. Several factors and features of new media communication interventions may help bridge the digital divide and effectively reach the underserved.

- Overall outcomes of mass media and new media programs should be evaluated in the context of the health communication intervention for which they have been designed. Still, it is important to understand and take into account qualitative and quantitative parameters that specifically apply to mass media and new media.

FOR DISCUSSION AND PRACTICE

1. You are pitching consumer publications (for example, women's magazines, local and national newspapers, online publications) with a story that aims at raising awareness of the importance of regular mammograms for breast cancer prevention in women over forty years of age. List some potential elements and angles for your story in order to attract reporters' attention and secure media coverage.

2. This chapter lists some of the key factors in designing ethical PR programs and also refers to existing guidelines. Share your reaction to each of these characteristics (see Table 5.5). Can you recall any examples to which they may apply? Can you think of examples that do the opposite? Is there anything else you would do to preserve public interest and ethics of PR while designing the PR component of a health communication program?

3. Review the *Street Fighters of Public Health* case study in Box 5.4. Discuss what, in your opinion, could be future directions in the use and potential impact of this kind of blog. Compare with similar blogs you may know.

4. Research and discuss examples of key features of a new media communication program intended to reach and engage vulnerable or underserved groups. Compare such features and program-specific factors to those discussed in this chapter.

5. List and discuss key objectives and preliminary or projected results of an mHealth program you may be familiar with or have researched.

6. Design, develop, and maintain a blog on a health-related topic of your interest. Discuss lessons learned within the context of the specific health issue as well as the approach and web-based platform you selected in developing your blog.

KEY TERMS

blog

communities

hits

keyword mentions

mass communication

mass media

media pitch

mHealth

page views

podcasts

public relations (PR)

responses to text messages

social media

social networking

text messaging readership

unique visitors

use of mobile interactive features

virtual newsrooms

visits

COMMUNITY MOBILIZATION AND CITIZEN ENGAGEMENT

"Ask Canadians what the name ParticipACTION conjures up, and the majority of adults will easily recall the 60-year-old Swede" (Costas-Bradstreet, 2004, p. S25). "Is it true that the average 30-year-old Canadian is only as fit as the average 60-year-old Swede?" (Canadian Public Health Association, 2004) was one of the many questions addressed by the early public service announcements of a health communication program that ran for more than thirty years and was established by ParticipACTION, a nonprofit organization.

Public service announcements were the main tool of ParticipACTION in the early days of its implementation. Once the program's name had been established and Canadians became increasingly aware of the importance of fitness, ParticipACTION also implemented innovative strategies to involve people at the community level. The program "used community mobilization as a way to empower communities and motivate individuals to get more active" (Costas-Bradstreet, 2004, p. S25).

Community mobilization efforts originally focused on the city of Saskatoon in central Canada. Soon the enthusiasm generated by ParticipACTION community events, including "Walk a Block a Day" and other mass participation activities, spread to several levels of Canadian society, including other cities and regions, as well as provincial, territorial, and national governments (Costas-Bradstreet, 2004).

In 1992 alone, ParticipACTION trained fifty community animators who "generated 21,000 registered community events involving over 1 million volunteer leaders" (Costas-Bradstreet, 2004, p. S26). Over the years, the program attracted volunteers from all segments of society, including health professionals, the media, business communities, ordinary people, and government officials. It also developed partnerships with the federal government, professional societies (for example, Ontario Physical and Health Education Association, College of Family Physicians), the commercial sector (for example, the Ontario Milk Marketing Board, Merck Frosst Canada), and major health organizations, such as the Canadian Public Health Association (Costas-Bradstreet, 2004). All partners contributed with funds, activities, and other resources that expanded the program's reach.

The long-term impact of this program, which closed its doors in 2002 and was relaunched in 2009, are being assessed vis-à-vis a set of indicators that include organizational capacity building for physical exercise, partnership development, funding process reform, and others (Faulkner and others, 2009). The growing prevalence of obesity in Canada (Canadian Public Health Association, 2004; Eisenberg and others, 2011) still points to the need for sustained efforts in this direction. Still, many of the success stories and lessons learned from ParticipACTION and other similar programs around the world demonstrate the importance of community mobilization as a fundamental strategy of health communication and, more broadly, public health, health care, and community development interventions.

CHAPTER OBJECTIVES

This chapter establishes community mobilization as a key area of health communication. It also reviews some of the current theoretical assumptions and topics in relation to this approach. Finally, it provides practical guidance on the key ingredients of community mobilization programs and the need for considering this approach as part of a multifaceted and multidisciplinary intervention. In doing so, the chapter also builds capacity and encourages readers to "develop strategies to motivate others for collaborative problem-solving, decision making, and evaluation" (Association of Schools of Public Health, 2007, p. 9), because these are critical elements of effective health communication interventions.

Community Mobilization and Citizen Engagement: A Bottom-Up Approach

Definitions often provide a useful framework for understanding the platform and the key assumptions of any given approach. In the case of community mobilization, the importance of community dialogue, participation, and self-reliance is emphasized in its theoretical definition and practical applications.

In fact, **community mobilization** is often defined as "empowering individuals to find their own solutions, whether or not the problem is solved" (Fishbein, Goldberg, and Middlestadt, 1997, p. 294). Although this definition does not and should not absolve community mobilization strategies from the pressure and responsibility of producing results, it clearly indicates that local leaders and ordinary people are the key participants in this approach. At the same time, it places in their hands the potential for involving other levels of society (for example, governments, professional organizations, grant-makers, and the private sector) in the solutions they have found. In this way, community mobilization is a bottom-up approach because it tends to rely on people's power to involve the upper hierarchical levels of society and to develop collaborative efforts to address community-specific issues.

For example, one of the main success factors of ParticipACTION was its community-driven approach, which helped secure "long-term government and sponsor support" (Costas-Bradstreet, 2004, p. S25). Similar conclusions were drawn in regard to a community mobilization project in Cameroon that aimed at increasing knowledge and use of family planning methods and reproductive health services (Babalola and others, 2001). Babalola and others also highlight that once innovations were spread throughout local associations (called Njangi), they continued "to spread throughout the larger community, making community mobilization an effective tool for large-scale behavioral change communication" (p. 476). Effective community mobilization fuses public health and social justice, and also seeks to change social norms to support behavioral and social results (Michau, 2012).

The term **community** can indicate a variety of social, ethnic, cultural, or geographical associations, and it can refer to a school, workplace, city, neighborhood, or organized patient or professional group, or association of peer leaders, to name a few. As another example, Njangi are local socioeconomic associations that are quite common in most of Africa and "are formed on a geographic basis, by family structure, or through shared professions" (Babalola and others, 2001, p. 461). Communities always tend to share similar values, beliefs, and overall objectives and priorities. According to UNAIDS (2012, p. 14), a community is a "group of people with diverse characteristics who are linked by common ties including shared interests, social interaction or geographical location." Communities are also made of groups of people from multiple sectors who share similar concerns and objectives and will act together in their common interest.

community mobilization
One of the key areas of health communication. A bottom-up and participatory process. Using multiple communication channels, it seeks to involve community leaders and the community at large in addressing a health issue, becoming part of the key steps to behavioral or social change or practicing a desired behavior.

community
A variety of social, ethnic, cultural, or geographical associations, for example, a school, workplace, city, neighborhood, organized patient or professional group, or association of peer leaders

When communities drive public health or health communication interventions, they are not merely consulted. They share power and decisions. Community mobilization may be initiated by leaders within the community or stimulated by external agencies, organizations, or consultants. Still, the role of external organizations, health communication practitioners, and other consultants is to facilitate and follow the mobilization process (Health Communication Partnership, 2006c).

In this context, one of the main objectives of health communication practitioners and other health professionals who may be involved in the community mobilization effort is to provide local leaders and their community with technical assistance to accomplish a number of goals:

- Find solutions that build on the community's strengths and fit well within its overall context (Fishbein, Goldberg, and Middlestadt, 1997; Costas-Bradstreet, 2004).

- Facilitate partnerships with other segments of society (Costas-Bradstreet, 2004).

- Become aware of potential obstacles and ways to overcome them.

- Resolve conflicts among community members and create a consensus on potential solutions.

- Establish a process for community involvement, including the development of communication strategies, messages, materials, and activities, which can ultimately lead to social and behavioral changes.

- Point to resources and approaches that may facilitate long-term sustainability of all interventions and health solutions.

- Design a rigorous evaluation process, including community-relevant indicators so that the community can check on its own progress and accommodate changing needs.

- Keep the community focused on what it wants to accomplish.

It's only by encouraging participation and ownership of the health communication process and its outcomes among community members and other key groups that communication interventions are likely to lead to sustainable behavioral and social results. This is why community mobilization is a core area of health communication.

Community Mobilization as a Social Process

The impact of community mobilization is greater when different communities interact with each other and create a social force for change. This concept is incorporated in the idea of social mobilization. Although some of the premises of social mobilization may be different from those of community mobilization, the two terms are closely related and are used here interchangeably. **Social mobilization** has been defined "as the process of bringing together multisectoral community partners to raise awareness, demand, and progress for the initiative's goals, processes and outcomes" (Patel, 2005, p. 53). This definition is in agreement with the key elements of community mobilization as discussed in this chapter.

In the context of health communication, community mobilization tends to be disease specific and addresses behavioral issues that may help reduce the morbidity and mortality of a given condition. Still, there are a number of cases in which community mobilization is a component of health communication programs that complement larger public health interventions, and aim to guarantee or expand community access to health services and products or address social issues. In fact, community mobilization may entail and refer to different kinds of actions, from people marching to demonstrate their discontent about the paucity of research funds dedicated to a specific disease area, to community members connecting with others about the importance of disease prevention and leading the behavior change process.

Mobilizing local leaders and their communities is a long process that may vary according to the community's makeup and needs. However, several success factors can be extrapolated from existing experiences and programs, and apply generally to this kind of effort:

> **social mobilization**
> The "process of bringing together multisectoral community partners to raise awareness, demand, and progress for the initiative's goals, processes and outcomes" (Patel, 2005, p. 53)

- Evidence-based information, which is critical to attract attention to a health issue and convince people to prioritize it within a community. Moreover, it can help communities identify strategies and approaches that are likely to involve their members as well as other communities in the health behavior change process.

- An in-depth understanding of other conflicting community priorities coupled with efforts to effectively address them or showcase linkages with a specific health or social issue.

- A comprehensive analysis of social norms, key determinants of health, factors, and conditions that may prevent people from adopting and sustaining recommended health or social behaviors.

- A behavior-centered mind-set. In other words, what is it that communities would like to do? What kind of progress indicators do they feel comfortable establishing and achieving toward their behavioral and social objectives?

- The inclusion of all influential groups in the planning, implementation, and evaluation of the community mobilization process.

- The quality of the technical assistance and training provided to local leaders and their communities by health communication practitioners and other key health professionals and facilitators. Outside support and technical assistance are critical to sustaining the effort over the long term (UNAIDS, 2005).

- The potential for community ownership and program sustainability.

- The existence of complementary interventions (for example, mass media campaigns, capacity building and training, widespread access to services) that reinforce community-based communication efforts, and encourage participants' adherence to the process of change.

Most of these factors are common to the overall field of health communication and public health. Still, it is worth mentioning them here because of their critical importance in community mobilization programs.

Finally, facilitating a community-driven intervention requires good listening skills, a firm belief in the "value of collective action" (Costas-Bradstreet, 2004, p. S29), enthusiasm for the health or social cause, and a strong ability to transmit it. It also requires the application of many of the skills and theories previously discussed in relation to interpersonal communication. As an example of the many different phases and steps of community mobilization, Box 6.1 features a case study from UNICEF on addressing oral polio vaccine refusal in northern Nigeria via the development and training of a community mobilizer network.

BOX 6.1. TACKLING ORAL POLIO VACCINE REFUSALS THROUGH VOLUNTEER COMMUNITY MOBILIZER NETWORK IN NORTHERN NIGERIA

Current Situation

Nigeria remains one of the three polio-endemic countries in the world along with Pakistan and Afghanistan. As of June 22, 2012, Nigeria had forty-five cases of wild poliovirus (WPV) in ten states compared to twenty-five cases in six states for the same period in 2011 (see Figure 6.1). In 2011, Nigeria had sixty-two cases of WPV in eight states compared to twenty-one cases in eight states in 2010. The number of cases in 2011 was three times higher than it was in 2010. Nigeria, however, experienced 95 percent reduction of WPV cases in 2010 compared to the 388 WPV cases in 2009. Further, the total number of circulating vaccine derived poliovirus (cVDPV2) was thirty-five in ten states in 2011 whereas only one cVDPV2 case has been reported so far in 2012.

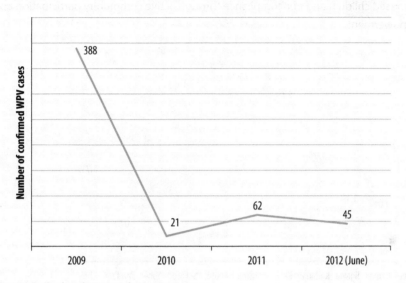

Figure 6.1 Number of WPV Cases by Year in Nigeria

As of June 2012 two national immunization plus days (IPDs) and one subnational IPD have been conducted covering ten very high-risk northern states. Four more IPDs are planned for this year in Nigeria along with mop-up campaigns (door-to-door immunization) to be implemented on detection of any new WPV cases. The proportion of missed children during campaigns has fluctuated over time due to a multitude of social, religious, and political reasons as well as campaign operational issues (June 2011—6.8 percent; November 2011—7.7 percent; and May 2012—7.2 percent). In terms of vaccine refusals, the goal is to keep actual noncompliance[1] (vaccine refusals) in high-risk states under 2 percent. Actual noncompliance was reduced to 1.7 percent in May 2012 from 2.1 percent in February (see Figure 6.2).

Intensified Ward Communication Strategy

Intensified ward communication strategy (IWCS) aims at addressing pockets of vaccine refusals among caregivers in northern Nigeria by using targeted, data-driven communication interventions through media, traditional institutions, religious leaders, and community volunteers in the most high-risk settlements. Traditional and religious leaders play a key role in addressing refusals driven by the men in the household, whereas different strategies need to be deployed to empower women.

In 2011, UNICEF piloted few community-based communication initiatives as part of its support to the IWCS in three northern states. These initiatives showed encouraging results by reducing missed children and noncompliance through active community participation and women's empowerment.

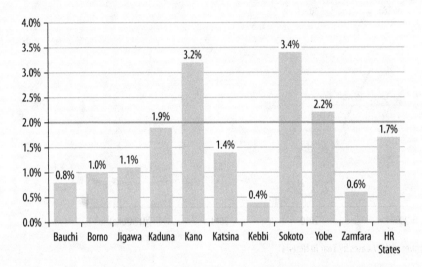

Figure 6.2   Proportion of Actual Noncompliance, High-Risk States, May 2012

With the support of Polio Eradication Initiative (PEI) partners and the Government of Nigeria, UNICEF is now spearheading a rapid scale-up of a volunteer community mobilizer network (VCM Net) targeting eight high-risk states: Kebbi, Kano, Sokoto, Zamfara, Jigawa, Yobe, Katsina, and Borno. In total, more than 2,150 settlement-level VCMs are being recruited, trained, equipped, and deployed in the settlements where missed children and refusals of oral polio vaccine are still persistent. These VCMs will reach out to over six hundred thousand households on a monthly basis to undertake communication interventions.

VCM Net is putting in place a targeted community-driven social mobilization effort and a house-to-house behavior change communication approach in high-risk settlements that is hoped to contribute to the reduction of the percentage of missed children in each campaign (see Figure 6.3).

Selected from their settlement, the VCMs have been trained to work as change agents in their respective communities. These women are trained to use simple pictorial materials to engage caregivers in a dialogue around key household practices as well as routine and polio immunization. It is hoped that the wider communication platform will create a positive environment in which routine and polio immunization can be more effectively promoted, eventually reversing the trend in vaccine refusals (see Figure 6.4).

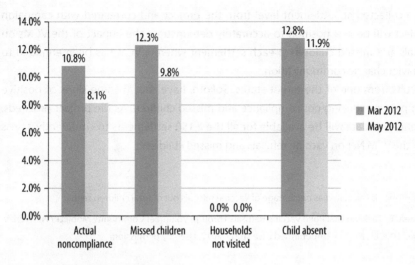

Figure 6.3 Preliminary Data, Sokoto VCMs

Note: Data are from forty-seven Sokoto settlements. HH stands for households.

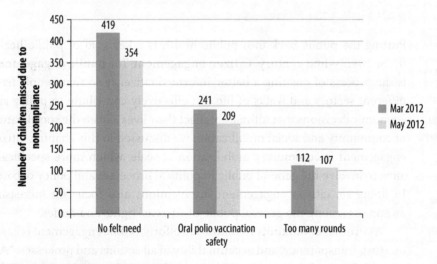

Figure 6.4 Main Reasons for Noncompliance

Note: Data are from forty-seven Sokoto settlements.

Volunteer supervisors are engaged to support clusters of VCMs (maximum ten) to make sure the mobilizers correctly use the IEC (information-education-communication) materials provided and are sufficiently skilled at engaging with caregivers in a behavior-changing dialogue. The supervisors also have to make sure all eligible children in the settlements are tracked and that the monthly monitoring tools are properly filled out.

With data collected at settlement level from the project and correlated with campaign data, the project will be in a position to accurately demonstrate the impact of the VCMs on vaccine refusals and missed children in each settlement where a VCM has been engaged to carry out behavior change communication.

Initial results from one of the target states, Sokoto, have shown some signs of positive results and impact in reducing noncompliance and missed children. As the project proceeds, more comprehensive data will be available for all the 2,150 settlements to confidently assess the impact of the VCM Net on vaccine refusals and missed children.

Note

[1] Actual noncompliance is calculated as percentage of vaccine refusals out of total children seen.

Source: Laulajainen, T. "Tackling Oral Polio Vaccine Refusals Through Volunteer Community Mobilizer Network in Northern Nigeria." UNICEF, Nigeria. Unpublished case study, 2012. Used by permission.

Engaging Citizens in Policy Debates and Political Processes

citizen engagement (or public engagement) The process of creating a better-informed citizenry so that people from different sectors and walks of life can effectively contribute to policy and economic decisions that ultimately affect their lives

Putting the public back into public health is a key goal of public health in the twenty-first century. **Citizen engagement** (or **public engagement**) is the process of creating a better-informed citizenry so that people from different sectors and walks of life can effectively contribute to policy and economic decisions that ultimately affect their lives. Given the social nature of community and social mobilization we discussed in this chapter, citizen engagement is community mobilization at scale, which more specifically aims to involve the general public in political processes and policy debates. In doing so, citizen engagement interventions also focus on increasing awareness among the general public of citizens' rights and duties.

As in other community mobilization efforts, public engagement is based on trust, transparency, and accountability of all actions and processes. "Accountability is often thought of in terms of government being accountable to citizens. In the context of mobilization, community members being accountable to each other is as important as government accountability. Those individuals elected to help lead projects are accountable to the wider community, their neighbors who are counting on them to implement projects in the best interest of everyone" (Mercy Corps, 2013, p. 8).

In community mobilization, every community and all citizens have the right to know the procedures, decision-making processes, and financial allocations and cash flow for programs, policies, and priorities that may affect all. Yet, as it relates to public health and health care systems, public engagement is strongly dependent on building capacity to increase health literacy and media literacy levels among average citizens. It is only by enabling people to understand, evaluate, and act on health information that citizen engagement is actually possible. So, health and media literacy are fundamental premises for public engagement, and more in general community mobilization (Schiavo, 2009d).

A key outcome indicator of community mobilization and public engagement is, or should be, sustainability, especially because it relates to citizens' ability to advocate for specific health policies or an equal distribution of resources, as well as to participate in political processes. As citizen engagement has proven to be effective in many different areas (see, for example, "The Case for Community Mobilization and Citizen Engagement in Risk and Emergency Communication" in this chapter), building capacity for mobilization should be a key priority in many countries and communities.

For example, a study conducted for UNICEF on community-based communication in pandemic flu settings revealed that identifying and building capacity of local social mobilization partners is one of the key priorities among UNICEF field staff, international organizations, and other professional groups so that local partners can effectively contribute to prepare and respond to epidemics (an infectious disease affecting many people at the same time and spreading from person to person within a community or city) and emerging disease outbreaks (Schiavo, 2009b; Schiavo and Kapil, 2009). Emerging diseases are either appearing for the first time in a region or evolving from other past diseases. Building the capacity of civil society and other local community-based organizations to become effective participants in community development and engagement is also one of the key steps followed by Mercy Corps (2013) as part of their community mobilization interventions. Other key elements of citizen engagement programming mirror the good practices and methods of community mobilization that are discussed later in this chapter, and include community and citizen dialogue to assess needs, preferences, and strategies for government accountability, public surveys, and local or national community meetings, among others.

As public engagement is increasingly valued within and outside health communication settings, several universities, for example, The New School for Public Engagement (2013), government initiatives (White House, 2013), and programs strive to address the need to involve citizens in policy debates and others. Although a lot of good work is in process, top-down approaches are sadly still too prominent even in areas such as reducing health disparities where community action and public engagement across sectors is key to advancing the health equity agenda. Therefore, it is a challenge and a great opportunity for public health, health care, and community development professionals in the twenty-first century to contribute to raising the influence of community and citizen voices on public matters.

Implications of Different Theoretical and Practical Perspectives for Community Mobilization and Citizen Engagement Programs

Over time, community mobilization has been influenced by many different fields (for example, behavioral and social sciences and social marketing) from both theoretical and practical perspectives. Yet, it is a different approach for behavioral and social change that perfectly fits the current emphasis on participatory strategies to communication.

For example, although community mobilization often uses social marketing strategies (see Chapter Two) as well as participatory research, "these terms are not synonymous" (Health Communication Partnership, 2006a). Community mobilization goes beyond participatory research, which involves key groups in the design, implementation, and analysis of research protocols and data related to the health issue and its audiences. Also, community mobilization is a different approach from social marketing.

Fishbein, Goldberg, and Middlestadt (1997) point to the definitions of social marketing and community mobilization in order to highlight their differences. Social marketing is designed to "influence the behavior of target audiences to improve their personal welfare and that of the society of which they are part" (Fishbein, Goldberg, and Middlestadt, 1997, p. 294; Andreasen, 1995, p. 7). Community mobilization seeks to promote community empowerment by developing skills that can be used beyond addressing the specific problem or health issue (Fishbein, Goldberg, and Middlestadt, 1997). It works toward a long-term change in community skills that can be replicated within different communities and segments of society as well as in addressing other kinds of health issues. Community and social mobilization principles are incorporated in several models and planning frameworks (for example, communication for development, COMBI, communication for social change) described in Chapter Two. Also, as previously mentioned (see Chapter Two) social marketing authors and practitioners increasingly emphasize social change as a key outcome of social marketing (Lefebvre, 2013).

In planning a community mobilization effort, community participants are likely to analyze the situation by trying to define the best way for the community to address the health issue. Social marketers are likely to think about the behaviors that need to be influenced for social good and the strategies to accomplish that (Fishbein, Goldberg, and Middlestadt, 1997).

However, even in a participatory and community-driven approach, helping communities to define potential behavioral and social outcomes allows community participants to frame the health issue in a way that will respond to community needs and effectively address it. "A behavioral science orientation can help design interventions aimed at influencing behavioral determinants" (Fishbein, Goldberg, and Middlestadt, 1997, p. 298).

In fact, the influence of marketing models on community mobilization efforts may help community members define and pursue the changes they want to address using a systematic approach. As in other areas of health communication, marketing's major implication for community mobilization is its research-based and structured approach to planning. Still, the emphasis of community mobilization efforts should be primarily on building the capacity of the community to address and prioritize its own problems.

Too often, it is possible to observe in the developing world the vacuum that is left when capacity building is not one of the key priorities of community mobilization as well as larger health communication or public health interventions. As soon as the outsiders leave, communities are left to manage programs and priorities they are not prepared to address. Many times circumstances revert to the original situation shortly after international agencies leave. This is exactly what well-designed and well-implemented community mobilization programs should try to avoid in both the developing and developed worlds. The recent emphasis on behavioral and social outcomes as well as increased community and key group participation in communication efforts is well positioned to accomplish that. As discussed in Chapter Two, several communication planning frameworks, such as UNICEF's Communication for Development (C4D) and Communication for Behavioral Impact (COMBI), emphasize the importance of community participation, ownership, and empowerment.

Moreover, models such as the community action cycle draw on several social change theories and are designed to help communities "acquire the skills and resources to plan, implement and evaluate health-related actions and policies" (Lavery and others, 2005, p. 611). Under the community action cycle, outcomes are defined in terms of changes in "social norms, policies, culture, and the supporting environment" (Health Communication Partnership, 2006a) so that results can be sustainable and lead to new social norms in support of health behaviors. Instead, under COMBI, the model for communication for behavioral impact adopted and refined by the World Health Organization [WHO] (2003), community mobilization efforts, which are also participatory and aim at building community skills, emphasize the importance of behavioral results as a key program outcome even when the program ultimately aims at social change.

Whether the emphasis is on behavioral or social outcomes should be determined by the unique characteristics of the health issue being addressed as well as those of the specific communities and audiences, and their existing health and social behaviors (see Chapter One). Yet, there are two important mantras to remember, which are strictly interconnected and somewhat cyclical:

- Social change occurs only as a result of gradual behavioral changes at different levels of society.

- Sustainable behavioral results at the individual, community, or population levels can be achieved only by addressing barriers to behavior adoption and implementation, social norms, and key determinants of health.

Ideally, all interventions should aim at creating permanent changes in social rules and community or health system structure. This is also in agreement with some of the key premises of the larger public health field of community health. In fact, "the movement called community health means more than just access to health care. It's strong families, good schools, safe neighborhoods, caring adults, and economic opportunities" (Emanoil, 2002, p. 16). Community health rightly regards disparities in health as going beyond individual behavior and actually being influenced by several socially determined factors as well as the kind of social support (or lack of) people receive throughout their lifetime, and more specifically at times of disease and crisis.

Box 6.2 offers a case study showing the correlation between behavior and disease burden and highlights how community mobilization can effectively address that. In reviewing this case study, readers should take into account that this intervention was aimed at reducing the impact of a sudden health crisis. Strategies used in this case may be different from more extensive interventions that would address and sustain a health behavior. Nevertheless, the case study provides a helpful example of the direct correlation among behavior, social engagement, and health outcomes, and how community mobilization, and, more generally, community-based interventions should be integrated also in epidemics, emerging diseases, and humanitarian emergency settings (see "The Case for Community Mobilization and Citizen Engagement in Risk and Emergency Communication" in this chapter for further discussion of this topic).

BOX 6.2. SOCIAL MOBILIZATION TO FIGHT EBOLA IN YAMBIO, SOUTHERN SUDAN

Controlling communicable diseases demands not only medical expertise but also social education. To meet this goal, WHO has adopted a type of social mobilization known as communication for behavioral impact (COMBI) that focuses on influencing behavior at the individual and community levels. This strategy was implemented in Yambio from late May to June 2004 during an outbreak of Ebola hemorrhagic fever that resulted in seventeen confirmed cases, including seven deaths.

In late May, WHO's social mobilization experts from the WHO Mediterranean Centre for Vulnerability Reduction (Tunis, Tunisia) were included among the international WHO-coordinated Ebola response team. On arrival in Yambio, their first task was to determine what changes in behavior were necessary to contain the Ebola outbreak.

The social mobilization team was immediately confronted with numerous misconceptions about the outbreak. For example, many people in Yambio were unconvinced that there was actually an Ebola outbreak, and others believed that blood and skin samples were being removed from patients and sold. There was also an unsubstantiated fear of the isolation ward, wariness of the surveillance teams, and other irrational beliefs. For example, some people refused to leave home between 5:00 and 7:00 pm, believing this would reduce their risk of contracting Ebola.

To counter these misconceptions, the social mobilization team, which included pastors, teachers, and community development workers (who wore uniforms to increase credibility), spoke to villagers daily at their homes, marketplaces, restaurants, churches, and schools. Simple measures were emphasized, such as asking sick individuals to contact the Ebola team within twenty-four hours of the onset of symptoms, recommending to people that they avoid direct contact with sick individuals, and suggesting that the community refrain from traditional practices of sleeping next to or touching dead bodies for the duration of the outbreak.

A key element of the team's strategy was the distribution of informational pamphlets, which answered basic Ebola questions, as well as dispelling common rumors. Recognizing the stigma that accompanies Ebola, the social mobilization team also worked to explain the need for the isolation ward at Yambio Hospital, and included pictures of the ward in the pamphlet, to show the local population that the fence around the ward was short enough for patients to see and talk to their family and friends from a safe distance.

By placing communities at the center of the social mobilization program, the rapid containment of the Ebola outbreak in Yambio can be attributed largely to the efforts of local people themselves. As WHO and partners gain more experience in identifying and responding to Ebola outbreaks, social mobilization will undoubtedly continue to play an important role in the successful containment of future outbreaks.

Source: World Health Organization. "Social Mobilization to Fight Ebola in Yambio, Southern Sudan." Action Against Infection, 2004c. http://wmc.who.int/pdf/Action_Against_Infection.pdf. Used by permission.

Community (or social) mobilization has been positioned by several authors and organizations as a key component of global health communication, especially in the context of behavior and social change models (WHO, 2003; Health Communication Partnership, 2006b; Patel, 2005; Renganthan and others, 2005; Obregon and Waisbord, 2010; Schiavo, 2010a; UNICEF, 2013a). For example, in Namibia, one of the core elements of the Health Communication Partnership (2006a) communication program is a community mobilization effort aimed at increasing HIV community awareness as well as the use of HIV preventive measures and competent health services.

Still, community mobilization is not an all-inclusive tool to address community health issues. Its likelihood for success is related to the use of an integrated multifaceted approach in which other tools and areas of communication are used to reinforce the community change process. Multiple channels (for example, mass media, new media, theater, interpersonal communication channels) should be used to share relevant information or reach out to specific key groups with tailored messages in order to create the kind of support needed for behavioral or social change within a community. Most important, community mobilization efforts should complement other relevant public health and community development interventions.

Impact of Community Mobilization on Health-Related Knowledge and Practices

As in other areas of health communication, community mobilization efforts aim to influence health behavior as well as social norms and policies that may have an impact on health outcomes. This section reviews some of the key aspects and potential outcomes of the process of influencing health-related knowledge and practices through community mobilization interventions.

Reliance on Community Members

Communicating ideas about health and behavior as well as social issues related to health outcomes is a long and difficult process. Using a peer-to-peer approach, such as relying on credible community members, to diffuse new ideas and prompt action may shorten this process (Babalola and others, 2001). For example, the Office of Minority Health Resource Center (OMHRC) of the Department of Health and Human Resources (DHHS) Office of Minority Health (OMH) has been successfully using a peer-to-peer communication approach for their preconception peer educator (PPE) program, which seeks to raise awareness of high rates of infant mortality among African Americans and to encourage the adoption of preconception health behaviors among trained PPEs (college and graduate students) and the communities they reach (Office of Minority Health, 2013; Schiavo, Gonzales-Flores, Ramesh, and Estrada-Portales, 2011; Schiavo, 2012b).

Because of the involvement and leadership of community members in the different phases of program planning, implementation, and scaling up, community mobilization can be a time-saving and effective approach to influence health-related knowledge and practices. When external organizations, health communicators, and other kinds of facilitators approach a community, they should always identify, engage, and train local leaders who have an interest in the issue as well as in involving their communities and carrying on the mobilization process. This may pass through many different stages, which include but are not limited to communication and disease-specific training. Several experiences have pointed to the importance of identifying an adequate number of social mobilization partners as well as training and engagement on interpersonal communication and community dialogue skills (Schiavo, 2009b; Schiavo and Kapil, 2009). Such partners can include women's groups, teachers, community and religious leaders, community health workers, local government officials, and many others who feel passionate about a specific issue, and care about the well-being of their community.

Sometimes people who are well suited to become community leaders because of personal characteristics and social status lack specific knowledge and understanding of the health problem's relevance within the community. Other times potential leaders need to go through a process of change themselves. Sometimes leaders already exist within a community and are ready to facilitate the process of change but may need technical assistance in the planning and implementation of the process (as in the case study featured in Box 6.1). Other times people may become leaders because of life events or the exposure to engaging communication tools and activities that influence their core beliefs and attitudes, prompt a personal change, and make them want to help others. The example in Box 6.3 shows the different phases of the process of personal growth, disease awareness, and commitment to the prevention of sexually transmitted diseases (STDs) that a young man in Kenya experienced after attending a few community theater sessions on the topic, and engaging in a series of discussions with the health communication staff and the local coordinators from the Program for Appropriate Technology in Health, an international health organization that had developed the theater sessions.

BOX 6.3. HOW BINGWA CHANGED HIS WAYS

At age twenty-four, Bingwa (not his real name) represents the typical Kenyan out-of-school youth: unemployed and hot-blooded, but generally hopeful and lively. He had been a regular attendee of the community theater sessions organized by Program for Appropriate Technology in Health (PATH), an international nonprofit organization, in collaboration with the local Rojo-Rojo troupe in Mumias, in Kenya's western province.

Between January and September 2002, Bingwa's life evolved dramatically. This very average young man—married, father of a fifteen-month-old son, sexually active outside his marriage but insulated by a sense that he was not at risk of any infection—became one of the first youths to be stimulated by Magnet Theatre to navigate a course to new personal behavior that has made him a community role model. He volunteered to go for voluntary counseling and testing (VCT), learned for himself that he was not infected, and took serious steps to reduce his sexual risk by taking charge of his personal life.

Bingwa made a living by taking care of his uncle's four rental houses and eked out his income by selling Coca-Cola and odds and ends from a kiosk. His buddies would hang around at the kiosk, talking about politics, football, jobs, and girls. Bingwa, married and with a child, was economically better off than his friends, and indeed the de facto group leader. There was a time, in his bachelor days, when his house used to be known as "The Butchery" in recognition of the fact that the young men in the estate would bring girls over there for sex. Bingwa was always happy to make his house available and disappear for a while.

Bingwa's first questions came on a Friday in January 2002, at the end of a session of community theater by the Rojo-Rojo Magnet Theatre troupe. PATH's theater coordinator, Madiang, was looking forward to the weekend and was packing up after a Magnet Theatre show.

Bingwa approached Madiang, and after a few moments of small talk, asked, "Say, is an STI [sexually transmitted infection] the same as AIDS?"

Madiang answered in the negative. But Bingwa became pensive and launched a second question: "Okay, then, if they are not the same, does an STI later become AIDS if it is not treated?"

Madiang explained to Bingwa the difference between STI and HIV, and that HIV is just one of various STIs. After citing some examples of other STIs, he offered an explanation on how some STIs can pave the way to infection with HIV.

Bingwa now asked, rather hesitantly, "So which STIs are treatable?"

As they spoke, Madiang was trying to understand why Bingwa was asking these questions. He came to several assumptions: Bingwa could be infected with an STI; he might be seeking treatment for that STI; he could be concerned about his HIV status. He possibly engaged in multipartner or unprotected sex.

Ironically, Bingwa believed that he was not at risk for HIV at that time, even though he was regularly having unprotected sex with multiple partners outside his marriage. Bingwa wrongly believed that one could get HIV only from a sex worker.

Three weeks later, Bingwa had more questions, this time about VCT, which had been the topic of the play. What was VCT? Does the test also check for the other STIs? Must someone undergo the counseling in order to be tested?

In truth, Bingwa had already heard about VCT but did not understand it well. He confessed that it was at the Magnet Theatre discussions that he had begun wondering if he might be a candidate for VCT. The enactments had led him to start reflecting on his former life. He had become convinced that he was probably infected with an STI and that it was only a matter of time before this issue came to light. VCT seemed to him an opportunity to check his STI status.

These questions also seem to have been a turning point in Bingwa's life. It was after asking these questions that he "sat back alone in the kiosk and really looked at his life." Every answer he received only confirmed his fear that he was already infected. It was around this point that he decided, in his words, to "stop engaging in sex, even with my wife. I was afraid!" Bingwa had never met anyone who had gone for VCT and even doubted whether anyone actually did.

Not long after, Bingwa decided to go for VCT. He spoke to Madiang in private for nearly one-and-a-half hours and asked him more questions than he ever had before. He would listen to the answers keenly, be quiet for a while, and then launch another question. Two days later, Bingwa became one of the first young men to go for VCT as a result of his exposure to the Magnet Theatre process.

Bingwa's life has not been the same since he went for VCT. He has already spoken out on a popular Kenyan radio serial drama produced by PATH, Kati Yetu, strongly urging others to go for VCT and reflect on their sexual lives and behaviors. Standing in front of his peers in a Magnet Theatre session, Bingwa pledged that he would no longer engage in multipartner sex. As of that year's end, Bingwa affirmed that he had had neither extramarital nor unprotected sex. That was six months after he adopted a new behavior. Today Bingwa has become a role model in his community and has helped innumerable numbers of his peers to also go for VCT. He is often asked to share his experience and the benefits of VCT, information he is always willing to give out.

And his house is no longer called "The Butchery."

Advancing Knowledge and Changing Practices

Regardless of how leaders decide to become engaged in the community mobilization process, this approach has proven to be effective in prompting changes in people's health knowledge and practices. For example, one of the most important lessons learned in the past few decades is that "a fully mobilized and supportive environment is a crucial element of effective HIV prevention" (Amoah, 2001, p. 1).

In the United States, gay activists have played a fundamental role in controlling the AIDS epidemic. By speaking up, they have helped break the cycle of misinformation, shame, and stigma that is still an issue in too much of society, but was even more relevant in the early years of the epidemic, and risked paralyzing any form of progress. AIDS activists not only have ensured that "HIV prevention, treatment and care stayed a global, national and local priority" (Gay Men's Health Crisis, 2006) but have also influenced disease awareness, drug approval regulations, work-related policies, prevention and treatment strategies, and access to medications, to name a few accomplishments. In doing so, the gay community, which started the overall AIDS activism movement in the United States, has involved different segments of society and contributed to show that AIDS is not only a gay disease. Box 6.4 presents a time line of AIDS events that summarizes some of the most important stages and results of this community mobilization process. The example also highlights that many of the policy and social changes were triggered by knowledge and behavioral changes at the legislative, general public, and scientific community levels.

BOX 6.4. GAY MEN'S HEALTH CRISIS HIV/AIDS TIME LINE

1981	CDC reports Kaposi's sarcoma in healthy gay men.
	New York Times announces "rare cancer" in forty-one gay men.
	Eighty men gather in New York to address "gay cancer" and raise money for research.
	CDC declares the new disease an epidemic.

1982   GMHC (Gay Men's Health Crisis) is officially established.

An answering machine, which acts as the world's first AIDS hotline, receives more than one hundred calls the first night.

GMHC holds its second AIDS fundraiser; produces and distributes fifty thousand free copies of its first newsletter to doctors, hospitals, clinics, and the Library of Congress and creates buddy program to assist PWAs (persons with AIDS).

CDC changes the name from *gay cancer* to *AIDS*.

1983   PWAs form National Association of People with AIDS (NAPWA).

GMHC funds litigation of first AIDS discrimination suit.

New York State (NYS) Department of Health AIDS Institute established.

1984   CDC requests GMHC's help to plan public conferences on AIDS.

GMHC publishes its first safer sex guidelines.

The human immunodeficiency virus (HIV) is isolated in France and later in the United States.

1985   Revelation that Rock Hudson, a US TV and movie star, has AIDS makes the disease a household word.

FDA approves first test to screen for antibodies to HIV.

The American Association of Blood Banks and the Red Cross begin screening blood for HIV antibodies and rejecting gay donors.

GMHC's art auction is world's first million-dollar AIDS fundraiser.

First international conference on AIDS held in Atlanta, Georgia.

CDC estimates one million HIV-infected people worldwide.

US military starts mandatory HIV testing.

First conference to discuss AIDS in communities of color held in New York City.

1986   New York City's first anonymous testing site opens.

GMHC's client base now includes heterosexual men and women, hemophiliacs, intravenous drug users, and children.

US surgeon general calls for AIDS education for children of all ages.

GMHC holds first AIDS walk in New York City.

Several states pass bills to ban PWAs from food-handling and educational jobs, making it a crime to transmit HIV, and force testing of prostitutes.

1987   AZT, the first drug approved to fight HIV, is marketed.

President Reagan uses the word *AIDS* in public for the first time.

CDC expands the definition of AIDS.

The United States shuts its doors to HIV-infected immigrants and travelers.

Political attacks against GMHC and educational efforts on safer sex that "encourage or promote homosexual sexual activity."

1988	Condom use is shown to be effective in HIV prevention.
	The first World AIDS Day held on December 1.
	Surgeon general mails 107 million copies of "Understanding AIDS" to every US household. The United States bans discrimination against federal workers with HIV.
1989	GMHC leads successful effort to draft and pass New York State's AIDS-Related Information Bill, ensuring confidentiality. GMHC and other AIDS organizations protest against US immigration policies.
1990	AIDS activist Ryan White's death points to need for urgent funding legislation.
	The Ryan White Comprehensive AIDS Resources Emergency (CARE) Act passes, authorizing $881 million in emergency relief.
	Americans with Disabilities Act (ADA) signed to protect people with disabilities, including people with HIV, from discrimination.
	The first book to talk about long-term survivors of AIDS is published.
	The first GMHC dance-a-thon raises over $1 million.
	US AIDS deaths pass the one hundred thousand mark.
1991	Earvin "Magic" Johnson announces he is HIV-positive, becoming the first celebrity to admit contracting HIV via heterosexual sex.
	Condoms become available in New York City high schools after months of debate.
	A Roper poll commissioned by GMHC finds that a majority of Americans believe that more explicit AIDS education is needed.
1992	In response to mounting activism and protest, FDA starts "accelerated approval" to get drugs to PWAs faster.
	A federal court strikes down proposed "offensiveness" restrictions on AIDS education materials.
	First time that a US president is elected on a campaign platform that also contains HIV and AIDS issues.
1993	CDC expands the definition of AIDS. New AIDS diagnoses expected to increase by as much as 100 percent as a result of the change.
	Over 13,800 PWAs have been clients of GMHC at this point.
	The CDC, NIH, and FDA jointly declare that condoms are "highly effective" for prevention of HIV infection.
1994	GMHC begins a New York City subway campaign aimed at gay, lesbian, and heterosexual young adults.
	WHO estimates 19.5 million HIV-infected people worldwide.

1995	CDC announces that AIDS is the leading cause of death among Americans aged twenty-five to forty-four.
	The FDA approves the first in a new class of drugs called protease inhibitors.
1996	The FDA approves the sale of first home HIV test kit.
	GMHC launches its first prevention campaign for HIV-negative men.
	The FDA approves HIV viral load test, used to track HIV progression and efficacy of combination therapy.
	Cover stories hailing AIDS breakthroughs and the "end" of the epidemic start appearing in major US publications.
1997	The first human trials of an AIDS vaccine begin.
	WHO estimates 30.6 million HIV-infected people worldwide.
	GMHC begins providing on-site HIV testing and counseling services.
1998	GMHC launches the largest survey of gay and bisexual men, "Beyond 2000 Sexual Health Survey."
	New York State HIV Reporting and Partner Notification Act signed, requiring that cases of HIV (not just AIDS) be reported to the Department of Health.
	A GMHC study reports that an estimated 69,000 people in New York State have HIV but remain unaware.
1999	First large-scale study of young gay men finds that large numbers have been infected in the last two years, many of them black men.
2000	As the result of years of lobbying by HIV/AIDS organizations, New York State passes legislation decriminalizing sale and possession of syringes without prescription.
	The CDC reports that black and Latino men now account for more AIDS cases among gay men than white men.
	The GMHC AIDS Hotline becomes accessible via e-mail.
2001	Twentieth year of AIDS epidemic.
	In response to the arrest of participants in needle exchange program, federal court rules that police may not interfere with public health initiatives that combat disease through education and prevention.
	UN General Assembly adopts global blueprint for action on HIV/AIDS and calls for creation of $7 to $10 billion global fund for the developing world.
	Abstinence-only HIV prevention programs begin to be promoted by US government.

2002	The FDA approves a new rapid HIV testing device.
	GMHC joins activists to protest US underfunding of domestic and global AIDS programs.
	GMHC begins offering on-site hepatitis C testing and launches new initiative looking at gay men's health in broader context.
2003	GMHC holds eighteenth annual New York AIDS Walk.
	US bill authorizing up to $15 billion for global AIDS, TB, and malaria treatment and prevention for twelve African and two Caribbean countries is signed.
	Activists express doubts about provision that assigns abstinence-only programs a third of USAID's prevention funding.
2004	GMHC launches a new women's institute to explore new approaches to HIV prevention, particularly for women of color.
2006	About 38.6 million people are estimated to be living with HIV and AIDS worldwide.
2009	President Obama and the Office of National AIDS Policy unveil the "9$\frac{1}{2}$ Minutes" campaign. Every nine-and-a-half minutes, someone in the United States becomes infected with HIV, equaling more than fifty-six thousand new infections each year.
2011	GMHC celebrate its thirtieth anniversary and is recognized by the White House as a pivotal organization in the HIV/AIDS field.
2012	AIDS Walk New York commemorates its twenty-seventh year as an event at the forefront of the fight against HIV/AIDS.

Source: Gay Men's Health Crisis. Gay Men's Health Crisis HIV/AIDS Timeline. New York: Gay Men's Health Crisis (GMHC), 2013. Used by permission.

As another example, in India and Armenia, a community mobilization effort that was implemented within a multichannel behavior change strategy was shown to improve knowledge and practices in many areas of childhood diseases management, including "improvements in births attended by skilled practitioners, exclusive breastfeeding, immunization, and HIV/AIDS awareness and prevention knowledge" (Baranick and Ricca, 2005). Efficient mobilization requires regular and efficient information exchange, and new media and mobile technology have provided low-cost options for information exchange in many settings.

The list of disease areas and health issues in which community mobilization has made or could make a difference is endless. By empowering people to take their lives and health in their own hands, community mobilization can produce long-lasting results in health behaviors and practices as part of a multidisciplinary and multifaceted approach.

Key Steps of Community Mobilization Programs

There are several models and frameworks that describe the key steps of community mobilization. Although some of the stages they describe may be different or use interchangeable terms, a few general criteria are common to all of them or reflect practical experience. These steps also apply to citizen engagement but need to be considered in a larger scale.

- The importance of understanding the community's key characteristics, structure, values, needs, attitudes, social norms, health behaviors, and priorities

- A cross-cultural communication approach through which health communicators and other community mobilizers should refrain from any form of cultural bias in exchanging information about health systems, beliefs, and behaviors, as well as other kinds of topics

- The need for engaging community members at the outset of the intervention, including during the community assessment or participatory research phase (and whenever possible, prior to that)

- A research-based planning process that should respond and evolve according to community needs and priorities

- An emphasis on capacity building and community autonomy, and ownership of the overall communication and goal-setting process

- An efficient information-exchange process that relies on culturally competent communication channels and venues

- A rigorous evaluation process that needs to be mutually agreed on by all community members and leaders, identifies behavioral or social outcomes as key evaluation parameters, and includes a number of other evaluation measurements to monitor progress and process at different stages

- The ability for the process to be replicated during the scaling-up phase (in which the program is expanded to reach other communities and regions) as well as to address similar issues within the community

Following are a few examples of models for community mobilization that incorporate all these criteria in different phases or by using slightly different terminologies. Methodologies used for most of these steps are common to the planning and implementation process of the overall field of health communication, and are described in further detail in Part Three of this book.

Common Terms and Steps in Community Mobilization

Community mobilization is a long-term process that relies on a variety of sequential yet interdependent steps and activities. Some of the most common terms and phases of community mobilization are described next, starting with how to select and engage community organizations and leaders.

Engaging Community Organizations and Leaders

Before conducting any community mobilization effort, health communicators and other community mobilizers need to identify communities that may have an interest in participating in such effort. The following key criteria should be considered:

- The community has expressed a preliminary interest in participating and places a high priority on the specific health issue.
- There are high rates of disease incidence, morbidity, and mortality within the community.
- Specific community characteristics can be used as a model for replication of the effort.
- The health issue is relevant to the community's health and development.
- There are relevant special needs or issues.

Engaging and equipping community leaders with potential new skills they may need to be effective participants in the overall communication process (including defining the key elements and initial steps of the intervention) are critical and should be part of the initial community engagement process.

This phase should be informed by preliminary formative research, including analysis of secondary data (literature, articles, and other information compiled by others) as well as stakeholders' interviews, which will inform health communicators about how to approach the community regarding the specific health issue. At this stage, key stakeholders may include representatives of local nongovernmental organizations (NGOs), companies, international health agencies, local churches, women's groups, government, and everyone who can provide initial information on the community's key characteristics, structure, and issues as well as existing interventions in the same health area. Formative research can also be instrumental in identifying potential community leaders.

Preliminary research findings and analysis should be shared with community members formally and informally. For example, as part of a joint malaria prevention effort in Angola by UNICEF and the local ministry of health, preliminary research findings were shared first with a team of government officers, and then with a larger group representing local NGOs, companies, universities, and other key stakeholders (Schiavo, 1998, 2000). This gave an opportunity to all participants to brainstorm about the findings, prioritize their relevance within the community, and develop preliminary strategies for a community outreach effort aimed at enhancing malaria awareness as well as the use of insecticide-treated mosquito nets for malaria protection (Schiavo and Robson, 1999). At the same time, this helped recruit and train community members for the participatory research effort and other phases of the program.

Of great importance in approaching any community to share information and to initiate a dialogue on a specific health issue is to take into account community needs, preferences, and existing priorities. For example, in approaching a refugee camp in any underserved region of the world to discuss malaria prevention and potential interventions, facilitators should be prepared to hear that the main concern among community members may not be malaria at all but actually food supplies, transportation, and others. Because these are very important priorities, health communication practitioners and community leaders should make all attempts to build trust, make sure community members feel they have been heard, provide links to resources and people who may address other priority issues, and make linkages between community-specific priorities and the health topic being discussed. Chances are that many different determinants of health, including those highlighted by the community, are contributing to disease severity and overall impact. For example, "malaria and poverty are intimately connected" (Gallup and Sachs, 2001, p. 85). Malaria exacerbates the impact of malnutrition, is a deterrent for foreign investment and tourism, and "has lifelong effects on cognitive development and education levels through the impact of chronic malaria-induced anemia and time lost or wasted in the classroom due to illness" (Gallup and Sachs, 2001, p. 85). As with other health conditions for which significant health disparities exist, malaria is a key determinant of socioeconomic development just as much as nutrition, transportation, education, and economic opportunities are key determinants of malaria severity and overall impact. This kind of analysis should be part of community-based conversations when approaching community members to share information on any kind of health issue.

Participatory Research

participatory research (community-driven assessment, participatory needs assessment, community-needs assessment)
A collaborative research effort that involves community members, researchers, community mobilizers, and interested agencies and organizations. It is a two-way dialogue that starts with the people, and through which the community understands and identifies key issues, priorities, and potential actions.

Participatory research, also referred to as **community-driven assessment, participatory needs assessment** (Centers for Disease Control [CDC], 2006i), and **community-needs assessment**, is a collaborative research effort that involves community members, researchers, community mobilizers, and interested agencies and organizations. It is a two-way dialogue that starts with the people, and through which the community understands and identifies key issues, priorities, and potential actions. Participatory research should inform and guide all phases of the community mobilization effort.

The US Agency for Healthcare Research and Quality (AHRQ) defines participatory research as "an approach to health and environmental research meant to increase the value of studies for both researchers and the community being studied" (Viswanathan and others, 2004, p. 1). Participatory research uses traditional research methodologies such as focus groups and one-on-one or group interviews. Another important method for participatory research is community dialogue, which is discussed in Chapter Four, because it is a form of interpersonal communication at scale.

Although the community should be involved in designing the research protocol and questions as well as recruiting research participants and analyzing research findings, experience shows that "participation levels vary" and depend on many factors, related to both the community and the health communication and research teams (Mercer, Potter, and Green, 2002). Also, the concept of participation may mean different things to different people and institutions.

Ideally, the community should be the main protagonist of this process. This phase should represent an opportunity to exchange information; understand community preferences, concerns, and priorities; and identify culturally appropriate communication activities, channels, messages, and spokespeople, as well as the behavioral or social outcomes that would need to be achieved through the intervention.

Community Group Meetings

Community group meetings involve larger segments of the community in addition to the original members who have been recruited for the participatory research phase. They can be existing meetings (for example, monthly administrative meetings of a women's group, hospital, or other kind of community) that are used to inform and engage community members in the community mobilization efforts. They can also be specifically organized for other reasons:

- Sharing participatory research findings and securing feedback from a larger number of community members
- Informing about the health issue, its relevance to the community, and potential behavioral or social changes that have been identified during formative or participatory research, and then securing feedback and suggestions on all elements
- Advancing understanding of the community's priorities and needs
- Promoting an ongoing dialogue among community members on the health issue and its potential solutions as well as other community priorities
- Motivating and engaging additional volunteers or community leaders to participate in the community mobilization effort
- Identifying roles and responsibilities of community members for program implementation
- Addressing other community- or issue-specific topics

Ideally, community leaders should conduct these meetings with the help, when necessary, of health communicators and other facilitators. Sometimes if local leaders are not ready or adequately trained to conduct such meetings, the community mobilization external team could take the lead, but only after discussing and agreeing on meeting strategies and agenda with relevant community leaders.

Partnership Meetings

Once the community has identified its key priorities and actions, partnership meetings can be held to define and start establishing collaborations among community members, agencies, and organizations that have participated so far in the process or to introduce them to potential new partners and organizations. These kinds of meetings should attempt to achieve several goals:

- Define the roles and responsibilities of all different partners
- Advance agreement on standard procedures and specific contributions to the community mobilization effort
- Develop strategies and action plans

- Define and mutually agree on evaluation parameters
- Discuss lessons learned
- Provide an update on progress

A discussion on establishing and maintaining partnerships is included in Chapter Eight of this book.

Mobilization Tools for Urban Communities

Although all the methods and tools discussed so far also apply to mobilization efforts in urban settings, some other methods may also be very helpful in mobilizing urban communities. Urban health settings present many similarities but also several distinguishing features from other geographical, cultural, and physical contexts. Several authors have dwelled on the key characteristics of urban environments and their implications for public health, health care, and community development interventions and outcomes. Although some of these factors include social determinants of health that are not unique to urban environments, they are often "transformed when viewed through the characteristics of cities such as size, density, diversity, and complexity" (Vlahov and others, 2007, p. 16) and contribute to health challenges that may be unique to, or exacerbated by, urban environments, including "poverty, violence, social exclusion, pollution, substandard housing, the unmet needs of elderly and young people, homeless people and migrants, unhealthy spatial planning, the lack of participatory practices and the need to seriously address inequality and sustainable development" (Waelkens and Greindl, 2001, p. 18).

In this context, mobilization tools may need to be expanded to be inclusive of different groups, to account for geographical distances, and to address perhaps higher levels of diversity than in smaller communities or rural areas. Some tools that may be helpful in urban settings include the following:

participatory influential road mapping
A participatory and community-driven process to identify key stakeholders and other influentials who need to be engaged as part of the community mobilization and citizen engagement process

- **Participatory influential road mapping**, a participatory and community-driven process to identify key stakeholders and other influentials who need to be engaged as part of the community mobilization and citizen engagement process. Although identifying key influentials is key to all kinds of mobilization efforts, it is perhaps even more relevant in urban settings where health communication practitioners and other team members may be faced with a large number of influencers that are specific to the different groups living in a given city.

- Strategic partnership training to make sure that different communities and professionals understand key success factors and the dos and don'ts of successful multisectoral partnership and are well equipped to plan and execute them. A more detailed discussion on strategic partnerships and constituency relations is included in Chapter Eight. This may be designed as preliminary to action planning and partnership meetings.

- **Consensus-building workshops**, which may be embedded as part of community meetings and facilitate the building of consensus as well as momentum on key priority issues and innovative ways to address them. These meetings should lead to a shared vision of the future that communities want to build for themselves and their children because it relates to a specific health or social issue.

consensus-building workshops
Workshops that facilitate the building of consensus as well as momentum on key priority issues and innovative ways to address them

Public Consultations

Public consultation is a process in which the general public is asked to provide input on policies or other matters that may affect them. An example of public consultation is the one conducted by the Canadian government in the prepandemic flu phase (prior to the H1NI flu outbreak of 2009) to assess citizen and stakeholders' priorities on pandemic flu mitigation, including antiviral stockpile and prophylaxis (Schiavo, 2009b). Such consultation was implemented via several delivered dialogue sessions with citizens and health and nonhealth stakeholders. **Delivered dialogue** is a method for public dialogue and consultation that usually relies on the use of specific discussion tools, including a discussion guide, sequence of questions, and briefing materials and instructions for dialogue facilitators. The consultation empowered the Canadian public on deciding fund allocations for different pandemic flu interventions, and revealed that citizens regarded public health communication as a means of prevention (to be supported by adequate funding), and preferred to invest funds in antiviral supplies only as stockpiles for treatment interventions and not as a preventive measure (prophylaxis) (Schiavo, 2009b).

Another example of public consultations is the **referendum** (a vote on a ballot question in which the entire electorate is asked to accept or reject a policy change). Referendums on specific policy issues are conducted in many countries, including Italy. Yet, public costs of referendums are prohibitive for many developed and developing countries, thus delivered dialogue may be a more cost-effective method for public consultation (in addition to enabling qualitative assessment of public needs and preferences).

public consultation
A process in which the general public is asked to provide input on policies or other matters that may affect them

delivered dialogue
A method for public dialogue and consultation that usually relies on the use of specific discussion tools, including a discussion guide, sequence of questions, and briefing materials and instructions for dialogue facilitators

referendum
A vote on a ballot question in which the entire electorate is asked to accept or reject a policy change

Culturally Competent Communication Approaches, Channels, and Messengers

Community mobilization is complemented by or relies on many different communication approaches and channels, such as theater, traditional media, new media, brochures, home visits, workshops, and rallies. (A detailed discussion about the development of communication messages and tools is included in Part Three of this book as part of the overall health communication planning and implementation processes.)

Nevertheless, it is important to note here that all strategies and action plans need to include community-based methodologies, channels, and venues (for example, existing meetings and communication vehicles), address community priorities and needs, and support behavioral or social outcomes. Most important, communication tools and messages need to be developed and delivered by and for the people.

All communication approaches, channels, and messengers or spokespeople should be carefully selected and evaluated vis-à-vis their cultural adequacy. As effective information exchange is key to the success of community mobilization efforts, communication channels should be culturally competent. Yet, of equal importance is that such channels are traditionally used to share health-related information and not only to communicate on other topics.

For example, traditional media such as community radio have been successfully used to announce community meetings and reinforce health messages. Radio is a popular communication vehicle in many developing countries (and is still quite popular in many Western countries), which has been traditionally used also for health communication programs. In the new media era, mobile technology, which is fast advancing also in developing countries, has been used to communicate in between regular community meetings, to share information in disaster or public health emergency settings as well as to build people's capacity to help each other, and to provide information to other team members on early signs and indicators that external factors may change and therefore affect programming (Mercy Corps, 2013). Although new media are valuable communication tools in community mobilization, in many parts of the world there is still no substitute for interpersonal communication venues and channels, because word-of-mouth, trusted community leaders and social mobilization partners, community-friendly venues, and ultimately human interactions continue to account for a large percentage of all kinds of communications on health and illness. Therefore, it is important to research and identify culturally competent communication channels to facilitate the exchange of information and ideas during the community mobilization or citizen engagement process.

Community Action Cycle or Model

Several versions of the community action model have evolved over time. Some of them include evaluation as one of the key steps (Health Communication Partnership, 2006c) whereas others consider evaluation a separate step from the overall cycle (Lavery and others, 2005). Some also include a scaling-up phase (Health Communication Partnership, 2006c), and others describe scaling up as a separate process. Including evaluation and scaling up as part of the overall planning and implementation cycle may signal the importance of these steps to inform and guide follow-up interventions as well as the replication of the same intervention in other communities at different times. Nevertheless, fundamental premises of this model remain the same and include community participation, emphasis on social outcomes, capacity building, and the importance of an ongoing dialogue among community members in relation to health issues (Health Communication Partnership, 2006c; Lavery and others, 2005).

Under this model, health communicators and other facilitators assist the community in "creating an environment in which the individuals can empower themselves to address their own and their community health issues" (Health Communication Partnership, 2006a). One of the versions for this model includes the following key steps (Health Communication Partnership, 2006c):

- "Organize the community for action" by identifying community leaders who have an interest in becoming engaged in the process, training them, and facilitating the discussion about issues that are important to the community.

- "Explore health issues and set priorities" using participatory research.

- "Plan together" to establish the community actions that need to be implemented to support social change and address the specific health issue. Actions need to be achievable, sustainable, and have the potential "to persuade groups, organizations or agencies to make policy changes" (Lavery and others, 2005, p. 615). They may include different kinds of activities such as lobbying with local governments, stakeholder presentations about a specific health issue, or organizing a health fair.

- "Act together" in the implementation of the actions previously defined.

- "Evaluate together" through a process of participatory evaluation in which all community members and program partners compare actual outcomes with the presumed social outcomes defined at the outset of the program.

The major difference of this model compared with other participatory models used by the World Health Organization (2003), the Centers for Disease Control (2006j, about the CDC's syphilis elimination effort), or other key organizations is its emphasis on social outcomes instead of behavioral outcomes. When the specific health situation as well as the community characteristics and level of preparedness allow for it, this model is well suited to address health disparities (Lavery and others, 2005) and other broader social issues related to health. Still, it is always important to remember that social change begins and ends with a series of behavioral changes at the individual, group, community, and policymaker levels and within multiple sectors of society, which in turn help create the right social, infrastructural, and policy conditions for health behaviors to be adopted and sustained.

The Case for Community Mobilization and Citizen Engagement in Risk and Emergency Communication

"The increased complexity of the public health and aid environments have been recently calling for a more systematic and theory-based approach for public health emergency and risk communication" (Schiavo, 2010a, p. 18). Within this context the case for integrating community mobilization and citizen engagement strategies with other communication areas, including mass media and new media communication, interpersonal communication, and others, has been made by both theoretical and practical experiences (Schiavo 2007b, 2009c; Schoch-Spana and others, 2006; Communication Initiative, 2008).

Public health emergency and risk communication within epidemics, emerging disease outbreaks, and humanitarian emergency settings (with the latter setting often leading to increased health risks and crises) present specific challenges. These include the need to communicate at times of uncertain science and certain deadlines; the clear danger or threat emergencies pose; and most important, the need to leave no one behind, avoid further harm, and concomitantly address people's emotional and psychological reactions to crisis that, along with social norms and culture, may prevent the adoption and sustainability of mitigation measures (Schiavo, 2009b, 2009c, 2010a). Yet, public health emergency and risk communication should be also grounded in theory and lessons learned from past experiences and inspired by the key characteristics of health communication in the twenty-first century (Schiavo, 2007b) as also described in Chapter One. Within this context, citizen engagement and community mobilization strategies have contributed to the following (Schiavo, 2009b, 2009c; Schoch-Spana and others, 2006; Communication Initiative, 2008):

- "Greater ability to govern and maintain trust during a crisis

- Ability to complement existing services or provide services that neither national authorities of the market can provide

- Increased feasibility of emergency plans and recommended behaviors and other mitigation measures," which as a result of community engagement can be tailored to reflect public needs, priorities, and judgments

- "Cultural and group-specific validation of communication strategies and expected results

- Impact on perceived or actual legitimacy of public policies and emergency measures

- Increased outreach to and inclusion of vulnerable and hard-to-reach populations

- Development of key constituency groups made of citizens and community members who are invested in the success of emergency response and related interventions, and work toward achieving positive outcomes and behavioral results in their communities" (Schiavo, 2009c)

As "an increased emphasis is being placed on *short-term and long-term behavioral and social results* of public health emergency and risk communication," community mobilization and citizen engagement are increasingly important. "While *short-term behaviors* apply to individual, community or social practices that we seek to see adopted by different groups during the acute phase of emergency response," long-term behaviors and social results refer to those "behaviors and social norms that need to be in place in order to be 'ready' to respond" to an emergency (Schiavo, 2010a, p. 21) and be considered and addressed both in the preparedness and readiness phases. This concept is reiterated in Figure 6.5, which calls for revisiting the traditional pre-during-post emergency scenario, in which lessons learned do not necessarily translate into communication readiness or readiness measures for future emergencies (some authors call this the "disaster management rut" [Kelman, 2004]), to the newly developed preparedness-readiness-response-evaluation-constant cycle (PRRECC) (in which lessons learned, cultural preferences, community needs, social norms, and existing behaviors, policies, and obstacles are researched, evaluated and addressed from a capacity-building standpoint in the preparedness phase, and "then used to address situation- and group-specific needs as well as existing individual and social behaviors to create *long-term readiness for communication response*") (Schiavo, 2009b, 2010a, p. 23). The PREECC model is an evolution of the RREEC model (Schiavo, 2009c, 2010a).

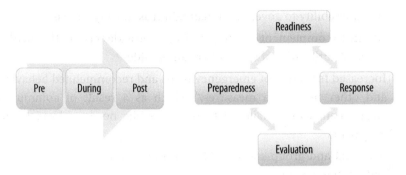

Figure 6.5 Moving from the Pre-During-Post Scenario to the Preparedness-Readiness Response-Evaluation-Constant Cycle (PRRECC)

Source: © Renata Schiavo. This model is an evolution of the RREEC (readiness-response-evaluation-constant cycle) model first developed and presented by the author at a 2009 WHO informal consultation (Schiavo, 2009c and 2010a; WHO, 2010).

PREECC refers to the following actions:

- *Preparedness* is a research and evaluation stage in the prepandemic or interpandemic periods, in which governments, international and local organizations, and local communities work together to assess lessons learned from previous disease outbreaks, and other relevant case studies as well as key factors and obstacles that may affect the implementation (or lack thereof) of different measures to mitigate the impact of and respond to potential future outbreaks of a given disease. As part of this step of the cycle, a comprehensive communication plan is developed, including building local capacity for its implementation, developing alliances and decision-making processes, addressing potential obstacles that pertain to the living and working environment of at-risk communities, engaging local communities, identifying special needs and risks of underserved groups, selecting social mobilization partners and other key actors and spokespeople, and reaching mutual agreement on preliminary progress and outcome indicators in case of a disease outbreak (among others). This phase is informed by evaluation data from previous pandemics and disease outbreaks.

- *Readiness* refers to developing interventions and local capacity to address community needs and overcome irrational fears or existing social norms and traditions that may influence behavioral readiness as it refers to the adoption and sustainability among different groups of specific behaviors recommended during an emergency. Behavior readiness is an established concept (Paek and others, 2008; Schiavo, 2009b, 2009c, 2010a; WHO, 2010) and is associated not only with people's beliefs, attitudes, and social norms vis-à-vis recommended behaviors in case of a public health emergency but also to the concept of self-efficacy (for example, "I am confident that during an emergency I can wash my hands or wear protective gears at critical times and for the recommended amount of time") (Schiavo, 2009c), and perceived response effectiveness (for example, I am confident that "washing my hands or wearing protective gears will increase my chance to stay healthy during this emergency situation," Schiavo, 2009c) (Paek and others, 2008). Whereas the readiness and preparedness stages of the model often overlap with each other, and ideally should be implemented at the same time, the readiness phase is more specifically correlated to behavioral indicators and results among different community groups than to other aspects of the overall communication plan (as, for example, advance agreement on issues of response coordination and decision-making processes, training of local spokespeople, and others). As such, this stage strongly relies on community participation and engagement to create the conditions for behavioral readiness to adopt recommended emergency measures. Because of the critical importance of behavioral results in emergency and risk communication (in which we often deal with life-or-death situations to which people need to promptly react), the readiness step is designed to provide additional emphasis and focus on behavioral outcomes.

- *Response* refers to all different measures to be implemented during a public health emergency (epidemic or disease outbreak) by local governments and their international and local partners. The scope of this book does not include a discussion of different components of emergency response in epidemics and disease outbreak settings.

- *Evaluation* refers to research, monitoring, and evaluation strategies, and community feedback mechanisms that need to be designed and implemented to collect data and evaluate results and lessons learned from all different phases of emergency or risk communication interventions during a disease outbreak or other emergency. As for other steps of this cycle, evaluation designs and tools always benefit from community participation and input. Evaluation data from a specific disease outbreak will inform future preparedness for similar situations, therefore creating a *constant cycle*.

The integration of community mobilization and community engagement strategies in emergency and risk communication along with mass media, new media, interpersonal, and other kinds of communication interventions is supported by several recent experiences and models (Paek and others, 2008; Reynolds, 2005). "A community and household consultation model that is participatory—but yet focused on specific individual, community, and social behavior outcomes—may help community members to reflect on past health emergencies and disease outbreaks as well as identify key factors and communication chains that may contribute to increasing community trust and perceived transparency of future communication activities while gaining knowledge" on the specific emergency issue. "A fundamental step in implementing this community consultation model is to empower and train community leaders, relevant groups, and communication and social mobilization partners on interpersonal communication skills, dialogue and group facilitation, and information management as well as overall communication planning and implementation strategies" (Schiavo, 2009b, p. 23).

Key Concepts

- Community mobilization is a key area of health communication that seeks to empower communities to make the changes needed for better health outcomes. It often starts with ordinary people and attempts to engage all different levels of society.

- Community mobilization describes different kinds of actions (behaviors), from people marching to demonstrate their discontent about the paucity of research funds dedicated to a specific disease area to community members communicating with others about the importance of disease prevention and leading the health behavior change and community development processes.

- In this chapter, the terms *community mobilization* and *social mobilization* are used interchangeably. One of the key premises of the definitions and case studies used in this chapter is that the potential impact of community mobilization is greater when several communities and multiple sectors come together and create a force for social change.

- Putting the public back into public health is a key goal of public health in the twenty-first century. Citizen engagement (or public engagement) is the process of creating a better informed citizenry so that people from different sectors and walks of life can effectively contribute to policy and economic decisions that ultimately affect their lives. Given the social nature of community and social mobilization we discussed in this chapter, citizen engagement is basically community mobilization at scale.

- As part of health communication interventions, community mobilization still tends to be disease focused but often also addresses or should address broader health and social issues, and key social determinants of health as well should complement other health communication, public health, and community development efforts.

- Community skills building as well as community participation and autonomy are fundamental aspects of community mobilization.

- The role of health communicators and others who may facilitate the community mobilization process should not take away from community autonomy and power. So-called community mobilizers should act only as consultants and technical experts in accompanying the process of community reflection and empowerment on relevant health issues.

- The effectiveness of community mobilization interventions increases when they are part of larger health communication programs and complement existing public health initiatives and strategies.

- Community mobilization has been influenced by several theoretical and practical models, including behavioral and social sciences, social marketing, and participatory research. Nevertheless, these terms are not synonymous.

- Several models describe key steps of community mobilization efforts. All of them focus on behavioral or social outcomes and share many common characteristics.

- Community mobilization and citizen engagement strategies are integral to public health emergency and risk communication interventions.

FOR DISCUSSION AND PRACTICE

1. Discuss your reaction to the Bingwa case study in Box 6.3. List all factors that, in your opinion, contributed to Bingwa's change and rank them in order of importance. Use role-play to imagine a potential conversation on the same topic (STDs and their prevention) you may have with your peers or someone like Bingwa.

2. Do you have any personal or professional experience with community mobilization? Did you ever participate in a community-based meeting or event? If yes, describe and apply key concepts from this chapter to your description wherever they are relevant.

3. Can you think of an example in which a series of behavioral changes led to a health-related social change as the result of community engagement and mobilization? Describe the sequence of events as well as the specific changes that occurred at different levels of the community or society. You can refer to examples that recently appeared in the news or to personal experiences. In the absence of specific examples, think of a desirable social change (for example, a new health policy in a specific health area or removal of the stigma associated with a specific disease), and identify the behaviors that may lead to social change.

4. Review the Gay Men's Health Crisis HIV/AIDS time line in Box 6.4. Identify cause-effects relationships between different elements of the time line and key milestones that were achieved in different years. Discuss sequential events as well as any other kinds of community mobilization and citizen engagement interventions you may have followed during a specific phase of the HIV/AIDS epidemic or nowadays.

5. Identify and review a case study on a recent disease outbreak or humanitarian emergency that also led to public health consequences. Discuss the case study in light of the models and concepts being covered in the "The Case for Community Mobilization and Citizen Engagement in Risk and Emergency Communication" section of this chapter. Focus on how you will attempt to apply such concepts and models in developing key questions and strategies for community consultation and mobilization within the context of the case study you have selected.

KEY TERMS

citizen engagement

community

community-driven assessment

community mobilization

community-needs assessment

consensus-building workshops

delivered dialogue

participatory influential road mapping

participatory needs assessment

participatory research

public consultation

public engagement

referendum

social mobilization

CHAPTER 7

PROFESSIONAL MEDICAL COMMUNICATIONS

Health care systems and, consequently the practice of medicine, have changed tremendously in the past few decades. For example, Fischer (2001) reports finding among the personal memorabilia of his father-in-law, a surgeon in Sioux City, Iowa, and a governor of the American College of Surgeons, a number of records showing that many of his patients did not actually pay him. Instead, "in-kind contributions of chickens, potatoes, knickknacks, etc., served sometimes as 'payment' for the care he delivered uncomplainingly for the better part of his 91 years" (pp. 71–72).

My own great-grandfather, who was a general practitioner in a small town in southern Italy, led a very different life from today's physicians and other health care providers. He died at the age of 102. One can speculate that good genes, a good diet, his passion for his work and long walks, and a relatively stress-free lifestyle all contributed to his long life. There are not many health care providers in this era of technological advances, malpractice suits, increased medical specialization, insurance-based health care, and other cost-cutting interventions who can say they lead a stress-free life.

Today, physicians and all other health care providers are faced with a number of additional day-to-day demands and tasks:

- Containing costs and being aware of the cost-effectiveness of the procedures and medications they recommend
- Keeping up with technological advances and the rapid evolution of medical standards and practices

- Being prepared to answer complex medical questions by increasingly informed patients

- Competing with other practices for patient retention

- Completing significant paperwork to satisfy billing and health insurance requirements

- Seeing an ever-increasing number of patients because of health workforce gaps in many areas and countries

- Addressing increasing diversity and determinants of health disparities as part of patient care

Professional communications can help health care providers meet their challenges with peer-to-peer information and tools that contribute to the effectiveness of their clinical practices and, ultimately, better health outcomes for their patients. The importance of this communication area is directly correlated to the need to ensure that "medical practice reflects state-of-the-art scientific knowledge" (Solomon, 1995 p. 28). This is also the rationale for the recent emphasis on behavioral and institutional change models that encourage physicians and other health care providers to adopt new behaviors and practices (Solomon, 1995; Bauchner, Simpson, and Chessare, 2001).

CHAPTER OBJECTIVES

This chapter defines medical professional communication and describes theoretical assumptions that influence this communication area. It also highlights key elements and commonly used activities and tools of professional communications programs. Finally, it establishes the context for professional communications and emphasizes how this approach can complement other strategies and areas of health communication in public health and health care settings.

Communicating with Health Care Providers: A Peer-to-Peer Approach

Scientific exchange was recognized as a need and an opportunity in the early history of medicine and other health care fields such as psychology and nursing. In most contexts and situations, peer-to-peer scientific exchange aims at advancing medical practices and advocating for the application of new standards of care. An everyday example of scientific exchange is the role of mentors, such as senior physicians and head nurses who train or advise younger health care practitioners on different areas.

The concept of scientific exchange can be traced to Hippocrates, the ancient Greek physician who is considered the father of modern medicine (Pikoulis, Waasdorp, Leppaniemi, and Burris, 1998). Hippocrates, a prolific writer of his ideas and findings, "recommended that physicians record their findings and their medicinal methods, so that these records may be passed down and employed by other physicians" (Crystalinks, 2006; Winau, 1994).

Professional medical communication has evolved from the concept of scientific exchange as a peer-to-peer communication approach intended for physicians, nurses, physician assistants, and all other health care providers, as shown in Table 7.1. **Professional medical communication** (also *professional clinical communication*) can be defined as the application of health communication theories, models, and practices to programs that seek to influence the behavior and the social context of these professionals directly responsible for administering health care. In other words, it is the process of planning, executing, and evaluating communication programs intended for

professional medical communication
A key health communication area that seeks to influence the behavior and the social contexts of these professionals directly responsible for administering health care

Table 7.1   Key Audiences of Professional Clinical Communications

Physicians

Physician assistants

Medical directors

Nurses
- Nurse practitioners
- School nurses
- Visiting nurses
- Camp nurses

Therapists
- Speech therapists
- Physical therapists
- Other therapists

Dentists

Nutritionists

Dietitians

Social workers

Psychologists

Thought leaders

Health sciences and medical librarians

Other health care providers

health care providers. This term is used interchangeably with *professional clinical communications*. Professional medical communications aim to (1) promote the adoption of best medical and health practices; (2) establish new concepts and standards of care; (3) publicize recent medical discoveries, beliefs, parameters, and policies; (4) change or establish new medical priorities; and (5) advance health policy changes.

In professional communications, the concept of peer describes professionals with similar education, training, and overall capacity. Some peers who are recognized by their community as thought leaders in a field or on a health issue tend to take the lead in communicating with other physicians or nurses about new information in their area of competence. Other times, professional associations and other organizations, which may be responsible for setting new standards of care or keeping their membership up to date on recent medical and scientific progress, act as peer leaders in a communication effort.

Health sciences and medical librarians also have a key role in professional clinical communication because of their training and access to tools that provide information on different aspects of a health issue or disease. Medical librarians are integral members of the health care team. They help physicians, nurses, and other professionals to stay abreast of new information that may affect patient outcomes. They also provide medical information to patients and other library users, therefore influencing provider-patient communication and helping patients ask the right questions of their health care providers. Therefore, they should always be included as a key group in professional clinical communication interventions because they are key influentials within health care teams. (For information on the role of health science librarians outside of clinical settings, including in health communication and public health, see the relevant case study in Chapter Fifteen.)

More recently, emerging needs (for example, increased urbanization and diversity of the patient population, health disparities, and global health workforce gaps) have been calling for increased collaborative efforts among the health care, public health, and community development fields so that scientific and medical progress, and its applications, are informed by population and key group-specific issues at the intersection of these fields.

Although physicians and other health care providers are just another important audience of health communication, and should be considered as such, some differences exist. In fact, professional communications relies on several specific tools and activities as well as specialized skills (for example, excellent science writing skills and the ability to speak in complex medical or clinical terms), which are not always used in addressing the needs of other audiences. This is why professional communications is considered a separate area of health communication in this book. This also reflects the actual practice of health communication. In fact, health communicators who facilitate the development of professional communications programs need to be able to relate to physicians and other health care providers and use medical and scientific terms. This requires an in-depth technical understanding of the health issue and a much higher level of knowledge about the peer-reviewed literature related to it. Similarly, science writers are often specialized members of the health communication team.

Professional medical communications is often an important component of health communication programs. This approach is instrumental in a number of ways:

- Promotes the adoption of best practices
- Establishes new concepts and standards of care
- Raises provider awareness of recent medical and scientific discoveries, beliefs, parameters, and policies
- Changes or establishes new clinical priorities
- Advances health policy changes by engaging thought leaders and professional organizations in advocating such changes
- Uses emerging technology to expand efficacy of clinical practices and address global health workforce gaps

Finally, professional clinical communications is an important component of multifaceted interventions that ultimately seek a behavioral or social change at the patient or public level. In fact, they are instrumental in creating a receptive environment for patient demand and increased use of health services.

Take the fictitious example of José, a Puerto Rican man who reads in the local newspaper about the higher risk for oral cancer among Puerto Ricans versus other ethnic groups (Hayes and others, 1999; Parkin and others, 1997; Suarez and others, 2009). At his next appointment, he asks his dentist whether he regularly performs oral cancer screening. If his dentist is not aware of the higher risk among Puerto Ricans or does not consider oral cancer screening one of the priorities of his practice, he may dismiss José's request and reassure him that he has nothing to worry about. In this case, any intervention directly intended for José and other Puerto Ricans may not be effective if it is not supported by efforts that involve dentists and other primary care physicians in prioritizing and performing oral cancer screening at routine visits.

Similarly, the mother of a nine-year-old boy who still wets the bed at night as the result of primary nocturnal enuresis (PNE), a common medical condition that is still highly misdiagnosed and misunderstood in the United States (Hodge-Gray and Caldamone, 1998; Mast and Smith, 2012), may be rebuffed by her son's pediatrician when she asks for help. The pediatrician may believe that wetting the bed is a behavioral problem, which has been shown to be irrelevant in the etiology and treatment of PNE (Cendron, 1999). This may lead to additional years of suffering and humiliation for the boy, who would be limited in his ability to participate and enjoy common childhood activities, such as summer camps and sleepovers (Hodge-Gray and Caldamone, 1998). The recurrence of this health problem will also continue to have a negative effect on family interactions and stress levels (Cendron, 1999).

These two examples confirm that professional medical communications efforts should be based, like all other communication interventions, on a true understanding of the audience's common beliefs, attitudes, practices, and needs. They should focus on changing the behavior of health care providers and, when necessary, the social norms and policies of the professional community to which they belong. Finally, they should engage health care providers in the design, implementation, and evaluation of such programs, and elicit among them feelings of ownership and leadership in the solution of the health issue.

Theoretical Assumptions in Professional Medical (Clinical) Communications

Planning and implementing professional communications interventions is not so different from planning interventions intended for other key groups. "Whether intended for physicians or others, there is a standard method for designing interventions that includes the selection of appropriate intended audiences, program goals, and messages as well as methods for delivery, implementation and evaluation" (Solomon, 1995, p. S28).

As in other areas of health communication, an important factor in the potential success of professional communications efforts is the participation and involvement of health care providers as well as the key institutions that represent or exert an influence on them. This process helps engage and build capacity of key opinion leaders in similar ways to those described in the chapter on community mobilization (see Chapter Six). After all, the medical and scientific community is still a community.

Sometimes taking an institutional approach to physician behavior change may help produce faster results (Solomon, 1995; Solomon and others, 1991, 2010). When reputable professional organizations take the lead in promoting change on the beliefs, priorities, and practices of their memberships or employees (for example, in the case of a hospital), they implicitly acknowledge and influence what Solomon (1995) calls the "social nature of decision making" (p. S30).

Although all shifts in policies and practices are gradual and require a systematic and step-by-step approach, chances are that attempting to change an institutional policy may help implement the kind of peer pressure that is sought at the individual health care provider level. Still, in order to change the policy of an institution or organization, a series of behavioral changes is needed at the different hierarchical levels of the institution. Sometimes it is an ordinary member who believes in the need for change and starts modifying his or her practice as well as discussing the changes with colleagues and other members of the organization, all the way to the top. At other times, the behavioral and institutional changes start with the vision and leadership of top management, which becomes convinced, because of professional communications programs, direct experience, or new scientific discovery, of the need for new policies and practices.

Regardless of the original approach to behavioral change, the overall aim of professional medical communications efforts is to make sure that the largest number of individual physicians and health care providers endorses and implements practices that result in the best patient outcomes. It all starts with the awareness that scientific and medical discovery is just one step in improving patient outcomes. Despite such progress, the practice of medicine in most countries varies from region to region, practice to practice, and physician to physician (Burstall, 1991; Woods and Kiely, 2000; Mercuri and Gafni, 2011).

In the United States, there are still common and widespread gaps in the quality of care patients receive (Institute of Medicine, 2001), which may be explained by differences in the use of state-of-the-art technologies or recommended medical practices as well as managed care restrictions (see Chapter Two). For example, "a review of 48 MEDLINE studies about US quality of care showed that 50% of recommended preventive care, 40% of recommended chronic care, and 30% of recommended acute care was not provided, whereas 20% to 30% of the care given was not recommended and so ranged from unnecessary to possibly harmful" (Grol, 2002, p. 245; Schuster, McGlynn, and Brook, 1998; Davis, Schoen, and Stremikis, 2010).

Closing the gaps and improving the overall quality of care is a step-by-step process that includes many of the stages highlighted by the behavioral and social change theories discussed in Chapter Two, and requires a systematic people-centered approach. As Grol (2002) highlights, several studies and experiences have shown that knowledge and more traditional educational activities are not sufficient to change physician behavior. "Activities and measures at different levels (individual, team, hospital, practice and the wider environment) are required to be successful" (p. 246). This is one of the fundamental and more general assumptions of well-designed and well-implemented health communication programs.

All theories and models that more generally apply to health communication are also relevant to professional clinical communications. As in other areas of health communication, theories and models should be selected because of their relevance to the specific health problem and customized to meet the needs and preferences of physicians and other health care providers. Still, there are a few more specific considerations and theoretical assumptions that may help explain why health care providers do what they do and how to influence behavior change in providers.

How to Influence Health Care Provider Behavior: A Theoretical Overview

Health care providers should be considered just another key group to be engaged in the health communication process. In designing communication interventions intended for them, their professional role as well as the key factors that influence provider behavior should be analyzed in the same way health communicators would do with any other audience.

Although there is a general lack of agreement on the theoretical basis for physician behavior or, more in general, health care provider behavior, many authors do agree about the relevance of behavioral and social change theories (Grimshaw, Eccles, Walker, and Thomas, 2002; Grol, 2002). Most of these theories were examined in Chapter Two and should be considered part of a tool kit used to guide the design of professional medical communications. Behavioral, institutional, and social outcomes of each professional intervention should be defined early in the process and used to measure the potential success of the professional communications effort.

Another theoretical perspective is the importance of finding the right balance between individual and organizational or community-based interventions (Grol, 2002). For example, Slotnick and Shershneva (2002) suggest that physicians learn in **communities of practice**, which they define as "a group of people who share interests in an aspect of human endeavor and who participate in collective learning activities that both educate and create bonds among those involved" (p. 198). This is not very different from other

communities of practice
"A group of people who share interests in an aspect of human endeavor and who participate in collective learning activities that both educate and create bonds among those involved" (Slotnick and Shershneva, 2002, p. 198)

community-based groups, which are usually influenced by the opinion and practices of their peers.

Well-designed professional medical communications use a strategic blend of activities and channels that aims at involving individual providers and professional organizations to which they belong. In planning the behavioral change process, health communicators and other professionals should ask at what levels the intervention should occur, and which kinds of actions are expected at each level. Not surprisingly, "usually, actions focusing on individuals should be complemented by those directed at teams, organizations and the wider environment" (Grol, 2002, p. 248).

Sporadic and single communication activities almost never produce long-term results. Professional communications should be viewed as a process that is in integration of many other interventions, such as mass media and new media communications, strategic policy communication, and clinician communication training.

Prior to designing any activities, it is important to understand providers' beliefs, attitudes, current behavior, and potential peer pressure about the health issue or practice being addressed. Of equal importance is the need to assess providers' level of comfort with addressing a specific health topic vis-à-vis their training, interests, and experience.

The analysis should consider more general social factors that influence providers' behavior and practices. These may include both personal factors, such as the overall level of satisfaction with their profession, and practice-related factors, such as medical priorities established within their practices, level of collaborations with other medical specialties or health care providers, policies and social norms that prevail in their communities, and managed care or other cost-related restrictions. The same analysis should be conducted on organizations or professionals who influence health care provider behavior and practices: professional organizations, insurance companies, medical schools, and hospitals, for example. Finally, serious consideration should be given to potential obstacles to the implementation of new practices as well as the strategies to remove them. Multifaceted interventions that also focus on addressing potential barriers tend to be more effective (Grimshaw, Eccles, Walker, and Thomas, 2002) and produce sustainable behavior change.

Table 7.2 lists some of the common obstacles to behavioral change among health care providers. This list is not all-inclusive and, in some cases, would need to be modified to address the specific health issue or provider's specialty.

Table 7.2   Key Obstacles to Clinician Change

Gaps in knowledge or specific skills
Time constraints
Conflicting priorities
Information overload
Insufficient facilities or medical equipment
Lack of financial incentives
Managed care restrictions or other cost-cutting interventions
Perception of clinician's role as limited to disease treatment

References: Grimshaw, J. M., Eccles, M. P., Walker, A. E., and Thomas, R. E. "Changing Physicians' Behavior: What Works and Thoughts on Getting More Things to Work." *Journal of Continuing Education in the Health Professions*, 2002, *22*, 237–243; Spickard Jr., A., and others. "Changes Made by Physicians Who Misprescribed Controlled Substances." Nashville: Vanderbilt University Medical Center. 2001. www.mc.vanderbilt.edu/root/vumc.php?site=cph&doc=1094.

Key Elements of Professional Medical Communications Programs

One of the most important elements of professional communications programs is their multidisciplinary and multifaceted nature. Only interventions that rely on a sustained effort as well as on multiple tools and activities have the potential to become effective elements for provider change.

A list of some of the key characteristics of professional communications programs, which are discussed in further detail in this section, follows. Interestingly, many of them also reflect the key elements of best clinical practices. In other words, best practices in professional communications planning often mirror the same key considerations that the health care and scientific communities consider in establishing best clinical practices. The asterisks in the following list indicate that these are also key elements of best clinical practices according to Steenholdt (2006):

- Evidence-based*
- Group-specific
- Behavior-centered
- Patient-centered*
- Practical*
- Easy to implement
- Multifaceted
- Consistent*

Evidence-Based

Health care providers are accustomed to basing their decisions on statistically significant data, scientific information, and professional guidelines.

Large-scale clinical trials, new scientific discoveries, and clinical experience, which often lead to the development of organizational or disease-specific guidelines, provide evidence to support the need for a new clinical practice or behavior.

Professional communication interventions should take into account the data-driven mind-set of physicians and other health care providers, and rely on reputable scientific evidence and well-documented case studies to advance the adoption of best clinical practices.

Group-Specific

As in all other areas of health communication, professional communication efforts should be tailored to specific medical specialties and health care providers. In fact, the level to which different providers may need to apply new clinical recommendations and practices can vary in relation to their level of competence and responsibility for a specific aspect of care.

For example, detailed information on how to reconstitute a vaccine from its powder formulation as well as storage conditions and vaccine appearance is particularly relevant for nurse practitioners, who are usually responsible for the actual administration of vaccines. However, because nurses are also on the front line with patients in addressing questions about the safety and efficacy of vaccines, as well as potential misconceptions and other social or patient-specific barriers to immunization, information on new vaccines and their characteristics should be as comprehensive as that discussed with physicians. In this way, provider-patient communications will be consistent and accurate, and all members of the health care team will be adequately equipped to influence patient outcomes and decisions.

Behavior-Centered

As always in health communication, behavioral outcomes should be clear at the outset of program planning and ideally discussed and decided together with members of the clinician's group who will be ultimately responsible for the adoption and sustainability of all changes. In other words, program planners should work together with clinicians and ask themselves what kinds of changes would ultimately help improve patient outcomes, and whether such changes are supported by the existing health care system and policy environment. All interventions should be designed to encourage such behaviors and changes in practices, and also tackle larger issues within the sociopolitical environment and the health system in which clinicians operate. This may require system-changing objectives and activities at the policy and health care system levels so that clinicians are supported in their intention to make changes to their existing practices.

Patient-Centered

Within clinical settings, the patient is at the center of health communication interventions. In fact, the ability of health care providers to digest and apply new medical and scientific information to day-to-day care or to communicate with patients effectively across different cultures, beliefs, and health literacy levels may have a fundamental impact on health outcomes. As a consequence, professional communications strategies, activities, and tools should always strive to remind health care providers of the connection between the information being presented and potential patient outcomes.

Whenever possible, information about specific diseases or new medical practices should be integrated with the discussion and modeling of approaches to improve provider-patient communication on that specific topic. This is particularly relevant in the case of chronic illnesses, behavioral health (for example, substance abuse), or other medical issues that have a long-term physical or psychological burden on the patient and are determined by several socially influenced factors within the patient's living or working environment. In many cases, provider-patient communication can be integrated with peer-to-peer communication strategies so that community leaders and family members can reinforce outside of clinical settings key information patients discuss with their health care providers. This strategy may also be instrumental in increasing the cultural competence of all patient-related communication by building capacity at the community level to discuss clinical information in the community's own words and culturally relevant terminology and promoting information and cultural exchanges among health care providers and the communities they serve. As a consequence, professional medical communication interventions should also focus on building capacity on cultural competence and cross-cultural health communication (see section in this chapter called "Prioritizing Health Disparities in Clinical Education to Improve Care: The Role of Cross-Cultural Health Communication").

Practical

Professional communications should always begin by asking, "So what?" Health care providers should leave all encounters and readings that are part of the professional communications intervention with a clear understanding of how the new information or its endorsement by a specific community of practice or organization apply to their day-to-day work. This is easier to accomplish if clinicians and their representatives have participated in the development of key elements of the professional communication intervention.

For example, in developing a workshop on malaria, professional communicators should first emphasize practical approaches about the disease diagnosis and treatment, and only later address the debate about the efficacy of different strategies for malaria prevention—for example, use of insecticide-treated mosquito nets versus house spraying or use of chloroquine (American Association for the Advancement of Science, 2006; Centers for Disease Control [CDC], 2006e; World Health Organization [WHO], 2006). Moreover, malaria should be discussed within the social and environmental context of most affected populations.

Easy to Implement

Time barriers, conflicting priorities, managed care restrictions (see Chapter Two), and other obstacles often limit providers' ability to change and implement new practices. Therefore, professional communications should strive to make it easy to sustain the adoption of such practices. As Grol (2002) writes, "Particularly important here is that the change activities are embedded within day-to-day activities as much as possible and that the change will not be seen as extra work" (p. 249). This could be achieved by developing disease-specific or practice-specific activities and tool kits that health care providers can use as a reference or with their patients.

For example, as part of a communication effort to improve recognition and management of mild traumatic brain injury (MTBI) or concussion, a condition that in the United States affects 1.1 million people and still is underdiagnosed and undertreated, the CDC (2006d) has developed a physician tool kit that includes "easy-to-use clinical information, patient information in English and Spanish [which physicians can distribute to their patients to complement or initiate in-office discussions], scientific literature, and a CD-ROM." Overall, traumatic brain injury (TBI), which ranges from mild to severe, is a serious problem in the United States that affects 1.7 million people (CDC, 2013c). The kit is aimed not only at improving the diagnosis and treatment of MTBI but also at providing physicians with the tools to communicate with patients and the community at large on how to prevent MTBI. The kit is complemented by other initiatives intended for the general public, state departments of health, and special key groups (for example, athletes' coaches) that aim at increasing awareness and prevention of MTBI. This includes two free online courses, one for health care professionals and another for youth and high school sport coaches, parents, and athletes (CDC, 2013b) so that they can be aware of and recognize early symptoms of a concussion. In this way, physician change is also supported by attempts to change health behaviors in the patient communities that physicians attend to.

Table 7.3 Communication Approaches and Tools and Their Effects: Analysis of Thirty-Six Systematic Reviews

Approaches and tools	Number of reviews	Effect of studies
Educational materials, journals, mailed information	Nine	Limited effects
Continuing medical education courses, conferences	Four	Limited effects
Interactive educational meetings, small group education	Four	Few studies; mostly effective
Educational outreach visits, facilitation, and support	Eight	Particularly effective for prescribing and prevention
Feedback on performance	Seven	Mixed effects
Use of opinion leaders	Three	Mixed effects
Combined and multifaceted interventions with education	Sixteen	Mostly (very) effective

Source: Adapted from Grol, R. "Changing Physicians' Competence and Performance: Finding the Balance Between the Individual and the Organization." *Journal of Continuing Education in the Health Professions*, 2002, *22*, 244–251. Used by permission.

Multifaceted

A multifaceted approach has been proven to be more effective than single and sporadic activities. Table 7.3 provides an analysis of thirty-six systematic reviews and compares different approaches in relation to their effect on changing clinical performance (Grol, 1997, 2002). As part of this analysis, the table shows that single approaches have limited or mixed effects, whereas multifaceted interventions are mostly very effective.

As another example, when the US National Foundation for Infectious Diseases (NFID) took over the leadership in advocating for policy and practice changes related to pediatric immunization against flu (see Box 7.1), it used a multifaceted approach that encouraged and supported the CDC recommendation for pediatric immunization as well as a widespread use of this practice.

BOX 7.1. NATIONAL FOUNDATION FOR INFECTIOUS DISEASES FLU FIGHT FOR KIDS: CASE STUDY

Research shows children under two years of age are hospitalized due to influenza infection at the same high rate as persons sixty-five years and older. In 2002, the CDC issued a new policy to encourage influenza vaccination of all children six to twenty-three months of age. Extensive research and communication with key pediatric influenza thought leaders, policymakers, and practicing physicians showed most physicians supported pediatric influenza immunization, but needed to overcome infrastructure barriers in their practices to implement annual flu vaccination programs. In addition, thought leaders and physicians identified several perceived barriers to six- to twenty-three-month-old influenza immunization.

In 2002, the National Foundation for Infectious Diseases (NFID) launched the Flu Fight for Kids initiative to stimulate discussion on the topic and to create a climate of receptivity for routine annual influenza vaccination of infants and children six to twenty-three months of age. Thought leaders and policymakers needed to be convinced that immunization of six- to twenty-three-month-old children was feasible. At the same time, parents needed to become aware of their children's risk for flu and ask their health care providers to vaccinate their children.

Key Actions

2002 Roundtable Meeting and Consensus Document

NFID convened a roundtable meeting with the participation of experts from many sectors, including public health, private practice, nursing, and infectious diseases. This was instrumental to reaching a consensus about the severity of pediatric influenza and highlight best practice models to help pediatric practices implement annual vaccination programs. A comprehensive consensus report, "Increasing Influenza Immunization Rates in Infants and Children: Putting Recommendations into Practice," summarized the meeting proceedings. The report outlines barriers to influenza vaccination as well as strategies to overcome them. It also provides best practice models for achieving optimal influenza vaccination rates. The document was widely distributed and presented to the CDC's Advisory Committee on Immunization Practices (ACIP) as a resource to demonstrate that annual influenza vaccination programs can be implemented in physician practices.

Media Outreach

Trade and consumer media outreach were conducted to communicate to the medical community, as well as to parents, the serious nature of influenza illness among children six to twenty-three months of age. Outreach also focused on strategies for immunizing this population within pediatric practices throughout the Flu Fight for Kids initiative. Key placements were secured in leading consumer and trade media throughout the campaign, including *USA Today*, *AAP News*, *Parents*, and *Child*.

Satellite Symposium at American Academy of Pediatrics (AAP) Annual Meeting

NFID sponsored a continuing medical education (CME) satellite symposium highlighting the proceedings from the roundtable meeting and report at the American Academy of Pediatrics annual meeting in November 2003. Hundreds of physicians attended the program on-site and several hundred more participated in an online CME program, which was made available following the event. The CME program provided information to help pediatricians prepare their practice for routine influenza vaccination of all children six to twenty-three months of age.

CDC Issues Full Pediatric Recommendation

During the campaign, two key meetings of the CDC's ACIP took place in June and October of 2003. Before both meetings, NFID invited key thought leaders to highlight the strategies from the roundtable meeting and consensus report. At the October meeting, NFID enrolled a practicing pediatrician to address the panel about his successful vaccination program.

Results—First Year of Routine Recommendation

On October 15, 2003, the CDC's advisory committee unanimously voted to recommend influenza vaccination for children six to twenty-three months of age, beginning in fall 2004. NFID's steady, year-long outreach to thought leaders, physicians, policymakers, and parents contributed to early adoption of the recommendations. Data from the first year of the full recommendation (2004–2005 influenza season) reported the new vaccination recommendations for all children six to twenty-three months of age resulted in a higher than expected 48 percent coverage rate. This is the most rapid uptake of any routine pediatric vaccine to date.

Continuing its efforts to help physicians implement the new recommendations and improve immunization rates in the population, NFID developed a comprehensive resource kit, Kids Need Flu Vaccine, Too! The kit helps health care providers establish in-practice influenza vaccination programs. The kit was issued in 2004 and updated with additional educational materials in 2005. Key objectives of the resource kit are supported by the American Academy of Pediatrics (AAP) and the National Influenza Vaccine Summit, which is cosponsored by the American Medical Association and the CDC.

Source: National Foundation for Infectious Diseases. "Flu Fight for Kids." Unpublished case study, 2005b. Copyright © 2005. National Foundation for Infectious Diseases. Used by permission.

Consistent

Communication messages should be consistent throughout the stages of the professional communications intervention. They should also be consistent with recent medical discoveries, best practices, and clinical guidelines.

Message consistency is a fundamental concept in communication and helps establish a clear path to change. Conflicting recommendations and messages may confuse key groups, hinder their willingness to change, and affect their overall perception about the quality of the communication program.

Overview of Key Communication Channels and Activities

Physicians and other health care providers have traditionally relied on peer-reviewed publications to communicate with their communities about scientific and medical discoveries as well as clinical practices. This remains an important evidence-based tool for credible scientific exchange about research findings. However, Grimshaw, Eccles, Walker, and Thomas (2002) identify a number of limitations of relying solely on this approach as well as its impact on translating new evidence to actual medical practice: (1) the limited time physicians dedicate to reading, which according to several polls is on average not more than one hour per week; (2) the fact that many physicians lack specific training to evaluate the quality of published research; and (3) the existence of several barriers to the application of evidence-based information to actual clinical practice. Well-designed and well-implemented professional communications programs rely on multiple channels and activities that do the following:

- Complement peer-reviewed publications
- Present information in an easy-to-digest and practical format
- Prioritize and highlight the weight of different research findings in relation to actual clinical practice
- Point to specific guidelines and best practices
- Provide guidance and tools to overcome existing barriers to the adoption of new clinical practices and behaviors
- Use emerging technology to provide new tools for professional communication and to facilitate provider-patient interactions

For example, more recently, physicians and other health care providers rely on the use of **tablets** (one-piece mobile computers, such as the iPad or the Kindle) that contain apps "to check drugs, or apps that allow them to share anatomical drawings with patients to explain procedures" (Dolan, 2013). "According to a study by the technology firm CDW, professionals generally gain about 1.1 hours in productivity per day by using a tablet computer" (Dolan, 2013). As another example, although many hospitals still use one-way pagers, an increasing number of facilities are turning to texting to communicate about situations that need immediate attention, such as emergencies or staffing needs (Sindel, 2009). Nurses have been adopting texting as a preferred communication method, both with other nurses and physicians (Sindel, 2009).

Table 7.4 sets out tools, activities, and channels that are traditionally used in professional communications, and specifically pertain to this

tablets
One-piece mobile computers, such as the iPad or the Kindle

Table 7.4   Key Communication Tools and Channels in Professional Communications

Communications venues and channels	Annual meetings, professional conferences
	Regional meetings, professional chapter meetings
	Institutional meetings (for example, hospital or patient conferences)
	Special events (roundtables, symposia, lecture series)
	Internet
	Professional and trade media
	Special communication tools
Key tools	
Print	*Monograph:* A document, book, or leaflet that is complete in itself and contains multiple articles or sections
	White paper: A type of monograph that is based on the discussion at a thought leader roundtable or working group
	Consensus document: A type of white paper to establish consensus on a health issue or practice, with conclusions voted on by all members of the working group or closed roundtable
	Call-to-action document: A type of consensus document that calls for specific actions to be implemented by different key groups in the medical and professional community; may help shape new health policies or practices
	Journal supplement: A compilation of scientific articles or meetings proceedings, usually packaged with the primary journal for distribution
	Trade publication article: An article being published by a thought leader or professional organization on publications that target specific professional audiences, including op-ed pieces and letters to the editors; standard editorial process, not peer reviewed
	Peer-reviewed journal article: Peer-reviewed article on original research data or new ideas on existing research
Online	*Websites*
	E-alerts: Issued by professional organizations to their membership and key constituencies to alert them to new medical practices, publications, events, and other information of interest
	Online discussions, live seminars, symposia, educational programs, workshops, and training courses
	Online tools
	Audio and video programs, including podcasts, videocasts, online proceedings of conferences and meetings
Mobile	Apps for a variety of clinical purposes (for example, diagnostic tools, patient-provider communication, disease or drug-related facts, etc.)
	Texting within hospitals settings or among health care providers to communicate about emergency situations, staffing needs, reporting on latest patient development
Audio and video programs	Training videos (online and CDs and DVDs)
	Spin-off of a primary program (for example, audiotaped conference, videotaped symposium)
	Videos and other media to support topic- and audience-specific presentations at conferences and meetings
Easy-to-implement tools	Tool kits: online, print, or electronic versions of materials that clinicians can use for a variety of issue-specific reasons: communication with patients, diagnostic tool, training sessions for all members of the clinical team, as a reminder of the importance of a new medical practice; may include brochures, fact sheets, videos, patient testimonials, case study discussions, relevant statistics, CD-ROMs

communication area. All of them—and many others—should be considered in identifying the strategic elements of issue-specific and audience-centered professional communications programs that seek to promote best clinical practices or new standards of care, or encourage the development of communities of practice as well as innovative solutions to medical problems, patient care, health workforce training, and scientific exchange. Among them, peer-reviewed or trade publication articles are usually written by opinion leaders and scientific advisors who are close to an organization's mission or are actually members of their scientific board of advisors. In fact, it is common practice for nonprofit and other private organizations to ask their scientific leaders to be directly involved in publicizing the data or ideas developed or advocated by the organization. Other times, the organization simply keeps track, in a publication plan, of all forthcoming articles on a specific topic and makes sure to extend the reach of the publication through other professional communication channels and activities. It is important to note here that most print peer-reviewed journals and trade publications now either have an online version or have completely migrated to being published only online.

Another important point is that serious consideration should be given to active approaches, such as interactive and online workshops and opinion leaders meetings, which should be designed to fit in the busy schedule of clinicians. Interactive approaches are more likely to be effective, even if they are more expensive (Grimshaw, Eccles, Walker, and Thomas, 2002; Spickard and others, 2001; Bauchner, Simpson, and Chessare, 2001). Practical experience has always confirmed this view.

Finally, professional communications activities and tools should respond to program strategies and be designed to transform "roadblocks into stepping stones" (Painter and Lemkau, 1992, p. 183) toward clinician change and, ultimately, better patient outcomes.

Using IT Innovation to Address Emerging Needs and Global Health Workforce Gap

The rapid advancement and uptake of information technology (IT) provides a unique opportunity to address emerging communication and training needs of health care providers across geographical areas and countries. This is of particular importance for underserved communities (such as rural areas in the United States, and low-income developing countries) where health care providers may not have access to the same kind of opportunities for interaction with colleagues as well as training events, courses, and certifications that exist for providers who work in urban settings or wealthy nations.

Information technology (including the use of videos, online resources, podcasts, and mobile technology) may help bridge gaps in health outcomes among affluent and underserved communities by empowering health care providers with information, tools, and knowledge to which they may not be exposed in some of the geographic areas or community settings where they operate. It can also help break down the cycle of professional isolation and limited opportunities for professional growth that still affects many providers in developing countries, and has contributed, among many other factors, to their large-scale emigration (also known as **brain drain**).

brain drain
The large-scale emigration of health workers from developing countries

The 2013 Global Education and Technology Health (GETHealth) Summit brought together professionals from multiple sectors and government agencies "to generate fresh knowledge, partnerships, and ideas that will more effectively leverage the three IT domains (infrastructure, devices, software) to address the critical health workforce gap" (GETHealth, 2013). Existing experiences already validate this approach. For example, the Center for Clinical Global Health Education at Johns Hopkins University has been using telemedicine and distance learning to share its expertise with providers from the neediest world's countries (GETHealth, 2013). In the United States, Project ECHO at the University of New Mexico "leverages teletechnology to train primary care doctors in rural and underserved areas to treat complex chronic illness. Through virtual grand rounds and other mentoring, providers and their care teams become part of a large knowledge network, experiencing real-time transfer of knowledge and best practices" (Robert Wood Johnson Foundation, 2013). Additional opportunities for these kinds of programs continue to exist given the increasing penetration of mobile technology among underserved communities in the United States and developing nations. Ultimately, using IT innovation as part of larger interventions may contribute to behavioral and social results that will foster global health equity among many underserved and vulnerable populations. IT innovation may contribute to increase the number of health care providers in areas where they are most needed; provide additional communication channels for professional development as well as dissemination of best clinical practices; and involve other health professionals (for example, social workers and community health workers) in providing information and services that reinforce health care provider recommendations.

Health communication is a key discipline in making progress toward this agenda. In fact, health communication professionals have pioneered the strategic use of new media and other emerging technologies as key components of comprehensive interventions that seek to improve public and patient health outcomes. As part of professional medical communication interventions, additional focus should be placed on the following:

- Encouraging multisectoral partnerships to address emerging needs in clinical settings

- Advocating for resources and political commitment to further the use of IT innovation

- Building health and media literacy capacity among health care providers

- Working closely with medical experts to devise simple and culturally competent solutions

- Making sure that essential skills, such as health literacy assessment, cultural competence, and cross-cultural communication, are efficiently integrated as part of all professional medical communication efforts

- Creating a critical mass in support of this overall endeavor by engaging professional and lay communities on the topic

Because multisectoral partnerships are at the core of addressing complex issues, further collaborations across different sectors are much needed to implement this agenda in different countries.

Prioritizing Health Disparities in Clinical Education to Improve Care: The Role of Cross-Cultural Health Communication

As urbanization continues to be a steady trend in population health, this is also changing the clinical landscape and contributing to increasing patient diversity in clinical settings. Such diversity is limited not only to culture, age, gender, language, and health beliefs but also includes the socioeconomic and political environment in which patients live, work, and age. Clinicians are increasingly confronted with having to apply the psychosocial model of health (see Chapter Two) and therefore to factor in and address the many social determinants of health, which are the root cause of health disparities and poor health outcomes among patients from vulnerable and underserved groups.

"Reducing inequities in healthcare will require broadening medical training to include health disparities education and research beyond the current focus on race and ethnicity to consider determinants such as socioeconomic status, environmental conditions, gender identity, sexual orientation, behavioral choices, and access to medical care" (New York Academy of Sciences, 2012). This should also extend to all other clinicians in charge of patient care and related interactions in order to maximize impact on patient outcomes.

Some programs already attempt to incorporate a health equity–based framework and mind-set to clinical care. For example, Health Leads helps connect patients with resources and services, including food, heat, and other important determinants of health, as prescribed by their health care providers (Health Leads, 2013).

Within this context, the role of cross-cultural health communication is key to advancing a health equity–inspired framework for clinical care. As recommended by the Institute of Medicine (IOM) report, *Unequal Treatment* (2003a), cultural competence training of health care providers is one of the key interventions to reduce health care disparities and improve patient outcomes. Cross-cultural health communication is grounded within a cultural competence framework, and is a field that has experienced great growth since the 2003 IOM report. Relevant cross-cultural health communication skills may enable health care providers to effectively bridge cultural, socioeconomic, and ethnic differences, and to provide the kind of social support that patients may need to actually implement and benefit from clinical recommendations. Knowledge of cross-cultural communication methods and strategies can also help practitioners to communicate effectively with colleagues from different cultural, ethnic, and racial backgrounds, given the increasing diversity of the global health workforce. As demonstrated by some existing experiences (Betancourt, 2008), e-learning and podcasts can provide a complementary training venue to more traditional in-person venues.

Increased diversity always drives or should drive change. Cross-cultural health communication interventions and training are a key component in the quest for health equity.

Key Concepts

• Professional medical communications is the application of health communication theories, models, and practices to programs that seek to influence the behavior and the social context of health professionals who are directly responsible for administering health care.

• Professional communications is a peer-to-peer approach directly related to the need to ensure that clinical practice always reflects state-of-the-art scientific evidence.

• Because of the influence of health care providers on patient outcomes and decisions, professional medical communications is a very important area of health communication. Often it is also a critical component of larger health communication programs that seek to encourage behavioral changes at the patient or public level, or advocate for a medical policy or practice change.

- Although physicians and other health care providers are just another group to be engaged in the health communication process, and should be considered as such, there are several specific skills (for example, advanced scientific writing ability) and tools that are used primarily or solely in professional communications. This creates the need for considering professional communications as a separate area of health communication.

- Although there is no consensus on theories and models for clinician change, great emphasis has been placed on the importance of behavioral and social change theories as well as many other constructs that are already part of the health communication theoretical toolbox (see Chapter Two).

- As in other areas of health communications, behavioral and social outcomes should be defined in advance and used to evaluate the intervention's effectiveness, ideally together with health care providers and their representatives. Ultimately, professional communications programs should aim to facilitate and encourage the adoption of best practices that may result in better health outcomes.

- The key characteristics and tools of effective professional communications programs should be considered in planning and implementing such interventions.

- Given the complexity of the health care environment, special consideration should be given to the following observations:
  - Professional communications programs that address existing barriers to clinician change are more likely to be effective.
  - Although more expensive, interactive approaches (whether offline or online) should be preferred because of their higher potential to motivate behavioral change among health care providers.
  - Multifaceted approaches are usually more effective than single or sporadic approaches in converting state-of-the-art scientific evidence in the adoption of new or best practices by clinicians.
  - Practical experience has validated the importance of using the right combination of individual and group strategies with institutional strategies.

- Innovation in information technology (IT) provides new opportunities to address emerging needs for capacity building among health care providers as well as the global health workforce gap. Health communication is an essential discipline in making progress on this public health and patient-centered agenda.

- Cross-cultural health communication in clinical settings plays a key role in improving care among underserved and vulnerable populations.

FOR DISCUSSION AND PRACTICE

1. In your opinion, in what circumstances may professional medical communications programs be an essential component of health communication interventions? Use specific examples or anecdotal experiences.

2. What are the key differences between professional medical communications and other areas of health communication? What are the key similarities?

3. How do health care providers' social networks and professional associations influence clinician behavior and practices? What are some implications of the providers' social context in professional medical communications?

4. Review Table 7.2, and rank, based on your opinion, the most important obstacles to clinician change. Explain your rank ordering and relate any personal or professional experiences that may support your selection.

5. What kind of technology does your physician, nurse, or other health care provider use? Describe what you have observed and how this may relate to and affect your own experience during clinical encounters (routine visits, sick visits, etc.). Provide your opinion on the pros and cons of the use of technology in clinical settings, and in relation to patient-provider communication.

6. A national nursing association launches a communication program to raise awareness of the reemergence of an infectious disease as well as recommended approaches to prevent it. Until then, the disease had been underestimated and underdiagnosed. In year one, the program's primary audience encompasses only health care professionals; in year two, the program's reach is extended to patients and the general public. List potential reasons for the association's decision to focus only on providers in the first year of the program, and discuss pros and cons of this approach.

KEY TERMS

brain drain

communities of practice

professional medical communication

tablets

CHAPTER 8

CONSTITUENCY RELATIONS AND STRATEGIC PARTNERSHIPS IN HEALTH COMMUNICATION

In most democratic societies, constituency relations is a structured approach that policymakers and elected government officials use "to consult, interact and exchange views and information with the public, so that citizens can express their preferences and provide their support for decisions that affects their lives and livelihood" (United Nations Development Programme, 2006). The general public as well as special groups and communities are the main constituents of policymakers.

At the same time, local government officials are a key constituency for public health. In fact, they influence the actions of local health departments as well as the allocation of funds and human resources to public health interventions and fields. Helping local government officials understand the true meaning of public health, which sometimes they regard only as the provision of specific health services and not as broad-based and community-centered interventions to improve public health outcomes, has been identified as an important role of public health managers. This helps gain visibility for public health (Lind and Finley, 2000) and enhances the chance that funding of public health interventions becomes a priority in a specific state or region.

These examples are only a few among the many contexts of constituency relations in which two different groups (policymakers and the general public, or local government officers and public health officials) can mutually influence each other. Constituency relations is an approach that is used in the public health, nonprofit, health care, community development, and commercial sectors to address a variety of health issues and situations, often in the context of health communication. It applies to different kinds of constituency groups that vary in function concerning the specific health issue.

CHAPTER OBJECTIVES

This chapter defines constituency relations and establishes its key contexts as well as "the importance of working collaboratively with diverse communities and constituencies (for example, researchers, practitioners, agencies and organizations)" (Association of Schools of Public Health, 2007, p. 11). It also provides examples of how the practice of constituency relations is relevant to the field of health communication and is also an integral approach of all communication action areas. Finally, it highlights examples, key steps, and dos and don'ts of this health communication area, as well as strategies to develop successful multisectoral partnerships.

Constituency Relations: A Practice-Based Definition

constituents

Individuals, communities, and groups that are influenced by or can influence a specific issue

constituency relations

The process of convening, exchanging information, and establishing and maintaining strategic relationships with key stakeholders, communities, and organizations with the intent of identifying common goals that can contribute to the outcomes of a specific communication program or health-related mission

Before defining constituency relations, it is important to understand what a constituency is. **Constituents** range from the body of voters who elect a specific policymaker or a political party or the board member of a professional organization to "groups of supporters or patrons" of different causes, or groups "served by an organization or institution" (*American Heritage Dictionary of the English Language*, 2004a). In public health and health care settings, they include patients, physicians, and other health care providers, hospital employees, professional and advocacy groups, nonprofit organizations, academia, health care–related companies, public health departments, the general public, and policymakers, to name just a few groups. These groups mutually influence each other. Depending on the specific health issue, situation, or setting, some of them may be more effective than others in helping advance public health causes, organizational missions and goals, or patient outcomes.

In health communication, **constituency relations** can be defined as the process of convening, exchanging information, and establishing and maintaining strategic relationships with key stakeholders, communities, and organizations with the intent of identifying common goals that can contribute to the outcomes of a specific communication program or mission. In fact, "communicating often involves reaching out to the audience first and building a constituency for the message" (Carter, 1994, p. 51). This process of establishing effective relationships and building key constituencies relies on all action areas of health communication (for example, interpersonal communication, strategic policy communication, new media communication). It is also an integral element of all of them and at the same time a communication area of its own. Often, constituency relations leads to strategic partnerships and coalitions.

Constituency relations has been used since the 1990s as a strategic area of communication in the private and commercial sectors. It has been employed to develop alliances to address public-policy issues as well as to extend political or marketing reach by corporations. In this context, key constituency groups are also called **third-party groups**, and include nonprofit, special interest, and advocacy organizations (Burson-Marsteller, 2006). Usually all parties in these relationships have shared goals that often can be achieved through collaboration, partnership, or interaction.

third-party groups
Key constituency groups in constituency relations, and include nonprofit, special interest, and advocacy organizations

In the corporate world as well as in many health care institutions such as private and public hospitals, constituency relations may be explained by looking at the stakeholder theory (Freeman, 1984). Originally developed to describe which groups in a corporation should receive management attention, the stakeholder theory recognizes that there are internal (for example, employers, investors) as well as external parties (customers, of course, but also political groups and communities) whose needs and wishes should be addressed as part of corporate decisions and initiatives. "A stakeholder in an organization is (by its definition) any group or individual who can affect or is affected by the achievement of the organization's objectives" (Freeman, 1984, p. 25; Scholl, 2001).

Other theoretical influences in the practice of constituency relations can be found in theories and models that look at the interrelation between different individual, group, or community factors, organizations, and levels of society, as well as their influence on health and social behavior (for example, the socioecological model mentioned in Chapter One and the ideation theory covered in Chapter Two). In general, constituency relations is a structured approach that can maximize the value of these connections and unleash the power of relationships to achieve health or social goals. Key principles of community and social mobilization and citizen engagement (see Chapter Six) can also be considered major influences in the practice of constituency relations.

In public health, several organizations and institutions increasingly recognize the role of constituency relations. For example, in 1999 the US National Institute of Mental Health launched the Constituency Outreach and Education Program, a nationwide initiative to "focus the energy of advocacy groups on merging science with service" and provide them with tools and information to develop health communication programs that will increase access to appropriate medical interventions by patients who suffer from mental illnesses (Cave, 2013). The program, now called the Outreach Partnership Program, has enlisted over the years "national and state organizations in partnerships to help bridge the gap between research and clinical practice by disseminating the latest scientific findings; informing the public about mental disorders, alcoholism, and drug addiction; and reducing the stigma and discrimination associated with these illnesses." The program also provides the National Institute of Mental Health with the opportunity to engage community groups across the United States in developing a national research agenda grounded in public health need (National Institute of Mental Health, 2013b). Recently, outreach partners have been conducting "targeted outreach activities to address mental disorders among children and adolescents and other populations identified to be at-risk, and mental health disparities that occur because of race, ethnicity, age (for example, older adults), education, income, disability status, geographic location, or risk status related to sex and gender. In addition, Outreach Partners promote volunteer participation in NIMH and NIH clinical trials and often collaborate with researchers to advance the research process" (National Institute of Mental Health, 2013a).

Constituency relations can help advance several disease-specific or social objectives within a health communication program. Some of the key areas or issues on which constituency relations can help are discussed further on in this chapter.

Recognizing the Legitimacy of All Constituency Groups

Positive relationships with organizations, communities, opinion leaders, and individuals who have a stake in a specific health issue often lead to the creation of a favorable and receptive environment for the strategies, messages, and activities of a health communication program. However, relationships should extend beyond groups or individuals who share common ideas and goals. Recognizing the legitimacy of all constituents, including groups that may have an opposite point of view, is an integral component of the practice of constituency relations (Burson-Marsteller, 2006).

Understanding opposing opinions as well as the key facts that may lead to them is one step toward anticipating and managing criticisms as well as gaining the respect of those who advocate opposite causes or solutions for the same health issue. In some cases, it may help find common ground, minimize differences, or identify solutions that may be acceptable to all parties, and consequently, sustainable.

Although it is not always possible to bridge different opinions, it is important to convey the impression of being for or against an issue and not against someone personally. At a minimum, contacts with opponents or information about their activities can guide communication efforts and tactics.

A relevant example is the ongoing debate on animal rights versus animal research that has been taking place for decades in Europe and the United States. Some of the animal rights organizations in the United States have long recognized that "an uncompromising, vegetarian-only, anti-medical-progress philosophy has a limited appeal" (Center for Consumer Freedom, 2013) with key constituencies, including the general public and policymakers. In some European countries, animal welfare organizations had to react to increasing support as well as petitions in favor of animal research by scientists, doctors, and reputable opinion leaders from the medical community. As a result, some of them have somewhat changed the focus or the tactics used in their efforts (Constance, 2005).

In recognizing the legitimacy of all constituencies, many of the skills and theoretical bases of interpersonal communication and other health communication areas come into play in managing criticisms as well as looking for common ground whenever possible. In fact, constituency relations use many of the tools and tactics of these communication areas (for example, public advocacy, one-on-one meetings, issues management, mass media and new media communication) to address criticisms as well as develop alliances with key constituency groups that share similar values and goals.

At the same time, constituency relations is an integral component of all the other areas of health communication. For example, public advocacy (see Chapter Nine) is often used to attract new constituents to a health issue. At the same time, establishing and maintaining relationships with key representatives of the mass media as well as building virtual communities in support of a specific issue are fundamental to media advocacy efforts and use many of the principles of constituency relations.

Constituency Relations: A Structured Approach

As with other areas of health communication, constituency relations is both an art and a science. Health and community development organizations that approach this field for the first time may require changes at the individual, team, and organizational levels in order to succeed in their constituency relations efforts. Still, as experience has shown, constituency relations and building are critical elements in the process for addressing existing and new public health and health care recommendations and challenges (Kimbrell, 2000). "An effective constituency-building practice allows public health leaders to develop relationships that facilitate community health improvement." Using this as an organizational practice, "public health leaders identify major public health constituents, delineate participation factors, develop and manage effective interactions with constituency groups, and apply strategies for evaluating and improving constituency engagement in public health initiatives" (Hatcher and Nicola, 2008, p. 443).

Organizations in public health and other fields and communication teams may want to consider building internal capabilities to establish and maintain relationships with key constituencies and, ideally, develop strategic partnerships and coalitions. This transformation usually starts with key management (for example, executive directors, board members, and communication directors) and extends to all levels of the organization. Encouraging a constituency relations and partnership-oriented mind-set among staff and consultants has these key components:

- Identifying constituency relations and outreach champions and, when resources allow, establishing professional positions or departments dedicated to this area. For example, the US National Institute of Mental Health has an Office of Constituency Relations and public liaison. Also, the Campaign for Tobacco-Free Kids, "a leading force in the fight to reduce tobacco use and its deadly toll in the United States and around the world" (Campaign for Tobacco Free Kids, 2013), has staff members dedicated to constituency relations.

- Emphasizing the importance of teamwork, listening, and negotiation skills, as well as balancing different needs and sharing credit for success with other organizations.

- Training staff members.

- Sharing results with other organizational departments.

In addition, organizations and health communication teams need to develop a long-term vision about key constituency groups as well as their key issues and priorities. They also need to establish and cultivate long-term relationships with all of these groups. Table 8.1 gives examples of the dos and don'ts of establishing and preserving relationships with key constituents.

Table 8.1   Guidelines for Establishing and Preserving Long-Term Relationships

DO	DON'T
Understand the mission, strategic priorities, and focus of key constituency groups	Look down at constituency groups if they are smaller in size or in favor of a different approach to a health issue
Reach out to these groups at the program's outset	
Keep an open mind in exchanging relevant information	Assume they will support every aspect of your cause or communication program
Consider their worries and concerns	Give the impression they are not accountable for their responsibilities if a partnership is established
Recognize and respect cultural, ethnic, or other kinds of differences	
Look for shared goals and priorities	Do their share of the work
Act to establish long-term relationships based on trust and mutual respect	Try to control or micromanage them
When of interest, address barriers to potential partnerships	
Keep assessing the value of the partnership to all partners vis-à-vis mutually agreed-on parameters	
If a partnership is established, honor deadlines, financial commitments, and mutually agreed-on procedures and roles	
Encourage and maximize participation by all partners in program design, implementation, and evaluation	

Developing Alliances to Address Health or Social Issues and to Expand Program Reach

One of the common outcomes of constituency relations is the development of partnerships, coalitions, or other kinds of collaborations. Coalitions often grow out of partnerships and require a more formal structure, including written memoranda of communication agreements, bylaws, a dedicated management team, and common tools, as well as a long-term commitment to the coalition's cause. A relevant example is the Coalition for Health Communication (2013), "an inter-organizational task force whose mission is to strengthen the identity and advance the field of health communication." The coalition, which includes several groups, associations, and US federal agencies, has a common website, a management team, and common activities and tools.

Regardless of their format, partnerships, coalitions, and other forms of collaborations can help advance health and social goals by strengthening the credibility and relevance of a specific issue; giving a structured voice to constituencies that can influence policymakers (see Chapter Nine), the press, and other key stakeholders; expanding the program's reach; or combining different resources and expertise. Box 8.1 features an interview with key staff members from Physicians for Human Rights, an international nonprofit organization, and provides a practical perspective on the importance of constituency relations.

BOX 8.1. HOW CONSTITUENCY RELATIONS CAN HELP ADVANCE AN ORGANIZATION'S MISSION: A PRACTICE-BASED PERSPECTIVE

The following perspective on constituency relations reflects a telephone interview and personal communications in 2006 with Gina Cummings and Nancy Marks, who at the time were respectively the deputy director of operations and the director of outreach for Physicians for Human Rights.

Physicians for Human Rights (PHR), founded in 1986, mobilizes health professionals to advance the health and dignity of all people through actions that promote respect for, protection of, and fulfillment of human rights. In 1997 PHR shared the Nobel Prize for Peace as a founding member of the Steering Committee of the International Campaign to Ban Landmines. PHR is a membership organization of physicians, nurses, public health experts, forensic scientists, human rights experts, and others dedicated to advancing health and human rights. Health care professionals are a reputable voice in society and have the power and credibility to advocate for human rights protection.

Over the past few decades, the organization has evolved in its mission and has made many changes to engage health care providers (including physicians, nurses, and medical, nursing, and public health students) from the United States and many other parts of the world in studying the impact of human right abuses on the health status of populations as well as advocating for change with policymakers and other relevant parties. PHR built a US-based professional constituency that provides expertise and documents abuse and advocates for new policies and practices. It also began to cultivate a similar constituency in Africa to work on issues related to the prevention of HIV/AIDS and treatment and care of HIV/AIDS patients.

Medical, nursing, and public health students are key constituencies in the organization. PHR believes that students represent the future of public health and human rights. Student volunteers raise awareness of health care disparities, persuade policymakers about the importance of viewing HIV/AIDS as a global crisis with an impact on health care and health care systems, and work to end the genocide in Darfur, Sudan.

PHR work has been focusing not only on building and supporting new constituencies but also on maintaining and cultivating relationships with existing constituency groups and other stakeholders, including US policymakers, ministries of health in developing countries, the World Health Organization [WHO], and other human rights organizations, including Amnesty International. PHR is often a resource for policymakers and other key constituencies; for example, it provides scientific content about human rights and health issues and proposes strategic solutions. PHR also acts as a convener of stakeholders in meetings, workshops, and summits that aim to establish consensus on potential solutions of health and human rights issues, as well as a clear path to achieve them.

For example, in recognizing that most health centers in rural Africa are attended by nurse practitioners, PHR partnered with the US Association of Nurses in AIDS Care to organize an HIV summit that included the participation of twenty-five to thirty nurses working with AIDS in Africa. These nurses not only had an opportunity to exchange information on best clinical practices in HIV/AIDS treatment and prevention but were also able to meet with US policymakers to address issues related to the funding of HIV prevention, care, and treatment in Africa. The summit also addressed the issue of the increasing shortage of health care professionals in developing countries due to deteriorating socioeconomic conditions. PHR gave to the project its expertise in human rights, whereas the nurses' association contributed technical competence and its wealth of knowledge in the HIV/AIDS field.

Building a constituency is often the result of speaking with organizations or people who understand the specific health or human rights problem and its potential solutions. It also requires a clear understanding of roles and responsibilities of different constituencies, expected outcomes of potential partnerships, the time frame of all joint efforts and collaborations, and the decision-making process that will be used for joint efforts.

Most people understand the nuances of the work required in constituency relations only after many years of practice. This is the kind of professional competence that one learns on the job. Nevertheless, it is important to become familiar with the values and key principles of this important area as part of formal education and training.

Strategies to Develop Successful Multisectoral Partnerships

Most health and social issues are complex and multisectoral in their nature or potential solutions. For example, in a community with high rates of obesity, the typical solution might appear to be focused on working with local grocery stores to provide healthy, affordable options. Yet, focusing only on local stores would demonstrate a lack of recognition that simultaneous initiatives must also be in place. For example, a more comprehensive approach would include working with city planners to create park space, bike lanes, and free running tracks, with statisticians to map which parts of a neighborhood have higher rates of obesity and to determine why, with health care providers to offer culturally competent nutritional counseling and information, with local businesses to offer exercises classes at worksites or incentives such as lower insurance premiums for individuals who lose weight, with community organizations to enhance their capacity to encourage community participation in devising local solutions or providing social support to less privileged groups, with local schools and radio programs on messaging, in addition to other key actors (Health Equity Initiative, 2012a). Our increasing understanding of the many social determinants of health, and vice versa, and the role health plays—along with many other factors—in community and social development no longer justifies any investment on strategies and programs that only bring to the table the narrow perspective of one organization, no matter how prominent that organization may be.

The practice of multisectoral strategic partnership management and development has flourished in recent times. It is supported by prominent organizations, as well as recommended core competencies in public health (Association of Schools of Public Health, 2007) and clinical settings (National League for Nursing, 2005; National CNS Competency Task Force, 2010; Partnership for Health in Aging, 2013); it is the focus of professional development trainings and resources (Health Equity Initiative, 2013c; Community Tool Box, 2013); and it is helping shape the content and reach of large international initiatives (for example, the Every Woman, Every Baby global campaign by UNICEF and its partners) within and outside the field of public health. Core competencies of nurse educators issued by the National League for Nursing (2005) identify creating and maintaining "community and clinical partnerships that support educational goals" as an important competency. Also, several medical associations, including the American Geriatric Association, include the ability to "communicate and collaborate with older adults, their caregivers, health care professionals, and direct-care workers to incorporate discipline-specific information into overall team care planning and implementation" (Partnership for Health in Aging Workgroup, 2008) as a core competency.

multisectoral partnerships
Partnerships that result when governments, nonprofit, private, and public organizations, academia, community groups, individual community members, and others "come together to solve problems that affect the whole community or a specific population" (Community Tool Box, 2013)

Multisectoral partnerships result when governments, nonprofit, private and public organizations, academia, community groups, individual community members, and others "come together to solve problems that affect the whole community or a specific population" (Community Tool Box, 2013). These kinds of partnerships are designed to address systemic public health, health care, and community development issues, are based on collaboration rather than competition, and should be considered a long-term enterprise. Ultimately, multisectoral partnerships should aim to encourage community action and ownership of health and social issues and their community-driven solutions. Other kinds of short-term partnerships can be considered to address specific aspects (for example, service delivery, community outreach, information dissemination) of a health communication program or larger public health or global health or community development intervention.

Building strategic partnerships requires hard work both in the exploratory and the maintenance phases. It is also a process that requires a well-thought and structured approach in order to increase the effectiveness of program efforts as well as to increase long-term sustainability of the partnership itself. It is important to identify potential partners early in the process (so they can effectively participate in intervention planning, implementation, and evaluation) as well as to be aware of organizational restrictions and administrative requirements of one's organization that may prevent or regulate partnerships.

The decision about developing partnerships should be made early in program development. In doing so, health organizations and communication teams should be aware of the potential drawbacks of partnerships and be prepared to address them efficiently (National Cancer Institute at the National Institutes of Health, 2002) as part of a participatory process that engages all partners on establishing relevant protocols, decision-making processes, and sample solutions at the outset of the partnership.

In general, most drawbacks can be successfully addressed if all partners have established and agreed on well-defined objectives for the specific partnership, standard procedures, shared workload, common goals, and a consensus-driven action plan. All of these elements are usually addressed as part of the partnership plan component of a health communication program (see Chapter Thirteen).

Nevertheless, partnerships take time and commitment. Being aware of some of the potential drawbacks is a step forward in overcoming barriers and preserving long-term relationships. Table 8.2 lists potential drawbacks. Some of them may be minimized by choosing the right partners, one of the many steps in building long-lasting and results-driven partnerships.

Table 8.2 Potential Drawbacks of Partnerships

Feelings of loss of control over program development

Time-consuming process

Partners who may go off strategy

Lack of partners' participation or real commitment to the project

Too many administrative roadblocks

The cost (economic or human resources) of maintaining and managing the partnership

Sources: National Cancer Institute at the National Institutes of Health. *Making Health Communication Programs Work.* Bethesda, MD: National Institutes of Health, 2002; Weinreich, N. K. *Hands-on Social Marketing: A Step-by-Step Guide.* Newbury Park, CA: Sage, 1999; Weinreich, N. K. *Hands-on Social Marketing: A Step-by-Step Guide to Designing Change for Good.* (2nd ed.) Thousand Oaks, CA: Sage, 2011.

Choosing the Right Partners

Because the list of potential partners is often quite long, the following criteria may help identify partners and organizations that are best suited to support and contribute to the health communication program or the mission of a specific health organization:

- Mutual mission and goals, which often starts with a common vision but sometimes can be the result of an engaging communication process in which common interests and solutions are identified, negotiated, and selected to the satisfaction of all potential partners

- Background and experience in relation to the specific health issue or group the program is seeking to address or engage; it also includes relevant experiences in different fields that may function as a model for new health communication interventions

- Access to intended audiences and stakeholders through existing programs, resources, and community outreach and mobilization efforts or because of the reputation of potential partners with key groups, the mass media, or other key stakeholders

- Preexisting relationships with your organization

- Access to additional resources and skills

- Ease of development in terms of the review process for program elements (for example, message development, materials) as well as lack of the kinds of standard protocols that may not be flexible enough to accommodate partners' working styles and routine procedures

- Costs (economic, time, and resources) that need to be dedicated to establishing and managing a specific partnership

- Enthusiasm about your mission or program's goal

In short, it is always better to identify partners that have organizational, professional, or mission-related objectives that in the long term can contribute to the achievement of the health communication program's goals and objectives. If and when partnerships with commercial companies are considered, most nonprofit organizations have written or informal criteria and policies that guide such partnerships. These criteria are set to preserve the nonprofit organization's credibility and independence, as well as the overall reputation of the partnership. Usually they are also welcomed and endorsed by most commercial entities.

Box 8.2 provides the US National Cancer Institute's guidelines for the evaluation of commercial partners that may participate in health communication interventions or other institute efforts. Specific criteria and steps also apply to other special kinds of partnerships such as coalitions, public-private partnerships, and **collaborative agreements** (such as those that involve universities, health care professionals, and organizations). Appendix A includes a select list of resources in relation to special kinds of partnerships.

collaborative agreements
A special kind of partnership involving universities, health care professionals, and organizations

BOX 8.2. NATIONAL CANCER INSTITUTE GUIDELINES FOR CONSIDERING COMMERCIAL PARTNERS

Policies

- The National Cancer Institute [NCI] will not consider any collaboration that endorses a specific commercial product, service, or enterprise.
- The National Cancer Institute name and logo may be used only in conjunction with approved projects and only with the written permission of NCI. NCI retains the right to review all copy (for example, advertising, publicity, or for any other intended use) prior to approval of the use of the NCI name and logo.
- The National Cancer Institute will formally review each proposal for partnership.
- No company will have an exclusive right to use the NCI name and logo, messages, or materials.
- Confidentiality cannot be guaranteed for any collaboration with a federal program.

Criteria for Reviewing Corporations Prior to Partnership Negotiations

- Company is not directly owned by a tobacco company and is not involved in producing, marketing, or promoting tobacco products.
- Company does not have any products, services, or promotional messages that conflict with NCI policies or programs (for example, the company does not market known carcinogens or market some other product that NCI would not consider medically or scientifically acceptable).
- Company is not currently in negotiation for a grant or contract with NCI.
- Company does not have any unresolved conflicts or disputes with NCI or NIH [National Institutes of Health].
- Establishing a partnership with this company will not create tensions/conflicts with another NCI partner or federal program.
- Company or institution satisfactorily conforms [to] standards of health or medical care.
- There is evidence that the company would be interested in becoming a partner with NCI.

Source: National Cancer Institute at the National Institutes of Health. *Making Health Communication Programs Work.* Bethesda, MD: National Institutes of Health, 2002, p. 37.

Building Long-Lasting and Results-Driven Partnerships

Building long-lasting and results-driven partnerships is all about maintaining the kind of momentum, enthusiasm, and commitment levels that brought different partners together at the outset of the partnership. It is not an easy task, but can become a bit easier with the help of careful planning, partner feedback mechanisms, and monitoring, evaluation, and reporting, not only in relation to the intervention's outcomes but also in regard to partners' motivation to stay in the partnership and overall satisfaction levels with key accomplishments and processes (Schiavo, 2006, 2007, 2012). It also requires great interpersonal skills, which may help partners to stick together at times of uncertainty, change, low funding levels, and other kinds of potentially difficult situations that characterize long-term partnerships.

Throughout the process of building and maintaining partnerships, it is important to remember that "partnerships are not painless. They often involve melding different cultures and always imply significant investment of time, and compromises. But when they work, they can generate better results for all parties" (United Nations Foundation, 2003, p. 4). In looking at different organizational cultures, it is also important to understand what is internally rewarded by different kinds of organizations. For example, some organizations focus on and reward individual achievement, others value team work, others are mission-driven or have specific financial or commercial objectives (with many different combinations of these and other characteristics that contribute to organizational cultures). Asking potential partners about what would make them succeed within their own organization as a reflection of their participation in the partnership-driven intervention is a way to get to know them and their organizations and start melding cultures.

Table 8.3 includes key partnership success factors as extrapolated from lessons learned from two different interventions: (1) the design and development of a multisectoral center for tropical diseases in Brazil, with the aim of contributing to the reduction of morbidity and mortality of malaria and leishmaniasis; and (2) a national communication campaign in the United States to raise awareness of key contributing factors to and build professional networks on primary nocturnal enuresis (PNE; bedwetting over age six) (Schiavo, personal files, 2012c, 2013). Many of these success factors apply across different kinds of partnership building and management efforts along with others that may be situation or issue specific.

Partners' satisfaction with the partnership's outcomes and processes as well as their sustained motivation to participate is key to the intervention's

Table 8.3   Sample Partnership Success Factors

Extensive upfront research on partners' needs, interests, and mission

Development of key selling points for each potential partner

Identification of key partnership champions for each organization

Early involvement of all partners in program design and implementation

Common vision and shared program goals

Shared spotlight on a rotational basis

Regular meetings to discuss next steps, assess results and processes

Project supervision by partnership board with coordination by one of the partners (for example, secretariat or coordination group)

Familiarity with each other's standard practices, beliefs, mission, and so on

Partners' appreciation of professional guidance of the overall partnership and program development process

Honesty, commitment, enthusiasm, respect of others

Source: Schiavo, personal files (2012c, 2013).

progress and outcomes. Because motivating factors as well as what people define as "success" may vary from person to person and from organization to organization, it is important to develop specific indicators to evaluate the success of the actual partnership outside of program-specific indicators. For example, as part of a recent experience on building capacity for the development of multisectoral task forces for infant mortality prevention in four US cities, participants in a two-day workshop and partnership plan development session in each city contributed and agreed on criteria they would use to evaluate the status and progress of the partnership (Schiavo, Estrada-Portales, Hoeppner, and Ormaza, 2012). This was instrumental in clarifying individual, professional, and organizational motivations to participate in the task force and to develop suitable indicators for the long-term evaluation of partners' satisfaction and motivation, among other factors (Schiavo, Estrada-Portales, Hoeppner, and Ormaza, 2012).

As collaborative endeavors require time and mentoring, the success of all partnerships is ultimately related to the existence of adequate mechanisms and communication tools that would enable partners to be supported in their efforts, discuss obstacles and common issues with implementing the partnership, and continuing to grow in their knowledge on key partnership strategies and success factors. As previously mentioned, this may start with creating a culture of collaboration with one's organization or community by identifying partnership champions; dedicating staff or organizational departments to constituency relations and partnership development; and providing staff and community members with opportunities for training and professional development on new trends, strategies, and processes in this area.

Different Types of Partnerships

Although the scope of this book does not include a comprehensive discussion of different kinds of collaborative efforts and structures, this section provides examples of select types of partnerships as well as key factors students and professionals may want to consider as they approach the development of strategic partnerships in health communication or other fields.

For example, working with small to medium-sized community-based organizations (CBOs) starts with taking into account that for them making a difference is key, because their staff is highly dedicated to their mission and often representative of the communities they serve. As CBOs are often juggling many different conflicting priorities in the face of limited economic and human resources, they are likely to partner with other organizations only on programs that they feel strongly about, that fit in their overall mission and with existing programs, and that are likely to be met with the approval of their key constituencies and the community members they serve (Community Tool Box, 2013; Schiavo, 2012). Setting clear goals—both for the intervention and the CBO's participation—is necessary to maximize the use of their limited human resources. Of equal importance is to consider the economic environment and the financial cycle in which the CBO operates. Very often CBOs need to prioritize activities in light of financial restrictions, and may need financial incentives, or alternatively, to wait for better times in order to engage in new programs and partnerships. Yet, CBOs are essential to creating connections with local communities, increase cultural competency of all interventions, and ultimately encourage community participation, so all efforts should be made to involve them in new or existing programs and initiatives.

Other examples of strategic partnerships are public-private partnerships (PPPs). A **public-private partnership** is "a collaboration between public bodies, such as central government or local authorities, and private companies" (*PPP Bulletin International*, 2012) or organizations. PPPs "involve at least one private for-profit organization and at least one not-for-profit or public organization" (Reich, 2002, p. 3).

Public-private partnerships aim to achieve long-term goals or institutionalize interventions at the public sector level. They focus on mutually agreed-on areas and need a formal structure, including leadership or steering committees, written memoranda of agreement or contracts for program implementation, clearly stated mission and goals, dedicated staff, frequent communication channels, member development and training, external resources, and a formal evaluation process, including members' level of accountability (Schiavo, 2012). Many of these requirements are not unique

public-private partnership
"A collaboration between public bodies, such as central government or local authorities, and private companies" (*PPP Bulletin International*, 2012) or organizations. PPPs "involve at least one private for-profit organization and at least one not-for-profit or public organization" (Reich, 2002, p. 3).

to PPPs but they are often more important, given the high level of senior commitment and capital that is required by PPPs. Most important, PPPs require all partners to embrace

> a view of the world for which we believe that in all sectors (public, policy, nonprofit, healthcare, private, etc.) the majority of people share a common sense of human decency and may want to leave a better world for their children. By avoiding any temptation to divide the world into good and evil, and starting to act as if no one has any choice other than contributing to health equity [or other health and social causes], we may achieve more than when we are less inclusive or too quick to assign labels. This is a communication challenge in itself, and one that resonates with the call to action for all sectors to help reduce disparities delivered by prominent leaders, such as WHO's Director General Dr. Margaret Chan. (Schiavo, 2011b, p. 68)

An example of a PPP is the Global Public-Private Partnership for Handwashing (PPPHW) with Soap, a coalition of thirteen international stakeholders, including UNICEF, USAID, Procter & Gamble, FHI360, London School of Hygiene and Tropical Medicine, Unilever, University of Buffalo, and the State University of New York, among others. "The PPPHW seeks to promote awareness, build political commitment, and trigger action" on proper hand washing with soap at critical times at local, national, and international levels.

The PPPHW adheres to the following principles:

- The public sector in each country takes the lead, with technical assistance and support from outside agencies.
- Political commitment is required.
- PPPHW programs are national in scale.
- Public-private partnerships are only a means to an end.
- The focus is on building and integrating existing water and sanitation, infrastructure, health, and school programs.
- The focus is on measuring the impact of large-scale hand-washing programs.
- Partnerships are inclusive. (PPPHW, 2013)

The PPPHW operates in several countries. Published results from an advanced intervention in Ghana "showed an increase in reported hand-washing rates by 13% after using the toilet and by 41% before eating" within a national sample skewed toward rural participants (Curtis, Garbrah-Aidoo, and Scott, 2007, p. 637), and with several ongoing interventions accounting toward additional progress both in Ghana and other countries. Other similar PPPs have been instrumental in advancing outcomes in very diverse fields, including obesity (Coalition for Healthy Children, 2013); oral health (Cohen, 2011); cancer treatment and prevention (Weir, DeGennaro, and Austin, 2012); health care access, quality, and efficiency (Sekhri, Feachem, and Ni, 2011); and neglected tropical diseases (Bush and Hopkins, 2011), among others.

In conclusion, the practice of constituency relations, as well as the potential for strategic partnerships or other kinds of collaborations that derive from this practice, is a valuable asset in all health communication areas, and more, in general, in the fields of public health, health care, and community development. For example, when planning the professional medical communications component of a health communication program, it is critical to understand and involve health organizations and groups that can influence physician behavioral change. At the same time, constituency relations rely on many of the theoretical assumptions and tools of other areas of communication (for example, interpersonal communication) and can be considered a strategic communication area of its own. Often new communication programs and approaches as well as the decision to focus on a specific health issue start with an informal meeting, an e-mail, or telephone call in which constituency groups are involved. From this starting point, the road to effective interactions, collaborations, and strategic partnerships is as complex and gradual as described in this chapter.

Key Concepts

- The importance of "working collaboratively with diverse communities and constituencies (for example researchers, practitioners, agencies and organizations)" (Association of Schools of Public Health, 2007, p. 11) has been established by several prominent organizations.

- Constituency relations is a key area of health communication as well as a critical component of all other action areas of communication.

- In health communication, constituency relations can be defined as the process of convening, exchanging information, establishing, and maintaining strategic relationships with key stakeholders, communities, and organizations with the intent of identifying common goals that can contribute to the outcomes of a specific communication program or organizational mission.

- Constituency relations is commonly used in the public health, non-profit, health care, and commercial sectors as a fundamental area of communication.

- One of the fundamental premises of constituency relations is the importance of recognizing the legitimacy of all constituency groups, including those that may have opposite opinions on or approaches to a health issue.

- Establishing and maintaining positive relationships with groups that share common values and goals depends on a number of factors.

- Most health and social issues are complex and multisectoral in their nature or potential solutions. Multisectoral partnership is a key tool in effectively addressing such issues.

- Multisectoral partnerships result when governments, nonprofit, private, and public organizations, academia, community groups, individual community members, and others "come together to solve problems that affect the whole community or a specific population" (Community Tool Box, 2013).

- Building a constituency around a health issue or building and maintaining strategic partnerships and collaborations requires hard work and several fundamental steps.

- These steps are usually summarized in the partnership plan component of a health communication program (see Chapter Thirteen) and are also introduced in this chapter along with key success factors of strategic partnerships and examples of different kinds of partnerships.

FOR DISCUSSION AND PRACTICE

1. Discuss examples of partnerships or coalitions of which you are aware and highlight their role in advancing public health or organizational goals.

2. Review Table 8.1 and describe a professional or personal experience in which any of the dos or don'ts in the table have influenced the process of establishing and preserving long-term relationships. Rank the dos and don'ts in the table in order of importance and provide a rationale for your ranking order.

3. How do constituency relations fit in health communication? Provide examples to illustrate key concepts explored in this chapter.

4. Research and discuss a case study on a health communication program that was developed thanks to the efforts of partners from multiple sectors. Highlight lessons learned and key success factors of this multisectoral partnership.

5. Think of two different organizations you may be familiar with and list key characteristics that contribute to their organizational culture. Identify what they have in common and what are some of the issues that may need to be addressed to blend cultures as part of any potential collaborative effort.

KEY TERMS

collaborative agreements

constituency relations

constituents

multisectoral partnerships

public-private partnerships

third-party groups

CHAPTER 9

POLICY COMMUNICATION AND PUBLIC ADVOCACY

Truly transformative leadership moments in public health or social development policy are always the result of hard work and long-term commitment by many people in order to achieve policy change and implementation. Yet, such moments have the potential to make a long-term impact on large populations as well as vulnerable and underserved groups. The image that comes to my mind is one of a taxi driver, a fun and hard-working immigrant who had lived in the United States for several decades with his family and was already in his late seventies. He drove me in a Florida city to a meeting that was taking place at a local community health center. "These people are great," he kept saying in describing the quality of care he received there. He also felt that community health centers are a life-saving option for people like himself, who have limited resources. He was truly grateful for their existence, and could not stop recounting clinical encounters and other situations in which he felt they saved his life or "put him quickly back to work."

"America's Health Centers owe their existence to a remarkable turn of events in US history, and to a few determined community health and civil rights activists working in low-income communities during the 1960s. Millions of Americans, living in inner-city neighborhoods and rural areas throughout the country suffered from deep poverty and a desperate need for health care. Among those determined to seek change was H. Jack Geiger, then a young doctor and civil rights activist. Geiger had studied in South Africa and witnessed how a pioneering community health model had wrought astonishing improvements in public health" (National Association of Community

Health Centers, 2013). The road from these early days of the Community Health Center Movement to the declaration of the "War on Poverty" by President Johnson, "which included the first proposal for the U.S. version of a Community Health Center," and finally, to the approval of funding "in 1965 for the first two neighborhood health center demonstration projects, one in Boston, Massachusetts, and the other in Mound Bayou, Mississippi" (National Association of Community Health Centers, 2013) was paved by policy communication and public advocacy efforts not only in communicating with policymakers and other key stakeholders but also in creating a critical mass of informed citizens in support of the health centers.

CHAPTER OBJECTIVES

This chapter focuses on approaches and strategies to communicate about health policy and management using appropriate channels (Association of Schools of Public Health, 2007), discuss communication methods to advocate for public health policies (Association of Schools of Public Health, 2007), and engage relevant groups and citizens in advocating for policy change and enforcement. The chapter defines and establishes policy communication and public advocacy as key integrated areas of health communication.

Policy Communication and Public Advocacy as Integrated Communication Areas

The main premise of this chapter is that all of us, regardless of whether we work in public health, health care, the private sector, community development, or other fields, find ourselves communicating often enough about policies and their management as part of our professional endeavors. Think, for example, of an academic instructor who communicates with students about the department's policy on internships or number of credits required to obtain a degree, or a clinical technician communicating with patients about the medical practice's policy on the release of health exam results, or a nonprofit organization communicating with the communities it serves on a national health policy it is contributing to implement at the local level, or a grant-maker speaking with potential grantees about the organization's grant policies in the public health field. At the same time, all of these professionals may be able to craft, demonstrate the need, and advocate for policy change within their organizations, and will need to secure the support of different publics (for example, peers, the communities they attend, and influential groups) in order to pass a new policy or implement an existing one. This should demonstrate that **policy communication** (communicating about health or scientific data in support of policy change, or a new or existing policy and its implementation and evaluation) and **public advocacy** (the strategic use of communication to affect changes in public opinion and attitudes so that it influences policymakers or other decision makers and promotes changes in behaviors, social norms, policies, and resource allocation to benefit a community, group, population, or organization) also find application outside the realm of elected officials and other politicians. Also, although organizational and local policies often have less of a broad impact on large populations than national policies, their cumulative effect is likely to touch the lives of many people and communities.

Yet, "the term 'advocacy' has multiple meanings depends on the context in which it is used. It broadly describes the influence of groups in shaping social and political outcomes in government and society. In law and regulation, advocacy refers to types of reportable activities, but regulatory agencies may differ on their use of the term. In research, advocacy may describe both the representational and participatory aspect of groups as intermediaries between citizens and decision makers, types of organizations and their capacity to advocate, and strategies of action in different venues" (Reid, 2013).

In most contexts, a fundamental component of public advocacy efforts is the use of the mass media, and new media, which is also called *media advocacy*, reflecting advocacy efforts that heavily relies on the strategic use of the mass media and new media.

Although communicating with policymakers has been, for a while, an essential competency in public health, health care, community development, and most fields in the public and private sectors, the past few decades and the advent of many new technologies have marked a significant increase in the practice of communicating about policy among different professional and lay groups. Policymakers are also increasingly jumping in the public discourse and using many of the tools from public advocacy to convey their perspective or support of specific policies on health and social issues. For example, the twentieth century has marked an increase in presidential policy communication, which has taken alternative forms outside of presidential rhetoric, including the use of newspapers, public letters (Hoffman, 2010), and, in the twenty-first century, websites and new media.

policy communication
Communicating about health or scientific data in support of policy change, or a new or existing policy and its implementation and evaluation

public advocacy
The strategic use of communication to affect changes in public opinion and attitudes so that it influences policy makers or other decision makers and promotes changes in behaviors, social norms, policies, and resource allocation to benefit a community, group, population, or organization

Policy communication and public advocacy are strictly interconnected and are integrated with many complementary, and sometimes overlapping, strategies, activities, and media. Policy communication rarely happens in a vacuum, and most times it is supported by public advocacy efforts that seek to engage the general public or specific communities or groups in backing up intended outcomes of conversations with policymakers and other stakeholders. As previously mentioned, the American Heart Association (2006b) defines public advocacy as "the act of influencing decision makers and promoting changes to laws and other government policies to advance the mission of a particular organization or group of people." In a way, this definition suggests that policy communication may be a component of public advocacy in the case of policy change when the role of adequately presenting research findings and health-related data is also key to advocating for new policies or resource allocation. Policy communication that is intended to further the reach or implementation of new or existing policies may be more distinctive from public advocacy, because it often does not require the same level of engagement of the general population or large segments of specific groups.

Several organizations have been working to create much-needed capacity on policy communication. For example, the Population Reference Bureau has a policy communication fellow program, which is open to "individuals from developing countries currently enrolled in academic institutions pursuing doctoral programs" and focuses on several health and social development areas, including family planning, reproductive health, poverty, health equity, and population growth (Population Reference Bureau, 2013). "The program aims to bridge the gap between research findings and the policy development process. Although research often has profound policy implications, it must be communicated effectively to a variety of nontechnical audiences in order to have an impact" (Population Reference Bureau, 2013).

Supporting the quest for policy change with scientific data is important for policy communication and public advocacy within the context of tailoring all communications to the cultural preferences, needs, "so-what" attitudes, and literacy levels of different groups. This is also true within the context of communicating about policy implementation and management in which several stakeholders and decision makers are asked to prioritize and reach out to their own constituencies to facilitate widespread enforcement and impact evaluation of a given policy. The sections that follow focus on relevant experiences and approaches for evidence-based policy communication and public advocacy.

Communicating with Policymakers and Other Key Stakeholders

As with all other influential and citizen groups, understanding your audience before engaging policymakers in any kind of conversation or public debate is key. For this purpose, looking at voting records on your issue, information on groups to which specific policymakers may belong, history of support of health and social issues, as well as the key components of political systems, agencies, and organizations; the rules and potential limitations of the specific office for which policymakers have been elected or serve into; and many other critical factors is a first step of all communications. No matter what you do, you need to prepare before talking about policy with any kind of decision maker.

For example, the Annual Health Education Advocacy Summit, organized by the Coalition of National Health Education Organizations and its partners, helps participants polish their "advocacy skills in just 48 hours. This event offers basic, intermediate, and advanced level advocacy training, and features issue-specific seminars by skilled government relations staff. The Summit culminates with visits with legislators or key staff on Capitol Hill—either individually or in state/district delegations" (Virginia Public Health Association, 2013; Health Education Advocate, 2013). It usually focuses only on two to three specific tasks that may benefit the general population, specific groups, or may help further advance the health education profession (Health Education Advocate, 2013). Participants are invited to prepare in advance and to attempt to schedule appointments with their senators or congress representatives. This is also a good opportunity for those new to policy communication and public advocacy to work together with and learn from experienced health advocates. Other organizations have also developed guides or specific training sessions to advance the policy communication and public advocacy skills of their key constituencies as well as other organizations in their same field (for example, Society for Neuroscience, 2006; American Heart Association, 2006b; Christopher and Dana Reeve Foundation, 2013).

Regardless of one's training, communicating with policymakers and other key decision makers within your organization, professional association, or community center is always influenced by personal styles, individual beliefs, passions, and experiences. Yet, there are a few fundamental mantras that may enhance the success and outcomes of all efforts (Population Reference Bureau, 2013; Health Education Advocate, 2013; National Association of Chain Drug Stores, 2013):

- *Make a meaningful connection.* Disclose and emphasize that you are a constituent of the policymakers you are approaching. Are you a voter in their state or district? Do you represent a specific group or association that carries weight on the specific health and social issue you seek to discuss? Are you bringing an innovative perspective that may resonate with the policymaker's key constituents? Are you an employee of a specific organization who has been affected by specific workplace-related policies?

- *Describe why you care about the health issue as it relates to your personal experience.* Are you a physician concerned about a potential new policy that may affect the quality of care you provide to patients? Are you a community member who seeks additional resource allocations to the local community health center for community engagement and informational activities that go beyond patient care? Are you the parent of a child who died of cancer and seeks increased funding for pediatric cancer research?

- *Define the problem and make the link with public health, medical, and scientific data.* Establish yourself as a resource for policymakers by discussing the specific problem within the context of relevant population and health studies, demographic surveys, market surveys, and any other research that may support your arguments. Tie this information with key points on the history of prior policy action or inaction, and bring it back to why it is important to address and prioritize this specific health or social issue.

- *Be concise and limit the number of issues discussed at each encounter.* Whether it is an in-person meeting for which you may have as little as two to five minutes, or an e-mail or phone conversation, keep it concise and simple, and avoid professional jargon. Also, try to focus on a limited number of issues in each communication.

- *Be prepared to answer potential questions in a meaningful way* related to the policymaker's knowledge and level of understanding of a specific issue. Do not try to answer questions for which you are not sure of the answer, and promise to get back with relevant information (use this as an additional opportunity for contact). Be helpful.

- *Listen,* and try to identify what really matters to the policymakers and what kind of opportunities and challenges may exist for further discussion of the issue and its potential solutions and future negotiations and communications. Take notes and share with other members of your group or organization.

* *"Always include a formal ask and thank you."* Whether you ask for general support on a specific issue or the policymaker's vote on an upcoming legislation or organizational policy, it is important to make your expectation clear. Too often, "one of the biggest reasons why policymakers do not assist is because they have never been asked" (National Association of Chain Drug Stores, 2013).

Although the "walk on the Hill" (Capitol Hill, in Washington, DC, where US senators, Representatives, and other policymakers have their offices) or other kinds of in-person meetings with policymakers and other decision makers—both in the US and international settings or within one's organization—are important and sometimes defining moments in the process of communicating with policymakers, several other communication channels and methods support, prepare, or sometimes substitute personal encounters. Many policy communications happen via phone calls, faxes, and e-mails. "Outside of face-to-face meetings, phone calls are the most influential way to communicate your position" (National Association of Chain Drug Stores, 2013). In the United States, there are a number of resources to find the phone number of a specific elected official in the House or Senate. Often, organizations involved with advocacy will provide their own members or constituent groups with contact information of relevant decision makers. You can also call the Capitol Hill switchboard in Washington, DC, and be connected with your policymaker's office by providing your ZIP Code. Similarly, by calling the switchboard of a prominent professional association or group you should be able to be connected to the office that handles a specific health issue and related policy. If you are seeking a policy change in your own organization, it should be easier to figure out the decision-making process and its key players.

Faxes and e-mails are also suitable ways of communicating to reach members of the House and Senate in the United States. Unless you have a different and more personal contact, faxes are usually addressed to the staff member in the policymaker's office who handle a specific health issue. Whether one uses faxes or e-mails, it is important to be concise and to the point, just as in face-to-face meetings. It is also important to call in advance to ask about preferred modes of communication. This also applies to other key decision makers from a variety of sectors in addition to elected officials.

Policy briefs (a concise summary of an issue of public interest, potential policy solutions, and some recommendations on what may be the best policy option) are another important communication tools in both policy communication and public advocacy. There are two basic types of policy

policy briefs
A concise summary of an issue of public interest, potential policy solutions, and some recommendations on what may be the best policy option

advocacy briefs
Policy briefs that "argue in favor of a specific course of action" (Food and Agricultural Organization, 2013, p. 143)

objective briefs
Policy briefs that only "give objective information for the policy maker to make up his or her mind" (Food and Agricultural Organization, 2013, p. 143)

briefs: **advocacy briefs**, which "argue in favor of a specific course of action," and **objective briefs**, which only "give objective information for the policy maker to make up his or her mind" (Food and Agricultural Organization, 2013, p. 143). Because policy briefs are used "to present the findings and recommendations of a research project to a non-specialist readership, they are often recommended as a key tool for communicating research findings to policy actors" (Jones and Walsh, 2008, p. 1), and for this reason, they may be suitable tools for public health, medical, and other kinds of researchers to influence public policy. As with other policy communication tools, policy briefs need to be concise, to the point, based on firm evidence from multiple experiences and studies, and deal with recommendations and the big picture, and not with issues such as the study's methods, or implementation details on the recommended course of action (Food and Agricultural Organization, 2013). The language of the policy brief needs to be catchy, engaging, and appeal to a nonspecialist readership in order to attract the attention of the policymakers to whom they are addressed. There are different formats of policy briefs, but essential elements to be included are featured in Table 9.1.

Policy briefs are succinct, and should not exceed two to three pages (including references). The use of tables, side boxes, figures, and other graphic elements increase the visual appeal of the policy brief and should always be considered. A list of online resources on how to develop a policy brief or find sample briefs and templates is included in Appendix A.

Table 9.1   Key Elements of a Policy Brief

Introduction or executive summary, highlighting the purpose of the brief, and in the case of an advocacy brief, its recommendations. In writing this section, ask yourself what the main points of the briefing are. In other words, if the policymaker had to read just this section, what would you like him or her to take away from it?

Nature and magnitude of the problem, including data and other evidence-based information to establish its relevance, both in general terms and among key constituency groups that are relevant to the policymaker.

Affected groups, populations, and communities. This section should prioritize most affected groups, relevant data, as well as affected groups of importance to the policymaker because the last may be a motivational factor for change.

Risk factors, including individual, community-specific, and environmental conditions or policies that may create risk among most affected groups or populations.

Economic and social consequences of the health issue, such as, for example, lack of ability of affected groups to connect with social opportunities, jobs, and other needed areas because of poor health outcomes; impact on lost work days; high cost of treatment and hospitalization versus preventive measures.

Potential policy solutions, which derive from the findings presented so far.

Recommended course of action, including priority action steps (only in the case of an advocacy brief).

References, because they relate to findings and other data discussed in the document.

As previously discussed, policy communication is complementary to public advocacy, which is instrumental in building and engaging key constituencies for or against a policy-related issue. As Paletz (1999) describes, congressional leaders and their staff review a variety of local and national newspapers, websites, journals, magazines, and other print, broadcast, and online media channels to monitor public response to legislative and policy matters. "Public opinion plays a number of important roles in a representative democracy. Leaders can take public opinion into account when making laws and formulating policy . . . Opinion polls provide a mechanism for succinctly presenting the views of the mass public to government leaders who are making decisions that will affect society" (Paletz, Owen, and Cook, 2012). Similarly, key decision makers and top executives in a variety of organizations, in both the public and private sectors, like to take the pulse of public opinion and to understand what matters to their constituencies. The tone and content of media coverage or the prominence of specific opinions on online resources and social media often shape their decisions and perspectives on a given issue, and may help create a receptive environment in which policymakers may be willing to listen to their constituents' ideas and concerns. Yet, no matter what kind of communication strategies and media we use, policy change does not occur overnight; only long-term and sustainable efforts can produce results.

The Media of Public Advocacy and Public Relations

In order to be effective, public advocacy relies on the strategic use of most of the communication areas we discussed so far (including mass media and new media communication, community mobilization and citizen engagement, interpersonal communication, and constituency relations) and related media. Table 9.2 includes sample areas to which public advocacy efforts contribute (Schiavo, 2007a).

Many organizations use public advocacy strategies to advance their agenda or preserve the interest of their key constituencies. For example, the Malaria Vaccine Initiative, which is part of the nonprofit organization PATH and seeks "to accelerate the development of promising malaria vaccines as well as to ensure their availability and accessibility in the developing world," developed a Malaria Vaccine Science & Society Fellowship Program (Blount, 2007). The program trains and promotes African scientists from several countries as "voices from the field" to influence the policy process in donor countries and to foster "understanding and support of clinical trials and introduction of malaria vaccines" as well as allocation of additional resources and research funds (Blount, 2007). Lessons learned from this

Table 9.2   Why Public Advocacy?

To gain public and policymaker support for policy and social goals

To create political willingness and help set the public debate and agenda

To provide public voice to key constituencies

To contribute to changes in social and organizational norms and practices

To create a critical mass in support of policy and social change

To engage and empower communities in the advocacy process

References: Schiavo, 2007a and 2007b; Hoover, 2005.

program, which seeks to enable fellows "to better engage the media and policymakers," include the critical importance of a three-day training workshop, one-on-one assessments on the overall advocacy experience with each fellow, as well as advance preparation by the trainees before the workshop. The training workshops focus on media and advocacy theory, message development, media and speaker training, and op-ed writing, among other skills (Blount, 2007).

Public advocacy strategies and tactics are also used to influence companies and other publics to change their policies or manufacturing practices. An example of public advocacy efforts targeted to the commercial sector is the HIV treatment access campaign by Doctors Without Borders and many other international organizations (Calmy, 2004; World Health Organization and Joint United Nations Programme on HIV/AIDS, 2005a) that have been advocating for a price reduction of essential HIV medications when sold in the developing world. Whereas treatment access is actually dependent on many other factors in addition to price, their efforts were successful in engaging several pharmaceutical companies in the public debate as well as in an attempt to find appropriate solutions. Similarly, consumer awareness of the potentially negative health effects of transfat acids has motivated many companies in the food industry to develop transfat-free products (MSNBC, 2006; FoodNavigatorUSA, 2005a, 2005b; Unilever, 2006).

Among other theoretical influences, public advocacy is also grounded in public relations, media theory, and practice. Public advocacy is very similar and uses the same tools as public affairs, a key PR function (see Chapter Five). In fact, PR, with its many media channels, is also a key component of government relations and policy communication because of its ability to influence legislators and other key decision makers.

Because of the power of the mass media to influence public opinion, local and national publications, community newsletters, broadcast media, the Internet, and new and social media can all be useful channels to advance public commitment to and awareness of a health issue or policy. They can help create the critical mass that is needed to motivate legislators or other decision makers to endorse the policy being advocated by their publics. Public relations thus becomes public advocacy when it seeks to influence health policies, laws, and practices.

Similar to policy communication, which, in the case of efforts driven by the need for policy change, overlaps with and is almost an area of public advocacy, public advocacy relies on multiple media and activities, including community or town hall meetings and one-on-one encounters with policy and decision makers. However, a fundamental component of public advocacy efforts is the use of the mass media and new media platforms. More recently, public advocacy that heavily relies on the strategic use of the mass media and new media is also called **media advocacy**. Media advocacy supports community and citizen engagement and mobilization to advance a social or policy initiative. In health communication, the scope of media advocacy is to help advance public health, health care, or social policies in support of improved public health outcomes.

Along with community mobilization and citizen engagement as well as constituency relations strategies (see Chapters Six and Eight), media advocacy contributes to creating a critical mass in support of policy or social change and its implementation. Figure 9.1 includes sample questions that should be asked in the planning phase of the media advocacy component of a public advocacy effort. With the exception of the media-specific questions, such questions also apply to the planning of the overall public advocacy intervention.

As with other health communication interventions, the media of public advocacy should be selected on the basis of the preferences and needs of the key groups we seek to influence. For example, people living with HIV/AIDS or suffering from rare disorders or parents of children with pediatric cancer have created strong online communities (hiv/aidstribe, 2013; Association of Cancer Online Resources, 2013) where it may be possible to reach out and engage them in public advocacy efforts. Local and national legislators and other elected officials may read completely different newspapers because they primarily value the news that most affects their key constituency groups (including voters). Rural communities in low-income country settings may be excluded from public advocacy processes in absence of culturally competent media, such as interpersonal communication channels, word-of-mouth, theater, radio, or other sources, which are specific to each community and literacy levels. Participatory photography (**photovoice**) has also been used to engage marginalized or

media advocacy
Consists of public advocacy strategies and activities that heavily rely on the use of the mass media and new media. Supports community and citizen engagement and mobilization to advance a social or policy initiative.

photovoice
Participatory photography

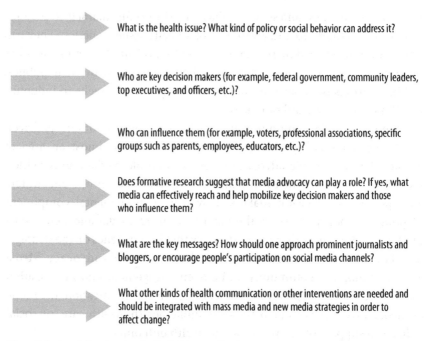

What is the health issue? What kind of policy or social behavior can address it?

Who are key decision makers (for example, federal government, community leaders, top executives, and officers, etc.)?

Who can influence them (for example, voters, professional associations, specific groups such as parents, employees, educators, etc.)?

Does formative research suggest that media advocacy can play a role? If yes, what media can effectively reach and help mobilize key decision makers and those who influence them?

What are the key messages? How should one approach prominent journalists and bloggers, or encourage people's participation on social media channels?

What other kinds of health communication or other interventions are needed and should be integrated with mass media and new media strategies in order to affect change?

Figure 9.1 Sample Key Questions for Media Advocacy Planning
References: Schiavo, 2007a and 2007b; Hoover, 2005.

issue-affected community in the advocacy process by allowing new voices to be heard, and combining documentary and personal voices (Photovoice, 2013; Wang, 1999) on topics including HIV/AIDS, women's health, and social determinants of health (Photovoice, 2013; Wang, 1999; Haque and Eng, 2011). Conversely, in Europe and the United States, op-ed pieces (see Chapter Five for definition) and letters to the editor in top newspapers or guest blogs are commonly used for public advocacy (even if one could argue that these media may be best suited to reach out to most affluent groups with high education levels, and that they leave out large segments of the population). So, once again, media selection is key group–specific, whether for public advocacy or other communication purposes.

Influencing Public Policy in the New Media Age

We live in an era of rapid technological advances, which have expanded the communicator's tool kit. This is the era of Twitter, Facebook, YouTube, LinkedIn, mHealth, blogs, websites, and tablets. By the time this book will be published there will be many other emerging media and ways to communicate. As previously discussed in Chapter Five, new media are an important channel in health communication, and also in the context of influencing public policy.

"Since the 1990s, there have been growing discussions of Internet activism and how new media have been used effectively by a variety of political movements" (Kahn and Kellner, 2004, p. 87; Best and Kellner, 2001; Couldry and Curran, 2003). Policymakers have also noticed this, and in fact, they are also on Twitter and other popular social media sites. This is no longer true only in developed nations (as, for example, in the case of President Obama and his staff and many senators and congressmen in the United States) but also in Africa and other low-income country settings, where "many younger Ministers are on Twitter, and this creates the possibility for direct contact with citizens" (Davidson, 2012). Yet, their staff runs many of elected officials' social media accounts, so there is still an indirect connection to consider because aides and other officers from the policymaker's team are quite influential both online and offline.

New media activism has also flourished on blogs and online news sites. Political bloggers have been able to influence policy and political campaigns by stirring controversy or publicizing arguments against opponents' opinion (Kahn and Kellner, 2004). Twitter is also another important tool to influence policy, whether you are an activist or a policymaker. As an example, at the time this book is being written, the debate about reducing gun violence in the United States by regulating gun access is taking place in several venues across the country including the new media setting. There are an average of seven to twelve tweets per hour, which include the hash tag #gunviolence (Twitter, 2013b) on any given day on Twitter, which represent opposite views and sides of the issue. Policymakers are also using this tool to create support for their opinion. For example, President Obama's request to endorse his plan to reduce gun violence was retweeted 728 times in less than 90 minutes, with 301 Twitter users adding his request to their favorite list in the same time period (Twitter, 2013a).

Yet, in most developing countries, there are still several limitations on working in the online space given the small percentages of people with online access and despite the expansion of mobile technology. As highlighted by a report on a 2012 panel on New Media and Activism organized in Africa as part of OpenForum2012, there is "a high proliferation of disparate small-scale donor-funded projects using mobile technology to help deliver services (such as m-health). [This is] all very exciting and innovative, but is seldom taken to scale and usually ending abruptly as soon as the initial donors lose interest" (Davidson, 2012). Also, in countries like Tanzania "online conversations are still limited to a tiny elite" (Davidson, 2012). As another example, in Kenya, "'you can't work online without also working offline' and that for all the hype about African tech innovation, the number of genuine online participants remains low." It may not be feasible to start the conversation on the online space but it may be possible "to continue it there" (Davidson, 2012).

Although access and use may increase over time among different key groups, the situation in Africa is not that different from the experience of vulnerable and underserved groups in developed countries. The question remains how communication interventions can also contribute to building capacity on health and new media literacy among nonelite users and disadvantaged groups at the same pace as that of constantly emerging new technological advances (see Chapter Five for further discussion of this topic).

In looking at how to incorporate new media in public advocacy and policy communication efforts, many of the strategies discussed in Chapter Five still apply to influencing policy via new media channels. Yet, in the case of public advocacy a few features of well-designed new media–based communication programs are even more important in shaping public opinion, engaging communities in the advocacy process, and influencing policymakers' decisions. These include the following:

- The power of storytelling and how to craft videos, photographs, and other visuals that are able to convey a powerful reason for action.

- The importance of diversified media for distribution on different social media channels and venues. For example, you may be able to make one video to educate and engage a legislator about a health issue and another video—with a completely different look and message—to engage a specific key group in advocacy efforts that put pressure on the policymaker.

- A comprehensive distribution strategy that relies on key influentials and channels, both online and offline.

- Message simplicity and consistency.

- The participation of key constituency groups both in social media outreach efforts as well as spokespeople or feature stories in visual media.

- The ability to translate online action to real life changes.

- The effective integration with interpersonal communication, community mobilization, mass media communication, and other areas and channels used in influencing and communicating about policy.

Of most importance is to start to develop more specific indicators and evaluation models that would help assess in rigorous terms the contribution of new and social media to policy communication and public advocacy as well as to other communication areas. Chapter Fourteen discusses trends and models for new media evaluation in health communication.

Key Concepts

- Truly transformative leadership moments that result in a new policy have the potential to make a long-term impact on large populations as well as vulnerable and underserved groups.

- The main premise of this chapter is that all of us, regardless of whether we work in public health, health care, the private sector, community development, or other fields, find ourselves communicating often enough about policies and their management as part of our professional endeavors. At the same time, different kinds of professionals may be able to craft, demonstrate the need, and advocate for policy change (and its management) within their organizations.

- Policy communication is about communicating with policymakers and other decision makers about health or scientific data in support of policy change or a new or existing policy and its implementation and evaluation.

- Public advocacy is the strategic use of communication to affect changes in public opinion and attitudes so that this will influence policymakers and other decision makers and affect changes in behaviors, social norms, policies, and resources allocation to benefit a community, group, population, or organization.

- Policy communication and public advocacy are strictly interconnected and are integrated communication areas with many complementary and sometimes overlapping strategies, activities, and media.

- There are several specific communication strategies, activities, and channels that are used in policy communication and public advocacy. Select examples are described in this chapter.

- In order to be effective, public advocacy relies on the strategic use of most of the communication areas we discussed so far (including mass media and new media communication, community mobilization and citizen engagement, interpersonal communication, and constituency relations, and related media). Media and activity selection is informed by key group–specific preferences and uses.

- Among other theoretical influences, public advocacy is also grounded in public relations and media theory and practice. Public advocacy is very similar and uses the same tools as public affairs, a key PR function (see Chapter Five).

- No matter what kind of communication strategies and media we use, policy change does not occur overnight; only long-term and sustainable efforts can produce results.

- New media activism as well as the use of new and social media for policy communication has been flourishing and providing new options for the communicator's tool kit. Yet, integration with other communication areas and channels is key to maximizing reach, and so is a rigorous evaluation of new media's contribution to policy communication and public advocacy.

FOR DISCUSSION AND PRACTICE

1. Analyze the newspapers, online sites, and social media you have been monitoring in recent times in relation to a prominent health policy issue being discussed in the media either in the United States or international settings. Discuss your impression of the efforts being conducted in favor or against a new health or social policy through the lens of both policy communication and public advocacy. Compile and discuss a list of groups that appear to be involved in policy communication and public advocacy on this specific issue.

2. Using the format discussed within this chapter, develop a policy brief concisely summarizing issues, policy alternatives, and key considerations for action on a public health or global health issue of your interest. For sample briefs and other resources, see links in Appendix A.

3. Identify and discuss examples of specific health or social policies that have directly affected you, your family, or your community.

KEY TERMS

advocacy briefs

media advocacy

objective briefs

photovoice

policy briefs

policy communication

public advocacy

PART THREE

PLANNING, IMPLEMENTING, AND EVALUATING A HEALTH COMMUNICATION INTERVENTION

This section provides a step-by-step guide to the development, implementation, and evaluation of health communication interventions. Each chapter covers specific steps of the health communication planning process or implementation and evaluation phases and provides practical guidance and examples. Chapter Ten provides an overview of the health communication cycle and planning process, as well as practical guidance on how to establish the overall program goal and outcome objectives (behavioral, social, and organizational) of your health communication intervention. Each of the other chapters focuses on other specific steps of the health communication planning process as defined in this text: situation and audience analysis (Chapter Eleven), identifying communication objectives and strategies (Chapter Twelve), designing and implementing an action plan (Chapter Thirteen), and evaluating outcomes of health communication interventions (Chapter Fourteen).

Case studies, practical tips, and specific examples aim to facilitate readers' understanding of the planning process, as well as to build technical skills in health communication planning and evaluation. Recent methodologies and trends in measuring and evaluating results of health communication programs are explored here and so are specific strategies and tools to evaluate new media–based interventions.

CHAPTER 10

OVERVIEW OF THE HEALTH COMMUNICATION PLANNING PROCESS

Most health organizations have or expect to have a communication plan to promote their mission or address a specific health issue at some point in their life cycle. However, many of them have difficulties converting plans into actions that have an impact on their constituencies, their mission, or the visibility of their organization, and most important, the people they serve or are accountable to. Most of the problems stem from a lack of understanding of the fundamental steps of a health communication plan and how to design communication interventions that fit the organization's mission, as well as the needs of its key constituencies and stakeholders. In other words, there is often a lack of clarity about what the plan should do for the organization (Adams, 2005) and the groups it wants to engage or serve.

A practical example is the use of mandated cigarette warnings as part of the US public policy strategy "to educate consumers about the risks of smoking" (Krugman, Fox, and Fischer, 1999, p. 95). However, the cigarette warnings implemented for more than three decades since they were required in the late 1960s were ineffective communication tools. Part of the problem is that they were designed as the result of negotiations between the US federal government and the tobacco industry and "neither developed nor implemented with specific communications goals in mind" (p. 95). More recently, the Family Smoking Prevention and Tobacco Control Act enacted in 2009 requires pictorial warnings that depict the negative consequences of smoking (Hammond, 2012). The impact of the new warnings will shed more light on the design and content of effective health warnings.

It is important that policymakers clearly understand and establish at the outset of the warning program what they expect warnings to accomplish. Should warnings be designed to communicate the risks associated with smoking or attempt to prevent smoking initiation? Did the current design and message length take into account how much time tobacco users would spend reading the warning? Did warnings aim to reach primarily adolescents or also other age groups? What about the graphic appeal of the warnings in contrast with the flashy images of tobacco industry ads? Were the warnings designed with the participation of tobacco users? Are warnings part of a larger program that addresses the social determinants of health of tobacco consumption and effectively provides support to communities to prevent smoking initiation or encourage cessation? Understanding all of these factors and many others that are not listed here may increase the efficacy of cigarette warnings if they become part of a comprehensive health communication program (Krugman, Fox, and Fischer, 1999; Hammond, 2012). "There is a need to monitor the impact of warnings over time and among various subpopulations. For example, to what extent does the impact of health warnings vary across socioeconomic status or other subgroups of smokers? What types of health messages or health effects are most effective among youth and young adults? Research is also required to monitor the 'wear out' of warnings over time and the ideal period for 'revising' the warnings. Finally, the impact of warnings may be enhanced through linkages to other media campaigns and tobacco control policies" (Hammond, 2012, p. 65).

This example reinforces several of the fundamental premises of this book: know your audience, be clear about behavioral and social results that will improve health outcomes, use a multifaceted and participatory approach to engage communities and other stakeholders, and help them own the change process. In health communication, planning is a rigorous evidence-based process. Health communication terminology is important in guiding the different planning and implementation steps.

CHAPTER OBJECTIVES

This chapter, the first in Part Three, which provides a step-by-step guide to health communication planning, implementation, and evaluation, discusses why planning is important and highlights the key steps of the health communication process. It provides an overview of this process and introduces "strategy-based communication principles" for health communication planning (Association of Schools of Public Health, 2007, p. 7; US Department of Health and

Human Services, 2012b), which will be discussed in further detail in the remaining chapters. Finally, using practical examples, this chapter defines the meaning of an overall program goal and provides practical guidance in establishing these goals at the outset of the program together with integrated behavioral, social, and organizational objectives.

Author note: In this chapter, as well as other sections of this book, the terms *audience* and *key group* (see definition and discussion in Chapter One) are used interchangeably because they are both terminologies widely used in different communication models and practices. As we use them in this book, they both imply a participatory approach to health communication planning, in which participation levels of different key groups may be related to their own cultural preferences and other specific factors as described in the "Approaches to Health Communication Planning" section of this chapter.

Why Planning Is Important

Too often, health organizations operate in emergency mode and use communication primarily as a tool to respond to emerging health needs or sudden crises. This frequently leads to difficulties in securing adequate funding or response to what appear to be last-minute needs. Establishing any health-related "issue" as such so it is prominent in the minds of donors and potential partners takes time, commitment, and adequate communication strategies from the real outset of trying to address it. The truth is that most needs can be anticipated and many crises averted if communication planning is one of the standard protocols and activities of an organization.

Communication planning is an evidence-based and research-driven process. An in-depth understanding of the health communication environment as well as the needs, preferences, and expectations of key audiences and stakeholders on a health issue may result in multifaceted and well-designed interventions that are far more effective than single, sporadic, and disconnected approaches to communication. Even when the health communication intervention is part of a larger public health, health care, or community development effort, which happens in most cases, "a plan specific to the health communication component is necessary" (National Cancer Institute at the National Institutes of Health, 2002, p. 16).

A health communication plan can help clarify how an organization can accomplish the following:

- Advance its mission
- Engage others in a health issue and its solutions

- Expand the reach and implementation of its ideas and practices or generate new ideas and solutions
- Encourage action and partnerships across sectors
- Ultimately support health and social change

Moreover, planning can help in other ways, too:

- Provide further knowledge on the health issue being addressed and key factors influencing its occurrence as well as potential solutions
- Develop a clear understanding of key audiences' characteristics, culture, preferences, needs, lifestyle, behavior, and social norms
- Engage key communities, groups, and stakeholders in the design and implementation of the health communication intervention, and create ownership of the process
- Clarify what the program is asking people to do and whether the proposed change is feasible
- Evaluate the strengths, weaknesses, and cost-effectiveness of different approaches that can be used to support change
- Set communication priorities
- Identify and engage potential partners
- Evaluate the organization's internal capability and resources to address the health issue
- Develop culturally appropriate materials and activities
- Define program time lines, roles, and responsibilities, as well as budget parameters
- Establish evaluation parameters designed to facilitate program assessment, refinement, and scale-up

An example illustrates one of the benefits of planning: gaining knowledge on the health issue. Imagine an organization that initially thought about launching a communication program to reduce sodium consumption among young women, with the ultimate goal of reducing the incidence and morbidity of hypertension in this age group. Before focusing exclusively on sodium consumption, the organization should explore the importance of sodium in the pathology of hypertension versus other contributing factors, as well as lessons learned from previous experiences that focused on only one element of a multifactorial condition. Cultural preferences, lifestyle, traditional diets, social norms, and living and working contexts—along with many other factors—should also be explored in partnership with communities and women's groups so that they can contribute to assessing and prioritizing the issue as well as to designing a suitable intervention. These are just a few of the many areas that should be addressed to gain understanding of the health issue and its potential solutions. Research, community engagement, and feedback will help the organization validate its original idea or, depending on key findings, may prove the need for a different and broader approach.

Approaches to Health Communication Planning

Although there may be variations in the number of phases different authors use to describe communication planning, the fundamental steps and principles of the overall planning process are always the same and are described in the next section of this chapter. However, from a theoretical perspective, there are many differences between the traditional approaches to planning and a more participatory approach (National Planning Council, Colombia, 2003).

In general, *traditional planning* is "centralized," "vertical (from the top to the bottom)," "technical (done by experts)," and "recognizes a certain population as an object that will benefit from the plan." By contrast, *participatory planning* is "decentralized," "horizontal and agreed upon (from the bottom to the top)," "dialogue-based," "democratic," and "recognizes social actors as active subjects in their own development" (National Planning Council, Colombia, 2003).

However, in looking at the characteristics of traditional planning versus participatory planning, it is important to remember that the word *participation* may have different meanings to different people, groups, or cultures. Ideally, key groups and stakeholders should be always involved in the research, planning, implementation, and evaluation of a health communication program. Behavioral and social changes are always more likely to occur if people are part of the process and feel a sense of ownership in prioritizing issues and shaping key interventions. "Social efficacy is a key concept in the field of health communication. For it to be achieved, groups' and persons' social skills must be made use of and influence program design" (Ader and others, 2001, p. 190).

Yet, participation levels as well as people's expectations and perceptions of participation may vary in different cultural and country settings. For example, critics of the participatory approach, especially in Asia, have highlighted that often "participatory models were premised on Western-styled ideas of democracy and participation that do not fit political cultures somewhere else" (Waisbord, 2001, p. 22). In other words, people from different communities and cultural groups may not always welcome participation, at least not to the same extent and with the same implications with which participation is conceptualized in the Western world. It is important to acknowledge that in some cases the community may not be interested in investing time in a democratic decision-making process and may have other priorities. In certain contexts, "recommendations for participation could be also seen as foreign and manipulative by local communities" (Waisbord, 2001, p. 22).

Moreover, there are situations in which one of the two approaches may be better suited to address a specific health issue or avert a crisis and limit its negative consequences. For example, "in some cases such as in epidemics and other public health crises, quick and top-down solutions could achieve positive results" (Waisbord, 2001, p. 21), when there is need to address the unexpected. Yet, even in these cases, advance participatory planning will help with the acceptance and adoption of recommended measures, especially if such a planning phase has been engaging relevant communities and stakeholders in deciding the protocol for decision making in case of unexpected information and needs that were not factored in by the plan. Overall, a participatory approach to planning is better positioned to achieve long-term and sustainable behavioral and social outcomes in most health and social development areas, and to prepare for public health emergencies and disease outbreaks. In other circumstances, characteristics of a specific planning process are mixed and matched from the two approaches.

There are also circumstances in which the proposed issue or health problem is not a key priority within the community or key group being approached. Take the example of a group of women who were living in a refugee camp in Angola some time during the twenty-seven-year civil war (1975–2002). Picture the refugee camp: people live in homes made of plastic sheets and sticks. Malnutrition is the norm. Starvation is more than common. Children run around playing with remains of whatever they find. Many adults have fevers, cough, undiagnosed and often untreated conditions. There are people everywhere living in the camp's relatively small area. Now, suppose you know that malaria may be responsible for many of the fevers. Suppose you approach the women's group to engage them in designing a program to protect them from malaria by sleeping under an insecticide-treated net. Do you expect them to jump to the offer or ask you for what they perceive as more important priorities: food, clothes, medications? And if the latter happens, as in most cases, how do you make sure these women are heard and feel respected in their lack of desire to participate?

Cases like this pose an ethical dilemma. You may know people may be dying of malaria but yet the community you seek to engage does not perceive this as a threat and is preoccupied with other equally important priorities. These are moments in which many of the theories that refer to health communication as process-oriented come to practice. These are moments in which you need to first address people's own priorities by pointing them to resources and programs that may help them. This is also an opportunity to listen, build trust, start conversations, and look for local champions who may be already speaking with others about malaria being an issue. Ultimately, if people decide to become engaged in malaria prevention, they will discover that disease prevention helps them stay stronger as well as enables them to develop sustainable solutions to their priority problems. But again, this is a process in which listening is key, just as it is key to take into account and attempt to address the many social norms and factors that contribute to any health issue.

In summary, some of the characteristics mentioned in this section as attributed to participatory and traditional planning models may vary from situation to situation and country to country in their practical application. Therefore, they should be interpreted only as general tendencies of these two approaches, which may diverge from the elements we discussed or should be customized to meet the needs of specific audiences, cultures, and situations. This is not very different from other aspects of health communication. In fact, theories, models, and approaches should always be considered part of a tool kit with multiple options.

The Health Communication Cycle and Strategic Planning Process

Different authors and models may describe the phases of communication planning or the general health communication cycle in divergent ways. However, the general premises and steps of the health communication cycle tend to stay the same:

* Understand how health communication can contribute to the resolution of a health problem or advance the mission of a health organization.

* Research the health communication environment and the key characteristics and needs of key groups and stakeholders via a combination of literature review, stakeholder in-depth interviews, participatory audience research, and other research methods.

- Establish a multidisciplinary team, which includes representatives of key program audiences.

- Determine the best approach and channels to reach intended audiences and involve them in the communication and behavioral and social change processes.

- Develop communication messages, materials, and activities, as well as identify key communication channels and media, and seek input from intended audiences before launching any elements of your program.

- Implement the health communication program.

- Evaluate program effectiveness in relation to behavioral, social, organizational, or other key outcomes and parameters that were set in advance and agreed to by all team members and partners.

- Refine or validate program elements in agreement with lessons learned and evaluation analysis.

Figure 10.1 describes the phases of health communication planning and shows how strategic planning is directly connected to the other two stages of the health communication cycle (program implementation and monitoring, and evaluation, feedback, and refinement). In fact, effective strategic planning influences the success of the implementation experience as well as the overall evaluation process and potential outcomes. In turn, planning is influenced by observations and lessons learned during the

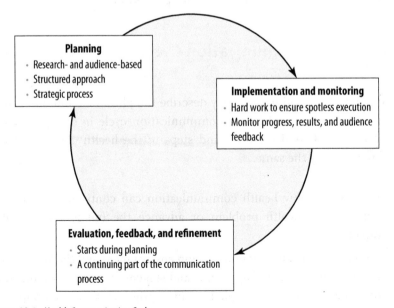

Figure 10.1   Health Communication Cycle

implementation and evaluation phases, which may validate or call for changes in all or some of the elements of the initial communication plan. Finally, all steps of the planning phase are interdependent. Failure to complete all steps may limit the program's ability to meet the expectations and needs of intended audiences as well as effectively address any given health issue.

Key Steps of Health Communication Planning

The steps listed in this section are key to effective strategic planning and reflect actual communication practice. All of them are described in further detail in the following chapters. Additional resources are also included in Appendix A, which includes worksheets and other practical information. Because health communication planning is a step-by-step process in which all phases are interdependent and each informs and guides the next one, following this sequence is important. Figure 10.2 shows the key steps of health communication planning, which are further described in the following sections.

Overall Program Goal

The goal is a brief description of the "overall health improvement" (National Cancer Institute at the National Institutes of Health, 2002, p. 22) that the health communication program is planning to achieve—for example, "contribute to the elimination of health disparities and improve overall health outcomes among African Americans," "reduce the morbidity and mortality associated with asthma among children under age ten," "help reduce the number of deaths associated with vaccine-preventable childhood diseases," or "improve the quality of people living with a mental health condition." The **overall program goal** always refers to an overall improvement on one of these parameters as they relate to a specific health condition:

overall program goal
Describes the overall "health improvement" (National Cancer Institute at the National Institutes of Health, 2002, p. 22) or "overall change in a health or social problem" (Weinreich, 1999, p. 67; 2011) that the program is seeking to achieve

- *Morbidity:* Another term for *illness. Comorbidities* refer to diseases occurring at the same time. *Morbidity rates* or *levels* are equivalent to prevalence rates of a given health condition.

- *Mortality:* Another term for *death. Mortality rate* is the number of deaths due to a given health condition or other specific causes—such as, for example, pregnancy-related causes for maternal mortality—in a specific population divided by the total number of people living with that condition.

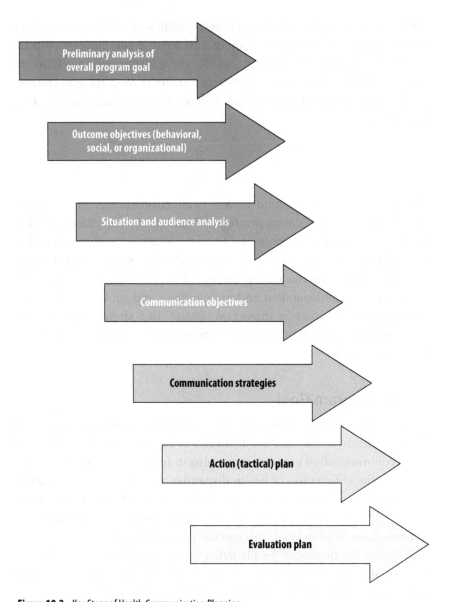

Figure 10.2   Key Steps of Health Communication Planning

- _Incidence:_ The number of newly diagnosed cases of a disease within a given population and a specific time period.
- _Prevalence:_ Total number of disease cases existing in a given population; also expressed in terms of the percentage of a given population suffering of a given disease.
- _Quality of life:_ The general well-being of individual, patients, and other key groups. Quality of life is a complex concept, which is linked to

cultural, age- and gender-specific values, and individual, key group, and social expectations of their position in life. In the context of people living with a health condition, quality of life is defined in relation to four different categories or domains: "physical, psychological, social, and environment" (Skevington, Lotfy, and O'Connell, 2004).

This goal should inspire and guide the design of the health communication intervention.

Outcome Objectives: Behavioral, Social, and Organizational

This is the statement of a specific behavioral, social, or organizational result that is sought by the program and supports the overall program's goal. Behavioral, social, or organizational objectives (**outcome objectives**) are the ultimate desired results of the health communication program. They complement the program's goal and should be validated by the research phase. They explicitly highlight what key audiences should do (**behavioral objectives**); what policy, social norm, or new practice should be implemented and institutionalized (**social objectives**); and how an organization should change in relation to a specific health issue or its mission (**organizational objectives**). Ideally, behavioral objectives (World Health Organization [WHO], 2003) and other kinds of outcome objectives should be time bound and measurable because they are often used as key indicators for program evaluation. Social and organizational objectives are usually achieved as a result of the attainment of a series of behavioral objectives. Therefore, behavioral change is a key milestone of any kind of change. At the same time, behavioral objectives may be difficult to achieve in the absence of policies, social norms, and other practices that may provide the critical social support needed for behavioral adoption and maintenance. Examples are "prompt US mothers of children under age two to immunize their children against flu" [behavioral objective—to be quantified with actual percentages of intended population and dates, whenever possible]; "promote adoption, by the year 2015, of a US health policy recommending pediatric flu immunization" [social change objective]; and "initiate and sustain a process of change that would make pediatric immunization the number one priority of KIDS TODAY [fictional name of organization] by the year 2018" [organizational objective].

Some authors (National Cancer Institute at the National Institutes of Health, 2002) consider behavioral, social, or organizational objectives as one type of communication objectives. Other authors and communication

outcome objectives
The desired outcomes the health communication program is seeking to achieve through behavioral, social, and organizational objectives

behavioral objectives
Outcome objectives that explicitly highlight what key audiences are expected to do as the result of the health communication program; can be synonymous with behavioral indicators

social objectives
Outcome objectives that highlight the policy, practice, or social change that the program is seeking to achieve or implement

organizational objectives
The change that should occur within an organization in terms of its focus, priorities, or structure in relation to the specific health issue addressed by a health communication intervention

models (WHO, 2003; Donovan, 1995) separate them from communication objectives, which are considered the intermediate steps to achieving behavioral and other kinds of outcome objectives. This chapter, as well as all other chapters in Part Three, is based on the latter models. Therefore, outcome objectives are distinguished from communication objectives. In practice, after establishing the overall program goals, there are some key questions that do or should resonate in communication planning meetings:

- What should key groups do as a result of the communication intervention? What are some of the key actions that may lead to a decrease in disease incidence, morbidity, or mortality?

- What kind of policy, social structure, or norm would support the overall program goal?

- What kind of change do we need to make in our organization to be able to implement a program that would serve our redefined mission or goals we have just established?

In general, a model that can be used in developing outcome objectives such as behavioral, social, and organizational objectives is SMART. Under SMART, objectives should be as follows (O'Sullivan, Yonkler, Morgan, and Merritt, 2003, p. 79; Annulis and Gaudet, 2010):

Specific	They describe who should do what.
Measurable	They are defined by quantitative parameters.
Appropriate	They reflect audience needs and preferences.
Realistic	They can be reasonably achieved.
Time bound	They can be achieved within a specific time frame.

SMART has been endorsed by several organizations and planning guides (UNICEF, 2006c; O'Sullivan, Yonkler, Morgan, and Merritt, 2003; Institute of Medicine, 2013; WHO, 2008). SMART can be a valuable framework for a participatory approach to planning in which key groups and stakeholders can use this model to provide structure and reach consensus vis-à-vis its key components.

Establishing outcome objectives early in program planning helps guide the development of key research questions for the initial planning steps as well as inform all other program elements. This is also instrumental for consensus among team members on what the program wants to achieve.

Situation and Audience Analysis

This step is a detailed and evidence-based description of all factors that influence a specific health issue and its potential solutions, as well as the adoption of new behaviors, clinical practices, and policies. It includes an in-depth analysis of the health communication environment as described in Chapter One (see Figure 1.1) in relation to the specific health issue and all related factors. The situation analysis is integrated by a comprehensive and research-based audience analysis for intended audiences as well as key stakeholders whose opinions or actions are most important to the success of the health communication intervention. Both the situation analysis and audience profile (a report on findings from the audience analysis) are developed on the basis of a comprehensive literature, case study, and document review in integration with surveys, stakeholder interviews, participatory audience research, focus groups, and other research methods.

Communication Objectives

These objectives describe the intermediate steps that must be taken to achieve the program's goals (UNICEF, 2001; National Cancer Institute, 2013). They may coincide with behavioral, social, or organizational objectives when the audience's readiness, the specific situation, or the overall lack of complexity of the health issue allows for simplified programs that expect to produce an immediate behavioral, social, or organizational change.

Typically communication objectives describe changes in knowledge, attitudes, and skills that, in support of the overall program's goal, can lead to behavioral, social, or organizational change. In these circumstances, they are the intermediate evaluation parameters of the potential effectiveness of a communication effort. Whenever possible, they should be measurable, and they are always audience-specific. Examples are "increase the awareness of HIV preventive measures and services among an additional 10 percent of young women in the United States by the year 2018," "fifteen percent of adolescents in the key group will report by the year 2016 that they know about the risk associated with using recreational drugs," "there will be an increase in clinician recognition of the importance of early diagnosis and treatment of primary nocturnal enuresis among 70 percent of health care providers in urology clinics in the United Kingdom," and "by the year 2020, there will be a 30 percent increase in the number of African American men who actively participate in preconception and prenatal health. Active participation is defined as . . . (explain what could be considered active participation, such as, for example, accompanying women on at least 75 percent of clinical visits)."

Communication Strategies

This step results in a broad statement on how the program will reach its outcome and communication objectives. Strategies are not tactical. In other words, they do not mention in detail flyers, brochures, media campaigns, workshops, or other tactical elements. They are conceptual descriptions of the communication actions that need to be undertaken to reach specific objectives. Strategies are audience specific—for example, "Promote among women aged eighteen to nineteen short-term family planning methods as well as their safety and efficacy via health care provider counseling" (O'Sullivan, Yonkler, Morgan, and Merritt, 2003), "leverage natural opportunities (for example, annual conferences) to highlight pertusis severity and cycle of transmission among physicians and other professional audiences," "create a social and professional network to support high-risk groups in their intention to seek screening for prostate cancer," "use peer-to-peer communication to mobilize at-risk communities on infant mortality prevention," and "focus on the impact of gun violence on children to increase women's participation in online forums on this topic."

Action (Tactical) Plan

The tactical plan provides a detailed description of all communication messages, materials, activities, and channels, as well as the methods that will be used to pretest them with key audiences. It is audience specific and usually consists of a strategic blend of different areas of health communication (for example, interpersonal communication, mass media and new media communication, citizen engagement) as described in this book. The tactical plan also includes a detailed time line for the program implementation, an itemized budget for each communication activity or material, and a partnership plan with roles and responsibilities that have been agreed on by all team members. (How to develop a tactical plan is addressed in detail in Chapter Thirteen.)

Evaluation Plan

The plan includes a detailed description of the behavioral, social, or organizational indicators as well as other evaluation parameters to be used for program assessment. Expected outcomes and other evaluation parameters need to be mutually agreed on by all team members and program partners. The plan should also describe methods for data collection, analysis, and reporting as well as related costs. (See Chapter Fourteen for a comprehensive discussion on how to develop and implement an evaluation plan as well as theories, models, and topics on the assessment of health communication programs, including new media–based interventions.)

Elements of an Effective Health Communication Program

Only well-planned and well-executed health communication campaigns have the potential to achieve long-term and sustainable results. Key elements of effective health communication interventions are listed in Table 10.1 and briefly discussed here.

Careful Analysis of the Situation, Opportunities, and Communication Needs

Health communication is a research-based discipline. Only a true understanding of the political, social, and market-related environments can lead to the design of optimal interventions. This analysis should rely on a variety of the approaches and research methods described in Chapter Eleven.

Understanding of Constituency and Audience Needs and Preferences

Because the audience is at the center of the health communication approach, its evolving needs and priorities should be understood and considered in communication planning and execution. Communicators should be open to redefining interventions on the basis of their understanding of the needs, preferences, and cultural values of key audiences and constituency groups (see Chapter Eight). This process, which starts with the development of an audience profile as part of communication research and planning, should be participatory—by including key groups and stakeholders in

Table 10.1   Key Elements of an Effective Health Communication Program

- Careful analysis of the situation, opportunities, and communication needs
- Understanding of constituency and audience needs and preferences
- Community and key stakeholders' participation
- Early agreement on expected outcomes and evaluation parameters
- Well-defined communication objectives
- Strategies designed to meet the objectives
- Multiple and audience-specific communication channels
- Adequate funding, commitment, and human resources

sharing information on their needs and preferences—and should continue throughout the communication process via the regular input and feedback from key stakeholders and representatives of interested communities.

Community and Key Stakeholders' Participation

As previously discussed, health communication planning is a participatory and audience-centered process. Engaging and encouraging community and key stakeholders' participation is key to the development of interventions that will resonate with local communities, and are likely to be sustainable in the long term. There is nothing more powerful than a group of engaged citizens who are invested in making change possible and work toward achieving it. For this reason, community participation and stakeholder engagement should be integral to health communication planning.

Early Agreement on Expected Outcomes and Evaluation Parameters

A question that is too often asked in the evaluation phase of communication interventions is, "Why were our donors [or clients or partners or the communities we serve] not satisfied with the results of our program even if we achieved the program's objectives?" A common answer to this kind of question is that partners, donors, constituencies, or communities were not involved in planning and defining of expected outcomes of the communication program.

Establishing mutually agreed-on outcome objectives and evaluation parameters with key stakeholders is the latest wisdom in evaluating health communication programs, at least in the private and commercial sectors, and is gradually expanding also to the nonprofit and public sectors. This allows the extended communication team to discuss and share early on their vision about expected outcomes as well as minimizes the potential for disappointment that may result in changes in program funding or a decrease in the level of commitment and participation by the program's partners. Moreover, early agreement on evaluation indicators and parameters informs and shapes the development of all other elements of health communication planning. As discussed in Chapter Six, community mobilization and citizen engagement are powerful strategies in health communication. In creating community and citizen ownership of health issues and their solutions, there is nothing more powerful than empowering them in defining success in their own terms so they may be invested in achieving the results they set for themselves.

Ideally, planning frameworks and evaluation models should stay consistent at least until the preliminary steps of the evaluation phase of a program are completed. This allows communicators to take advantage of lessons learned and redefine theoretical constructs and communication objectives by comparing program outcomes with those that were anticipated in the planning phase.

Well-Defined Communication Objectives

Communication objectives need to respond to the audience's needs. For example, if the audience is not aware of being at high risk for oral cancer, communication efforts should address the need to raise awareness of that risk. If instead the audience is aware of the high risk for oral cancer but does not know how to prevent it, communication efforts should focus on, for example, key risk factors and how to make lifestyle changes or how to discuss with dentists and other primary health care providers the importance of regular oral cancer screening. Sometimes several communication objectives can be defined and achieved in the same time frame. At other times, communicators need a more gradual, step-by-step approach in which different objectives are achieved at different times. These kinds of decisions need to be based on an in-depth analysis of the audience's needs and levels of receptivity to the communication effort (see Chapter Eleven).

Communication objectives are intermediate steps toward achieving outcome objectives (behavioral, social, and organizational). As with outcome objectives and evaluation parameters, communication objectives also need to be discussed and mutually agreed on with representatives of intended audiences, key constituencies, and partners. In this way, all members of the extended communication team will have in mind similar program outcomes and can work toward achieving them (see Chapter Eleven for a more comprehensive discussion).

Strategies Designed to Meet the Objectives

There may be many good ideas in health communication, but just a few of them may actually support communication objectives. Because communication strategies represent how communication objectives are met, they should always support objectives and represent a creative and cost-effective solution to reach them.

Multiple and Audience-Specific Communication Channels

Creating and identifying multiple and audience-specific communication channels, media, and messages are among the keys to the success of well-planned health communication programs. Messages and channels need to respond to audience needs, cultural preferences, and literacy levels. Messages and channels intended for lay audiences are often different from messages on the same topic that are intended for key opinion leaders, policymakers, or health care providers. For example, in many countries in the developing world, theater and puppet shows that travel from village to village to spread AIDS prevention or immunization-related messages have been effective media to reach the general public in areas where low literacy levels and the absence of more sophisticated communication outlets may jeopardize the use of alternative channels. At the same time, communication efforts have been engaging health care providers via more traditional venues and channels, such as professional meetings, peer-reviewed journals, and online forums and audio files that are specific to health professionals.

Adequate Funding, Commitment, and Human Resources

Too often, well-designed communication programs fail to achieve projected outcomes because of insufficient funds or human resources. An adequate budget and human resources estimate is an important component of effective planning. Budget estimates should also include contingency funds for potential crises or changes in plans that may become necessary to meet emerging needs or other specific circumstances. Failure in estimating adequate funds or human resources may affect the program's quality as well as the perception of the overall effectiveness of health communication interventions in the eyes of partners, constituencies, or funding agencies.

This leads to the next point on this topic: the role of health communication professionals in advocating for adequate funding of communication interventions by proving their added value in the public health, health care, and community development fields. In fact, "despite the proven success of communication programs, communication activities often do not receive adequate funding. They are often considered optional and, therefore, vulnerable to being cut in budget shortages" (Waisbord and Larson, 2005, p. 2).

Unfortunately, this happens also in clinical areas, such as childhood immunization, where several studies have shown "a positive association between communication campaigns and behavior" (Waisbord and Larson, 2005, p. 2). In the United States, the recent emphasis on health communication by federal agencies and reputable organizations and sources such as *Healthy People 2020* (and, before, *Healthy People 2010*) may contribute to improve funding resources for health communication interventions in the nonprofit and public health sectors. Still, program planning is one of the most important opportunities to argue for the value of communication interventions by showing their strategic connection with health outcomes.

Establishing the Overall Program Goal: A Practical Perspective

In establishing health communication among its priorities, *Healthy People 2010* set the goal to "use communication strategically to improve health" (US Department of Health and Human Services, 2005, p. 11-13). *Healthy People 2020* further expanded this mandate to make sure that vulnerable and underserved populations are not left out from the potential impact of well-designed communication interventions. Under *Healthy People 2020*, the goal for health communication is "to improve population health outcomes and health care quality, and to achieve health equity" (US Department of Health and Human Services, 2012b). Improving health is a strategic goal of health communication and is reflected in the definition of the overall program's goal in communication planning. In fact, program goals are developed to reflect and meet a specific need. They express the reason that a program is considered, initiated, and developed. They should be viewed as the rationale for seeking funds or asking a health organization to invest in communication. They are meant to reduce the impact or occurrence of a given health condition and improve the quality of life of people who suffer from it.

As with the other elements of health communication planning, the program goal is evidence-based. At the time program goals are developed, the communication team should already have conducted some preliminary research (for example, a literature review or one-on-one conversations with key stakeholders, representatives of key audiences, community members, potential partners, or organizational departments), or received a briefing on the health issue, or engaged communities in preliminary observations or dialogue that allows them to state the need to address a specific health problem. In this phase, the situation analysis and audience profile may still need to be completed and, most important, validated (or not) with interested communities and stakeholders.

Still, a preliminary goal can be established by keeping in mind the initial research findings or briefing. As previously stated, the program goal highlights the health improvement or "the overall change in the health or social problem" (Weinreich, 1999, p. 67; 2011; Centers for Disease Control and Prevention [CDC], 2013c) the program is seeking to attain. At this stage, the program goal is preliminarily defined and will need to be validated and clearly stated once a comprehensive situation analysis and audience profile (see Chapter Eleven) is finalized. Among the practical examples of program goals are the following:

* Contribute to decrease HIV incidence rates among Hispanic men

- Help limit the impact of women's depression on family and work-related settings

- Decrease the incidence of mild traumatic brain injury among young people in the United States

- Decrease infant mortality rates among African Americans and other at-risk communities

Health communication interventions are almost always part of larger public health, health care, or corporate initiatives. Therefore, using words such as *contribute* or *help* may serve to acknowledge that change is always the result of comprehensive efforts, of which communication is an important element but nevertheless just one element. It may also help the communication team and its audiences focus on what communication can and cannot do (see Chapter One for a discussion of this topic) so that program design is based on realistic expectations and seeks achievable results.

At this stage, the health communication team in research settings may have already selected the theoretical framework or model that will guide their key assumptions and logical thinking throughout program planning or at least for some of its phases (for example, applying the steps of a behavior change theory to the development of the audience profile). Although this approach may not be rigorously applied in other contexts (for example, in the nonprofit, public, or commercial sectors), it is still important to use consistent models and assumptions throughout program planning and evaluation.

Outcome Objectives: Behavioral, Social, and Organizational

Outcome objectives (behavioral, social, and organizational) complement the program goal and should be initially established after the preliminary research or briefing on the health issue. As with the program goal, these objectives would need to be refined and validated by the key findings of the situation analysis and audience profile (see Chapter Eleven). Still, stating the potential behavior, social, or organizational change objectives at the outset of the planning process helps focus all research efforts (for example, literature review, one-on-one interviews, focus groups, questions to be addressed by participatory audience research) that lead to the situation analysis and audience profile and, ultimately, the development of adequate communication objectives. The communication objectives should support the program goal and help achieve the behavioral, social, or organizational change that is sought by the program (National Cancer Institute at the National Institutes of Health, 2002, 2013). In fact, "the early stages of any communication planning model should explicitly link the overall program's broad goals, specific outcome objectives, and individual behavior change objectives to the communication component of the program" (Donovan, 1995, p. 215). Such objectives should be established in partnership with outside experts and facilitators and intended communities and stakeholders depending on the nature of the health communication intervention.

Behavioral objectives refer to what key groups and stakeholders should do in relation to a specific health issue or situation, social change objectives highlight the policy or social change that the program is seeking to achieve, and organizational objectives refer to the change that should occur within an organization in terms of its focus, priorities, or structure in order to address a specific health and social issue. Key program outcomes will be measured against these outcome objectives as well as other intermediate parameters that may correspond to the communication objectives or be specifically identified and agreed on by the health communication team. Still, this assumes that all these objectives support the attainment of the overall program goal and are critical to it.

Outcome objectives should be measurable and realistic. Setting the right expectations is critical in defining the percentage of the population or key group in which any change is expected. Human behavior is difficult to change, so expecting 30, 40, or 50 percent of the intended audience to make a change is quite unrealistic. Sound objectives may look at a 3 to 5 percent change in a realistic time frame that may extend for several years (E. Rogers, cited in Atkin and Schiller, 2002; Health Communication Unit, 2003c; National Cancer Institute at the National Institutes of Health, 2002). This time frame as well as the percentage of people being affected by a health communication intervention may vary according to the health issue or program. Many of the methods and considerations that go into developing communication objectives (see Chapter Twelve) also apply to the definition of outcome objectives.

Most important, behavioral, organizational, or social change in health communication should be considered instrumental to a reduction of the burden of disease and the mitigation of the social and political factors that contribute to it. Therefore, behavior, social, and organizational objectives should refer to changes that make possible the attainment of the overall program goal.

Additional examples of behavioral, social, or organizational change objectives are included in Exhibit 10.1 and refer to the prevention of asthma severity and mortality in inner cities in the United States. Asthma is "the third leading cause of hospitalization among children under the age of 15" (American Lung Association, 2012). It is a condition that can be aggravated by several indoor triggers, for example, dust or mold

(Ad Council, 2006a, 2006b; CDC, 2006a). In addition, lack of medical insurance or inadequate knowledge may jeopardize the prevention and management of asthma attacks (Lara, Allen, and Lange, 1999; Halterman, Montes, Shone, and Szilagyi, 2008). "Many children with asthma have unmet health care needs and poor access to consistent primary care, and lack of continuous health insurance coverage may play an important role. Efforts are needed to ensure uninterrupted coverage for these children" (Halterman, Montes, Shone, and Szilagyi, 2008, p. 43).

EXHIBIT 10.1. EXAMPLES OF OUTCOME OBJECTIVES FOR A PROGRAM ON PEDIATRIC ASTHMA

Overall program goal

Reduce the severity and mortality of asthma among children fifteen years old and younger who live in inner cities in the United States

Behavioral objectives	Social objectives	Organizational objectives
Within three years from program launch, prompt XX percent of parents or caretakers of asthmatic children in target neighborhoods to	By the year 2015, increase social acceptance within XX percent of families and schools on the role of children as key agents of change in providing support and ideas for asthma prevention in their communities (effectively establishing a new social norm).	By the year 2020, become a leading medical professional organization in pediatric asthma management as recognized by XX percent of health care providers, donors, and other key stakeholders in the field (for example, in the case of a professional organization that has a new vision; believes in its potential to contribute to the overall program goal; wants to develop and disseminate new solutions or guidelines;
• Recognize early signs of an asthma attack		
• Go immediately to the emergency room		
By the year 2020, persuade XX percent of parents or caretakers in the intended group to		
• Get rid of triggers (for example, mold, dust mites, cats, and dogs) of child asthma attacks in their homes		

(continued)

Behavioral objectives	Social objectives	Organizational objectives
• Keep their health care providers abreast of progress	Remove by the year 2020 existing health insurance policy–related barriers to adequate access to services and medications for asthmatic children in inner cities via local and national policies.	and understands that its reputation in the field is instrumental to its cause).
Within the next year, prompt XX medical practices in target neighborhoods to discuss pediatric asthma with children and their families		By the year 2015, develop organizational capacity to train and support XX number of health professionals in adopting and sustaining best clinical practices (to be specifically defined) in the prevention and treatment of pediatric asthma.
• At routine visits		
• Using bilingual materials and interpreters, when needed		
• Recommending community resources and social support groups on this topic		
• Identifying and discussing with children and their families key obstacles to asthma attack prevention and management		

Note: The goals and objectives in this exhibit are an example. The definition of actual goals and objectives for a program on pediatric asthma in inner cities should be based on an in-depth situation analysis and audience profile, which are developed with the participation and engagement of communities and groups they are intended for.

Key Concepts

• Health communication planning is an evidence-based and strategic process that is necessary to the effectiveness of health communication interventions.

- Planning is a fundamental stage of the communication cycle, which also includes implementation and evaluation, feedback, and refinement.

- Strategic planning helps clarify what health communication programs should do for an organization and its audiences and stakeholders.

- There are variations in some of the stages and categories that different authors or organizations use to describe the health communication cycle as well as the planning process. Still, the overall general premises tend to stay the same and describe the overall function of each step or stage in the process.

- The key elements of a health communication plan are
  - Overall program goal
  - Behavioral, social, and organizational objectives (outcome objectives)
  - Situation and audience analysis
  - Communication objectives
  - Communication strategies
  - Action (tactical) plan (including communication messages, channels, activities, and materials)
  - Evaluation plan

- The key elements are research-based and interdependent. Each affects decisions in relation to the others.

- Health communication planning terms serve to increase clarity about the different steps of communication planning.

- The overall program goal is evidence based and describes the overall "health improvement" (National Cancer Institute at the National Institutes of Health, 2002, p. 22) or "overall change in a health or social problem" (Weinreich, 1999, p. 67; 2011) that the program is seeking to achieve.

- Behavior, social, and organizational change objectives (outcome objectives) complement the overall program goal and should be defined early in program planning. They help focus the research phase and initial community engagement and dialogue phases, which lead to the next steps of the planning process as well as to the development of adequate communication objectives.

- Program outcomes should be measured against outcome objectives as well as other intermediate evaluation parameters, which are refined and finalized on the basis of the key findings of the situation analysis and audience profile (see Chapter Eleven).

FOR DISCUSSION AND PRACTICE

1. In your opinion, why is planning important? List and discuss what you see as the top three reasons for a structured and rigorous approach to planning in health communication.

2. Luciana is a nineteen-year-old Italian woman who loves spending time at the beach and is unaware of the risk for skin cancer associated with prolonged sun exposure. (For additional detail on Luciana's beliefs, behavior, and social context, see Box 2.1 in Chapter Two.) Apply the core definitions in this chapter to the following:
   - Establish the preliminary overall program goal of a health communication program intended to engage Luciana and her peer group.
   - Identify key groups and stakeholders who should become engaged and provide input on health communication planning on this topic.
   - Develop measurable outcome objectives (behavioral, social, and organizational) for this program. For organizational objectives, think of professional or consumer organizations that may have an interest in participating in a program on skin cancer prevention.

3. Imagine you are a health communication consultant who has been hired to develop a health communication plan. Identify the steps in your planning process using (a) a traditional, expert-led approach to planning and (b) a more participatory approach involving intended audiences and key stakeholders. Discuss the pros and cons of the two approaches and the steps you have envisioned. Analyze the impact of these two potential approaches as they relate to issues of program sustainability and potential effectiveness.

4. Research case studies and other examples of community and stakeholder participation in health communication planning on a topic of your choice. Extrapolate and discuss key lessons learned.

5. Identify, research, and discuss examples of key social and political factors (as they relate to the environment in which people live and work) that contribute to a health issue of your choice or to either chronic diseases or mental health in your city. Prioritize top factors and explain how they may relate to future health communication planning on the topic.

KEY TERMS

behavioral objectives

organizational objectives

outcome objectives

overall program goal

social objectives

CHAPTER 11

SITUATION AND AUDIENCE ANALYSIS

Health communication planning can be compared to a tower with many building blocks. Think about the potential verbal or written briefing that health communication teams may receive from an organization, funding, or government agency, relevant communities, or other groups that seek to address HIV/AIDS prevention among young women in the United States. This briefing can be regarded as the first building block that allows communicators to establish, share, and discuss the preliminary program goals, as well as the potential behavioral, social, or organizational objectives with team members and other key program stakeholders. Most likely the briefing has been complemented by some preliminary research, including a few conversations with key opinion leaders in the HIV/AIDS field, an initial literature review, or conversations with representatives of relevant communities and other groups.

Still, the foundation of the health communication tower is not yet solid. The team members will have many gaps in their understanding of the issue that they will have to address in order to implement the health communication program. These gaps may include the team's actual understanding of the extent and severity of HIV/AIDS among young women, as well as all factors contributing to higher incidence rates and limited use of preventive measures. The tower's foundation will be built only by using a comprehensive situation analysis, including audience analysis for all key groups and communities the program intends to reach and engage. This analysis should enlist the participation of key groups and stakeholders in defining and prioritizing the health issue and its potential solutions within the context of their living and working environments.

The situation analysis is a fundamental building block in the communication tower and its actual foundation. A well-executed and solid situation analysis informs and guides all the other steps of health communication planning. It also makes sure that all the building blocks in the tower are not at risk of falling for lack of the evidence- and audience-based glue that holds them together.

CHAPTER OBJECTIVES

This chapter focuses on how to build a solid foundation for health communication programs by developing an in-depth situation analysis and audience profile (the report summarizing audience analysis). In doing so, it provides a step-by-step guide on how to research and analyze all key factors contributing to a health problem, as well as to select and prioritize the information that is instrumental to the development of health communication objectives and strategies. The chapter also emphasizes the importance of a participatory approach to research in assessing key groups' needs and preferences. This information is complemented by a detailed worksheet included in Appendix A (see "A1: Situation and Audience Analysis Worksheet: Sample Questions and Topics").

How to Develop a Comprehensive Situation and Audience Analysis

The term *situation analysis* has different meanings in different contexts. In this book, it is used as a planning term and describes the analysis of all individual, community, social, political, and behavior-related factors that can affect attitudes, behaviors, social norms, and policies about a health or social issue and its potential solutions. This analysis is integral to the development of communication objectives and strategies.

The participatory situation analysis is not just a compilation of data and statistics. It is an analytical and selective process—and related report—on the health communication environment (see Figure 1.1 in Chapter One) and all audience-related factors. It helps communicators gain an in-depth understanding of how these factors influence the health issue and how health communication can affect the environment. All topics in the situation analysis's report are selected, prioritized, and covered only to the extent that they are relevant to a specific health issue and its audiences and stakeholders.

Ultimately the situation analysis helps identify what may work and what has not worked. For example, in Nigeria, a situation analysis report on the government's efforts to prevent sexually transmitted infections (STIs) showed that "past actions have lacked coordination, failed to establish linkages between projects and actions, and suffered from insufficient financial allocations" (Soul Beat Africa, 2006). The report also identified the lack of involvement of many key sectors of society in previous initiatives as well as the absence of critical information on key audiences.

Some authors distinguish the situation analysis from the audience analysis and consider them to be two separate steps. In this book, the **audience profile** (an analytical report on key findings from audience-related research and data analysis) is described as one of the key sections of the situation analysis. This also reflects actual health communication practice as well as the need for engaging key groups and stakeholders in all different phases of communication planning both in assessing the health issue as well as individual, community, social, and political factors that may contribute to it.

audience profile
An analytical report on key findings from audience-related research (also called audience analysis) and one of the key sections of the situation analysis

The audience profile focuses only on the audience's characteristics, demographics, needs, values, social norms, attitudes, lifestyle, and behavior. These descriptive factors are also used to segment key audiences. However, practical experience has shown that often many of the issues pertaining to a group are also related to the health communication environment described within the situation analysis. For example, the social stigma that in many countries is attached to certain health conditions such as HIV/AIDS should be analyzed not only as part of the social environment of a community or group but also as part of the audience profile. Fear, poor knowledge of HIV transmission modalities, and a lack of empathy for a disease that may appear to be self-inflicted (International Center for Research on Women, 2003; Sengupta and others, 2011) may feed social conventions and at the same time be reinforced by them. Social norms, policies, and key group beliefs, attitudes, and behaviors are all mutually influenced. When the audience profile is part of the situation analysis, this connection and mutual interdependence may become easier to understand. For this reason, the audience profile, which refers to a detailed description of the key program's audiences as well as groups that influence them, is included in this book as part of the situation analysis.

These practical tips may help in developing a situation analysis:

* Never feel as though you have spoken with too many people about a health issue or condition. Gathering multiple perspectives is essential to the planning process.

- Use a team approach in collecting data and relevant information. Brainstorm in advance about research needs and methods, as well as potential difficulties and strategies to overcome them.

- Use participatory research methods and community dialogue to engage and encourage ownership of the communication process among key groups and stakeholders. Involve representatives of key audiences across the various research and analysis phases!

- Do not get discouraged if it is difficult to find a specific piece of information (O'Sullivan, Yonkler, Morgan, and Merritt, 2003). Be persistent.

- Share and solicit feedback on research findings as well as the final situation analysis from key audiences and as many people as possible in your organization or team.

- Use data strategically to develop sound communication objectives and strategies, but do not jump ahead. Do not include communication objectives and strategies as part of the situation analysis. Develop communication objectives and strategies only after reviewing, discussing, and analyzing key findings (see Chapter Twelve) with key groups, team members, and partners.

- Look for signs suggesting there is sufficient information in support of a basic framework of understanding of the specific health issue and its key groups and stakeholders. Examples are the emergence of recurring trends or multiple data from different sources that point to similar conclusions or community members reaching consensus on the contribution of a specific topic to the health issue.

- Incorporate a social-determinants-of-health-driven mind-set in all of your research steps and analysis. Understand key factors (socioeconomics, race, gender, age, access to services, transportation, education, etc.) that may contribute to the health issue or health disparities within specific groups.

All of these points provide practical guidance in completing the steps of a situation analysis as illustrated in Figure 11.1.

Define and Understand the Health Issue

The first step in developing a situation analysis is to gain an in-depth understanding of the health issue: its medical causes as well as the socially determined factors that may contribute to it, its severity, risk factors, and statistical significance among different audiences and groups. This step

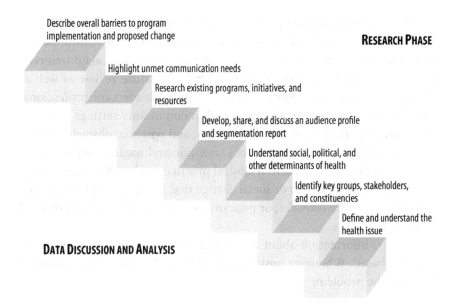

Describe overall barriers to program
implementation and proposed change

RESEARCH PHASE

Highlight unmet communication needs

Research existing programs, initiatives, and
resources

Develop, share, and discuss an audience profile
and segmentation report

Understand social, political, and
other determinants of health

Identify key groups, stakeholders,
and constituencies

Define and understand the
health issue

DATA DISCUSSION AND ANALYSIS

Figure 11.1 Key Steps of Situation Analysis

leads to identifying the populations or audience segments the program
would prioritize because they are ultimately most affected by the issue.

For example, key decisions about intervention design as well as key
groups to be engaged in a communication intervention that seeks to
address sudden infant death syndrome (SIDS), a condition that has been
associated with many risk factors, including improper infant sleeping
position (National Institutes of Health, 2003; Centers for Disease Control
[CDC], 2002) and infant-parent bed sharing (Kelmanson, 2011), may be
influenced by the higher mortality rates among African American children
than among other US children (National SIDS/Infant Death Resource
Center, 2006; National Institute of Child Health and Human Development,
2005; Moon, Oden, Joyner, and Ajao, 2010). If economic and human
resources limit the program's ability to reach multiple groups or the
general public, it may make sense to focus all resources on engaging
African Americans, where the risk for SIDS deaths is higher. Of course,
these decisions are influenced by many factors, including the organizational
competence to address the needs of a specific group or population.

Other important information pieces to include in this first step of
the situation analysis are data and opinions on current treatment and
prevention strategies, recent scientific progress, anticipated preventive or
therapeutic options, best clinical practices, existing guidelines, social barriers to the adoption of preventive behaviors, and other relevant obstacles.
If a new health product or service is involved, information about its major

advantages and disadvantages as well as how they compare with existing products or services should be obtained at this stage along with information on key factors that may increase access among vulnerable and underserved populations. Such data can be obtained by a literature review as well as telephone or in-person interviews with key opinion leaders and professional organizations, and further discussed within community settings to gather information on people's needs, preferences, and potential obstacles as they relate to their ability to benefit from scientific and medical advances and services. Understanding current clinical practices and available tools helps shed light on the behavior or social change that needs to be addressed at a patient, health care provider, or policymaker level, to name a few potential audiences.

Finally, information about the health issue or condition needs to be evidence based. Whenever possible, use statistically significant parameters to define the problem:

- *Incidence:* The number of new cases of a health condition that are occurring or are expected to occur in a given population within a specific time frame—for example, "HIV/AIDS cases in Africa are expected to increase by X percent in the next five years."

- *Prevalence:* The total number of cases of disease in a given population at a specific time, often expressed as a percentage of the population—for example, "X percent of US children age six and over have suffered from primary nocturnal enuresis at any time during the past five years."

- *Mortality:* The total number of people who died of a health condition during a specific time frame—for example, "In 2002, there were X deaths due to pertussis in the United States."

- *Morbidity:* The number of people who present with severe symptoms of a disease and are either temporarily or permanently disabled as a result—for example, "In 2010, X percent of US adults forty to fifty years old who were severely obese were hospitalized for longer than one week."

- *Cost of the health condition* to individuals, health organizations, communities, groups, or the society as a whole—for example, "In 2011, depression accounted for X number of lost workdays, which resulted in X dollars in lost earnings among people suffering from depression."

- *Morbidity or mortality of other conditions associated with the primary health condition or issue*—for example, "Serious head injuries as a result of falls among Alzheimer's patients is a common disease complication and occurs in X percent of patients."

- *Percentage of people who received or had access to adequate preventive or treatment options*—for example, "In 2010, X percent of Canadian children received all the immunizations in the recommended childhood immunization schedule."

- *Impact of key social determinants of health on a specific health condition*—for example, "By 2020, it's estimated that X percent of elderly people living with chronic conditions won't be able to access essential clinical services because of the lack of adequate and age-friendly transportation systems in their cities."

Ideally, all of these parameters should be explored and defined by age, gender, and ethnic and cultural group or other relevant variations at the population level. Peer-reviewed publications, organizational websites, and other relevant literature can be used to gather specific information related to this step.

Identify Key Groups, Stakeholders, and Constituencies

This step entails identifying key groups and stakeholders (the primary and secondary audiences) that would need to be engaged in the health communication intervention. Stakeholders are all individuals and groups who have an interest or share responsibilities in a given health issue. They may represent the primary audience (for example, AIDS activist groups or breast cancer survivors' groups, or community leaders and members, or a group of engaged citizens) or influence them.

The *primary audiences* of a health communication program are the people who may benefit the most from the health communication intervention and behavior and social change, for example, the people who are at risk for a certain medical condition or are suffering from it, and parents or caregivers who are responsible for pediatric care decisions for their children. In some cases, the primary audience may also include other audiences (for example, health care providers and policymakers) when programs are small and tailored only to a specific group or constituency we seek to engage (for example, through professional communications or government relations). *Secondary audiences* are all individuals, groups, communities, and organizations that have an influence on the decisions and behaviors of the primary audiences. In other words, secondary audiences include those people who can help reach the primary audience. They are the grandmothers who may suggest how to put a baby to sleep, or the community leaders who influence gender roles as they relate to health and social issues, or the health care providers whose cross-cultural communication skills may help convince a patient to exercise and eat healthy, just to name a few examples. Behavioral and social change starts with the support provided by these key influential groups, which often may need to make changes of their own or reinforce their current behaviors and practices (for example, community group leaders may need to become more supportive of and provide resources and guidance to peers who may attempt to quit smoking). Primary and secondary audiences can change or switch over time when, for example, some of the program objectives are achieved and the program focus is redefined by all program partners and key groups and stakeholders.

No matter what, key stakeholders need to be identified, cultivated, and engaged in the early phases of program planning. Planning together with key constituency groups as well as effectively addressing criticisms and different viewpoints held by key influential groups are important components of the health communication process and should be a key priority in the planning phase.

For example, in designing a program that aims to reduce flu transmission from health workers to patients by promoting immunization of nurse practitioners and other health workers, it makes sense to engage with organizations that represent nurse practitioners. In doing so, the communication team can solicit their feedback on key research findings about current beliefs, attitudes, social norms, and behaviors, as well as potential communication objectives and strategies. Moreover, brainstorming with them about communication activities and their involvement in the program provides invaluable insight into the design of the communication intervention and increases the likelihood that the program will effectively reach nurse practitioners.

As another example of how to identify different groups, think of the prevention of human papilloma virus (HPV), which is a sexually transmitted infection and can present with almost no symptoms (Weinstock, Berman, and Cates, 2004). Persistent HPV infection with specific types of the virus has been described as one of the leading causes of cervical cancer (Sellors and others, 2003). In 2006, the US Food and Drug Administration (FDA) approved the first vaccine against HPV. Depending on the specific vaccine, immunization is recommended for use in women as well as men nine to twenty-six years of age (US Food and Drug Administration, 2006, 2009). Primary audiences of a health communication program to reduce HPV incidence by getting people vaccinated might include adolescents and young adults, as well as parents of children nine to twelve years old who can influence their preteens' decision to be immunized. The decision to select one of these two groups (or both of them) as the primary audience of a health communication intervention should be based on a number of factors, including audience risk for HPV, organizational competence to address an audience's needs, current policies and medical practices, and the chance for success in convincing people to comply with immunization. Most important, the decision should be taken via a participatory approach in which at-risk communities and parents identify areas of needs as well as specific groups that should be prioritized by the intervention.

Secondary audiences should be identified by using a similar process and include all groups (for example, family members, health care providers, peers, student associations, community centers, religious leaders, and others) that may have an influence on the primary audiences. In the case of HPV, one obvious secondary audience is health care providers, including pediatricians (when the primary audience consists of parents of children ten to twelve years old), as well as family practitioners, gynecologists, nurses, and family planning counselors. In fact, health care providers are a credible source of information on vaccine-preventable diseases, and are used to discuss immunization issues because they relate to key benefits and safety inquiries.

While identifying potential audiences, both primary and secondary, it is important to start analyzing and segmenting them by their preferences and needs, age, professional associations, cultural or ethnic factors, religious beliefs, gender, current attitudes, practices, behaviors, as well as other distinguishing characteristics that contribute to the makeup of a specific group or community. This information will be used and analyzed to complete the audience profile and segmentation.

Moreover, this information is also important within the context of the initial focus groups or conversations with community members and key stakeholders. For example, tweens (nine to twelve years old) may feel uncomfortable discussing any kind of issue within a group that includes older teens or parents. Similarly, parents may prefer an initial forum where they discuss their concerns among themselves and not within a group that also includes health care providers. Yet, community dialogue sessions (see Chapter Four) should also be organized and encouraged, because most of the times the best ideas come from the collective thinking of a given community whose members work together across sectors, age groups, and other segmentation parameters.

Understand Social, Political, and Other Determinants of Health

Once the health problem has been defined and potential audiences identified and engaged in the communication planning process, the next step is to understand the social and political factors that influence the current situation or may represent a challenge or opportunity for change. This phase takes into account the social nature of human interactions and decision making. Individual decisions are usually influenced by peers, institutions, social norms, and policies. Medical practices and government policies are often shaped by the communities to which legislators or health care providers belong, as well as their constituencies and the public at large. People's ability to adopt and sustain a health or social behavior is greatly influenced by the social and political environment in which they live, work, and age; the level of social support they may receive by peers, family, community members, and others; as well as by adequate access to a variety of services (for example, health services and information, transportation, parks, recreational facilities), and goods (for example, fruit and vegetables, medications).

Consider the fictional example of Adriana, a forty-five-year-old Italian woman who takes care of her brother, Mario, who has suffered from schizophrenia since age twenty. He is now thirty-five years old and lives with his seventy-year-old mother. Adriana is married with four children but spends her time between her own home and her mother's home.

Similar to her brother, she lives in a small town where family values are strong and dictate people's involvement in the care of less-fortunate family members. Still, the community is also dominated by a lack of understanding of mental illness and feelings of fear about anyone who suffers from it. Adriana's work colleagues and many friends have isolated her and her family and seem to expect that she may also become "crazy" at any moment. In a way, the community values are contradictory: on the one hand, Adriana is supposed to take care of her family, and on the other hand, almost no one is able to offer the emotional and social support she and her brother need.

Over time Adriana and her mother have been influenced by social prejudice against mental illness. They kept Mario's illness a secret for a long time, and Mario avoided treatment and counseling at the local mental health clinic for fear of being seen there by his neighbors and friends. He accepted professional help only at a late stage of his illness. Overall, the lack of social support and the high level of family stress this created affect Mario's ability to comply with treatment and have had a negative impact on his health. This also prevents him from holding a steady job or performing other regular daily activities.

Unfortunately, most countries and communities are still overridden with social prejudice against mental illness. People tend to believe that mentally ill patients are dangerous (Corrigan, 2004) and "twice as likely today than they were in 1950 to believe that mentally ill people tend to be violent" (Dingfelder, 2009, p. 56). However, many of them are in a middle group: "struggling with mental illness [yet] living on their own with a full-time job" (Medscape, 2004).

Prejudice may be reinforced by or, in some cases, lead to specific local policies and practices. For instance, "voters with mental disabilities . . . face a particularly insidious barrier to equal participation in the electoral process—discriminatory rules and procedures applied only to them" (National Network for Election Reform, 2013). Discrimination may also apply to the quality of health care mentally ill patients receive. For example, people with mental illness appear to be less likely to receive cardiac care (Medscape, 2004; Druss and others, 2000). Finally, additional disadvantages in health insurance policies "also reflect the stigmatization of people with mental illness" (Gaebel, Baumann, and Phil, 2003, p. 657).

In the case of schizophrenia, "delayed intervention leads to greater secondary morbidity" (Hustig and Norrie, 1998, p. 58; Vancouver/Richmond Early Psychosis Intervention, 2013). A social, medical, and policy environment that does not encourage early intervention and instead contributes to family and patient stress may have a negative impact on patient outcomes.

This mental illness example shows why social norms and medical practices as well as existing policies and regulations need to be analyzed and included as part of the situation analysis of a health communication program. Stigma is only one of many elements that are influenced by multiple interdependent factors. Others include the following:

- People's beliefs, attitudes, and behaviors
- Cultural, ethnic, gender, religious, and age influences
- Social norms, policies, and regulations
- Health insurance policies or other practices related to the health care system
- Overall ideas of health and illness within a specific population or subgroup
- Market- or media-related considerations, such as the way a disease is portrayed by the media
- Living and working environment, including access to key services and information (not only limited to health care)
- Disease-related stereotypes

This step of the situation analysis focuses primarily on analyzing all relevant external factors related to the social, scientific, market, media, and policy environment, including these aspects that may be specific to a given health issue, community, or region of the world. In completing this step, it is important to take into account how people are influenced by these factors, as well as how the communication intervention can help them shape the environment in which they live.

Develop, Share, and Discuss an Audience Profile and Segmentation Report

Developing the audience profile and segmentation in groups with similar characteristics and behavioral stages is one of the most significant steps of the situation and audience analysis. "Know your audience" is probably the most important mantra of health communication. In fact, no one can attempt to engage and influence people without making an effort to know them first. The analytical research report we refer to as *audience profile* is grounded in an in-depth understanding of key groups and stakeholders and comprehensive audience research.

Only health communication interventions that are based on a true understanding of their key groups and stakeholders have an actual chance of succeeding and meeting expected outcomes. Depending on the type of health communication intervention, either representatives of key groups or large segments of the community should be involved and complement expert efforts to profile and analyze key findings about the needs, preferences, characteristics, beliefs, attitudes, social norms, and behaviors of intended audiences.

In most cases, profiling an audience also includes segmenting it into groups with similar characteristics and needs. This helps make sense of the audience's complexity and guides the allocation of resources as well as the development of adequate communication objectives and strategies for each segment, as recommended by members of such groups. Audience segmentation may lead to several different combinations of attributes for each segment. However, there are cases in which segmentation is not necessary because the audience presents with similar characteristics and behavioral and social stages.

A number of obvious categories should be used in profiling, grouping, and segmenting an audience as part of participatory and traditional research methods, and literature, case study and document review:

- *Demographic characteristics*, including age, gender, race, ethnic background, language, marital status, number of children, and literacy level

- *Common beliefs, attitudes, social norms, and behavior* in relation to the health issue, including perceived or existing barriers to the adoption of new behaviors or the use of new health services and products

- *Geographical factors,* such as location, rural versus urban environment, size of city or county, climate, and means of transportation

- *Socioeconomic factors,* such as income level, education, and professional and social status

- *Lifestyle and cultural characteristics,* such as preferred pastimes, risk behaviors, work versus family balance, cultural values, ideas about health and illness, religious beliefs, media habits, and preferred media channels

- *Physical or medical factors,* such as health status, medical history, comorbidities, and group and individual risk factors

- *Living and working environment* as it relates to access to health services and information, adequate transportation, jobs, and other socioeconomic opportunities, recreational facilities and parks, nutritious food, and other key social determinants of health

- *Other factors that may be issue or audience specific*

Sometimes all of these categories apply to the health issue being analyzed. At other times, only a few of them may be more significant. For example, an analysis of the transportation system of a specific region may be relevant in northeast Brazil, where there are large distances and very few well-equipped health centers (Stock-Iwamoto and Korte, 1993; Tannebaum, 2006). By contrast, transportation issues and related audience preferences will not be relevant to interventions intended to promote screening for breast cancer among US women under age fifty who live in metropolitan areas, where public transportation and access to health care facilities are generally diverse and widespread. Yet, transportation issues may be relevant in other US settings, such as in the case of underserved communities or vulnerable populations (for example, the elderly or people living with disability).

One of the most important parameters for audience segmentation is the stage of the audience's beliefs, attitudes, and health and social behaviors that are relevant to the health issue being addressed. How far are policymakers from passing legislation that would increase the number of available public health clinics? Are they convinced about the importance of this issue? Do they feel it is important to their constituencies? Do they care? Are they usually empathetic about the rights of underserved and underprivileged people? Are there any social norms that influence their beliefs, attitudes, and behaviors, and those of the people who influence them?

Some authors (Weinreich, 2011) suggest using the stages of behavior change model (see Chapter Two) to segment key audiences on the basis of their attitudes and behavior. The five steps of this theory (precontemplation, contemplation, preparation, action, and maintenance) are described in Chapter Two.

In general, if we think about human behavior and the reason that people may decide to immunize their child, use condoms on a regular basis, or protect their skin from the risk for cancer, the main reasons for adopting or not adopting a recommended behavior can be summarized in the following categories of people: "Don't know; know, but see too many obstacles; know, don't see obstacles, but don't see benefits; know, don't see too many obstacles, see benefits, but don't care" (Southwest Center for the Application of Prevention Technology, 2001); and "know, don't see too many obstacles, see benefits, care" but only later realize that they don't have the time, resources, tools, or support to implement the change. The last category includes the optimistic, the people who commit to adopt or maintain specific health-related behaviors but then realize they don't have the time or resources to implement them, or the people who, once they start implementing their decision, suddenly discover that their neighborhoods lack essential services or infrastructure that would enable them to succeed in making the changes they seek.

Interventions tailored to each of these segments may be quite different and will need to take into account the other characteristics of each segment (for example, socioeconomic factors, age, lifestyle, social norms). Sometimes because of the diversity of the approaches that are required to reach different segments or subgroups of a population, health communication teams (including representatives of key groups and stakeholders) may decide to focus on only one group or include other groups gradually. Exhibit 11.1 shows a practical example of audience segmentation that uses the categories set out here.

EXHIBIT 11.1. AUDIENCE SEGMENTATION EXAMPLE

Audience: US women over age fifty-five who suffer from type 2 diabetes and are severely overweight or obese

Stage of knowledge, attitude, or behavior	Examples of potential segments
Don't know	Women who are not aware of the association between obesity and type 2 diabetes. They may attribute diabetes to other causes or consider it a normal part of aging.
Know, but see too many obstacles	Women who know about the association between obesity and type 2 diabetes. However, they feel they will never succeed in losing weight because of one or all of the following obstacles: • Peer and family pressure to eat fast food or other kinds of unhealthy food • Lack of time to cook or implement lifestyle changes • Insufficient health club or gym presence in their neighborhood or prohibitive cost of membership • Overall feelings of being unable to make a change • Others
Know, don't see many obstacles, but don't see benefits	Women who know about the association between obesity and type 2 diabetes, don't see many obstacles or are confident they can overcome them. Still, they don't believe that at this point losing weight would make any difference in regard to their diabetes or any other comorbidities of obesity. For example, they may regard diabetes as a lifetime condition on which nothing can have an impact.
Know, don't see many obstacles, see benefits, but don't care	Women who know about the obesity-diabetes association, don't see many obstacles to change, see benefits, but don't care for any of the following potential reasons: • They currently are able to control diabetes with medications, so, what's the big deal?

(continued)

Stage of knowledge, attitude, or behavior	Examples of potential segments
	• They have a fatalistic view of health and illness and feel they cannot do anything about it (whatever it is, it is).
	• They are influenced by social norms that support their attitudes toward potentially taking care of their weight or diabetes.
	• They have many other conflicting priorities in their life and feel this is not one of them.
	• Others
Know, don't see many obstacles, see benefits, care, but then realize later they don't have the time, resources, tools, or support to implement change	Women who know about the obesity-diabetes link don't see obstacles to change and see benefits and care. They consider losing weight one of their top priorities but once they start implementing new behaviors are overwhelmed by the process and realize, for example, they may need help, social support, or tools to do any of the following:
	• Learn how to integrate exercise into their busy lifestyle or find cost-effective options for physical activity
	• Engage peers and family in their lifestyle change
	• Ask the right questions of their health care providers about weight loss
	• Become aware of quick recipes for healthy meals they can prepare after work
	• Find the right weight-loss program
	• Partner with local organizations, coworkers, and others to find solutions to the lack of services and community infrastructure they recently learned about, so to facilitate behavioral adoption and sustainability
	• Others

Source: With the exception of the last stage in this exhibit, the stages of knowledge, attitude, or behavior are from Southwest Center for the Application of Prevention Technologies. "Community Based Social Marketing." 2001. http://captus.samhsa.gov/southwest/resources/documents/307,12, Slide12. All examples in the right column have been developed for this text.

Once the segments have been defined, there are some general criteria and questions that can help prioritize audience segments and allocate appropriate resources:

- Is the segment at greatest risk for the health condition (Weinreich, 2011)?

- Can it be influenced given the current level of organizational competence to address the audience's needs and the specific health situation?

- Does change in a particular segment need to happen before focusing on other audience segments because of the group's ability to lead the process of change and influence social norms?

- Is the segment ready to make a behavior change (Weinreich, 2011; Hornik, 2003) or would this require economic and human resources that go beyond the current program estimate?

- What is the segment size (Hornik, 2003)? Is it worth a large investment or should resources be proportional to its size?

- Could the segment realistically adopt or sustain recommended health behaviors given their current living and working environment? If not, should the intervention first focus on addressing social, political, and economic barriers to behavioral and social change and involve community members in finding adequate solutions toward progress?

Secondary audiences should be profiled using a similar process and the same categories described previously in this section. In addition, there are a few specific criteria that apply to the process of profiling and segmenting secondary audiences: the level of influence exerted on the primary groups (in other words, do primary audiences listen to them?), potential benefits (for example, visibility, mission fulfillment) that secondary audiences may derive from their involvement in the program, and barriers to their involvement (Weinreich, 2011). Other criteria should include the level of difficulty in working with them, the audience commitment to the health issue, and existing opportunities (for example, ongoing communication channels, annual venues) that have been developed by secondary audiences and may expand program reach.

Box 11.1 is an example of audience profiling and segmentation. This example refers to the CDC (2006c) campaign "Got a Minute? Give It to Your Kids!" which sought to engage less-involved parents and uses social marketing as a planning framework and theoretical model to provide social support and parenting resources to this group.

BOX 11.1. AUDIENCE PROFILE: GOT A MINUTE? GIVE IT TO YOUR KIDS!

The Audience

The intended audience for this campaign is parents who are less involved with their nine- to twelve-year-old children—that is, those who are less likely to eat dinner with those children, know where those children are during the day, help those children with homework, or otherwise be involved in those children's lives. These are parents who need to become more involved if they are to help their children reject the lure of tobacco.

Why Are We Addressing Only Less-Involved Parents?

Segmenting or identifying a group of people who have enough in common that you can reach them or motivate them in the same way is an essential component of a successful social marketing campaign. The more precisely we can describe a group, the stronger our campaign can become. After all, the goal is to influence behavior among the largest number possible with the available resources.

We identified less-involved parents as our target audience after looking at extensive research: in 1998, CDC hosted sixty parenting experts at a meeting to determine how parents should be characterized. After that we looked at consumer data from sources such as Healthstyles and Prizm and conducted focus groups with parents. Our analysis showed us a distinction among three main clusters of parenting attitudes and behaviors:

- On-target parents—those doing all the right things according to the research
- Nonenforcers—those who were involved with their children and set clear rules but then failed to enforce those rules
- Less-involved parents—the group targeted with the Got a Minute? campaign

Who Are Less-Involved Parents?

It is not hard to empathize with less-involved parents. Parenting preteens is not easy. As they age through this period, children who were once running to their parents for help are suddenly running away, seeking independence. Parents can feel they have lost control. For our target audience, this is especially true. Less-involved parents want to be involved with their children, but they don't know how, when, or what to do. And as their children enter adolescence, the distance between parent and child often grows, placing these preteens at greater risk for tobacco, drug, and alcohol use.

Compared with the other groups, less-involved parents are overwhelmed. Time that may have been set aside for their children is quickly absorbed in household chores, work, or just trying to find a moment to relax. Although they work similar hours as other parents, our target audience can't find enough time to get organized and plan activities with their preteens or even with other adults. In short, for less-involved parents, efficiently managing their time is one of the largest barriers to participating in activities with their children.

The lack of time and general organization for less-involved parents is not due to involvement in activities without their children. This group seldom visits friends. They are typically not members of social clubs, churches, or volunteer organizations. In fact, nearly half would call themselves "couch potatoes" and most (62 percent) consider television their primary form of entertainment.

A powerless feeling is a defining characteristic of less-involved parents. They reported the lowest self-efficacy on a wide range of behaviors. They are often aware of a need to change unhealthy habits and daily patterns, but they don't believe they can.

Regarding parenting, our intended audience knows they should spend time with their children but believe they are unable to change current behavior patterns. They are less confident about protecting their children from behavioral risks than other groups of parents and are less likely to create, develop, and enforce rules with their children.

Snapshot of Less-Involved Parents

- 69 percent indicated consistently feeling a great deal of pressure.

- 43 percent see their home as chaotic.

- 90 percent feel they work very hard.

- 39 percent do not have their children do chores on a regular basis.

- 43 percent reported household incomes over $50,000.

What Do Less-Involved Parents Look Like?

Our intended audience can be found anywhere. They cross lines of ethnicity, education level, socioeconomic status, and marital status. Less-involved parents can be blue- or white-collar workers. They are more likely than the other groups to be part of a parenting dyad (nearly one-quarter of less-involved parents are likely to be separated, divorced, or never married). Most also fall within the low-middle to upper-middle household income levels. Not unlike the other groups, they want to be perceived as ambitious (75 percent), hardworking (98 percent), and courageous (88 percent), and they want their children to exceed their current socioeconomic status.

What Are Their Current Parenting Behaviors?

Although our intended audience wants to spend time with their children, they are not able to identify possible activities or actions they can take to increase or improve their time together. For example, a majority (54 percent) of less-involved parents do not usually eat dinner together as a family. They think food preparation should take as little time as possible and are less likely to feel guilty about serving convenience food.

Concerning rule enforcement and monitoring of children's activities, many parents in our intended audience are not requiring that their children do chores on a regular basis, and their children are usually not checking in with them regarding their after-school or weekend activities.

Overall, less-involved parents are not satisfied with how their lives are currently going (52 percent)—including their relationships with their children. They feel overwhelmed with obligations, have low self-confidence, and feel like they are never going to get a grasp on their parenting obligations.

How Do We Reach Them?

Our intended audience is open to ideas on how to improve their parenting behaviors. They are willing to listen to various communications channels and are not that selective about the messenger. If it seems like a good idea, they will try it. However, they are likely to resent messages that do not provide a choice or that criticize their current behaviors. One subtle distinction goes to the heart of this: they want ideas, not advice.

Thus, the Got a Minute? campaign is designed to offer help, not issue orders or encourage guilt. At its core, the campaign simply provides ideas about how to connect with their children—just what less-involved parents are seeking.

Source: Centers for Disease Control and Prevention. "Got a Minute? Give It to Your Kid: Audience Profile." www.cdc.gov/tobacco/parenting/audience.htm. Retrieved Feb. 2006c. Used by permission.

Finally, once the audience analysis and segmentation process has reached a stage in which information has been confirmed by multiple sources, research methods, and conversations, it should be shared with all members of the enlarged health communication team. This is an opportunity for all partners, stakeholders, and members of key groups to review the evidence and decide on adequate strategies and objectives as well as to discuss in detail whether the evidence-based prioritization of key segments that emerged from the research conducted for the participatory audience analysis and segmentation actually responds to the needs and preferences of those most affected by the health issue and their key influencers or other data should be collected. As the team moves forward with its strategic decisions, the audience profile and segmentation report should be finalized by also including a detailed analysis of preferred communication channels, media, and venues for each of the segments the intervention seeks to engage.

Preferred Communication Channels, Media, and Venues

Health communication interventions are specific to each key group and stakeholder. Understanding the media habits and preferences for different kinds of communication channels of each primary and secondary audience is an integral part of the audience profile section of the situation analysis. Special consideration should also be given to specific venues, such as annual conferences or existing community or chapter meetings that have a broad appeal among key groups and stakeholders.

In this book, the term *communication channel* refers to the means and the path selected to reach the intended audience with health communication messages and materials. Communication channels can be divided into five broad categories:

- **Mass media channels**: print and broadcast media, the Internet, and more established new media

- **New media channels**: social media, social networking sites, mobile technology, and others

- **Interpersonal channels**, such as counseling, one-on-one meetings, provider-patient encounters, peer education, stakeholder-led meetings, or other interactive channels

- Other **community-specific channels and venues**, such as local or traditional media, poetry, traditional folk media, theater, existing community meetings, churches, local markets, or conferences

- **Professional channels and venues**, professional conferences and summits, online forums dedicated to a specific profession, and organizational communication channels (such as those of a professional association)

The US Agency for International Development (1999) analyzes benefits and challenges of diverse communication channels on the basis of three key parameters: ease of message control, interactivity, and ease of boundary control. In this model, radio and television are the least interactive channels, and peer education and counseling are considered the most interactive. Interactivity is considered more likely to influence a group to take action. New media have definitely contributed to expanding on this concept and enabled groups who previously may have acted in isolation to connect and interact.

mass media channels
Print and broadcast media, the Internet, and other new media

new media channels
Social media, social networking sites, mobile technology, and others

interpersonal channels
Counseling, one-on-one meetings, peer-to-peer trainings, provider-patient encounters, stakeholder-led meetings, or other interactive channels and venues that are used for interpersonal communication

community-specific channels
Local or traditional media, poetry, traditional folk media, theater, churches, local markets, and existing community meetings, for example

professional channels and venues
Professional conferences and summits, online forums dedicated to a specific profession, organizational communication channels (such as those of a professional association)

In general, the most appropriate channels for a given health communication program are audience specific, reflect the audience's preferences, and depend on several criteria that should inform research objectives on this topic as well as the analysis of relevant findings:

- *Message content and complexity.* Complex messages cannot rely only on the use of the mass media; they also need to be delivered using interpersonal and new media channels and other community-specific media to reinforce mass media messages. Consider, for example, the mother of a twelve-year-old boy who may have read in a national newspaper about the recent increase in US pertussis incidence (CDC, 2013d). She may be aware of the need to immunize adolescents to protect them from contracting the disease and transmitting it to more vulnerable segments of the population such as infants and young children (CDC, 2006h). However, the decision to immunize her child would need to be supported by her physician as well as her peer group (both offline and online). This would be particularly important in the absence of school mandates and other specific regulation in her community. Health communication programs in this field should also include the use of interpersonal channels and tools to facilitate peer-to-peer interactions as well as provider-parent communications. Ideally, interpersonal channels such as one-on-one meetings or community-specific channels such as local government newsletters and meetings could also be used to support the introduction of school-based mandates at the local government level. Moreover, social media and social networking sites as well as online parenting forums, websites, and blogs should also be considered to encourage dialogue and provide support and resources to parents on immunization issues.

- *Audience reach.* A commonly used criterion in selecting communication channels is the number of people a channel can reach. In the case of print and broadcast media, this number is expressed in terms of audience circulation. Similarly, in the case of websites and other online resources audience reach is expressed in terms of visitors (new or recurring) and other metrics discussed in Chapter Five. In other cases, it may be the number of people from key groups that a workshop or community meeting is estimated to attract. These numbers are important to define the most suitable and effective channels to reach the largest percentage of key groups and relevant populations. Audience reach is one of the key parameters to consider in designing cost-effective interventions.

- *Cultural and issue appropriateness.* Even within the variety of channels that are specific to a given audience, a distinction needs to be made in selecting those that are culturally appropriate for discussing or breaking news about a specific health issue. For example, Bernhardt and others (2002) reported that African American and European American men who participated in a study on Internet-based health communication on human genetics were interested in the great potential for Internet communication but "voiced concerns about the credibility and accuracy of on-line information, lack of trust in many websites, and fear of safeguarding privacy" (p. 325). Conversely, people coping with HIV infection appear to regard the Internet as a source of empowerment that "augments social support and facilitates helping others" (Reeves, 2000, p. 47), as well as of overall coping skills (Mo and Coulson, 2012). Cultural differences influence communication, behavior, social norms, and values. For example, "there are differences in the way that people who identify with different cultures, based on both national identity and gender, manage their communicative behaviors within SNSs [social network sites]" (Sawyer, 2011, p. 3; Rosen, Stefanone, and Lackaff, 2010). Because social networking sites are increasingly used to connect with others who suffer from the same health condition, it's important to continue to observe how people use them in relation not only to a specific or social issue but also within different cultural, gender, age, and ethnic groups.

- *Cost-effectiveness.* Because cost-effectiveness is one of the key elements of health communication (see Chapter One), possible channels need to be assessed on the basis of budget parameters and priorities. Cost-effectiveness assessments should be based on a cost comparison of options that will lead to comparable results. This analysis should also include an evaluation of existing programs and resources as potential channels to expand on program reach. Cost-effectiveness assessment naturally leads to the next step of the situation analysis (existing programs, initiatives, and resources) and is one of the many reasons for researching past and ongoing programs.

Even within the same kind of communication channel (for example, interpersonal channels), it is important to consider the impact on health and social behavior that different people, speakers, or messengers may have on communicating with and engaging intended audiences. For example, studies have shown differences in the impact of parent communications versus peer communications on HIV/AIDS among high school students (Holtzman and Rubinson, 1995; Powell and Segrin, 2004). In fact, "young women were influenced more by HIV discussions with parents, while young men were influenced more by discussions with peers" (Holtzman and Rubinson, 1995, p. 235). Peer discussions were more likely to lead to multiple partners and unprotected sexual intercourse.

Once the key stakeholder analysis has been completed, further consideration should be given to the stakeholder access, level of comfort, and effectiveness with different communication channels. This analysis intersects with the assessment of key communication channels and may influence resource allocation for the development of tools, materials, or activities specific to a given channel.

The analysis of communication channels is one of the last steps of the audience profile section of the situation analysis. Of course, other group- or issue-specific factors may not be included in this book's description.

Once channels have been researched and analyzed, it is important to understand overall preferences and reactions to different communication vehicles among key groups. In health communication, the term **communication vehicles** refers to the specific means or tools that are used to deliver a message using communication channels (Health Communication Unit, 2003b). It includes communication activities, events, and materials. For example, if the communication channel is print media, such as a consumer magazine, potential vehicles include feature articles and advertorials. If the communication channel is new media, a virtual town hall is an example of a communication vehicle. Communication vehicles are audience and channel specific. All criteria that apply to the analysis of which kinds of communication channels to select also apply to communication vehicles. In health communication practice, the terms *vehicles* and *channels* are sometimes used interchangeably, which may lead to confusion. In order to avoid confusion, the term **tactics** in this book is primarily used to indicate the same category (for example, activities, materials, and events developed to serve the intervention's strategies and objectives) (see the Glossary and Chapter Thirteen).

communication vehicles
A category that includes materials, events, activities, or other tools for delivering a message using communication channels (Health Communication Unit, 2003b)

tactics
Refer to different components of a plan of action (tactical plan) that includes communication messages, activities, media, materials, and channels and is developed to serve the program's strategies and objectives

Research Existing Programs, Initiatives, and Resources

There are several reasons to research and analyze past and existing programs, initiatives, and resources:

- Lessons learned and key success factors of past and ongoing programs.
- Opportunities for partnerships, expanded program outreach, and enhanced access to key groups and stakeholders.

- Existing communication channels that may complement those used by the new program; capitalizing on existing activities and channels may reduce the new program's costs for material development and relevant outreach efforts.

- Knowledge of programs or approaches that may be in opposition to the health communication program goal and objectives; for example, if the program being developed is in support of animal research, it may be helpful to understand the rationale and key elements of health communication programs that advocate against animal research.

- Opportunities to build on existing results and other programs' achievements.

These should all be considered key components of this analysis. Key resources to collect information on past or existing programs and initiatives include the Internet, communication or public affairs or program directors of relevant organizations, health communication listservs, blogs and online forums, mass media articles, new media, peer-reviewed literature, field experts, and community leaders.

Highlight Unmet Communication Needs

This step complements and expands on the analysis of existing programs. In fact, the previous step may help identify unmet communication needs that have not been addressed by past or current programs or may help distinguish a program, and succeed in engaging key groups on other aspects of a health or social issue. However, this analysis is often integrated by information collected through interviews with key stakeholders and representatives of key groups, community dialogue, focus groups, literature review, or other research methods, which should contribute to highlighting specific communication needs and priorities for each audience.

Describe Overall Barriers to Program Implementation and Proposed Change

Health communication programs that are poised to address potential barriers to behavioral or social change or program implementation are more likely to achieve expected outcomes (Grimshaw, Eccles, Walker, and Thomas, 2002). Therefore, a description of barriers should be included in the situation analysis along with an initial vision for how to address and overcome them. This vision should be defined using the input of representatives of key audiences, stakeholders, and constituency groups, or, depending on the program characteristics and planning needs, the community at large.

Among the potential barriers are these:

- Cost, which is the actual financial cost of a potential product the program asks people to use or the human cost or sacrifices in terms of time, lifestyle, or supportive relationships needed to adopt a new behavior, policy, or practice

- Lack of adequate resources and tools to facilitate the integration of the proposed behavior into people's lifestyle

- Lack of capacity or technical competence that, for example, may help people become independent in adopting a new behavior (for example, lack of knowledge on how to perform a breast cancer self-exam) or advocating for a new policy

- Poor or inadequate local infrastructure that limits access to the recommended health behavior—for example, lack of health services or adequate transportation to reach such services in a region that is asked to become more proactive in using family planning methods or lack of hospitals that perform HIV screening within a certain geographical distance

- Lack of clear guidelines or clinical standards

- Time constraints

- Inadequate policies

- Individual, group, or community factors such as social norms, lack of communication training, existing prejudices, stigma, or language barriers

- Lack of organizational commitment to health communication and its funding

- Inadequate economic or human resources

- Other barriers that may be issue or key group specific

As an example, a study and research report to UNICEF on "Mapping & Review of Existing Guidance and Plans for Community- and Household-Based Communication to Prepare and Respond to Pandemic Flu" revealed that common issues and obstacles to pandemic flu communication planning and implementation included (among many others): "low awareness and knowledge on pandemic flu risk," "conflicting priorities," "limited knowledge on how marginalized groups may react, and/or should be reached and cared for during a pandemic," health workers shortage, "existing social norms and socio-economic conditions," "lack of communication training," influence of religious leaders, limited knowledge and mapping of high-risk groups, "irrational behaviors" and "other psychological reactions to crisis," and "limited funds and human resources" (Schiavo, 2009b, p. 10-12).

All barriers should be analyzed by reviewing key findings of the situation analysis and listing all factors and data that may point to potential issues as they relate to program execution or the achievement of expected results. There are circumstances in which existing barriers require a significant economic or human resource commitment for their removal. In these cases, it may be advisable to prioritize health communication efforts and initial resource allocations on minimizing or removing such obstacles. This will still require a behavior- and society-oriented mind-set. In fact, the focus of this initial barrier-conscious intervention would be, for instance, convincing local health authorities to improve access to health services or products; or changing existing social norms and removing prejudice within a community; or attracting additional funds and resources to the program's mission and overall goal. As part of the research and community engagement phase, key groups and stakeholders could also develop progress and outcome indicators that are obstacle driven (in other words, they seek to address and remove existing barriers to behavioral and social results).

Organizing, Sharing, and Reporting on Research Findings

Once the research phase of the situation analysis has been completed, the next step is to prioritize, share, present, and discuss findings with team members, representatives of key groups, health organizations, organizational departments, and, depending on the nature of the program, everyone who has a stake in the health communication intervention. Because not all of the data being collected are likely to be relevant to the program, the first step is to select and expand on the information that will lead to the development of communication objectives and strategies. This tends to be all information that has been confirmed as relevant by multiple sources and appears to meet key groups' needs and preferences in relation to the behavioral, social, or organizational outcomes that are sought by the program. This also represents the core briefing for the development of communication objectives and strategies.

In organizing, sharing, and presenting key findings and related conclusions, it may be helpful to divide the situation analysis in the categories described in this book for its different steps (see "A1: Situation and Audience Analysis Worksheet: Sample Questions and Topics" in Appendix A). Other logical categories should be added if they improve the overall organization and clarity of the analysis. Another practical tip is to think in terms of key issues—in other words, the facts, data, or information that are critical to the health issue and its audiences as well as to the achievement of outcome objectives.

A common practice in the private and commercial sector is the use of a SWOT (strengths, weaknesses, opportunities, and threats) analysis to organize the information about a particular product, behavior, social, or organizational change. Other authors have already suggested a much broader use of this tool in health communication planning (O'Sullivan, Yonkler, Morgan, and Merritt, 2003). SWOT analyses help in gaining a clear understanding of the situation and present it in an easy-to-digest format to share with partners and team members. Exhibit 11.2 includes a practical example of a SWOT analysis.

EXHIBIT 11.2. SWOT ANALYSIS FOR THE CARIBBEAN CERVICAL CANCER PREVENTION AND CONTROL PROJECT

Strengths	Weaknesses
1. Communication system that allows wide reach	1. Gaps in information
2. Previous initiatives to build and improve on	2. Limited resources
3. Dedicated workers	3. Limited reach and understanding of the message and material
4. Enabling environment for use of media	4. Deficiencies in academic curriculum for health workers
5. Established culture of health communication	5. Lack of control over media placement (when message will be aired)
6. Media houses with space and time dedicated for health	6. Conflicting message at all levels and in all sectors
7. Access to performing arts for health communication	7. Inadequate monitoring and evaluation
	8. Lack of a sustainable communication program
	9. Limitations of access to services promoted
	10. Inadequate social-marketing expertise

Opportunities	Threats
1. Destigmatization of cancer	1. Myths in the society
2. Ability to link with other programs	2. Gender roles and patterns
3. A fertile environment for the cervical cancer program	3. Differences in interpretation or presentation
4. Several potential partners in health CBOs, NGOs, private sector, opinion leaders, and so on	4. Multichannel media making reach more difficult and costly
5. Greater access to creative skills	5. Loss of human resources from public to private sector and overseas (brain drain)
6. Capacity for networking among countries, agencies, and programs	6. Limited buy in from health professionals

Source: Adapted from Caribbean Epidemiology Center. "Report of Communication Advisory Committee Meeting, Sub-Committee of the Technical Advisory Group." 2003. www.carec.org/documents/cccpcp/communication_advisory_report.doc. Used by permission.

The situation analysis leads to communication objectives and strategies. Still, it would be premature to develop communication objectives without first validating the initial program's goal as well as key behavioral, social, and organizational objectives, with the input of key groups, stakeholders, partners, and donors. Consider the example of the program goal of an asthma program that was originally established on the basis of preliminary data pointing to a higher disease incidence in a specific group. The overall program goal was to reduce the incidence and morbidity of asthma in that group. Yet more conclusive evidence has shown that asthma incidence in that group is actually comparable to rates for the general population. The key health issue is not asthma incidence but the disease severity and mortality because of the lack of knowledge and communication tools to help prevent and manage severe asthma attacks in that community. Observations and other feedback by community members also point to several obstacles and social factors that are preventing families from adequately managing asthma attacks and fatalities. Therefore, the final program goal should reflect the conclusions of the situation analysis and be restated as following: "Reduce the severity and mortality rates of asthma in a given group." Outcome objectives should be established to meet such a goal.

Common Research Methodologies: An Overview

Health communication practitioners and students need to be aware of key research strategies and methods in order to complete the research phase of the situation and audience analysis, as well as some other steps of the health communication process. This is equally important for cases in which more formal research is needed. As a consequence, in practice settings, the health communication team may need to interview, hire, and supervise the work of a communication research firm or engage colleagues from academia or other research organizations to provide technical input in research design and implementation.

Before moving to the definition of core methodologies, it is important to make a distinction between *market research* and *marketing research*. Although these terms are often used interchangeably, *market research* defines the process of gathering information about a market and its dynamics, and *marketing research* is a systematic approach to research that includes more than a description of market factors and dynamics and applies to much broader research needs, including audience profile and segmentation (QuickMBA, 2006). As discussed in Chapter Two, this systematic, rigorous, and analytical approach to research is one of the most important contributions marketing has made to the health communication field and heavily influences communication research.

Another important distinction is between participatory and expert-led research methods. Participatory research implies community and stakeholder engagement in the design, implementation, and analysis of research questions and related data. It requires great skills and competencies in interpersonal communication and relies on several different methods for **participatory research** (a process for collective analysis of key issues, which ultimately empowers people to establish key priorities for action as well as progress and outcome indicators of any given intervention in the health and social fields). Participatory audience research is also referred to in various planning frameworks as **community-driven assessment** or **participatory-needs assessment** or **community-needs assessment**. Community-driven assessment relies on several traditional methods of inquiry, including in-depth interviews, focus groups, photovoice, and many other methods. Community dialogue (see Chapter Four) can also be used as a method in participatory research. Within a participatory framework, research methods are used in a manner that positions audience members not as research subjects but as co-researchers engaged in a process of exploring, examining, and uncovering the detail and meaning of their own experience as it relates to health or social issues and their root causes. This is true regardless of a specific methodology. Participatory audience research is set to increase sustainability of all interventions by creating ownership as well as key groups' and stakeholders' commitment to achieving those milestones and results they have themselves established and also consider feasible.

participatory research
A collaborative research effort that involves community members, researchers, community mobilizers, and interested agencies and organizations. It is a two-way dialogue that starts with the people, and through which the community understands and identifies key issues, priorities, and potential actions.

A third important distinction is between qualitative and quantitative research. **Qualitative research** refers to research methods for data collection and analysis that are usually used within small-group settings. Qualitative data are not statistically significant, yet they add a wealth of significant information on themes, trends, and key factors that are relevant to participant groups and stakeholders. They shed light on emotions and feelings. Qualitative research is often used at the outset of the research phase to establish initial program goals and behavioral objectives, and also tends to provide in-depth details on motivations, attitudes, and behaviors. It is also frequently used to assess the format and needs for quantitative data. Qualitative research sometimes can include approximate numbers (for example, percentages) of a trend, opinion, or behavior. Yet, qualitative research's most important contribution is about revealing themes, emerging trends, and contributing factors the researcher may not have anticipated or considered important. Finally, qualitative research deals with understanding the worldview of the research system in which we operate through understanding other people's experiences. It is a very important method in health communication research because health communication influences and is influenced by several sociopolitical systems.

qualitative research
Research methods and approaches that are used to collect data in relatively small groups

Quantitative research refers to research methods and data that are statistically significant and are usually collected from large samples. Regardless of its focus (for example, health behaviors, media habits of intended audiences, frequency of physician-patient encounters on a health issue, or level of awareness about a medical condition), the aim of quantitative research is to provide the health communication team with exact numbers about different kinds of audience- or environment-related factors.

quantitative research
Research methods and data that are statistically significant and are usually collected from large samples

Many health communication programs rely solely on well-planned and well-executed qualitative research, but there are cases in which it is necessary to collect statistically significant data (for example, when statistically significant data are needed to convince key stakeholders of the relevance of a specific health issue and the significance of the health communication intervention). Conversely, programs that rely only on quantitative data may miss on important audience- or issue-related nuances and factors influencing a specific health and social issue. Table 11.1 lists some of the key characteristics of qualitative versus quantitative research, which further illustrate how these two kinds of research are complementary. In fact, qualitative and quantitative methods can clarify important aspects of a health or social issue and behavior. Therefore, the use of mixed methods as part of different research phases of health communication programming should be always encouraged.

Table 11.1   Qualitative Versus Quantitative Research Methods

Qualitative	Quantitative
Provides depth of understanding	Measures level of occurrence
Asks "why?"	Asks "how many?" and "how often?"
Studies motivations	Studies actions
Is subjective; probes individual reactions to discover underlying motivations	Is objective; asks questions without revealing a point of view
Enables discovery	Provides proof
Is exploratory	Is definitive
Allows insights into behavior and trends	Measures levels of actions and trends
Interprets	Describes

Source: From *Methodological Review: A Handbook for Excellence in Focus Group Research* by M. Debus. Copyright 1988 by The Academy for Educational Development, Washington, DC. Reprinted with permission.

This section provides a brief overview of key communication research methodologies for qualitative and quantitative research, as well as practical advice on how to select and use them. It also examines key principles in identifying and selecting a suitable communication research partner (whether a university, a research firm, or other research organization) to provide technical assistance with the research process in case this is needed (for example, in practice-related settings where different organizations may not have research capabilities or staff). Because a comprehensive discussion of different research methods is outside the scope of this book, this section provides only a brief overview of select methods. Formal instruction on research and evaluation methods is part of most graduate programs in public health, global health, health communication, communication sciences, medicine, nursing, social work, and many other relevant programs. Emerging and well-established health communication professionals should also strive to access resources and training on research and evaluation methods.

All methodologies described here apply at least to a certain extent to all research phases of the health communication process (Freimuth, Cole, and Kirby, 2000):

pretesting
An essential phase of formative research that uses several research methods to assess whether communication concepts, messages, media, and materials meet the needs of intended audiences, are culturally appropriate, and are easily understood

- *Formative research*, which consists of all research efforts that precede program design and implementation: the research conducted for the situation analysis and audience profile in order to assess the health communication environment and the key needs, preferences, and characteristics of all key groups and stakeholders, and the **pretesting** of messages, materials, media, and activities with intended audiences (discussed in further detail in Chapter Thirteen). A pretest is an analysis of people's reactions that takes place prior to the dissemination and implementation of messages, materials, and activities or the selection of specific media as main communication channels.

- *Process-related research*, which aims at assessing and monitoring the implementation phase of a health communication program. This process often relies on marketing research methodologies and means of contacts, such as stakeholder interviews and surveys, to secure audience feedback and input on program elements and their execution. Yet, community dialogue and **panel studies** (the same representatives of key groups or stakeholders are asked to provide input or observed over time) are also valuable methods to take the pulse of how a program is doing.

- *Summative research*, which refers to the research conducted as part of the evaluation phase of the program to assess the effectiveness of the program's strategies, the overall program reach, and its impact on the program's goals and key behavioral, social, or organizational objectives. This phase is also called *outcome* or *impact research* or *evaluation*.

panel studies
A research method that consists of creating a panel of representatives of key groups or stakeholders, and then contacting them at various and regular times during the research and program evaluation phases (for example, every six months or every year)

Depending on the nature of the health communication program, all research phases may be completed by the health communication team and their research partners or by the community itself with the guidance and technical assistance of outside research professionals and facilitators. As previously mentioned, the latter option is at the core of participatory research, which involves and gives authority to key groups and stakeholders for the design, implementation, and analysis of research efforts. Although the degree of participation of key audiences in research design and implementation may vary, this book advocates for the inclusion of at least key stakeholders and representatives of key groups in the process of sharing information, as well as providing feedback and analyzing research findings. Similarly, key communities and stakeholders should also be involved in all other research phases. Finally, summative research (outcome evaluation) should always engage outside experts and organizations that are different from those that participated in program design and implementation, so they can work collaboratively with key stakeholders and preserve the objectivity of evaluation findings.

Secondary Data

Secondary data are all information that has been collected, published, or reported by others in different formats (for example, unpublished reports, existing presentations, posters, websites, mass media articles, public health reports, guidelines, peer-reviewed articles) and in relation to different programs. The individuals or groups who analyze and use the data are not involved with the initial design and implementation of the research.

Potential examples of secondary data that may be relevant to a specific health communication program include information about key audiences' demographics and cultural beliefs, religious beliefs, and social norms, other countries' or programs' experiences in relation to the same health issue, and data from surveys or focus groups related to similar topics, groups, or health behaviors (to name a few examples).

Several authors (Saunders, Lewis, and Thornhill, 2003; Andreasen, 1995) have already highlighted many of the limitations that apply to the use of secondary data. However, all of them also agree on the value of secondary data at least in the initial research phase. Among the limitations are the following:

- Secondary data are gathered for different projects and purposes and may be incomplete in exploring topics critical to the health communication program.

- The credibility of secondary data varies and should be carefully assessed (for example, in relation to the credibility and reputation of specific websites and other online or new media–based resources).

- Secondary data may be difficult to interpret in the absence of the original research design or protocol.

- Secondary data can be outdated.

- Secondary data might include questions important to your study, but ask them to the wrong group of people (Vartanian, 2011).

"In many ways, users of secondary data trade control over the conditions and quality of data collection for accessibility, convenience, and reduced costs in time, money, and inconvenience to participants" (Vartanian, 2011, pp. 16–17).

Nevertheless, secondary data are important in the exploratory research phase to help gather critical background knowledge on the health issue and its audiences and to identify key questions that need to be further explored via a variety of research methods. Sometimes secondary data are current and relevant to a given health communication program. At all times, they need to be supplemented by some new research. For example, it is advisable to gather additional information at least through one-on-one interviews with key stakeholders and representatives of key groups. Secondary data will provide a valuable framework to develop key questions and engage key stakeholders and groups during the interview or community dialogue process.

The following sections look briefly at several sources and methods to research secondary data.

Literature, Case Studies, and Document Review

A review of existing literature, case studies, and relevant documents (for example, the national communication plan for public health emergencies in a given country, guidelines on patient-provider communication issued by a prominent professional association, reports on community dialogue sessions) can include peer-reviewed journals, press clips, broadcast segments, trade journals, unpublished reports, PowerPoint presentations, annual reports, and other types of publications by local and international health organizations, among others.

University and public libraries are good places to start a search. They also provide access to databases and online journals that may save time and facilitate the research process. However, health organizations now have the internal capability to conduct these searches from their offices.

In most countries where computer and Internet use are widespread, searches for existing literature or other secondary data can take place over the Internet (within some of the limitations described in Chapter Two relating to access and quality of Internet services in several developing countries). In most parts of the world, the number of online publications and virtual libraries has rapidly increased and includes countless peer-reviewed journals, magazines, newspapers, newsletters, and other kinds of publications.

The Internet also eases access to PowerPoint presentations, health organizations' annual reports, program descriptions, meetings proceedings, clinical guidelines, and a wealth of additional information. There are a huge number of available databases and search engines.

Search engines catalogue information from the public, private, news media, and academic sectors. Most people try more than one search engine or database when researching a specific kind of information. In the United States, Google, Yahoo!, and Bing are three of the most popular search engines (Search Engine Land, 2011).

Relevant databases for health communication research include Medline, the online database of the US National Library of Medicine; Ingenta-Connect, a large online resource of scholarly publications; and many other searchable archives and commercial databases of US and international magazines, newspapers, business, and legal documents to which users can subscribe or access using a public library system.

Users who are searching the Internet for data compilation and analysis must use objective criteria to evaluate information credibility. The information source (the author or organization, for example) is one of the key parameters to assess credibility (Montecino, 1998; Jitaru, Moisil, and Jitaru, 1999). "Yet, anonymous and multiple authors make the concept of 'source' difficult to understand or authenticate and, as such, users know little about the expertise, qualifications, and potential biases that may be infused into the information they obtain from these types of resources (Fritch and Cromwell, 2001; Sundar, 2008). Recently, the credibility of *Wikipedia* information has been debated due precisely to these problems, and opinions vary about the degree to which information found in such environments can be trusted (*BBC News*, 2007)" (Metzger, Flanagin, and Medders, 2010, p. 415).

Within these limitations, the ability to discern among different sources for health information is one of the key components of media literacy, and therefore source credibility continues to be an important parameter to assess information quality. Questions to consider include (University of British Columbia, 2012), is an author clearly identified? Does the author have necessary credentials (such as a university or organization affiliation) to write on the specific topic? Is the author's contact information stated? In case of health-related information, was the information reviewed by a medical expert, if not written by a health care professional (FamilyDoctor.org, 2010)? Is the author published in reputable journals and outlets or does he or she have a substantial number of publications? Does he or she have practical experience on the subject? Do other organizations or stakeholders recognize the credibility and authority of the organization that endorsed or publicized specific health data or information? Did the author or organization have any personal or group interest to support a given viewpoint? If the website appears to contain opinions and not facts, are they from a qualified person or organization (FamilyDoctor.org, 2010)? These are only some of the key questions that should be asked about the information source.

Other key criteria for the evaluation of online information include the editorial review process (Does the editorial board include recognized experts in the field?) and currency (Does the information reflect current data and trends?). How often does the information appear to be updated (FamilyDoctor.org, 2010)? Finally, websites that clearly disclose the author's or organization's intent or mission are likely to be more credible.

Websites of professional organizations, patient groups, government agencies, universities, and other groups may be also valuable sources for information on existing health communications programs or other

Table 11.2 Sample Criteria for a Credibility Assessment of Health-Related Websites

Source (Does it disclose source, authorship, and authority in a specific health field?)

Currency of relevant information (For example, what is the frequency and quality of updates, date of original information, posting date, accurate representation of different facts and opinions on a current issue?)

Evidence ranking (For example, is the information more prominently displayed on the site also supported by the largest number of studies or by studies conducted in a large percentage of a given population?)

Relevance (Does the information correspond to the aims advertised for the site?)

Review process (Is the information peer reviewed by an editorial board or scientific committee? Does the website include tools for audience feedback and rating of all information? Does the site have a seal of approval or accreditation from relevant organization or accrediting body?)

Accuracy (Is the information accurate and adequately referenced?)

Use of disclaimers and conflict disclosures (For example, is there information on grants, sponsorships, copyrights, as well as disclaimers suggesting that the site provides information and cannot replace medical or other professional advice?)

References: Kim, et al., 1999; Kunst, et al., 2002; Schiavo, 2008; Dalhousie University, 2011.

initiatives, case studies, potential partners, and best clinical practices, to name a few topics. They may also be helpful in identifying key stakeholders in a specific health field, who usually tend to be part of advisory boards or are mentioned frequently on reputable websites. The same criteria that apply to assessing the credibility of other online information are also relevant to websites and should be used to evaluate them. Table 11.2 includes sample criteria for the evaluation of health-related websites.

One-on-One Contacts and Interviews

In regions where the use of online libraries and information is less widespread (for example, in some developing countries because of poor Internet access, quality and speed of Internet connections, or high costs (World Health Organization [WHO], 2007), gathering secondary data may be challenging. A good way to start is by contacting university researchers, local public health departments, nonprofit organizations, government officers, corporations, and all other stakeholders who can point to the existence of previous reports, documents, and data, and perhaps share them together with their own professional experience. Although this approach is extremely valuable in situations in which Internet research is less of an easy option, contact with those in the field should be sought in all cases to confirm the validity of secondary research findings, supplement other data and professional experiences, and make sure that potential or actual stakeholders can have an opportunity to contribute to analyzing them.

Primary Data

Primary data include all information gathered specifically to address the research needs of a given health communication program. Such data are collected directly by the enlarged health communication team or its research partners by direct observation of specific facts and behaviors, or using systematic research approaches as described so far in this chapter. Primary research can be quantitative or qualitative or use mixed methods.

Because they are collected specifically for the purpose of informing and shaping program decisions, primary data are the most valuable resource in program planning. In the case of participatory research, which this book supports, members of key audiences or the community at large are also involved in most steps of research design, implementation, and analysis.

Overview of Qualitative Versus Quantitative Research Methods

Primary research relies on direct communication methodologies, which include all means of contact researchers use to gather data by communicating directly with research subjects "either in person, through others, or through a document such as a questionnaire" (Joppe, 2006).

The following techniques are common in qualitative research:

- *One-on-one in-depth interviews.* These can be telephone or in-person interviews with internal and external stakeholders, members of key audiences, or representatives of relevant health organizations. Whenever possible, it is preferable to conduct in-depth interviews in person.

- *Focus groups.* One of the most common research methodologies, a focus group consists of a small-group discussion. Participants are usually representatives of key groups that have a potential stake in the communication intervention (for example, mother of children under two years of age, African American men who are over forty-five years old, or emergency room physicians who work in metropolitan areas).

- *Case study analysis.* This method yields a detailed description and analysis of experiences and programs that are related to a given health communication program. It goes a step further than finding and reviewing a case study. It relies on a combination of in-depth interviews with representatives of the organization in which the experience, or "case," took place, with an analysis of secondary data, such as existing literature, press reports, evaluation findings, and unpublished data (if available).

- *Photovoice.* A research method used in public health, community development, and several other fields that combines photography, storytelling, and community action. Participants in photovoice projects are asked to take pictures that represent their specific opinions on a health or social issue and then discuss them by developing stories and other kinds of narratives, as well as reaching out to communities and peers. This methodology is particularly suited for low literacy and low health literacy groups. See Chapter Sixteen for a case study that discusses photovoice.

- *Panel studies.* This research method consists of creating a panel of representatives of key groups or stakeholders, and then contacting them at various and regular times during the research and program evaluation phases (for example, every six months or every year). Limitations of this approach include potential bias of research data because panelists are exposed to different phases of program design and implementation and become acquainted with information that may influence their answers and that the groups they represent may not know. Yet, this needs to be evaluated on a case-by-case basis.

Quantitative research relies primarily on survey-based studies that involve a large percentage of key groups or the general population, which can be conducted by telephone, online, distributed by mail, or at meetings or other venues. Many surveys tend to be self-administered by respondents. Following is a closer look at basic considerations and parameters in using qualitative and quantitative research methods.

One-on-One In-Depth Interviews

Stakeholder interviews, the most common form of in-depth interview, as well as other kinds of one-on-one encounters, require specific skills, advance preparation, and the ability to create rapport with the individuals being interviewed. It is always a good idea to precede the interview with a preliminary conversation, e-mail, or other form of communication that addresses the overall focus and purpose of the interview. Advance preparation should also include a list of key questions and a review of some background information on the organization, community, or group that the interviewee may represent. In today's competitive and busy work environment, wasting anyone's time for lack of preparation is not a good way to encourage their interest in helping with a specific health issue.

Often one-on-one interviews may become the forum to discuss the potential for partnerships or other topics that may digress from the initial focus but are still relevant to the specific health communication program. In general, in-person interviews are preferable to telephone interviews. However, telephone interviews are very common and help break down barriers related to lack of time or geographical distance. Also, Skype.com (which uses a videoconference system with webcam to connect people from computer to computer) has emerged as an additional tool for in-depth interviews and, more in general, for qualitative research. In a way, having multiple options also allows researchers to accommodate specific media preferences of the people being interviewed and make it convenient for them. Regardless of the media setting being used, the average in-depth interview lasts 30 to 120 minutes.

Some general criteria apply to the process of interviewing and may help establish a rapport with the person being interviewed. Although these criteria are particularly important in the case of one-on-one interviews, they generally apply to other research methods, such as focus groups and telephone surveys.

For example, it is important to ask general and nonintrusive questions first. Breaking the ice by making a joke or telling something about oneself helps create feelings of comfort among people being interviewed. Confrontational questions (for example, about an article the interviewer read that supports opposite views about the work of the interviewee) should always be asked toward the end of the interview. By then, the interviewee trusts the interviewer and may feel more comfortable addressing controversial topics. Also, whenever possible, it is a good idea to repeat and summarize some of the key points raised by the interviewee. This may help correct potential misunderstandings as well as organize the information once the interview has been completed. Following are other practical tips that can help the interview proceed smoothly:

- List the questions in a logical order.
- Use simple language and avoid technical words.
- Start with questions that may allow you to understand the background and interests of the person being interviewed as it relates to the specific health or social issue.
- Divide a complex question into multiple questions.

- Avoid leading questions, such as questions requiring a yes or no answer.

- Follow leads that emerge from some of the answers and ask if it would be all right to explore a specific point in more detail.

- Do not ask about statistics and other data that can be otherwise found in existing literature.

- Use the interview's time strategically to gain new insights and perspectives on a specific issue.

All interviewers, regardless of whether they are involved in one-on-one interviews, focus groups, or telephone surveys, should be trained and become familiar with all questions and potential follow-up inquiries in advance of the actual research implementation. As with all other qualitative methodologies, the use of summaries, including key points that emerge from the in-depth interviews; self-memos, which allow you to record ideas that may emerge as you think about the information you just discussed or next steps and tasks to complete; and research diaries, in which you take note of the overall research process, is helpful in facilitating recording and analysis of qualitative data.

Focus Groups

Focus groups are facilitated group discussions. They are not group interviews because the group dynamics influence the way participants interact with each other and decide (or not) to participate in the discussion. In the case of focus groups, the facilitator and interviewer, who is usually called a moderator, needs to be aware of group dynamics in order to make sure that all participants feel comfortable and encouraged to contribute to the discussion.

Focus groups are one of the most common means of contact in communication research. They are used to gather data for the situation analysis and audience profile; test the words and questions of a survey's questionnaire; secure the audience's feedback on the message and graphic concepts of communication materials and activities; and understand key groups' reaction to a specific health product, service, or behavior, and assess program results, to name a few applications. They may reveal unexpected details about audience preferences, beliefs, and main concerns.

For example, a focus group study on the use of insecticide-treated nets for malaria protection in Angola revealed that users would prefer nets to be in bright colors (yellow, orange, and pink) instead of white because of concerns with white nets, which can become visibly dirty shortly after installation (Schiavo, 1998, 2000). In another example, focus groups that were conducted as part of the assessment of a national program for infant mortality prevention validated quantitative findings and contributed to the identification of several key themes to be addressed by future interventions, such as, for example, the significance of community involvement, the importance of an expanded role for health care providers and men in preconception health and care, and the contribution of stress—as it relates to social discrimination—to infant mortality rates (Schiavo, Gonzales-Flores, Ramesh, and Estrada-Portales, 2011).

As with other research methods, focus groups are regulated by several codes of ethics (Office for Human Research Protections, 2006; National Institutes of Health, 2006) to protect participants in the research and make sure that they are fully informed about the research methodology and objectives. Although focus group participants usually receive and sign a consent form, which should include a description of the research's purpose and methodology, the meeting should begin by reviewing this information. The focus group moderator should do the following:

- Facilitate introductions and provide the rules for interactions within the group.
- Avoid asking leading or questions requiring only yes or no answers. Questions should be open-ended.
- Have a clear understanding of the research goals and the kind of information that is essential to discuss.
- Monitor topics to make sure the discussion stays focused on the research topic, but at the same time, builds on leads for questions on additional issues of relevance.
- Show respect for all participants and their opinions.
- Make sure everyone understands there is no right or wrong answer (National Cancer Institute at the National Institutes of Health, 2002).
- Shield shy participants from more verbal or aggressive panelists (Hester, 1996).
- Make sure everyone has an opportunity to express his or her opinion.

In participatory research, a community member may act as the moderator of the focus group. He or she may be a representative of a local organization, a member of the intended audience, or a local government officer, for example. In this case, a health communication research professional will likely be present at the focus group and only provide technical assistance. The research professional may be also responsible to train the community member for the moderator role well in advance of the focus group. A troubleshooting session to identify potential pitfalls and difficult situations that may arise during the focus group, as well as how to address them, should be included in the training.

Surveys

Surveys are a common technique used in collecting quantitative data. There are two primary types of surveys: telephone and self-administered. Among self-administered surveys, computerized and online surveys are gaining prominence in Western countries, given the proliferation of online survey software and research tools such as SurveyMonkey.com. Some authors (Joppe, 2006; National Cancer Institute at the National Institutes of Health, 2002) also mention in-person surveys, but these are used more sparingly because of their high cost, with the exception of household surveys, which continue to be relatively common especially for large studies.

Household surveys are a kind of in-person survey that have been used for a while by the United Nations, governments, and public health departments in many countries to collect data from all members of a household. They have been used in India since the 1940s (Lay, 2013). Household surveys are usually administered by trained staff who go from house to house with the aid of a computer laptop for notes and data input. They have been used for census data and several other topics, and they are a valuable survey method to reach out to underserved, marginalized, isolated, and other hard-to-reach populations.

Well-designed and implemented surveys are an excellent and accurate method to acquire information about a given population. Also, surveys rely on standard questionnaires that in some cases can be applied to different subgroups of the same population. This allows researchers to compare attitudes, behaviors, beliefs, social norms, and other information of one group to another. Moreover, using standard questionnaires ensures higher reliability and accuracy of the information being collected because the findings are not influenced by differences in interviewers' styles or other subjective parameters that can influence qualitative research findings.

The survey sample needs to be clearly defined early in the survey design phase. This needs to be representative (in terms of percentage) of the intended population (for example, parents of six- to eleven-year-old children, women under thirty-five years of age). If different racial and ethnic groups are included, as they should be, it may be worth defining in advance the percentage of the total sample each group should represent. In the case of a health issue that is quite widespread in the general population, for example, the epidemic of childhood obesity in the United States (Kaur, Hyder, and Poston, 2003) but is more prevalent among some at-risk groups, it makes sense to oversample these specific key groups or run a specific survey just for them.

Self-administered surveys require respondents to complete the questionnaire by themselves and in their own time, without any interaction with an actual interviewer. Self-administered questionnaires are usually distributed at professional meetings, by direct mail, posted online on relevant websites, or e-mailed as a weblink. In general, the response rate of self-administered surveys tends to be lower than that of telephone surveys (Wiggins and Deeb-Sossa, 2000; Wallace Foundation, 2013). For example, even with telephone reminder calls, mail surveys have a lower response rate than telephone surveys (Ngo-Metzger and others, 2004). Although some of these facts always change with the rise of caller ID, cellular phones, and other technological advances, telephone surveys are still one of the best methods for quantitative research.

Other elements contribute to response rates for both self-administered and telephone surveys. These include the clarity, length, and organization of the survey, the relevance of the topic it addresses, and other audience-related factors. For example, if the survey targets working parents of children younger than ten years of age, the time at which a telephone survey is administered may affect the response rate (Dillman, Sinclair, and Clark, 1993; Bogen, 2006). Weekends may be the best time to reach these parents because in the morning they are at work and in the evenings are probably busy with the children, dinner, and household chores.

Telephone surveys are commonly used and offer the advantage of quick methods for sample randomization. Random sampling facilitates "the extrapolation of characteristics from the sample to the population as a whole" (Joppe, 2006). One of the most common randomization methods is random digit dialing: all numbers are selected randomly on the basis of the last four digits or first three numbers of a telephone prefix, which are chosen by the interviewers.

Online surveys are usually administered via online survey software and programs (for example, SurveyMonkey.com), which also include data processing and analysis tools. Average response rate varies and depends on the nature and topic of the survey as well as methods for survey delivery (embedded in an existing website or e-newsletter or distributed via e-mail), intended population characteristics, ease of use, survey's sponsor, and other factors (Vovici, 2010).

Finally, survey questionnaires need to be developed by keeping in mind the limited time participants may have to reply to all questions, as well as literacy and health literacy levels and the importance of language clarity and simplicity. In addition to initial demographic questions (to confirm the respondent's age, sex, and other key information), the survey questionnaire can include different types of questions such as yes and no questions, scale questions (for example, "On a scale from 1 to 5, how do you rate this specific health service?"), and multiple-choice questions. Also of great importance within large surveys is to include a few open-ended questions, which may add insights and provide further explanations into the why of statistically significant data (Schiavo, Gonzalez-Flores, Ramesh, and Estrada-Portales, 2011). A comment box is one method but sometimes may not be enough. Open-ended questions should be designed carefully to encourage respondents to use a bullet-point format in their answers and to make a maximum of two to three points.

Working with Research Organizations and Professionals: Tips for Health Communication Practitioners

Health communication professionals who work in academia and other research organizations are also highly skilled researchers and very knowledgeable about research and evaluation methods as well as their theories. In practice settings, the health communication team sometimes does not have the expertise, time, or human resources to conduct formal research. In this situation, selecting a communication research firm or consultant may be the best option. Reaching out to colleagues from academia or nonprofit research organizations for a potential partnership is also another way to expand on core competencies of the health communication team.

In selecting a research partner, you should start by providing a detailed briefing. If you are planning to use a communication research or marketing firm, you should send the briefing to multiple companies and invite them to respond with recommendations and an estimated budget on the basis of this key information. This briefing can be delivered in person at an initial meeting or in writing. If instead, you would like to partner with colleagues in academia the briefing is more of a framework for an informal discussion and to assess whether this is indeed a good fit in terms of meeting mutual interests. In this latter case, it is likely that the budget will be developed and itemized in the grant-writing phase by all involved.

Written briefings are better to ensure that all potential research partners who have an interest in the project have access to the same information and are clear about the project's specifications and needs. Regardless of its format, the briefing should ideally include these components:

- A brief description of the health issue

- Overall program goals

- Key research and information needs

- The research sample being envisioned

- Key groups and stakeholders who will participate in research design and implementation (for participatory research)

- Preferred research methods

- Total available budget

- All other program- or audience-related information that may be relevant to research efforts

- What is expected from the research consultant, partner, or firm

The last point is extremely important in establishing the right relationship from the start. A communication research firm or consultant can be hired for different purposes, which may include helping with the research design, the actual research implementation and fieldwork, data analysis and reporting, or technical assistance throughout the process. For example, in the case of community-led participatory research, chances are that the research organization or consultant would help facilitate the overall process and provide technical assistance. Other times, they will conduct the entire research study or participate only in data analysis. Similar issues arise if you decide to engage research partners outside of the commercial sector.

Key parameters in selecting research partners are reputation (it is important to ask for references), previous experience in health communication research (which should be an ideal prerequisite) or the specific health issue, compliance with current codes of ethics and research parameters, affordability, dedicated staff (in case of large projects), professionalism, and others that vary from case to case. Yet, regardless of the kind of research partner selected, the health communication team should stay close to the overall research process, actively participating in all or most of its phases, and make sure key groups and stakeholders stay engaged as key participants.

Of great importance is to make sure that all primary research phases that involve the participation of human subjects are reviewed and approved by an **institutional review board (IRB)** (a group of research experts who are faculty members of an academic institution or research hospital or are part of an independent IRB) in light of the need to protect research participants. Important aspects to be reviewed by the IRB include the way you inform participants about the purpose as well as potential benefits and risks of your research, their ability to give their informed consent to participate on the basis of the information you provide, and other ethical considerations and

institutional review board (IRB)
A group of research experts who are faculty members of an academic institution or research hospital or are part of an independent IRB. IRBs review research protocols and methods to ensure protection of human subjects.

issues of privacy and confidentiality of personal information. Most universities have their own IRB training and testing process to make sure researchers and students comply with the university's ethical standards. Yet, the Collaborative Institutional Training Initiative (CITI—www.citiprogram.org) is a widely used subscription service that provides research ethics education and testing to any member of the research community who is affiliated with a CITI-participating organization.

Key Concepts

- The situation analysis is a fundamental step in program planning and should be the foundation of health communication programs. In fact, health communication is a research-based field.

- In this book, *situation analysis* is used as a planning term. It describes the analysis of all individual, community, social, political, and behavior-related factors that can affect attitudes, behaviors, social norms, and policies about a health or social issue and its potential solutions. The situation analysis has a number of steps, which are described in this chapter.

- Some authors distinguish the situation analysis from the audience analysis and consider them as two separate steps. In this book, the audience profile is described as one of the key sections of the situation analysis. This also reflects actual health communication practice as well as the need for engaging key groups and stakeholders in all different phases of communication planning in assessing the health issue as well as individual, community, social, and political factors that may contribute to it.

- Audience segmentation in groups with similar characteristics and behavioral stages is required for most programs. This is a process that requires the engagement of key groups and stakeholders and may influence communication priorities and resource allocation.

- There are several communication and marketing research methodologies. This chapter highlights the difference between market research and marketing research, participatory versus expert-led research, qualitative versus quantitative research, secondary and primary data as well as frequently used research methods (one-on-one in-depth interviews, focus groups, and surveys). Practical suggestions on how to use common research methodologies or to select research partners (for those organizations and professionals that focus on health communication practice and do not have significant research capability) are also included.

- This book advocates for a participatory approach to issue- and audience-related research, in which key groups and stakeholders are involved in all phases of research design, implementation, and evaluation, and also participate in defining suitable progress and outcome indicators for all communication efforts.

FOR DISCUSSION AND PRACTICE

1. Using again the fictional example of Luciana, the nineteen-year-old Italian woman who spends a lot of time at the beach and is unaware of the risk for skin cancer (see Box 2.1), list and discuss questions that need to be addressed as part of the situation and audience analysis of a program intended to engage her and her peer group. The worksheet in Appendix A (see "A1: Situation and Audience Analysis Worksheet: Sample Questions and Topics") provides additional guidance.

2. Provide situations in which you would use qualitative research methods versus quantitative methods. List all factors that may influence your decision to use a specific research method. Discuss what, in your opinion, could be key benefits of mixed methods.

3. Review key concepts in this chapter and discuss what, in your opinion, links the situation analysis to the other steps of health communication planning.

4. Research a health issue of your choice and conduct three to four in-depth interviews with key stakeholders or representatives of organizations who work in the field. Present key findings and lessons learned on existing communication programs and experiences.

KEY TERMS

audience profile

communication vehicles

community-driven assessment

community-needs assessment

community-specific channels

institutional review board (IRB)

interpersonal channels

mass media channels

new media channels

panel studies

participatory-needs assessment

participatory research

pretesting

professional channels

qualitative research

quantitative research

tactics

CHAPTER 12

IDENTIFYING COMMUNICATION OBJECTIVES AND STRATEGIES

The communication objective of a health communication program by Radio Salankoloto, a local radio station in Burkina Faso, Africa, is to tackle HIV/AIDS by increasing knowledge and understanding of HIV/AIDS preventive measures (Fisher, 2003). In the United States, one of the key objectives of the communication component of *Healthy People 2020*, the US public health agenda, is to improve the health literacy of the population (US Department of Health and Human Services, 2012b).

In both cases, the objectives support the overall goal of the health communication program or public health intervention as well as the behavioral and social objectives that the two programs try to achieve. In the case of HIV/AIDS in Burkina Faso, the overall goal of the health communication intervention is to help reduce the increasing incidence of HIV/AIDS in that country (Fisher, 2003) by prompting people to use preventive measures (behavioral objective). In the case of *Healthy People 2020*, improving health literacy is considered instrumental to "longer life, improved quality of life, and reduction of chronic diseases and health disparities" (National Institutes of Health, 2005), which are all key goals of the US public health agenda. In order to achieve these goals, people need to be able to act on health information (behavioral objective) of which health literacy is a fundamental premise.

Several strategies have been developed or suggested by Radio Salankoloto and *Healthy People 2020* in support of communication objectives and have highlighted not only the focus of the intervention but also the strategic use of communication approaches and tools to reach such objectives. In Burkina Faso, Radio Salankoloto uses popular forms of expression (radio drama) to reach its program's objectives and help people identify with the story. *Healthy People 2020* identified several health literacy–related areas for improvement, especially within the provider-patient setting (US Department of Health and Human Services, 2012b).

CHAPTER OBJECTIVES

This chapter focuses on defining communication objectives and strategies and highlighting the connection of these two important steps to other phases of the planning process that precede or follow them. By providing a practical guide on the dos and don'ts of establishing communication objectives and strategies, this chapter helps build knowledge of the technical skills that are needed to complete this step of health communication planning.

How to Develop and Validate Communication Objectives

communication objectives
The intermediate steps that need to be achieved in order to meet the overall program goals as complemented by specific behavioral, social, and organizational objectives

Communication objectives are the intermediate steps (National Cancer Institute at the National Institutes of Health, 2002) that need to be attained in order to meet the overall program goals as complemented by specific behavioral, social, and organizational objectives. Often communication objectives are expressed as follows:

"To raise awareness"

"To increase knowledge"

"To break the cycle of misinformation"

"To change attitudes"

"To facilitate interactions"

"To help build expertise or skills"

The outcomes highlighted by communication objectives all refer to the different components of the process of change that communication can affect. In fact, communication objectives are often about changes in knowledge, attitudes, beliefs, motivation, and human interactions (Colle and Roman, 2003), which are all intermediate and critical steps in the achievement of behavioral, social, or organizational objectives and, ultimately, the overall program's goal. Such changes can take place at the individual, group, organizational, or societal level as the result of communication interventions with well-defined objectives. In most cases, communication objectives address intermediate steps that lead to behavioral outcomes. For example, in the case of breast cancer prevention, some communication objectives could be "to raise awareness among Latino women over age forty of the need for annual mammograms" or "to facilitate supportive provider-patient interactions on breast cancer–related questions." Both objectives support the behavioral (outcome) objective that aims at prompting women to have annual mammograms.

Sometimes communication objectives are written to emphasize the role of a specific group in making the change. For example, the first of the two objectives on breast cancer screening can be stated as follows: "Latino women over forty years of age will report to be aware of the need for annual mammograms."

Whenever possible, communication objectives should include specific measurable parameters that can be used in the program evaluation phase to assess the success (or lack of) of the communication strategy in support of such objectives. Many authors agree that communication objectives should describe "who will do or change what by when and by how much" (Weinreich, 2011, p. 80). As previously mentioned, this rule also applies to outcome objectives such as behavioral, social, and organizational objectives.

Under this rule the possible communication objectives of breast cancer screening can be restated:

- "To raise awareness by the year 2010 of the need for annual mammograms among X percent of Latino women over forty years of age who live in a specific neighborhoods" (or, for broader programs, in the United States).

- "To facilitate by the year 2012 supportive provider-patient communications on breast cancer as reported by X percent of health care providers in fifteen selected medical practices in the target neighborhood." The word *supportive* is intended as reported by women in referring to their interaction with their health care provider(s).

In practice, especially in the private sector, including commercial and nonprofit organizations, communication objectives rarely specify quantitative measurements (for example, by "how much" and "when"). Sometimes they may include an approximate estimate of how long it may take to achieve them. This overall tendency is motivated by perceived difficulties and limitations of measurement, which also require the allocation of adequate funds.

In many corporations and nonprofit organizations, communication departments simply do not get funded to perform measurement. The culture of too many health organizations supports the idea of measurement but often does not justify or provide a means of paying for it. Other parameters, primarily process oriented, activity specific, or financial, are used to assess the success of a program. When changes in knowledge, beliefs, attitudes, or health and social behavior are measured, it is usually on a qualitative basis, by stakeholder interviews that are conducted before and after the intervention. In academic settings, by contrast, measurement of the quantitative parameters used to define outcome and communication objectives tends to be a standard practice for research-based efforts and other kinds of interventions in health communication.

Although it is true that all quantitative measurements of outcome and communication objectives require in-depth pre- and postintervention analyses in concentrated geographical areas and time periods (see Chapter Fourteen), setting measurable objectives is still an excellent practice for health communication. Measurable objectives are important for program evaluation (after all, communication objectives are the intermediate milestones of the program); creating agreement among team members, partners, and other key stakeholders on success factors and parameters; and helping focus the extended health communication team on what communication can do and by when. However, health communicators, partners, donors, and key stakeholders should always take into account that measurement in health communication faces several limitations, which are discussed in detail in Chapters Thirteen and Fourteen and relate to many of the points introduced in this section.

As for outcome objectives (behavioral, social, and organizational), SMART is a suitable model also to develop measurable communication objectives. Exhibit 12.1 shows the sample communication objectives that relate to a specific program goal as well as to a specific behavioral objective. Of note, changes in individual or social behavior and norms are more difficult to achieve than changes in knowledge, attitudes, or skills. Therefore, it is always more likely that in a given time frame outcome objectives will be attained within a smaller percentage of intended audiences when compared to changes in knowledge, attitudes, or skills that are defined by communication objectives.

EXHIBIT 12.1. SAMPLE COMMUNICATION OBJECTIVES: UNDERSTANDING
THE CONNECTION WITH OTHER PROGRAM ELEMENTS

Overall Program Goal: Reduce the incidence and mortality of adult melanoma cases associated with early and excessive sun exposure during childhood (by the year 2020)

Behavioral objective: By the year 2016, 10 percent of US parents who live in Florida will
use sunscreen, sun hats, and other preventive measures to protect their children from the
damaging effects of prolonged and excessive sun exposure.

Communication objectives (if all relevant to the specific stages of key group's beliefs,
attitudes, skills, and behaviors, they should be implemented in different program phases
because they are in excess of the recommended limit of two to three objectives per key group):
By the year 2015, 40 percent of US parents who live in Florida

- Will be aware of the association between excessive sun exposure during childhood and the
  risk for adult melanoma
- Will be able to define "excessive sun exposure"
- Will report having conversations with their health care provider about preventive measures
- Will know how to protect their children from excessive sun exposure and feel capable of
  doing so
- Will advocate within their community for the widespread use of sun-protection measures
- Will report having had conversations with their peers about how much they like to wear a
  hat when they are exposed to the sun
- Will report having easy access to sun protection products and information
- Will feel satisfied with the level and quality of communication and social support they receive
  from their health care providers, children's schools, and others as it relates to sun-protection
  measures

Setting Communication Objectives

The first step in setting communication objectives is to consider, share,
and discuss all data that have been gathered for the situation and audience
analysis with team members, partners, and stakeholders. It is important
to prioritize findings that point to a specific communication or audience

need or preference. Research findings should also be carefully analyzed in reference to the behavioral stages of the primary audiences as well as secondary audiences (individuals, groups, or stakeholders who may exert an influence on primary audiences). Communication objectives need to reflect and be consistent with the information gathered on these topics.

Before establishing communication objectives, it is important to validate the overall program goal, as well as the behavioral, social, and organizational objectives that were determined on the basis of the preliminary briefing or literature review. The framework for this validation should be provided by data from the situation analysis and audience profile, which should have been finalized by now. This will ensure that communication objectives are set to meet realistic and accurate program goals and outcome objectives. Once this preliminary step has been completed, the health communication team can start brainstorming to set and prioritize communication objectives. The following sections discuss practical tips and examples on how to develop adequate communication objectives.

Make Sure Communication Objectives Are Specific to Each Key Group and Stakeholder

Consider again the case of a program that aims to reduce the incidence of pertussis, a vaccine-preventable childhood disease that, in its severe forms, is characterized by a prolonged cough with a typical whoop. As with other vaccine-preventable childhood diseases, it is possible that young health care providers in the United States may have never seen a case of pertussis and may feel it is no longer a priority in their practice. Still, the disease is on the rise (Centers for Disease Control and Prevention [CDC], 2013d), and there have been a number of deaths among infants and young children from this disease. If interviews with key opinion leaders in this medical area show that there is low physician awareness of pertussis and its potential life-threatening consequences, as well as on how infants and young children can contract it (Cherry and others, 2005; Tan, 2005; Greenberg, von Konig, and Heininger, 2005), one of the communication objectives should address the need for increasing knowledge of pertussis, its cycle of transmission, and key characteristics among health care providers in the pediatric and primary care settings. The communication objectives that may be set for parents may be completely different and address other kinds of needs that can be highlighted by research findings. Most important, such objectives need to be set in partnership with members of these two key groups and other key stakeholders to increase the likelihood that they may be achieved and sustained over time.

Do Not Include Tactical Elements

A good practice in developing communication objectives is to leave out information related to tactical elements, such as communication activities, media, materials, and channels. At this point, program planners should focus on what communication should accomplish and not worry whether the program would use mass media, online events, interpersonal channels, new media, or any specific activity. All of these elements will be defined as part of the tactical plan and guided by the communication strategy.

Limit the Number of Communication Objectives

Too many communication objectives often result in too many messages. Because behavioral and social change is a gradual process, having too many objectives (and related strategies and messages) may be confusing for key groups and stakeholders. When research findings point to multiple communication needs, it is critical to prioritize communication objectives that are more likely to lead to the achievement of the program's goal. Another possibility is to distribute them over time in a logical sequence that addresses first the most important communication needs as identified by key groups and stakeholders participating in the process. Therefore, even if it is appropriate to start brainstorming about multiple objectives, the final communication objectives should not include more than two or three objectives per key group.

Identify and Prioritize Objectives

Consider existing levels of knowledge as well as attitudes and common beliefs. Look at existing policies and social norms, as well as past and ongoing programs that address individual behavior and community needs. Think about what kinds of attitudes, beliefs, skills, policies, or norms need to be in existence to attain the behavioral, social, or organizational objectives that have been established and validated in support of the program goal. Think about the existing situation and how communication can help.

These steps should lead to identifying the most important communication objectives, which usually correspond to the key steps of the logical, behavioral, and social processes of change. For example, an audience segment might be teenagers who are unaware of the health risks associated with smoking and have just started smoking. If awareness of smoking-related risk is low among teenagers, the decision to focus on increasing knowledge about smoking cessation methods and programs may leave out a large percentage of teenagers. In fact, communicating about how to quit smoking is of lower priority in the absence of a high level of key group awareness on the health damages caused by smoking. Although there are cases in which both objectives could be met at the same time (it is always a good idea to provide solutions while alerting people of specific health risks), focusing on smoking cessation methods without raising awareness of the health consequences of smoking is unlikely to lead to results in this audience segment. Also, another potential communication objective should address the need for facilitating conversations and social support for and among teens who may decide to quit smoking as they become aware of its risks.

Selecting and applying one of the behavioral or social theories described in Chapter Two can help identify and prioritize communication objectives. In fact, these theories can provide a logical framework to organize one's thoughts and prioritize communication objectives by taking into account the key steps of behavioral or social change.

Analyze Existing Barriers, Social Norms, and Potential Success Factors

After prioritizing and selecting communication objectives, program planners should analyze potential barriers that may delay or jeopardize the attainment of these objectives. It is possible that additional communication objectives would need to be established and focus on removing such barriers. In a case in which smoking cessation may be perceived as a very low priority because the community or the country's cultural and policy context supports it, potential communication objectives are (1) to persuade policymakers about the relevance of a smoke-free environment for some of their key constituencies or (2) to inform them about the risks associated with smoking and their responsibility to protect the communities they govern. This may help remove some of the barriers to change. For example, in January 2005, "the Italian government banned smoking in all indoor public places" (Gallus and others, 2006, p. 346). Until then, the only smoke-free areas had been selected public spaces such as airports and libraries, but not necessarily restaurants, bars, or offices. Preliminary analyses on the impact of the ban on smoking habits showed that the new policy was associated with a decrease of 8 percent in tobacco consumption (Gallus and others, 2006). Yet, the ban may have had limited impact on smoking disparities and prevalence in the long term (Federico, Mackenbach, Eikemo, and Kunst, 2012).

In similar cases, several issues need to be addressed to promote people's compliance with smoking bans. In fact, smoking bans and regulations are not always readily enforced (Godfrey, 2005; European Network for

Smoking Prevention, 2005; Borg, 2004; Partnership at Drugfree.org, 2008; Roll Call, 2012).

Of course, if social objectives had been established at the outset of program planning, policy changes should be part of the overall plan. Existing social norms should also be considered and addressed to create the kind of change that may be needed to move away from cultural values and norms that support smoking and may focus on its perceived "coolness" toward new social norms under which smoking initiation is prevented and cessation is supported. Peer and social support for smoking cessation may also be another important factor especially among vulnerable and underserved populations. Still, it is worth taking an additional look at all barriers in the context of the development of communication objectives. This will help establish the time sequence and priority of the changes that need to happen, and set realistic expectations about the overall behavioral, social, or organizational change process.

Success factors in achieving communication objectives should also be analyzed vis-à-vis community and key groups' experiences as well as lessons learned from past interventions. However, the analysis of these factors is relevant primarily to the development of communication strategies and tactical plans (see the next section as well as Chapter Thirteen). In fact, an analysis of estimated success factors may point to the key strategic approaches or activities that may lead to achieving the communication objectives.

Define Time Frames

This step is related to establishing the time frame within which a communication objective can be achieved. Many factors can affect this time frame. In addition to external factors (for example, existing behaviors, policies, specific circumstances, clinical practices, or potential barriers), which are usually highlighted by the situation analysis and audience profile, there are several program- or organization-related factors that can influence the overall time frame for the attainment of communication objectives:

- Available funds, which determine the program reach as well as the speed with which materials and activities (both offline and online) can be implemented

- Human resources, which need to be adequate in all phases of program implementation, monitoring, and evaluation

- Organizational competence and experience in a specific health field or in reaching its key groups; organizations with limited experience or reputation in a health field may need longer to achieve communication objectives because of the need to establish themselves with a specific group or on a given health area

- A clear understanding of team members' roles and responsibilities as well as core contributions by program's partners

- The level of participation and endorsement of the communication plan by key groups and stakeholders

- A specific time line that is shared with and endorsed by all team members and partners

- Overall program span, which may condition the interval between activities as well as the timing of specific communication objectives; for example, in public health or patient emergency situations, communication objectives need to be achieved much more rapidly than in the case of interventions that attempt to tackle chronic situations or diseases

Moving to the Next Step

Because all elements of health communication planning and the health communication process itself are interconnected and dependent on each other, communication objectives set the stage for the development of communication strategies. Well-designed communication objectives influence and guide the rationale used in the next steps of communication planning as well as in the allocation of resources.

Outlining a Communication Strategy

communication strategy
A statement describing the overall approach (the "how") used to accomplish communication objectives

A **communication strategy** is a statement describing the overall approach (the "how") used to accomplish the communication objectives. It highlights how people can become aware of a disease risk, gain knowledge about prevention methods, or improve patient-provider communications on sensitive health issues, among others.

Communication strategies shape the tactical elements of a health communication program; they are directly connected to and serve the overall program goal and the behavioral, social, organizational, and communication objectives. In fact, communication strategies are often highlighted as part of a strategy plan that includes all of these other elements. This approach showcases the evidence and logical sequence that has led to specific communication strategies.

Similar to the objectives, communication strategies are key group specific and research based. They are developed with the participation of key communities, groups, and stakeholders. Consider again the example of teenagers who are not aware of the health risks associated with smoking and have just started smoking. In this case, a potential communication objective is "to raise awareness of the health risks associated with smoking among 5 percent of teenagers from thirteen to nineteen years of age who live in the United States." This communication objective has been established to support the overall program goal of reducing the incidence of smoking-related morbidity among US teenagers. The communication objective also supports the behavioral objective of prompting teenagers to quit smoking.

A number of potential strategies, which are highlighted in the following in italics, can support this objective:

- *Use teenage role models* to highlight the risks of smoking.

- *Create a peer support network* to facilitate discussion of smoking risks.

- *Engage high schools* in establishing smoking risk-awareness programs.

- *Use natural opportunities and venues* (for example, teen meetings, publications, concerts) to raise awareness of the health risks of smoking.

- *Provide tools to parents* to speak with teenagers about health risks associated with smoking.

- *Develop core communication materials and activities* on smoking health risks that can be easily distributed, shared on social media and other new media, and customized by primary and secondary audiences.

- *Establish partnerships with local youth organizations* to include discussion of smoking risks in their agenda and enhance program reach.

- Promote smoking risk awareness *through one-on-one counseling in clinical settings.*

- *Create a safe space for peer-to-peer communication* where teens can discuss smoking.

- *Focus on the limitations that smoking poses to physical performance and excellence in sports.*

None of these examples of potential strategies mentions any tactical elements such as flyers, brochures, blogs, press releases, virtual town halls, infographics, or workshops. In fact, a communication strategy is an overall concept and describes in general terms how to achieve objectives. It is the guiding framework under which messages and tactics will be established. Communication strategies identify and describe in broad terms the right combination of communication channels, media, messengers, and settings, and guide message development.

Key Principles of Strategy Development

As described so far in this chapter, once health communicators have analyzed all findings from the situation analysis and audience profile and established sound outcome and communication objectives, they usually move to consider several strategic approaches that may resonate and have been discussed and evaluated with key groups and stakeholders. The process of identifying, rating, prioritizing, and selecting communication strategies relies on many steps, which are described next.

Review Key Evidence

The first step in strategy development is a careful review of the situation analysis and audience profile. This step is common to all phases of planning that follow the initial research steps. In the case of strategy development, research findings should be shared with partners, donors, key groups, and stakeholders, and analyzed to identify the most suitable group- or situation-specific approaches that would help meet the communication objectives. Audience preferences for specific communication channels, media, and messengers should be considered and analyzed as part of this additional data review.

Make Sure All Communication Strategies Are Specific to Key Groups

Similar to objectives, communication strategies are key group specific. Usually different strategies are needed for different groups. Also, multiple strategies are often needed to attain the communication objectives within a specific key group.

Evidence-based strategies always include a rationale for their development that is likely to be used as a framework to present, discuss, and develop the intervention with partners, perspective donors, key groups, and stakeholders (O'Sullivan, Yonkler, Morgan, and Merritt, 2003; Fielding, 2011). It is therefore important that the rationale for the development of a specific strategy is clear to all members of the extended communication team, including partners and key stakeholders.

A logical approach in developing a communication strategy is to have a people-centered mind-set so the strategy will be established in response to key groups' needs, preferences, pastimes, and influencing factors. Sound strategies should also consider strengths, weaknesses, opportunities, and threats (SWOT) as identified as part of the situation analysis, and discussed with key partners, groups, and stakeholders. For instance, the examples of strategies provided in this chapter support awareness of the health risks associated with smoking among teenagers in these ways:

- Relying on teenagers' needs or preferences (create a peer support network; use teenager role models)

- Tapping into the work, credibility, and networks of existing organizations (establish partnerships with local youth organizations)

- Reaching teenagers where they actually are and hang out (exploiting natural opportunities and venues)

- Identifying potential communication angles that may be relevant to teenagers (focus on the limitations that smoking poses to physical performance and excellence in sports)

- Identifying secondary audiences or settings that can exert an influence on teenagers (provide parents with tools, engage high schools, develop a safe space for peer-to-peer communication, one-on-one counseling in clinical settings)

Other categories can be chosen in relation to specific health or social issues or services and corresponding key groups and stakeholders. Among them, strategies that focus on identifying potential communication angles that may be relevant to and motivate key groups to action are particularly important in message development. In fact, this category helps define all attributes of a specific health behavior, social norm, policy, health service, or product that should be incorporated in communication messages so they may appeal to key groups and stakeholders. Obviously this should be complemented by awareness-, risk-, or action-oriented messages. This strategic category, as well as the specific message development process that this influences, is part of positioning, a core concept that communication borrows from marketing and social marketing. **Positioning** identifies the fit between what key groups are seeking and what the product (whether tangible or intangible such as a health behavior or social norm) could actually deliver or represent for them (Kotler and Roberto, 1989; Lefebvre, 2013). It has to do with the long-term identity of a behavior, health service, social norm, policy, or product that would make it desirable to intended audiences and facilitate the change process related to its acceptance and adoption (O'Sullivan, Yonkler, Morgan, and Merritt, 2003). "In general, a positioning statement might take this form 'We want [*our priority group*] to see [*the desired behavior*] as [*descriptive phrase*] and as more important and valuable to them than [*the competitive behavior or point of differentiation*].' An example of a positioning statement comes from the VERB™ campaign,

positioning
The fit between what key groups are seeking and what the product (whether tangible or intangible such as a health behavior or social norm) could actually deliver or represent for them (Kotler and Roberto, 1989; Lefebvre, 2013)

which addresses twelve- to thirteen-year old *tweens*: 'We want tweens to see regular physical activity as something that is cool and fun and better than just sitting around and watching TV or playing video games all the time'" (Lefebvre, 2013, p. 251). (See Chapter Fifteen for a case study of the VERB campaign.) In a way, positioning also deals with changing social norms by addressing the social appeal of different and sometimes competing behaviors.

In health communication, the concept of identifying and focusing on communication angles and topics that are relevant and resonate with key groups is often an organizing principle for individuals, groups, communities, and key stakeholders to get together about a health problem. For example, in the case of smoking cessation, many parents and teenagers agree about the benefits and rewards of a physically active life (CDC, 2001, 2006g). Sports and athletic competitions have been used as a motivating factor for keeping children away from smoking, drugs, and risky behaviors by many kinds of programs and interventions (Castrucci, Gerlach, Kaufman, and Orleans, 2004). The sense of pride that goes with practicing a sport or seeing a loved one excel in his or her performance motivates communities around the world to create athletic clubs, programs, and facilities where children can play and be together. Because the long-term effects of smoking include a reduction in physical fitness (American Heart Association, 2006b), focusing on this health consequence may become an organizing principle for communities and interested groups.

In summary, the rationale of a communication strategy should always state the reason why the strategy has been established and selected over other approaches (O'Sullivan, Yonkler, Morgan, and Merritt, 2003). Box 12.1 includes an example on how shifting to evidence-based communication strategies as well as involving key communities and different stakeholders in health communication planning and strategy development contributed to making progress toward polio eradication in Egypt.

BOX 12.1. MAINTAINING EGYPT POLIO FREE: HOW COMMUNICATION MADE IT HAPPEN!

After more than three thousand years of struggle, children of Egypt became safe from polio virus, but only in 2006. Egypt represented a special challenge in eradicating polio because of its high population density, tropical climate, the high mobility of its population, and suboptimal sanitation conditions. Integral to the struggle was the need to change public attitudes and health practices.

The Ministry of Health, assisted by UNICEF, WHO, and a number of national and international donors and partners, helped create a social movement across all segments of the society. As a result, public trust and cooperation with health teams was hence created and every home with a child under five years was reached. Key factors that catapulted Egypt were the shift to door-to-door immunization campaigns instead of fixed posts and the use of evidence-based communication for development (C4D) strategies. This shift in strategy led to increasing immunization coverage by 20 percent and reaching eleven million children under the age of five.

Findings of the 2002 national communication baseline survey supported designing a communication strategy that effectively addressed misconceptions and knowledge gaps. Findings of studies also helped to better target children who were consistently missed by every polio campaign. The communication strategy was based on the diffusion theory. Focus was to change the attitudes of those caretakers who repeatedly missed immunizing their children in addition to maintaining existing universal immunization coverage. Two major pillars included a comprehensive national media campaign and community outreach especially in slum areas where majority of missed children were better reached. The use of credible public figures and celebrities and local religious leaders who spoke out in mosques and churches to build needed trust toward the vaccinators was an effective tool. TV spots were aired as many as 650 times during a designated year. Additionally, targeting young caretakers (twenty-five to thirty-nine years old) in slum areas to adopt immunization practices included the high use of local media and music TV channels and FM radio to reach those groups. Megaphones and more than five thousand recruited youth volunteers spread the awareness messages prior to each polio campaign.

National communication surveys from year to year provided evidence of the steady improvement of communication campaigns. In 2002, for example, those who knew that a child can be vaccinated as young as one-day-old was 46 percent, compared with 92 percent in 2005. In 2005, the communication survey indicated that 98 percent of caretakers had listened to or seen any polio media material that informed them about the fact that a national immunization campaign was upcoming in the following week. Of those, 67 percent were able to recall in an unassisted manner the correct dates of the polio campaign. TV spots that broadcast polio campaigns were the most mentioned source of information by caretakers, followed by megaphones, billboards and fliers or posters, and radio. The majority of caretakers (91 percent) who watched TV spots indicated that they immunized their children at the last campaign after watching these spots.

An important knowledge indicator was the ability of the caretaker to report the correct age for polio immunization schedules. In 2002, three-quarters (75 percent) of Egyptian mothers (nationally) were able to report this although in upper Egypt, it was 64 percent. Both figures improved to 90 percent in 2005. Whereas only 46 percent were able to correctly report the minimum age for polio vaccination in 2002, the figure dramatically increased to 92 percent in

2005. The proportion of caregivers who believed that polio vaccine had a side effect decreased from 27 percent in 2002 to 10 percent in 2005.

The most compelling evidence for the continued maintenance of attitudes (see Figure 12.1.) and health practices that are pro mass immunization was the success of the most recent 2011 and 2012 polio national immunization campaign. In spite of the limited advertising that preceded the polio campaigns and the difficult security situation after the Egyptian revolution, universal coverage of the targeted twelve million under-five-year-old children was achieved. However, polio threat remains given the possible importation from the surrounding countries. This makes the role of communication always critical.

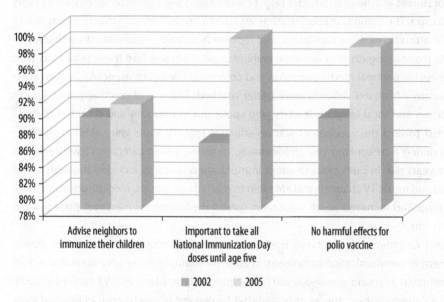

Figure 12.1   Changes in Attitudes Toward Polio Virus and Immunization

Reference: UNICEF. National Immunization Day for the Eradication of Polio in Egypt: Post Assessment. Final Report. Egypt: UNICEF, 2006a.

Source: Hegazi, S. Maintaining Egypt Polio Free: How Communication Made it Happen. Egypt: UNICEF, 2012b.

Rate, Prioritize, and Select Strategic Approaches

Different strategies have the potential of supporting a communication objective; however, some of them may be best suited to achieve communication objectives in an efficient, time-saving, cost-effective, and culturally competent way. In evaluating communication strategies, serious consideration should be given to the strategy's long-term sustainability, credibility, and strategic fit with suggestions and preferences of key groups and stake-holders, and implementation costs and barriers. Other factors may be issue or audience specific and include whether the strategy can accommodate an adequate and integrated blend of media and activities; is innovative and suited to secure people's attention and engagement, especially in relation to issues for which many programs may already exist; experiments with new and promising models; and is best suited to meet key groups' needs.

In the end, this kind of analysis aims at selecting strategies that are best positioned to meet the program's goals and objectives. This analysis should be conducted for each of the strategies under consideration.

The process of ranking and selecting adequate communication strategies can be organized to address the following issues and categories, for example:

- Key benefits: Can accommodate an integrated use of tools and activities
- Disadvantages: Lengthy implementation time needed
- Potential barriers to implementation: A lack of existing policies that support the strategy or the existence of social stigma that would prevent patients or survivors to be involved in the program
- Process: Community and stakeholder-driven design to increase the likelihood of key groups' commitment and endorsement
- Available resources, which should be adequate to strategy implementation
- Organizational capability and competence in executing the strategy

Appendix A includes a worksheet, "A2: Ranking and Selecting Communication Strategies: Sample Criteria," that incorporates all of these categories and can be used as a model to rank and select communication strategies.

Bringing the Steps Together

All elements of health communication planning are interconnected. In fact, in the early phases, most of the efforts are concentrated on linking the overall program goal with outcome objectives (behavioral, social, or organizational) and, in turn, with communication objectives and strategies. As discussed so far, the situation analysis and participatory audience analysis inform and guide all of these evidence-based steps.

Prior to the development of the tactical and evaluation plans, it is helpful to take a look at the progress in establishing these important foundations of the health communication program, as well as to appreciate the link and interdependence of all of these elements. Finally, the potential success of effective communication objectives and strategies is dependent on the quality and execution of the tactical plan that will be developed to execute them. This reinforces the concept of a health communication cycle in which key steps are interdependent, and all rely on the participation of key groups and stakeholders.

Key Concepts

- Communication objectives and strategies are interdependent and connected with all other components of the health communication program.

- Communication objectives are the intermediate steps or changes that are needed to achieve behavioral, social, and organizational objectives as well as the overall program goal.

- Communication strategies are designed to serve the communication objectives of the program as well as its outcome objectives (behavioral, social, and organizational).

- Communication strategies describe the approach (the "how") that would be used to meet the objectives. In other words, they focus on how the changes sought by the communication objectives will be attained.

- Neither communication objectives nor strategies focus on or describe tactical elements. Communication strategies inform and guide the development of the tactical plan (including communication messages, channels, media, materials, and activities).

FOR DISCUSSION AND PRACTICE

1. Discuss the difference between outcome objectives (behavioral, social, and organizational) and communication objectives. Use practical examples.

2. Using again the fictional example of Luciana in relation to skin cancer prevention among her peer group (see Box 2.1 as well as the discussion sections of previous chapters in Part Three), think of suitable communication objectives and strategies, and state them according to the methods and concepts included in this chapter.

3. Rank in order of importance and suitability all strategies you have developed for the previous question (for additional guidance on ranking key strategies, see "A2: Ranking and Selecting Communication Strategies: Sample Criteria" in Appendix A).

4. Research a case study in which communication objectives and strategies were developed via a participatory approach that was inclusive of key communities, groups, and stakeholders. Analyze key elements that may have contributed to community commitment to the planning process as well as its results.

KEY TERMS

communication objectives   positioning

communication strategy

DESIGNING AND IMPLEMENTING AN ACTION PLAN

This is the phase of health communication planning that most people really enjoy because they have an opportunity to unleash their creativity. This is the moment in which you can start thinking about all of these ideas for activities, media, and materials you have been holding onto so far. What kind of community-based forum should we organize to allow people to exchange information and experiences about a specific health issue? Or which celebrity should participate in our mass media campaign? Or what should be the content, title, and location of the interpersonal communication training workshops we need to organize for our community mobilization partners? Or what kind of topics, graphics, and interactive features should we incorporate in our social media sites to reflect what we have learned so far through our research efforts and the development of communication strategies and objectives? Creativity comes into play in this phase of planning, which relates to selecting a strategic blend of messages, channels, media, activities, and materials in support of the program strategies and objectives.

All elements of the action (tactical) plan are related to the different communication areas as defined in this book. For example, the action plan of a comprehensive intervention by the Centers for Disease Control and Prevention (CDC) that aims at reducing colorectal cancer deaths by encouraging screening and early detection includes public service announcements (PSAs), celebrity-driven messaging, online informational materials, community-based events and guides for local program implementation, social media sites, partnerships with multiple states and tribes in the United States to encourage community action and support population-based screening efforts, and many other communication activities, media, and materials (CDC, 2004/2005, 2006c, 2013b). The tactics in this program are related to different communication areas (for example, mass media and new media communication, professional communications, community mobilization) and support communication objectives and strategies.

Key premises of this chapter are that the selection of communication areas and tactics should be inspired by much more than creativity and effectively execute and support the program's strategies and objectives.

CHAPTER OBJECTIVES

This chapter focuses on some of the key attributes of strategic action plans as well as the key steps in developing them. It also discusses the integration of partnership and action plans in light of the partnership-based nature of most health communication interventions.

Definition of an Action (Tactical) Plan

tactics
Refer to different components of a plan of action (tactical plan) that includes communication messages, activities, media, materials, and channels and is developed to serve the program's strategies and objectives

One of the fundamental premises of this book is the critical role health communication should play in encouraging community and key groups' action in identifying and developing suitable solutions to health and social issues in collaboration with professionals from multiple sectors. Therefore, the title of this chapter is directly linked to the origins and literal meanings of the two key words of this important step of communication planning: action and tactics.

Action "is doing something toward a goal" (Microsoft Word Dictionary, 2013). *Tactics* are defined as a "procedure or set of maneuvers engaged in to achieve an end, an aim, or a goal" (*American Heritage Dictionary of the English Language*, 2004c). Although the term may evoke military procedures, **tactics** refers to different components of a plan of action that includes communication messages, activities, media, materials, and channels and is developed to serve the program's strategies and objectives. In other words, tactics are instrumental to put a plan or idea into action. Other authors and models (World Health Organization [WHO], 2003) use the term *action plan* to define this program component. **Tactical plan** or **implementation plan** are alternative words to **action plan** to describe actionable items of a health communication intervention, including the following:

action plan
A detailed, actionable, and strategic description of all communication messages, materials, activities, media, and channels, as well as the methods that will be used to pretest them with key audiences

- Key group– and stakeholder-specific messages, activities, materials, and related channels (including program launch activities and materials) that should be developed and implemented as part of the health communication intervention with the participation of such groups

- A detailed pretesting plan that should describe key research methods (for example, focus groups, in-depth interviews, community dialogue, participatory audience research) and questions that will be used to secure key group and stakeholder feedback on **communication concepts** ("ways of presenting information to intended audiences," National Cancer Institute at the National Institutes of Health, 2002, p. 55; as well as the overall content-related and visual appeal key groups and stakeholders may connect with) as well as draft messages, materials, media, and activities

- A partnership plan that summarizes all of these items of the action plan as decided by key partners, groups, and stakeholders, and also lists all partners, their roles and responsibilities, relevant contact information, partnership-specific evaluation parameters, and decision-making and internal communication processes

- A program time line for each activity

- A budget estimate for each activity, including evaluation activities (see Chapter Fourteen for additional information on how to develop an evaluation plan) and all materials and media

communication concepts
Concepts that describe "ways of presenting the information to intended audiences" (National Cancer Institute at the National Institutes of Health, 2002, p. 55) as well as the overall content-related and visual appeal (fear, hope, action, progress) key groups and stakeholders may connect with

Further consideration should be given here to the term *strategic* in the context of action plans. In fact, the action plan is a detailed extension of the broad outline for action established by communication strategies. It describes how to accomplish key objectives on a level of tactical details that strategies do not address. However, the action plan is still supportive of the same objectives that have been established for the program and the development of key strategies. In other words, the health communication cycle never ends.

Consider the example of a communication program that aims to reduce the impact of depression on self-esteem, feelings of happiness, work performance, and family interactions among women over forty-five years of age. The behavioral objectives of the program are to prompt women to (1) seek help when they feel depression is affecting their overall feelings of happiness and self-worth as well as their work and family lives and (2) comply with recommended practices in the prevention, treatment, and management of depression. If depression is still stigmatized in a specific population or country, as it is for example in Australia (Barney, Griffiths, Jorm, and Christensen, 2006) and among African Americans (Das, Olfson, McCurtis, and Weissman, 2006), a social objective may be to foster a change in social attitudes and norms toward depression so that this condition can be accepted and discussed in social and professional contexts by the year 2020. The program has set the following communication objectives and strategies:

Communication Objectives

- Raise awareness of strategies and methods to cope with depression among women over forty-five years of age who suffer from depression or are at high risk for this condition (quantitative parameters to be included).

- Increase understanding (include quantitative parameters) of depression as a medical condition within the US general public.

- Increase the number of people (include quantitative parameters) who report to have the intention of providing support to people living with depression and effectively integrating them in communities where this disorder is still stigmatized.

Communication Strategies

- Create a social and peer support network that will rely on women who successfully manage to minimize the impact of depression on work performance and family interactions.

- Use women role models to personalize depression and show the human face of this condition.

- Use traditional media and community-based venues to discuss depression within communities and ethnic groups in which this still may be stigmatized.

There are many ways to execute each of these strategies:

- Establish peer-to-peer communications meetings at local health clinics, major hospitals, and other community-based venues.

- Train women spokespeople, and create a media speaker bureau to react to and offer perspectives on recent news on depression as well as encourage media coverage of strategies and messages to cope with depression.

- Conduct outreach through women's magazines.

- Develop radio and TV PSAs pointing to a website for professional help and peer-support meetings.

- Organize Internet chats on top women's websites.

- Develop a new social networking site dedicated to discuss depression and its impact on women.

- Create a community bulletin board where members of local community centers can share resources and a calendar of events on depression-related topics.

- Organize several delivered dialogue sessions to discuss priority actions to reduce the stigma associated with the depression within community settings.

- Develop and stage specific programming on women and depression in partnership with local poetry clubs and theaters.

Because tactics are people and strategy specific, some of these activities may be better suited to support and execute one of the three strategies. Others may support all of them or perhaps should be discarded if they are not as effective as other options in serving the communication strategies. For example, the first of the tactics, "establish peer-to-peer communication meetings," may be suited to execute the first strategy, whereas the others may be used to support multiple strategies but may have unequal effectiveness. The selection of specific messages, activities, materials, media, and channels is related to research findings and key group–specific preferences, as well as many criteria that are related to the health issue and its environment.

Key Elements of an Action (Tactical) Plan

The success of a tactical plan is highly dependent on several elements that should guide its development. This section examines the most important features of well-designed action plans.

Integrated Approach

In designing an action plan that supports core communication strategies and objectives, multiple approaches and channels from different areas of health communication are likely needed to address a given health or social issue. The concept of an integrated approach, in which all tactical elements support and are complementary to each other, is commonly used in commercial marketing. Integrated marketing communications (IMC) is "a planning concept 'that recognizes the added value of a comprehensive plan that evaluates the strategic roles of a variety of communication disciplines and combines these disciplines to provide clarity, consistency and maximum communications impact' (Belch and Belch, 2004), as applied to social development challenges" (Hosein, Parks, and Schiavo, 2009, p. 537).

The concept of an integrated approach to communication is well established in health communication practice and incorporated at different levels in communication models for behavior and social change. In fact, IMC is one of the many influencing disciplines and factors of the communication for behavioral impact (COMBI) model (see Chapter Two) for health and social change (Renganathan and others, 2005; Hosein, Parks, and Schiavo, 2009) that has been used by WHO, several other United Nations agencies, and governments of many countries. Similarly, the communication for social change model (see Chapter Two) is defined as "an integrated model for measuring the process and its outcomes" (Figueroa, Kincaid, Rani, and Lewis, 2002, p. ii). Other examples include UNICEF's communication for development (C4D) framework, which integrates different human rights principles and communication tools, channels, and approaches (UNICEF, 2012); the overall field of development communication, which combines strategic communication with community and social development strategies (World Bank, 2013); and many of the objectives highlighted by *Healthy People 2020*, which, in order to be achieved, would need to rely on a multimedia and multicomponent approach to communication.

Similar to other characteristics of health communication and its planning process, the concept of integrated communications draws on everyday life. Communication, and more specifically health communication, is a common part of social exchanges and contexts, from personal and professional encounters to the mass media and traditional forms of expression such as theater and poetry, as well as informal conversations in barber shops, churches, restaurants, markets, and other public places (Exchange, 2006). Action plans should reflect this diversity of communication venues and channels to match how communication actually takes place. "What works in communicating about health depends on the context, and the way different communication processes and approaches are linked together or remain separate" (Exchange, 2006). Depending on how communication is used, different approaches can help "build momentum around some issues, but also isolate some social groups and conversations" (Exchange, 2006). A well-designed, well-integrated, and multifaceted action plan can help bridge gaps between current beliefs, attitudes, social norms, and behaviors and the kinds of changes that are needed at the individual, community, key group, stakeholder, and sociopolitical levels to achieve or maintain behavioral and social results.

Creativity in Support of Strategy

This book supports the role of health communication practitioners to redefine the theory and practice of health communication by incorporating lessons learned, trends, and effective strategies that worked well in related programs. Yet, health communication needs to be strategic. This means that great ideas are acceptable only as long as they support communication strategies and objectives and are connected to the other elements of the planning cycle.

Many professionals can recall colleagues who were in favor of a specific communication activity, channel, or media and used it in all interventions. And communication consultants or vendors who specialize in specific media or activities (for example, PSAs and videos, social media development) may have a partial view of the infinite possibilities for strategic tactics. Making videos for the sake of making videos does not help advance the communication goal and objectives the intervention is seeking to achieve, no matter how innovative and well designed the video may be. It is better to discard all great ideas that do not support communication strategies.

Cost-Effectiveness

Cost-effectiveness should be one of the parameters to guide the comparison of different tactical approaches. Ultimately this kind of analysis should still aim to select the best approach, but in the case of multiple options, it may provide an objective criterion to prioritize and rank different tactics with similar effectiveness. This type of analysis needs to address a number of questions, such as the following examples:

- How do different tactics compare in serving core communication strategies? If they all serve the strategy with similar effectiveness, is there any difference in their cost, including economic cost and the investment of time and human resources?

- Are there any existing programs or resources that could be used as a communication vehicle in support of communication strategies?

- Is there any potential for partnerships or collaborations with other organizational departments or external players that may save costs or time for the implementation of a specific communication activity?

- Were the tactics identified with the participation of key groups, partners, and stakeholders, and therefore may have a higher chance for success, given these groups' ownership, commitment, and endorsement of the overall planning process?

Saving costs and using human resources strategically are important not only in the case of limited funds or resources. Even when resources or costs do not appear to be an issue, which is almost never the case in health communication, there is no reason to waste them. The careful allocation of resources is one of the key elements of strategic health communication and related action plans.

Imagination

In developing an action plan, it is important to envision how communication messages, channels, and activities can be executed and ultimately have an impact on program strategies. Careful consideration should also be given to potential barriers in implementing all tactics so that these can be addressed, prevented, or minimized. Understanding key obstacles should also include careful consideration of living, working, and aging conditions, and key determinants of health, as highlighted by the situation and audience analysis. As in all other steps of communication planning (see Chapter Ten), communication models, theories, case studies, and past experiences, if adequately selected and interpreted vis-à-vis their relevance to the current intervention, can help develop this vision. In the case of the action plan, case studies and past experience are fundamental to foresee potential drawbacks, barriers to implementation, as well as estimated impact on program goals and objectives, and the kind of investment (time, costs, and human resources) that may be needed. Still, there is also an intuitive quality to imagining and visualizing future activities and potential drawbacks that is developed over time as a result of experience.

Culturally Competent and Issue-Driven Communication Messages, Channels, and Activities

Many observations throughout this book establish the influence of cultural, ethnic, geographical, socioeconomic, age, and gender-related factors on people's lifestyle, preferences, concepts of health and illness, reaction to illness, and overall health outcomes (see Chapter Three). The information gathered as part of the situation and audience analysis should also guide the selection of messages, channels, and activities that reflect the cultural characteristics and preferences as defined by key groups and stakeholders. Selecting culturally competent communication materials, media, and activities that also reflect the preferences of the people for whom they are intended is critical to the potential success of a health communication intervention.

For example, focus groups conducted in two geographical regions of Angola in sub-Saharan Africa with members of the local communities showed that interpersonal channels such as home visits and school- or church-based meetings were strongly favored by study participants because they are grounded in traditional and community-based practices. In one of the regions, strong preference was given to television versus radio when mass media were considered among potential channels. Finally, printed materials such as posters and brochures were excluded because of the high level of illiteracy among intended audiences. Focus group findings suggested that if printed materials were considered at all, they should rely more on graphics than words (Schiavo, 2000).

As another example, a preliminary assessment of a national program by the US Office of Minority Health (OMH) of the Department of Health and Human Resources (DHHS) on infant mortality prevention in the United States indicated that health care providers and related settings, school-based channels (for example, courses), and the Internet were preferred sources of information on infant mortality and preconception care among college and graduate students who had been trained by the Office of Minority Health Resource Center (OMHRC) to become preconception peer educators (PPEs) and participated in the program evaluation research (Schiavo, Gonzalez-Flores, Ramesh, and Estrada-Portales, 2011). *Preconception care* is a comprehensive intervention that identifies and reduces reproductive risks before conception, and has been associated with infant mortality prevention (Jack and Culpepper, 1990; Burns, 2005; Besculides and Laraque, 2005; Frey, Navarro, Kotelchuc, and Lu, 2008).

Equally important is to recognize and address, as part of all materials, media, and activities, existing social norms and potential obstacles to behavioral and social change as they relate to a specific health issue. For example, in developing a maternal and child health program in rural Ghana, which may seek to increase pregnant women's use of health services during pregnancy and at delivery, particular consideration needs to be given to issues such as existing gender roles, access to and quality of transportation, electricity, Internet, and other essential services (AudienceScapes, 2013), just to make a few examples of potential obstacles to behavioral and social results. Communication activities, media, and channels should attempt to address such obstacles by executing communication strategies that encourage community action and partnerships across sectors, as well as policy communication and public advocacy strategies in support of improvements within local systems. In addition, incorporating such issues in all materials, media, and activities will help recognize the legitimacy of people's feelings and perceptions about different obstacles that make it difficult for them to implement and sustain key health and social behaviors. This may increase the likelihood that key groups connect with and participate in the overall communication intervention.

In developing communication messages, materials, and activities, it is important to remember that it is almost never possible to use any kind of one-size-fits-all communication strategy and related tactics anywhere in the world. For example, communication materials or messages that have been translated from English to Spanish can be confusing to Spanish speakers and audiences. And the literal meaning of expressions adapted from English may be perceived as offensive. Therefore, communication messages and materials intended for Hispanic audiences should be developed directly in Spanish and tested with members of these audiences.

Similarly, media literacy levels (see Chapter Five or the Glossary for definition) of key groups and stakeholders are another important factor to be considered. Media literacy levels influence not only people's preferences on different types of media and their use but also their ability to use them to search for, relate to, trust, and act on health information. All communication interventions—no matter what the health or social issue they seek to address—should also attempt to incorporate resources and tools to improve on current media literacy levels of key groups and stakeholders.

Finally, in developing the graphic content of printed, online, or broadcast materials that address health issues of large public interest, it is important for different ethnic groups to be represented among the models featured in all images so that people are able to recognize themselves and feel included in the message. In selecting photos and other kind of imagery, health communicators should be aware that many stock photos (collections of photography and other kinds of images that can be purchased, used, and reused for design purposes by publishers, graphic designers, and health communication teams) tend to reinforce common stereotypes and misconceptions, and need to be analyzed in detail. Key groups or members of organizations who serve or represent them should contribute to select adequate imaging and photos, so this may help avoid or minimize the possibility of offending the people for whom the communication materials are meant.

The first step in developing communication concepts, messages, materials, media, and activities is to keep an open mind and not to assume that a specific message, workshop, social media site, or brochure may work for all. Participatory research, community-driven assessment, and audience feedback mechanisms in the formative and program implementation phases should guide the development of the action plan, which should be further validated by pretesting with representatives of key groups and stakeholders.

Concept Development

In health communication, *concepts* are preliminary to message and material development. They describe "ways of presenting the information to intended audiences" (National Cancer Institute at the National Institutes of Health, 2002, p. 55) as well as the overall kind of appeal (for example, fear, hope, action, progress) that will be used in reaching such groups as discussed and preferred by key groups themselves.

Communication concepts apply to actual messages as well as the content and graphic format of key materials, media, and activities. For example, the logo of a health communication program that aims at prompting health workers to get immunized against flu can evoke fear or a strict command that requires compliance (for example, a stop sign that crosses out the word *flu*) or wellness (a smiley face with a "feeling well" message around it). If such a logo is intended for use both online and within print materials it would be important to consider options that may adequately convey the core communication concept within these two kinds of media and their audiences. As another example, a communication campaign aimed at reaching drug abusers and convincing them to embrace the path to recovery can focus on eliciting fear for the life-threatening consequences of drug abuse or appeal to the sense of responsibility drug users may have for their children or other loved ones. Of course, both examples highlight only partial aspects of complex problems that need to be addressed by multiple interventions and messages.

A number of categories of communication concepts are commonly used in message development, such as the following examples (National Cancer Institute at the National Institutes of Health, 2002; R. W. Rogers, 1975, 1983; Witte and Allen, 2000):

- *Fear appeal:* Concepts developed to evoke fear and refer to an emotional response

- *Action step:* Specific recommended actions

- *Rewards or benefits:* Highlighting key advantages associated with recommended change

- *Perceived threat:* Influencing existing perception about group-specific risk levels for a specific health condition; attempts to elicit the kind of rationale response that is information based

- *Perceived efficacy:* People's perceptions about their own ability to perform recommended actions and behavior, as well as the impact of such actions on the actual threat

- *Hope:* This concept conveys that following the recommended behavior will enable people to achieve the kinds of milestones or changes they may hope for

Table 13.1 lists examples of concepts for a health communication intervention on childhood immunization that is intended for and seeks to engage parents. Similar to all other kinds of concepts, these are raw messages. Final messages should be selected to reflect key issues and informational needs that have been highlighted by research data, cultural values, parents' preferences, as well as their reactions to each of these possibilities. Notably, Table 13.1 includes a concept category of barriers, which refers to presenting information in a way that (1) may show that perceived or existing barriers to behavioral or social change can be addressed and eliminated or (2) proposes potential solutions and action plans for their elimination. The example in Table 13.1 refers to the first of the two potential connotations of a barriers-focused concept.

Prior experiences and research studies should also guide the selection process and provide information on the overall effectiveness of specific concepts. For example, fear appeal has been studied and applied over the years. Many health communication practitioners and researchers believe that "fear appeals backfire," but at the same time some analyses of communication interventions have suggested that "strong fear appeals produce high levels of perceived severity and susceptibility, and are more persuasive than low or weak fear appeal messages" (Witte and Allen, 2000, p. 591). "An example of fear appeal in the 90s is the 'Brain on Drugs' campaign,

Table 13.1 Examples of Communication Concepts for a Communication Intervention on Childhood Immunization

Benefits	Immunization protects children from severe childhood diseases. Vaccines save lives, and keep children healthy.
Benefits	Vaccines have a long-lasting protective effect on children and the communities in which they live and play.
Barriers	Childhood vaccines are safe and effective. The benefits of immunization are by far larger than the risk for side effects.
Consequences	Vaccine-preventable childhood diseases can have long-term effects on a child's physical and mental development.
Action steps	Immunize your child. Talk to your health care provider about vaccines.

where a fried egg represented the damaging effects of drugs on teenagers' brains" (Mayfield, 2006).

Today, we are witnessing an increased use of fear appeal by advertising agencies. For example, an antismoking public advertisement campaign of the New York City Department of Health to reduce smoking among Asian Americans features ads that include "photographic evidence, displaying nauseating pictures of esophageal cancer, stomach cancer, and pancreatic cancer. The tagline: 'Quitting is much less painful'" (Wu, 2012). A similar public advertisement campaign also in New York City, "'Suffering Every Minute,' includes two new television, Internet, and print ads depicting the devastation and suffering caused by smoking-related illness" (New York City Department of Health and Mental Hygiene, 2012). Yet, despite an increase in its use, especially in the context of advertising and mass media communication programs and some success stories, the effectiveness of fear appeal in health communication is still a controversial and much debated topic, with some authors (Robberson and Rogers, 2006, p. 277) concluding "that mass media health campaigns should use both negative and positive appeals."

Positive appeals to self-esteem also appear to be instrumental in influencing people to "adopt healthy lifestyles for reasons other than health per se (i.e., to enhance self-esteem)" (Robberson and Rogers, 2006, p. 277). Positive appeals—including role modeling and benefit-oriented imagery and messages—have also been used by mass media communication interventions and within other kinds of communication areas over many years. For example, Sesame Workshop, the nonprofit educational organization behind *Sesame Street*, has been using *Sesame Street*'s beloved characters to model and discuss key benefits of healthy behaviors to encourage children to make healthy food choices or brush their teeth, among other actions (Betancourt, 2008; Sesame Workshop, 2013). UNICEF has also used positive imagery in supporting the disability movement and positively portraying people with disability as part of action-oriented media and activities (UNICEF, 2013b). One of the benefits of positive appeals is the fact that they are strongly grounded in a human rights' perspective of health communication, and therefore convey hope and avoid displaying people's suffering, which at times may be in bad taste.

In practice, the use of different kinds of appeals is research based and specific to the groups we intend to reach. Their preferences and reactions (both emotional and rational) to different kinds of appeals should guide the selection of specific modalities. Regardless of the communication concept and appeal used by any given intervention, any discussion of a health or social issue should always be coupled with messages and resources that help build people's skills as well as confidence that they can succeed on their own. There is nothing worse than informing people about potential risks or health conditions without providing them with information and resources to prevent or manage them.

Recall the example of the parents of a nine-year-old boy who still wets the bed at night as the result of primary nocturnal enuresis, a common medical condition. Once the parents become aware that this is actually a medical condition and not a character flaw or behavioral problem (Cendron, 1999), they are likely to want to do something about it. They have already gone through many months of stress and shame and may feel relieved that help may be on the way. Suggesting they talk to a health care provider or go to a specialized health center is an important element of effective communication.

Similarly, think about the case of Maristela, the mother of five children who lives in a small village in northeast Brazil. She recently heard about the death of a child who used to play with her children. Apparently, the child had visceral leishmaniasis, which is also known as kalazar, a parasitic disease spread by the bite of infected sand flies and is found in Central and South America, Africa, and some Asian countries. Kalazar presents with vague symptoms such as fever, weight loss, fatigue, and an enlarged spleen and liver (CDC, 2006f), and is also known as *pot belly*. Rapid diagnosis, which starts with the initial suspicion of the disease in the presence of a pot belly, is critical to saving lives and is usually part of emergency control plans (Arias, Monteiro, and Zicker, 1996).

Maristela is scared of kalazar, does not understand it, and feels powerless about the possibility that her children might contract it. A health communication intervention intended to address the needs and concerns of Maristela and other parents in her village is likely to be more successful if, in addition to raising awareness of the disease and its early symptoms, incorporates action steps and self-efficacy concepts and messages, and is grounded in people's preferences and suggestions for action. Among others, key messages could encourage disease suspicion (when a child has a pot belly) and prompt early intervention (such as rushing to the closest health care facility) and inquiry to health care providers about the possibility that the child may have kalazar. The overall communication intervention should also help remove potential barriers to a prompt diagnosis. For example, communication efforts could focus on advocating for adequate transportation to connect people from remote communities with local health centers or using professional medical communication strategies to increase kalazar suspicion and training among local clinicians.

All of the examples in this section establish that communication concepts and messages are research based and should address specific needs and characteristics of key groups and stakeholders. Whenever possible, they should also be designed to show the path to behavioral or social change by highlighting a series of steps or actions leading to that. Most important, they should be validated one more time by intended audiences through pretesting methods and analysis.

Box 13.1 presents a case study by the US National Cancer Institute (NCI) that shows how communication messages were developed from a variety of initial communication concepts and on the basis of audience feedback. Practical tips on message development and an overview of pretesting methods and principles are addressed in the following sections.

BOX 13.1. NCI'S CANCER RESEARCH AWARENESS INITIATIVE: FROM MESSAGE CONCEPTS TO FINAL MESSAGE

In 1996, the NCI's Office of Communications (OC), then the Office of Cancer Communications, launched the Cancer Research Awareness Initiative to increase the public's understanding of the process of medical discoveries and the relevance of discoveries to people's lives. OC's concept development and message testing for this initiative included the following activities.

Three values of medical research were selected for concept development:

- Progress (e.g., we are achieving breakthroughs)

- Benefits (e.g., prevention, detection, and treatment research are benefiting all of us)

- Hope (e.g., we are hopeful that today's research will yield tomorrow's breakthroughs)

Based on these values, the following message concepts were developed and explored in focus groups with intended audience members:

- Research has led to real progress in the detection, diagnosis, treatment, and prevention of cancer.

- Everyone benefits from cancer research in some fashion.

- Cancer research is conducted in universities and medical schools across the country.

- Cancer research gives hope.

- At the broadest level, research priorities are determined by societal problems and concerns; at the project level, research priorities are driven primarily by past research successes and current opportunities.

The following messages were crafted after listening to intended audience members' reactions and their language and ideas about the importance of medical research:

A. "Cancer Research: Discovering Answers for All of Us"

B. "Cancer Research: Because Cancer Touches Us All"

C. "Cancer Research: Discovering More Answers Every Day"

D. "Cancer Research: Because Lives Depend on It"

E. "Cancer Research: Only Research Cures Cancer"

Mall intercept interviews were conducted to pretest them. Based on responses from the intended audience in these interviews, message D was selected as the program theme.

Source: National Cancer Institute at the National Institutes of Health. *Making Health Communication Programs Work.* Bethesda, MD: National Institutes of Health, 2002, p. 56.

Message Development and Health Literacy Assessment

Once the type of message and concept appeal has been selected, messages should be developed and pretested with intended audiences or their representatives (National Cancer Institute at the National Institutes of Health, 2002). Several factors can influence message efficacy and need to be considered in message development:

- *Concise and to the point.* There should be no more than two or three messages per audience; too many messages may be confusing.

- *Credible.* They are evidence based and delivered using reputable media and spokespeople.

- *Relevant to the key groups and stakeholders* as assessed by them. They need to address the "so what?" and "what is in there for me?" questions.

- *Consistent* throughout the communication activities and materials as well as over reasonable periods of time.

- *Simple.* They should not use jargon or technical terms and should take into account health literacy levels of key groups and stakeholders.

- *Descriptive.* Even when messages are simple they should be descriptive enough to make clear what kinds of actions people should undertake and why.

- *Easy to remember.* Whenever possible, they should include catchy language and evoke culturally relevant and traditional imagery and meanings.

- *Inclusive of social determinants of health.* Messages should acknowledge and address potential barriers to behavior, social, or organizational change, and key determinants of health.

If a health communication program has more than one message per key group, the most important message should be mentioned at the beginning and the end of each communication and activity. Communication trainers usually use a simple ten- to twelve-word exercise to prove this point. If a group hears a list of ten to twelve related words and then is asked to recall the list in order, chances are that most people remember the first and the last word and fewer people remember the words in between. This is also quite important in interpersonal communication and community mobilization efforts.

Message retention is also another important topic in communication. Message frequency, vocal variety and depth (in the case of interpersonal communication or live events), and a multimedia approach to message delivery, which creates the so-called resonance effect, can all have a positive influence on message retention by key groups. A common model for information retention is Ebbinghaus's curve of forgetfulness, based on the work of Hermann Ebbinghaus, a pioneer researcher of the psychology of human memory who studied message retention in the late 1800s (Perlotto, 2005). Ebbinghaus's curve demonstrates that "75% of information learned in week one, and not reinforced afterwards, is forgotten in week two. 90% of it is gone in week three, and so on" (Nuzum, 2004, p. 23). This supports the importance of message repetition and consistency, a common practice in effective health communication.

Assessing and understanding health literacy levels is also key to message and media efficacy. "The low health literacy of millions of adults in the USA has been referred to as a 'silent killer'" (Zarcadoolas, 2011, p. 338), so it is important for people to be able to understand and act on health information and messaging. Appendix A includes several online resources for health literacy assessment of communication materials and activities. Yet, as previously stated, health literacy is a complex construct that influences and is influenced by health communication. Language needs to be simple but not oversimplified. "Cultural appropriateness, relevancy and context are needed to close the gaps between health messages, health messengers and patients/the public" (Zarcadoolas, 2011, p. 338). A cross-cultural approach to message development that incorporates key groups' and stakeholders' feedback can improve the chances that messages will be understood, retained, remembered, and implemented.

Selecting Communication Channels and Vehicles

As a reminder, *communication channels* refer to the path that is used to reach out to and exchange relevant health information with key groups and stakeholders. *Communication vehicles* are materials, events, media, activities, or other means used to convey a message through communication channels. This category (materials, events, and activities) is also called *tactics*. Communication channels and vehicles are audience specific and should be researched as part of the situation and audience analysis (see Chapter Eleven).

Selecting appropriate and culturally competent channels and vehicles is extremely important in making sure that specific health communication messages or programs stand out and are actionable. Formative participatory research should set the stage for and guide the selection of adequate and audience-specific communication channels and tactics. At this point in program planning, the health communication team should have a clear understanding of key groups' preferences for channels and vehicles that are best suited to share information, ideas, and potential solutions. Moreover, health communication teams should stay informed of new options and trends in the use of communication channels and vehicles, as well as trends in their acceptance and use by different key groups. Media coverage, peer-reviewed studies, online resources, social media monitoring, and informal conversations with colleagues and representatives of relevant organizations are all excellent ways to stay informed. (Appendix A includes a sample menu of communication channels and venues as well as examples of related vehicles. See "A3: Sample Communication Channels and Venues and Examples of Related Vehicles (Tactics).")

Some of the criteria that guide the selection of group-specific channels and vehicles are message content and complexity, audience reach, cultural and issue appropriateness, and cost-effectiveness (see Chapter Eleven). The efficacy of specific communication vehicles also depends on their ability to grab people's attention (Health Communication Unit, 2003b), which is often related to the graphic and visual appeal of the vehicles (as it applies, for example, to the case of printed materials, social media sites, videos, or broadcast segments) as well as the credibility and appeal of key spokespeople. For example, the use of celebrities, well-known physicians, peer leaders, community leaders, or other role models may enhance the ability of communication vehicles to capture key groups' attention.

Effective vehicles should also be easy to reproduce and disseminate (Health Communication Unit, 2003b). Because message consistency and repetition are key factors in message development and dissemination, communication vehicles should reflect and accommodate these attributes of effective messages and be selected to ensure widespread message circulation.

Ultimately, the final word on clear and culturally appropriate messages, channels, and vehicles is determined by the key groups or their representatives, who should be involved in the development and pretesting of these essential communication tools. Box 13.2 features a case study by the Program for Appropriate Technology in Health (PATH) that highlights how the selection of culturally appropriate and research-based messages, media channels, and vehicles can influence changes in knowledge, attitudes, and behavior. The intervention featured in this case study relies primarily on the strategic use of traditional (for example, theater) and interpersonal media channels in integration with print media and others.

BOX 13.2. COMMUNITY THEATER IN BENIN: TAKING THE SHOW ON THE ROAD

Spacing births or limiting the number of children reduces risks to mothers' and children's health. Yet, women in northern Benin have an average of six children, and 20 percent of them have children dangerously close together—fewer than two years apart. Five women for every thousand children who are born die of complications from pregnancy and childbirth. Contraception prevents unwanted and high-risk pregnancies and can save women's health. Still, only 7 percent of families used it.

PATH, an international nonprofit organization, has found that theater is a highly effective way to address health issues—and even to begin to change social norms. In villages with no access to television or cinema, and in which many people cannot read, it's relatively easy to gather a large crowd—often up to three hundred people—for a performance. The lack of competing media makes the play even more efficient at spreading ideas and getting youth, parents, and elders thinking and talking about the health topic.

PATH designed the play "Spacing Our Children" to instigate discussion and raise villagers' awareness of modern family planning methods. In the first year, more than sixty-five thousand people in 232 villages in northern Benin attended the play, which was in the local Bariba language.

Constructing the Set

In preparation for the play, PATH assessed knowledge and attitudes of villagers. Research showed that men, who control the purse strings, often oppose their wives' wishes to use contraception. As a result, the play emphasized the husband's responsibility in family planning and the economic benefits of well-spaced, healthy children. The two central characters were brothers with divergent views and life situations. One had carefully nurtured his small family. The other had a large family that had fallen into poverty, disarray, and ill health.

An existing African theater troupe, Troupe Bio Guerra, helped PATH create and tour the production. Project staff trained the actors to administer oral surveys before and after the play and to hold short discussion groups with the villagers after each performance. The discussion groups, which were segmented by age and sex, were the first chance for villagers to freely exchange stories with their peers, ask questions, and clarify what they learned. The play's messages were reinforced by radio shows, printed materials, and home visits by community health volunteers.

Results

Data from surveys of villagers before and after the play indicated dramatic increases in the number of villagers who did the following:

- Were able to describe several contraceptive methods
- Said they would discuss contraception with their spouses
- Said they planned to have no more than four children

Use of contraceptives by married women increased from 7 percent prevalence in 2000 to 11 percent in 2002. The project continued to work to increase this percentage in 2003–2005. However, national statistics were not available at the time this case study was first published.

Source: Program for Appropriate Technology in Health Program for Appropriate Technology in Health. "Community Theater in Benin: Taking the Show on the Road." Unpublished case study, 2005a. Funding for this project was provided by the US Agency for International Development through an award to University Research Co., LLC. Copyright © 2005b, Program for Appropriate Technology in Health (PATH), www.path.org. All rights reserved. The material in this case study may be freely used for educational or noncommercial purposes, provided that the material is accompanied by this acknowledgment line. Used by permission.

Planning for Program Launch Activities, Media, and Materials

The action plan should also include a section that highlights the timing and the kinds of activities and materials that would be used to kick off the overall health communication intervention and introduce its key components to the general public and key groups and stakeholders. The program launch plan should be determined by formative research (also including participatory methods and community-driven assessment) findings. Launch messages should be the same as for the overall health communication program. Messages should be consistent until the evaluation and feedback phase is completed or has gathered significant results that point to the need for message refinement.

Launch activities and materials aim to spread the word about the intervention's core messages, resources, and services and implement its activities, potential services, and resources. A few practical suggestions can be used to develop effective launch plans:

- Make sure that program launch activities are key group, channel, and venue specific.

- Select communication channels and venues for maximum audience outreach. For example, if the audience is the general public, the mass media are effective channels, especially in developed countries. If health care professionals are a key group of the communication intervention, medical meetings and conferences as well as trade and medical publications are adequate venues or channels for launch activities. In the United States, a large percentage of patient groups and other kinds of stakeholders can also be reached at meetings and conferences. In the developing world, traditional communication channels (for example, theater) and venues (for example, the local village square or market) may be suitable for a crowd of community members to gather (see the example in Box 13.2) and participate in discussing their feelings, opinions, preferences, opportunities, and challenges as they relate to a specific health or social issue.

- Be creative. Program launch activities should be designed to attract the attention of key groups, as well as key **gatekeepers**, such as journalists, bloggers, professional organizations, and other individuals and groups that may provide access to them.

  gatekeepers
  All individuals, groups, or organizations that may provide access to intended audiences

- Whenever possible, involve celebrities, community leaders, role models, or other well-known opinion leaders who are recognizable and respected by key groups to speak on the health or social issue as well as key program components at program launch as well as during follow-up activities.

- In all launch activities, media, and materials, include information about where and how to obtain additional information or help about the specific health issue. For example, provide telephone numbers, website links, and the names and addresses of specific community centers or health centers or organizations. Ask people to become involved in the solution of the health issue or specific program-related activities.

- Avoid scheduling launch activities in conjunction with other presentations or events that may be of greater interest to key groups and stakeholders. Other research activities, news, and events that may interfere with the intervention launch and deflect attention from its core messages.

Special considerations apply to each communication channel, media, venue, and country. For example, in designing communication activities and tools for a health communication program that relies on the mass media for its launch activities, communicators must consider different options for their cost-effectiveness and efficacy in achieving media coverage. In the United States, press conferences are an adequate communication vehicle for program launch only in the case of breakthrough news or the participation of extremely well-known political figures and celebrities. Competition for media coverage is fierce. Journalists do not attend press conferences or in-person media briefings unless there is breakthrough news or a celebrity is participating. If these criteria cannot be met, traditional and emerging media relations tactics such as a virtual newsroom, press release, and a media alert announcing speaker availability for one-on-one telephone or in-person interviews may be a cost-effective option to secure coverage on the intervention's content and key messages.

Pretesting Communication Concepts, Messages, and Materials

Pretesting should be used to assess one more time whether communication concepts, messages, media, and materials meet the preferences and needs of key groups and stakeholders and are culturally appropriate. As defined in Chapter Eleven, pretesting is considered an essential part of formative research and is participatory in its nature. As in other phases of formative research, if intended audiences are multicultural, they should all be represented in pretesting studies.

Outside academia, many health organizations in the commercial and nonprofit sectors consider pretesting a costly and avoidable step in communication planning. This common misperception (National Cancer Institute at the National Institutes of Health, 2002, 2013) may result in messages and materials that do not support key objectives and strategies and fail to meet key groups' preferences and needs. In fact, "pre-testing answers questions about whether your materials [and messages] are understandable, relevant, attention getting, attractive, credible, and acceptable to the target audiences" (Washington State Department of Health, 2000; Doak, Doak, and Root, 1995). In other words, pretesting helps assess if all the criteria that inspired the development of draft concepts, messages, and materials have been met.

Pretesting starts within the immediate environment of the health communication team. Colleagues, program partners, representatives of key groups, and professional acquaintances can provide initial feedback on draft concepts and materials. Actual pretesting with members of key groups and stakeholders usually relies on marketing and communication research methods, participatory audience research, and community-based research methods (see Chapter Eleven), including focus groups, community dialogue, one-on-one interviews, expert or gatekeeper interviews, and surveys. Methods should be selected according to materials format, size of intended audiences, cost-effectiveness, and cultural preferences, to name a few criteria. Focus groups and one-on-one interviews tend to be most commonly used in pretesting.

Pretesting needs to be cost-effective. Obviously the cost should never exceed the cost of materials and activity development. A number of solutions can accommodate limited budgets and time concerns and make pretesting more affordable; examples are conducting stakeholder, expert, or gatekeeper interviews to validate program elements and adapting pretesting questions from previous studies.

In pretesting, "some of the most significant sample questions are: 'What can the readers do after reading this that they could not do before?'" (Washington State Department of Health, 2000). For example, what kinds of strategies to address key determinants of health in relation to a specific health or social issue can key groups effectively implement in their community or neighborhood after participating in this event or online forum? Messages and materials are more likely to encourage behavioral and social change when they are simple and do not try to accomplish too many objectives at the same time.

Finally, pretesting is important in assessing the overall level of comprehension of messages and materials by key groups. Low health literacy is a widespread issue in developed and developing countries (see Chapter Two). A good communication practice is to write in simple and clear terms for low-literacy audiences. Communication messages and materials should be designed for the reading level of intended audiences, but "most materials should be written for no higher than sixth grade reading skills" (Washington State Department of Health, 2000). (For resources on readability tests as well as examples of pretesting questions, see Appendix A: "Health Literacy Resources" and "A4: Pretesting Messages, Materials, and Activities: Sample Questions.")

Program Time Line and Budget Estimate

The action plan should include a program time line and budget estimate for each communication activity as well as the development of all communication materials. Budget estimates should include grants to partners, community groups, and other program associates for their work on the communication intervention; community incentives; research, monitoring, and evaluation costs; actual price quotes from printers, graphic designers, creative or communication agencies; research firms or consultants; other kinds of consultants or vendors; and also include funds for contingency plans and potential crises. It is also helpful to include an estimate for each activity about the time members of the communication team and their partners would be spending on implementing different aspects of the communication intervention. (Sample time lines and budget estimates are included in Appendix A. See examples 1 and 2 of "A5: Program Time Line: Sample Forms" and "A6: Budget Sample Form.")

Integrating Partnership and Action Plans

We live in a complex world where health issues are equally complex and require multisectoral solutions. It is almost impossible for any given organization or institution or community—no matter how competent, well-intentioned, passionate or well-connected its officers, representatives, or members may be—to be able to address the complexity of today's health issues and their root causes without engaging with partners from multiple sectors. Moreover, multisectoral partnerships have the added benefit of being grounded in multiple perspectives on issues of interest. They are also likely to create the kind of effect for which everyone—and not only most affected families or community members—may start caring about high rates of childhood obesity or infant mortality in a given community. See Chapter Eight for a discussion of constituency relations and strategic partnerships in health communication as well as Chapters Fifteen and Sixteen, which also include case studies that involve multiple partners.

Even if there are sufficient funds or human resources for program implementation, it is always important to consider partnering with other organizations and stakeholders to maximize impact of all interventions and build their long-term sustainability. Partners can increase the possibilities for program reach and add organizational skills competency in a specific area of implementation, credibility, technical and medical expertise, spokespeople, or other knowledge and skills that can contribute to the intervention's outcomes. Other authors and publications support the importance of sound partnership plans as a key component of health communication planning (National Cancer Institute at the National Institutes of Health, 2002; O'Sullivan, Yonkler, Morgan, and Merritt, 2003).

partnership plan
A summary of the collective efforts that result in the creation of a strategic partnership on a given intervention, as well as roles and responsibilities and expectations of all partners and related time lines

The list of potential partners to be considered or involved in a health communication program is issue and key group specific. Potential partners range from public health departments to voluntary organizations, from state or national professional organizations to patient groups, from corporations and local businesses to universities and other educational institutions, from student associations to many other kinds of organizations and stakeholders. Partnerships, coalitions, and other forms of collaborative efforts often arise from good relationships, as well as organized constituency relations efforts or kick-off partnerships meetings. The **partnership plan** is a way to summarize the collective efforts that result in the creation of a strategic partnership on a given intervention, as well as roles and responsibilities and expectations of all partners and related time lines.

In general, there are two phases in developing partnership plans. Phase one is part of the situation and audience analysis and continues with engaging potential partners in preliminary conversations and meetings to assess their interest in participating as well as the kinds of competencies, skills, and resources they may bring to the table. These preliminary interactions are also an opportunity to discuss organizational procedures and potential constraints, barriers, and issues that should be considered prior to engaging in a formal partnership.

Phase two is the actual partnership plan, which should be as comprehensive as possible in stating information about the health issue as well as the overall goal and outcome objectives of a potential intervention as well as highlight roles and responsibilities, time lines for project completion, processes, and budgets as they refer to all partners and their specific commitments within the partnership's structure (see Table 13.2). This phase should be completed while already working collaboratively on the design of the health communication intervention and its different elements. It is fundamental to the success of all partnerships to involve potential partners early in the planning process. The actual partnership plan is a way to formalize and record discussions and negotiations that should take place

Table 13.2   Key Elements of a Partnership Plan

Phase one	Phase two
• Project title	• Action plan (key activities, events, materials, and media) to be implemented by the partners
• Overall program goal and outcomes objectives	
• Key groups and stakeholders	• Steps to secure additional partners (if or when needed)
• Benefits of potential partnership	
• List of potential partners	• Names of partners' representatives
• Organizational constraints and policies	• Assigned roles and responsibilities (for each partner)
• Administrative issues	• Frequency of and methods (for example, partnership meetings, calls) for progress update and other routine communications among partners
• Potential drawbacks of partnerships	
	• Standard protocol for decision making and issue management
	• Expected program outcomes and intermediate milestones
	• Measures for program success as well as partnership viability and long-term sustainability

throughout the overall health communication process. Table 13.2 is an evolution and modified version of a very similar table from the first edition of this book (Table 12.2), which was also tailored and used for implementation in building capacity in four US cities for the development of community-campus partnerships for infant mortality prevention (Schiavo, Estrada-Portales, Hoeppner, and Ormaza, 2012).

An important component of phase two is to develop and describe a standard process for ongoing communications among partners (for example, a weekly phone call or scheduled meetings). All partners must understand the process, as well as how decisions will be made, and agree to it in order to preserve transparency and trust throughout the process. Mutual understanding and agreement on expected outcomes of these joint efforts as well as related measurement parameters will keep the partnership healthy by minimizing misunderstandings, and setting and managing realistic expectations among all partners. Finally, partnership management requires funds and human resources that should be considered as part of the overall program budget and resource allocation.

Planning for a Successful Program Implementation

Planning for a spotless program execution as well as the sustainability of the overall communication intervention also entails several steps that are related to establishing and maintaining standard practices for the management of funds, human resources, specific activities (for example, monitoring and data collection), and internal communications among all members of the extended health communication team. It is also related to anticipating and preparing for potential issues that may arise during program implementation and affect expected outcomes. A team-oriented mind-set, as well as attention to detail, is critical to the implementation of all practices and steps described in this section.

Human Resource Allocation and Budget Monitoring

The action plan should include a detailed budget estimate as well as a description of the roles and responsibilities of specific team members and partners. This should ideally incorporate an approximate evaluation of the time each team member is committing to the program. Action plans should also identify the program's management team. However, sometimes communication interventions get funded long after they were planned and call for a reassessment of these elements.

The first step in program implementation is to make sure that no changes in the original intervention's team are necessary in the light of recent career moves, loss of interest in the project, or conflicting and unexpected priorities. Program staff substitutions should be strategic and look at the specific skills and contribution the original team member or partner was bringing to the communication intervention. Perhaps a patient group that is well known for its research and advocacy work in the field of mental illness decides to withdraw from a specific health communication program for a variety of reasons. In this case, program managers should identify another organization with similar or complementary reputation, skills, interests, expertise, and constituencies in the same health area. In other words, human resources are allocated to a program on the basis of the skills, experience, and the kind of innovative thinking people may bring to the overall effort. The same principle should apply to potential substitutions or integration of partners and staff.

Finally, the health communication team should include or designate specific individuals who are responsible for budget monitoring, that is, making sure that all program tactics are implemented within the budget that has been estimated and allocated for each of them. This is usually the responsibility of the management team with the help of one or two additional team members. Budget reports, which include itemized expenditures and remaining amounts, may be a useful tool to record and share budget status. Budget reports also increase the transparency of all management processes and can be shared at regular intervals with key partners.

Establishing Monitoring Teams

Monitoring is an essential function in program implementation and is related primarily to four areas: (1) program activities and related process; (2) ongoing feedback by key groups and stakeholders on the intervention's key elements, overall content, messages, and progress-related updates; (3) news and trends about the specific health areas, key policies, changes in relevant socially determined factors, intended audiences, and other relevant facts and events; and (4) the collection and analysis of evaluation data. Different skills and collection methods are required for each of these areas. For example, monitoring key activities, which is part of process evaluation and serves to assess whether program implementation occurs within the parameters envisioned by the action plan, is frequently a management function. However, it also involves the participation of all team members dedicated to a specific activity. If a team member has strong relationships with, for example, the HIV patient and advocacy community, he or she is the best candidate to secure ongoing input and feedback on the intervention's key elements and contents from this key

monitoring
Monitoring is an essential function in program implementation and evaluation and is related primarily to four areas: (1) program activities and related process; (2) ongoing feedback by key groups and stakeholders on the intervention's key elements, overall content, messages, and progress-related updates; (3) news and trends about the specific health areas, key policies, intended audiences, and other relevant facts and events; and (4) the collection and analysis of evaluation data

group. Finally, evaluation data should be monitored and collected on the basis of the indicators and methods described in the evaluation plan. Early in program implementation, specific team members should be assigned to each of these areas of monitoring. See Chapter Fourteen for a detailed discussion on monitoring as an essential element of project implementation and evaluation.

Technical Support and Advisory Groups

If the program has the funds and the need to hire a specialized health communication research firm or consultant, event facilitator, or creative agency, chances are that these agencies and consultants have also been involved in program planning. In fact, involving agencies and consultants early in the process, and in any case not later than during the strategy development phase, is good practice in health communication and helps maximize the strategic contribution and dedication of all consultants.

Early in program implementation, all agencies that have participated in program planning should be invited to a team meeting to define the implementation process, confirm the program's time line, and develop a checklist of all logistics related to the execution of all activities. Finally, it is possible that additional consultants (for example, printers or mailing services) may need to be interviewed and hired in this phase of the program. Obviously, funds for hiring other consultants who are not part of the strategic communication process should have been included in the original budget estimate.

If specific needs arise or preliminary conversations with key stake-holders have confirmed the importance of a specific advisory group that could lend additional technical support to the intervention, these groups should be established and involved as early as possible. Advisory groups can serve multiple functions. For example, the Macy Initiative, a collaborative effort to enhance physician communication skills between the University of Massachusetts Medical School and the schools of medicine of New York University and Case Western Reserve University, have established an advisory group of faculty involved with the teaching and curriculum planning for the initiative (UMass Medical School, 2006). In Zambia, a youth advisory group "consisting of 35–40 young people from 11 youth organizations" advised the program's design team and developed communication objectives and abstinence messages for the HEART (Helping Each Other Act Responsibly Together) program, an HIV/AIDS initiative intended for young adults (Health Communication Partnership, 2004; Development Communication and Media Advocacy, 2009).

Advisory groups and consultants should also be involved in program implementation. In fact, they can be a valuable source of expertise and, in some cases, can function as a link with a specific key group to continue securing audience feedback and encouraging participation on all program elements.

Process Definition

The process needed for program implementation should be defined in the first few team meetings of this phase. This should include a plan of all logistics—for example, who will be the main contact with key stakeholders or responsible to coordinate the review process of key communication materials and related time lines, travel arrangements for workshops or other in-person communication activities, or contact local radio stations, or to share information on data collection processes for the evaluation report. Roles and responsibilities should be clear to each team member, who should also be aware of activity and logistic-specific deadlines. A specific time line should be developed for each activity and materials and be updated with new information and progress at periodic time intervals established by the overall team.

The implementation process should identify exact dates for team meetings and other kinds of in-person, telephone, Skype-based, or online communications that will be used for progress reporting, problem solving, or brainstorming with partners, team members, stakeholders, and representative of key groups.

Issue Management

Several chapters in this book have discussed issue management in the context of specific health communication areas (for example, constituency relations). However, issue management and the concept of preparedness that inspire this practice apply to the entire health communication cycle and have particular relevance in project implementation.

The issues that may arise in program implementation range from logistical issues (for example, the flight of a key speaker for a workshop is cancelled and the speaker is not able to attend the event; the materials intended for distribution at a local conference do not arrive on time) to more substantial and critical issues (for example, an article in a major newspaper attacks some of the fundamental premises of the intervention's approach; one of the key program partners withdraws a few days before the launch). It is important that the communication team is prepared to effectively address and manage potential issues, is clear about the decision-making process that would be used in facing them (in other words, who should be involved or would have the final say on how the issue is addressed), and knows who is ultimately responsible to manage them to everyone's satisfaction.

As part of the process of considering potential issues and ways to address them, key program spokespeople should be identified to address issues that involve the mass media or other public forums, as well as for communications with key partners and stakeholders in case of potential crises.

Key Concepts

Action Plan

* The action plan encompasses the communication messages, channels, media, materials, and activities that are designed to serve and execute core communication strategies.

* All elements of the action plan are informed and guided by research findings of the situation and audience analysis. Messages, channels, and activities are key group specific and should be developed and tested with the input and participation of such groups. When multiple tactics can serve the same communication strategies and objectives, it is important to rank and prioritize them on the basis of several parameters that are discussed in this chapter (for example, message complexity, audience reach, cost-effectiveness).

Program Implementation

* The implementation of a health communication program is a combination of human resources and funds management with monitoring program activities and impact. It requires hard work, perseverance, and problem-solving skills.

* A spotless execution is a key attribute of the implementation and monitoring phase of the health communication cycle. Even well-designed interventions can fail to achieve expected results if they are not adequately implemented.

* Several actions contribute to effective program implementation as well as the definition of the process that would be followed at different stages of implementation and monitoring.

FOR DISCUSSION AND PRACTICE

1. Describe the key steps you would take to evaluate the cost-effectiveness of two different tactics you are considering to influence the behavior of young adults and therefore to reduce the use of drugs and alcohol consumption in this age group (for example, a mass media campaign targeted to consumer media and college newspapers and publications versus a peer-to-peer series of interactive workshops at local colleges and universities). Focus only on cost-effectiveness parameters (for example, financial cost, human resources, time), and assume that key groups and stakeholders have already discussed and validated both tactics in terms of audience suitability, needs, preferences, and cultural relevance.

2. If you completed questions 2 and 3 of the "For Discussion and Practice" section of Chapter Twelve, think of examples of core communication concepts, messages, media channels, and tactics to address the issue of skin cancer prevention among Luciana and her peers.

3. Think of recent health communication materials (print or online) or social media sites you may have seen. Describe their content, key messages, visual appearance and appeal, key features, as well as what you believe are the key groups the materials seek to reach and engage. Identify core questions of a potential focus group to pretest these materials or social media sites with representatives of key groups.

4. Identify a local community organization in your city or neighborhood. Contact the organization to learn in advance about any upcoming health communication intervention it may be planning, and whether it is organizing any meetings with the groups it serves and community members to secure their participation and input on program elements. Ask to attend the meeting and analyze and report on your observations about the process of community engagement and participation in the development of different elements of the action plan. Alternatively, research and review two to three case studies on the same topic and summarize lessons learned.

KEY TERMS

action plan

communication concepts

gatekeepers

implementation plan

monitoring

partnership plan

tactical plan

tactics

CHAPTER 14

EVALUATING OUTCOMES OF HEALTH COMMUNICATION INTERVENTIONS

The assessment of health communication interventions is an integral component of health communication in the twenty-first century. Not only is evaluation a much-emphasized topic in health communication nowadays, it is also directly connected to the issues of accountability and resource allocation within a variety of sectors. Health communication is accountable to the people whose health and social outcomes we seek to improve, to the lives we know we can save via prevention and system-changing strategies, to our partners, donors, and other key stakeholders. Evaluation allows us to recognize innovation for what it is and understand what its impact may be on a variety of health and social issues. It also allows us to harness the lessons learned from previous communication interventions and well-established principles and strategies so they can guide us in our attempt to address similar or relevant issues. Evaluation continues to be a much-debated and ever-evolving topic in health communication and many other fields. Yet sound evaluation practices and related evidence are what should guide us in our attempt to make a difference in people's health and lives.

CHAPTER OBJECTIVES

This chapter establishes the need to develop a detailed evaluation plan as part of the action plan (and prior to program implementation). It provides an overview of trends and strategies in program evaluation as well as practical guidance in developing evaluation strategies and plans that reflect key assumptions, goals, and objectives of the health communication intervention.

Evaluation as a Key Element of Health Communication Planning

Although most authors, organizations, and experiences support the importance of developing evaluation parameters and plans prior to program implementation and early in the planning process (National Cancer Institute at the National Institutes of Health, 2002; World Health Organization [WHO], 2003; O'Sullivan, Yonkler, Morgan, and Merritt, 2003), too often measurement is considered only toward the end of a health communication program. This frequently leads to confusion and disagreement about the measures of success, and also has a potential negative impact on the ability of health communication teams to advocate for any kinds of scale-up phase or similar intervention. For example, if activity-related outcomes are being evaluated for an online discussion, sample measurement parameters can include the number of participants, the quality and significance of the questions and opinions they expressed, or the overall contribution of the discussion to addressing key research questions for future programs or policies or changes in knowledge, attitudes, social norms, and behavior among key groups and stakeholders. All of these may be valuable evaluation parameters, but different team members and partners may have different ideas about what can be called a successful online discussion.

Including an evaluation plan early in program planning helps health communication teams and partners to focus on the intervention's ultimate goals and objectives, agree on expected outcomes, and combine their efforts to achieve them. This is only one of the many important benefits of early evaluation plans.

evaluation plans
Detailed descriptions of the behavioral, social, or organizational indicators as well as other parameters for assessing program outcomes

Sound **evaluation plans** should include a comprehensive description of key measurement parameters and expected short-term and long-term outcomes of the health communication intervention, as well as the methods that will be used to collect and analyze data in relation to these parameters.

This format applies to the different phases of evaluation (formative, process, and summative) as defined and described in this chapter, as well as to related research methods (see Chapter Eleven).

Finally, further insights into the importance of evaluation and early definition of key parameters and methods are provided by the literal meaning of the word *evaluate*, which is defined as "to ascertain or fix the value or worth of [something]" (*American Heritage Dictionary of the English Language*, 2004b). People tend to ascertain the value of things they intend to buy or to which they are considering committing significant personal or professional time well in advance of moving ahead with their final decisions. For example, it is likely that house buyers will conduct some research on current prices for comparable houses in the same neighborhood. This information helps them determine what they are willing to pay for the house they are considering and whether it is worth their investment. Why should it be different for health communication planning? The worth of financial, human resources, and time investments should be evaluated prior to the use of these resources.

One of the fundamental premises of this book is that health communication is an intrinsic part of everyone's life (du Pré, 2000). As in other aspects of life, health communication interventions should establish early in the process the worth of each investment in relation to specific outcomes and measurement parameters. This practice is also critical in establishing the overall value of the health communication field in the public health, health care, community development, and private sectors as well as in the context of intervention-driven multisectoral partnerships. In fact, the inclusion of an evaluation plan at the outset of the intervention can help avoid, or at least minimize, potential disappointments among key stakeholders, partners, donors, supervisors, and clients about the return of their investment. However, it is important to recognize the limitations and costs associated with the evaluation of health communication programs, another of the key topics of this chapter.

Overview of Key Evaluation Trends and Strategies: Why, What, and How We Measure

This section provides an overview of evaluation trends, strategies, and topics in regard to their application to the field of health communication. It also includes a brief discussion of selected frameworks and models used to measure the outcomes of health communication programs.

Evaluation plans should be developed at the same time as action plans and should refer to the outcome (behavioral, social, or organizational) and communication objectives as well as the overall program goals that have been established. In fact, in designing messages, activities, media, and materials, health communication teams should always ask themselves how these elements support the program's goals and objectives. Do they serve the communication strategy? What were the theoretical assumptions and models that informed program planning, and how do they influence evaluation?

This kind of questioning lays the groundwork for a detailed evaluation plan in which all elements are interconnected and considered. In this phase, it's also important to be aware of the limitations and costs of the evaluation process in health communication so that all decisions made will contribute to the objectivity of evaluation parameters.

Why We Measure

Measurement in health communication is needed for more than satisfying the requirements of donors, clients, partners, or other key stakeholders in a specific health issue or program. In fact, it is instrumental for a number of other reasons:

- Focusing health communication staff, partners, and intended audiences on shared goals
- Clarifying the overall program goal and objectives
- Identifying and comparing effective health communication practices
- Improving service delivery (for example, in the case of health communication interventions that also offer specific public or community services or communication consultants and agencies)
- Adjusting the program in progress by refining strategies and messages
- Assessing the overall cost-effectiveness of the program
- Determining program reproducibility and sustainability, as well as opportunities for a scaling-up phase
- Communicating results to key groups and stakeholders
- Implementing lessons learned from new models and strategies in future interventions
- Competing for economic and human resources

In short, measurement is a valuable tool not only in assessing results but also in achieving those results. Through different phases, research and evaluation methods help inform, focus, and refine health communication programs.

The Language of Evaluation and What We Measure

Measurement, specifically mathematics, is the language of science. We use mathematics and related measurement parameters in everyday life to evaluate quantity, size, shapes, relationships, and personal and professional achievements. Health communication incorporates mathematical principles in many evaluation models and metrics, and also integrates them with qualitative principles that focus on people's perspectives on the root causes of health and social issues as well as their evolution over time. Although this book does not go into the details of specific mathematical or qualitative models used in health communication, we define common terms in evaluation:

- **Evaluation**: The science and process of appraising the value or worth of a health communication intervention

- **Program assessment**: A general term used to indicate program-specific evaluation

- **Metrics**: Another term for *evaluation parameters.* Metrics should be quantifiable and define a system of parameters to assess periodically specific program elements or outcomes (for example, process-related results or changes in attitude and behavior).

- **Return on investment (ROI)**: The economic benefits that may derive from having invested funds and other resources (for example, human resources, time) in a program or activity. This parameter is commonly used in the commercial sector to assess the impact of marketing and communication activities on product sales. In public health and community development, it may be useful in assessing the benefits of specific communication interventions. For example, the return could be calculated in terms of the percentage of people who changed knowledge, attitude, or behavior or benefited from a specific change in social norms, policies, and related practices or the cost-saving benefits of interventions that promote preventive measures. This terminology is increasingly used in the nonprofit field (including public health). For example, the theme of the 2013 National Public Health Week focuses is called "Public Health Is ROI: Save Lives, Save Money," and seeks to "raise awareness about the importance of investing in a strong public health system" even at "times of uncertain funding and declining resources" (American Public Health Association, 2012).

- **Outcomes**: A general term describing changes in knowledge, comprehension, attitudes, skills, behavior, policies, or social norms as

evaluation
The science and process of appraising the value or worth of a health communication intervention

program assessment
A general term used to indicate program-specific evaluation

metrics
Metrics should be quantifiable and define a system of parameters to assess periodically specific program elements or outcomes (for example, process-related results or changes in attitude and behavior)

return on investment (ROI)
The economic benefits that may derive from having invested funds and other resources (for example, human resources, time) in a program or activity

outcomes
A general term describing changes in knowledge, comprehension, attitudes, skills, behavior, policies, or social norms as established by the program's outcome and communication objectives (Coffman, 2002; Freimuth, Cole, and Kirby, 2000)

impact

An outcome in relation to a specific change or, alternatively, the long-term change influenced by a program in relation to the overall program goal

behavioral impact

The specific behavioral results of a health communication program; measured in relation to specific behavioral indicators that have been established at the onset of planning

social change indicators and social impact

Indicators—and their impact—that measure changes in social interactions, norms, policies, and practices, as well as changes in the issues of concern (for example, poverty reduction, HIV/AIDS rates) (Rockefeller Foundation Communication and Social Change Network, 2001) or any of the key social determinants of health (for example, the living, working, and aging environment of key groups, access to services or information)

established by the program's outcome and communication objectives (Coffman, 2002; Freimuth, Cole, and Kirby, 2000). Outcomes are measured in relation to the estimated influence the health communication program had on each change. *Short-term outcomes* are usually related to process indicators as well as intermediate steps and key milestones as those set by the communication objectives (for example, changes in awareness, knowledge, skills). *Long-term outcomes* are the ultimate results of health communication programs and relate to the achievement of behavioral, social, and organizational objectives (outcome objectives).

• **Impact**: Sometimes refers to outcome in relation to a specific change (for example, behavioral impact) influenced by a health communication intervention or activity. In other models (Coffman, 2002), it is used to refer only to the long-term change influenced by a program in relation to the overall program goal, such as changes in disease incidence, which are almost never directly used as an evaluation parameter in actual communication practice because it tends to be the result of multiple interventions. This term may also have other connotations in different models (Bertrand, 2005).

• **Behavioral impact**: The specific behavioral results of a health communication program. This is measured in relation to specific behavioral indicators that have been established at the outset of planning.

• **Social change indicators and social impact**: Measures of changes in social norms, policies, and practices, as well as changes in the issues of concern (for example, poverty reduction, HIV/AIDS rates) (Rockefeller Foundation Communication and Social Change Network, 2001) or any of the key social determinants of health (for example, the living, working, and aging environment of key groups, access to services or information). Social indicators for evaluation are issue and key group specific. They are also a consequence of behavioral change within different groups and communities. For example, if the social indicator is the establishment of a new policy, this is likely to be the result of changes in the beliefs and behavior of policymakers, which led them to support and pass a new policy, and ultimately to raise their hands in favor of the new policy (which is a behavior). As previously mentioned, social change (or social impact as defined in some models) is a complex construct, and relies on behavioral changes at different levels of society. Such behavioral results tend to be interconnected (although they may be sequential or happening at different times, or as a result of different interventions, which often makes the social change process a long-term endeavor) and

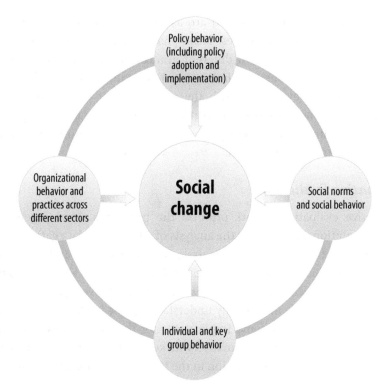

Figure 14.1   Social Change and Behavioral Indicators

supportive of each other in order to achieve long-lasting social results. Figure 14.1 describes social change in terms of the different kinds of behavioral results at multiple levels of society that may contribute to it. Several other types of behavioral indicators (in addition to those in the figure) may contribute to social change, and are health issue, key group, community, and stakeholder specific.

As these terms demonstrate, there are a variety of definitions as well as potential significances attributed to them. Using consistent theoretical assumptions and models throughout the planning and evaluation phases helps ensure the accuracy of measurement and limits the possibility of misunderstandings on evaluation parameters and terminology.

What We Measure in Different Evaluation Phases

Several authors (Bertrand, 2005; Freimuth, Cole, and Kirby, 2000; Hornick, 2002) identify three phases in the evaluation of health communication interventions: formative, process, and summative (the last is also called *outcome* or *impact evaluation*). These correspond to the research phases described in Chapter Eleven and are usually incorporated into effective health communication practices. These phases have evolved over time and may take different names in different evaluation models or incorporate a different set of evaluation indicators. For example, in this book, we combine process evaluation with the assessment of intermediate steps and key milestones (**progress indicators**) because these are all important steps in monitoring the progression of the communication intervention throughout its implementation.

progress indicators
Include intermediate steps and key milestones, which are assessed as part of progress evaluation

Formative Evaluation

Formative evaluation occurs prior to the program's development and implementation and includes the analysis of all research data gathered and shared as part of the situation analysis, audience profile, and pretesting. Formative evaluation informs, guides, and helps validate all elements of a health communication program. This is the phase of investigative research in which the focus is on (1) truly understanding the health or social topic as well as its root causes and implications for the well-being of intended communities, (2) sharing information with key groups and stakeholders, and (3) encouraging their participation in the health communication process.

Process Evaluation and Progress Evaluation

process evaluation
Used to compare key steps of the program's implementation with the original program plan and to measure expected results for specific activities, materials, media, and messages

Process evaluation is used to compare key steps of the program's implementation with the original program plan. Frequently process evaluation is also used to measure expected results for specific activities, materials, and messages. It refers to parameters such as audience reach, attendance, quality and tone of media coverage, message retention, ability to create alliances, newly formed partnerships, circulation numbers for key materials, page views for websites, number of followers on social media sites, and community or stakeholder endorsement of the program's key concepts and content.

As part of the evaluation phase, it is also important to monitor the intervention's impact vis-à-vis intermediate steps and key milestones, which we call here progress indicators. Sample progress indicators include short-term changes in awareness, knowledge, attitudes, skills, community participation levels, or other intermediate steps that may occur as a result of specific communication messages, activities, media, or materials. For example, some parameters for process evaluation of a communication workshop intended for health care providers may include the number of attendees, message retention, and attendees' feedback on and level of interest in the workshop's content. Sample progress indicators may include increased short-term awareness on the topic and the provider's intention to translate new information into actual clinical practice or to engage in effective dialogue with patients on this specific topic. These parameters can be assessed with various tools, for example, a questionnaire or evaluation form distributed to workshop attendees. Box 14.1 includes an example of how process evaluation was used to refine an entertainment-education program (a kind of health communication intervention; Freimuth and Quinn, 2004) to reach adolescents in Bolivia.

BOX 14.1. USING PROCESS EVALUATION DATA TO REFINE AN ENTERTAINMENT-EDUCATION PROGRAM IN BOLIVIA

In 1996, a Bolivian TV series on gender issues titled "Naked Dialogue" was produced and broadcast in twelve one-hour episodes on Saturday nights from March through May. The TV series targeted adolescents aged fifteen to nineteen with a talk-show format and was produced on a very small budget of US$12,000.

The evaluation team led by Johns Hopkins University/Population Communication Services developed an inexpensive research plan that consisted of two hundred randomly selected household interviews conducted midway and at the end of the broadcast period. In addition, four focus groups and forty-two in-depth interviews were conducted with low-income Bolivians before and after the series was broadcast.

The results of the midway survey shed light on the strengths and weaknesses of the script, broadcast schedule, and advertising strategy of the TV series. The research showed that the audience was interested on the issues addressed in "Naked Dialogue" (domestic violence, alcohol abuse, "machismo," reproductive health, homosexuality), but they did not like the talk-show format. Instead, the audience liked most the fictional segments of the TV series, which prompted them to identify with the characters portrayed.

The process evaluation also revealed that the Saturday night schedule was not the most appropriate for this young audience. Although TV shows broadcast on Saturday nights used to reach a considerable number of individuals among the general population, it did not have a high reach among members of the specific age group fifteen to nineteen. Actually, many of the individuals of the target audience were spending time with friends, and not watching TV at this particular time. The audience suggested broadcasting the TV show on a weekday evening.

Another important finding from this midway evaluation was the poor impact of the advertising strategy of the TV series. The production team had made a considerable investment in TV ads and newspapers ads. However, research showed that these ads did not reach the intended audience or did not prompt them to watch the show. Instead, the main source of awareness about the TV series was spontaneous tuning of the particular TV station before or during the TV series broadcast and word of mouth from friends and peers.

Changes were made, and in 1997, "Naked Dialogue" was renamed "Moon Skin" (Heimann, 2002). The new TV series adopted an all-fictional style similar to popular soap operas; it was broadcast on Thursday evenings; the investment in paid advertising was reduced, focusing the promotion of the new TV show in youth events to take full advantage of word-of-mouth communication among peers. "Moon Skin" became the second most popular program on Bolivian TV reaching 1,045,480 people. It won the first prize in the 1998 Latin American Festival of Videos Directed by Women.

Conducting midway surveys to monitor and evaluate entertainment-education programs increases the likelihood of success. Although these studies were designed initially to document program impact, the research results provided important information for program redesign and reformulation.

References

Heimann, D. "Reaching Youth Worldwide: Part III—JHU/CCP Programmes—Latin America." The Communication Initiative Network, www.comminit.com/node/1772. Retrieved Sept. 2002.

Valente, T. *Evaluating Health Communication Programs*. Oxford University Press, 2002), 80.

Source: Saba, W. "Using Process Evaluation Data to Refine an Entertainment-Education Program in Bolivia." Unpublished case study, 2012b. Used by permission.

Process and progress evaluation helps health communication teams keep track of the overall quality of the program's implementation as well as its progress toward outcome objectives. This is directly connected to the need for spotless execution, which is one of the key characteristics of effective implementation and monitoring of the health communication process.

Finally, progress evaluation should not be used to assess the direct impact of specific activities, media, or materials on long-term changes in knowledge, attitudes, skills, or behavior. This direct cause-and-effect relationship is somewhat difficult to establish in health communication because "change does not often occur as a result of just one specific activity" (National Cancer Institute at the National Institutes of Health, 2002, p. 45), and requires that we mirror the multiple ways communication on health and social issues actually takes place in everyday life.

summative evaluation
A phase of evaluation that measures the program's efficacy in relation to the outcome and communication objectives initially established by the program

Summative Evaluation (Outcome or Impact Evaluation in Different Models)

Summative evaluation measures program efficacy in relation to the outcome (behavioral, social, and organizational) and communication objectives initially established by the program. In other words, it "measures the extent to which change occurs. In health communication programs, the primary objective is usually a health-related behavior" (Bertrand, 2005). Behavioral impact is also the key evaluation parameter of communication for behavioral impact (COMBI) programs (WHO, 2003; see also Chapter Two). Behavioral change at different levels of society is also a key indicator—along with social change—of communication for development (C4D) (see Chapter Two). See also Figure 14.1 for a visual representation of how behavioral change at different levels of society may influence social change. The framework for analysis and intervention planning proposed in Figure 14.1 assumes that social change is sustainable only when different levels of society are affected by the health communication intervention. In fact, continuing to focus only on individual and community behavior may not be sufficient to address health and social issues, which often require changes in the behaviors of key influentials (for example, policymakers, philanthropists, clinicians) and their organizations. This is likely to have an impact on the social and policy environment and therefore on intersecting issues of equity, determinants of health and socioeconomic development, and public health outcomes.

With that in mind, often the primary objective may be a specific social or organizational outcome that addresses existing barriers to behavioral results. Yet, because social or organizational outcomes are the result of gradual behavioral changes by key stakeholders, communities, policymakers, and professionals from different sectors and levels of society, behavioral outcomes are still a key measurement. Changes in behaviors that may lead to social, policy or organizational change, as well as long-term changes in other indicators (for example, awareness, knowledge, attitudes, or skills) that have been established by outcome or communication objectives, should also be measured as part of summative evaluation. The latter (long-term changes vis-à-vis communication objectives) should be analyzed to understand and document the process that leads to behavioral, social, and organizational results, and help demonstrate linkages (or lack of) between such results and the health communication intervention. See "Linking Outcomes to a Specific Health Communication Intervention" in this chapter.

Moreover, summative evaluation, and related outcomes, should include an analysis of the kinds of results that are poised to improve the social, living, and working environments of key groups and relevant communities. For example, did policymakers and lead urban planners commit to design or already design an improved transportation system for an underserved neighborhood? Or did large chain stores start to offer nutritious food such as fruit and vegetables within so-called food deserts? Or did local philanthropists pledge funds for the development of a community-based recreational facility? Or did health care providers who attend patients in a specific ZIP Code start to provide social support and health information at an adequate health literacy level, as reported by their patients? Or did local public officials distribute city resources on the basis of need and not of privilege in implementing a new biking program or establishing new public parks? The program's impact on key social determinants of health and the behaviors of those stakeholders who can positively affect them is an important parameter in summative evaluation. This is an additional example of how social change is the result of multiple and cumulative behavioral changes at different levels of society (see Figure 14.1).

Finally, in some mass media health communication campaigns, audience reach is part of summative evaluation. In this book, audience reach is considered one of the measurement parameters of process evaluation.

Key Facts and Trends on Evaluating Health Communication Outcomes

Evaluation is considered an essential step by health communication theorists and practitioners. However, too many health organizations do not conduct evaluation of health communication programs. For example, "a study of 50 published nutrition and/or physical activity campaigns" showed that "fewer than 1/3 of the campaigns expressed goals in measurable terms" (Health Communication Unit, 2003a, pp. 28–29). Moreover, "goals were rarely formulated on the basis of data descriptive of target audiences" (p. 29). Similar findings also applied to audience segmentation, consumer research, and theory-based communication approaches. In fact, although the campaigns often mentioned social marketing as a planning framework, social marketing or behavioral theories concepts were rarely integrated into planning (Health Communication Unit, 2003b; Alcalay and Bell, 2000). No matter what the planning framework or theoretical field may be, lack of consistency and the absence of clearly defined objectives are not well poised to achieve long-term results.

In practice, most organizations are pressed for results and would like to conduct some kind of measurement. Many also firmly believe in the importance of evaluation. Still, only rarely do annual budgets include funds for evaluating health communication interventions or training human resources, which in the long term may positively influence the cost-effectiveness of the evaluation process. When evaluation is part of program planning, it tends to be formative evaluation. Process, progress, and summative evaluations are often perceived as too costly or inconclusive. In addition, lack of adequate training and understanding of evaluation tools

Table 14.1   Drawbacks of Evaluation

• Cost

• Time

• Chance of measuring the wrong variables and indicators

• Questionable accuracy for interventions with limited scope, reach, and duration

• Potential bias in evaluation methods or tools

• Hard to do if not planned ahead

• Results may be affected by independent influences on program's outcomes

and methods may result in a series of barriers to evaluation that may be perceived as insurmountable.

Evaluation has several drawbacks (Table 14.1), some of which are more difficult to overcome than others. Recognizing evaluation barriers and drawbacks helps set realistic expectations among team members, partners, donors, clients, and key stakeholders about the program's results and the overall evaluation process.

A major limitation in the evaluation of health communication interventions is related to the complexity of human behavior. Health communication efforts attempt to achieve behavioral or social change. However, because all people are influenced by multiple sources of information and social networks (both offline and online), as well as personal and professional experiences, it may be difficult to make a direct connection between the actual health communication program (or, even more difficult, specific communication activities) and the behavioral or social outcome. It is important to remember that "communication programs generally occur in a real-world setting, where there are many other influences on the intended audiences. [In many cases], it can be impossible to isolate the effect of a particular communication activity, or even the effect of a communication program on a specific intended audience" (National Cancer Institute at the National Institutes of Health, 2002, p. 45).

Say that a woman who is forty-five years old suddenly decides to change her previous behavior and see her physician for annual breast cancer screenings. It may be challenging to define with certainty to which degree her behavior has been influenced by an ongoing health communication intervention on this topic or that her best friend was just diagnosed with advanced breast cancer at age forty-three. Similarly, when a new law is passed to ban workplace discrimination against people who suffer from a specific medical condition, it may be difficult to ascertain which factors have weighed more in the legislators' decision: ongoing mass media and advocacy efforts, direct experiences of loved ones, professional observations, personal ambition, or something else. In both examples, chances are that all of these factors influenced the outcome. Being aware of the challenges of evaluation is fundamental to the design of adequate evaluation plans, which should include a combination of quantifiable parameters and qualitative analyses and sometimes rely on intermediate steps and other quantifiable measures to assess progress- and program-related results. This also helps link outcomes to the actual intervention.

In spite of potential limitations, ignoring this fundamental step of health communication planning may harm the overall perception of the field's efficacy and contribution, as well as the ability to secure funds and resources for subsequent health communication interventions. Most important, it will leave health communication teams without adequate instruments to evaluate the significance of their efforts.

Health organizations should find the optimal balance of evaluation, cost, and other factors that are related to measurement. This balance may vary from organization to organization. "Small nongovernmental organizations (NGOs) with limited resources may opt to perform only one of these types of evaluation [formative, process, or summative], whereas a major communication program with national scope would be remiss to exclude any of them" (Bertrand, 2005).

Still, in defining evaluation parameters, it is important to set realistic expectations. For example, impact measurement (if impact is defined as the effect of the program on the overall program goal, such as changes in disease incidence or mortality) may be difficult and take a long time to assess. Outcome evaluation such as behavioral and social impact or changes in knowledge, attitudes, and skills may include more realistic parameters. Therefore, it is important to select indicators that are strongly linked to the achievement of the overall program goal. This is already a common practice in many fields. For example, "increased immunization levels predict decreased child mortality. Increasing numbers of girls in school is often cited as a predictor of economic progress" (Rockefeller Foundation Communication and Social Change Network, 2001).

Because health communication is a cycle, this brings us back to several of the initial questions of communication planning. What should people do as a result of the communication intervention? Should they immunize their children? Send their girls to school and be proud of them? What are some of the social and political barriers to recommended behaviors and what kinds of stakeholders should the intervention engage to remove such barriers and promote equity in health and social outcomes? What are the intermediate steps to encourage these behaviors, and were they met by the program? Was the program well executed in relation to activities that supported intermediate objectives? Did the program reach the number of people originally estimated? Can you quantify the actual behavioral impact of the program? What about its social impact?

In health communication, behavioral change at different levels of society is the ideal standard measurement. However, evaluation needs to set realistic parameters that vary from program to program and case to case. In doing so, it is important to take into account that the complexity of evaluation increases with the complexity of the parameter being measured (Freimuth, Cole, and Kirby, 2000). Key evaluation parameters need to be mutually agreed on with all program partners, team members, donors, clients, or other key stakeholders.

Finally, participatory evaluation, which complements and includes the practice of participatory research (described in Chapters Six and Eleven), is an important evaluation approach (Bertrand, 2005) as compared with more traditional evaluation methodologies that usually rely on expert evaluation. In participatory evaluation, key audiences or their representatives lead or are part of the evaluation team. They contribute to the design of the evaluation plan and the analysis of key results as well as overall feedback. This approach is part of the participatory model of communication planning (see Chapter Ten).

Opportunities for participation of key groups and relevant communities should be always explored. For example, a 2008 study in the United States revealed that communities are dissatisfied with the lack of participation of community members in local research efforts (Cargo and Mercer, 2008) and other interventions. The appropriate level of participation by key groups, communities, and stakeholders, as well as the degree of expert input and involvement, are likely to be influenced by several factors, including cultural preferences and the specific characteristics of the health issue, audience, or country. In general, even with more traditional approaches, it should be common practice of effective health communication to establish and analyze measurement parameters with representatives of key groups, community members, and program partners. This is frequently accomplished by involving or soliciting the opinion of professional organizations, community groups, patient groups, and other constituency groups that attend or represent intended audiences. Finally, it is important to be aware that "participatory evaluation may not meet the methodical rigor of the scientific community to measure effectiveness" (Bertrand, 2005). Therefore, the participation of health communication practitioners, research experts, and other professionals to provide process facilitation and technical assistance may be critical to preserve such rigor.

Use of Logic Models for the Evaluation of Health Communication Interventions

The theoretical assumptions or planning framework of the health communication intervention can be summarized together with its components (key factors contributing to the health or social issue as highlighted by the situation and audience analysis, goal, objectives, strategies, tactics, and others) as part of a logic model. Logic models link program goals, objectives, strategies, activities, and outcomes with different indicators and monitoring, research, and evaluation phases (MR&E). Logic models are tools to provide a framework for the health communication intervention and its evaluation (see Chapter Two for a more detailed discussion and an example of logic models). For example, the theory of reasoned action (see Chapter Two) "is one of the most frequently used in campaign evaluation" (Coffman, 2002, p. 18). Logic models are increasingly used in the evaluation of health communication programs to organize and connect various program components with the program's outcomes (Coffman, 2002; University of Wisconsin, 2005; US Department of Health and Human Services, Office of Minority Health, 2010; Schiavo, Gonzalez-Flores, Ramesh, and Estrada-Portales, 2011; Parks, Shrestha, and Chitnis, 2008; WHO, 2012c).

Logic models rely on various terminologies and may emphasize different aspects of program planning, implementation, and evaluation. Yet, their basic purpose is to provide a logical structure for program planning and monitoring, research, and evaluation. Appendix A includes a list of online resources of how to develop a logic model (including different kinds of logic model templates as applied to various health areas). An example of logic model, as applied to the evaluation of a national infant mortality prevention program, is also included in Chapter Two.

How We Measure: Quantitative, Qualitative, and Mixed Methods

Measurement for each of the three types of evaluation uses traditional marketing, communication, and participatory research methodologies. Some of these are described in Chapter Eleven as part of the formative research phase that is needed to complete the situation and audience analysis.

For complex analyses, it is likely that many health organizations—as well as the communities and groups they may engage in the evaluation process—may need the help of evaluation experts. For example, assessing changes in attitudes and behaviors requires intensive efforts in a specific geographical area and period of time. Pre- and postintervention studies are needed to assess the baseline (in terms of frequent health behaviors or attitudes) as well as the impact of the communication program on such parameters. Because these studies require a significant financial commitment and specific skills, health organizations often turn to evaluation experts or research organizations from both the public and private sectors. This is also important to preserve the objectivity of evaluation findings. Within the context of participatory research, such experts work primarily to facilitate the overall process and to provide technical assistance to organizations, communities, key groups, and stakeholders as they work together to evaluate the intervention's results.

As part of all kinds of evaluation efforts, it's important to remember that behavioral and social change occur only over time. Only long-term efforts can generate sustainable behavioral results, which may also lead to social change. Therefore, measuring too soon after the program's launch may show some modest changes but will not guarantee that these changes can be sustained over time. Ideally, measurement should take place at various intervals using tracking surveys or other methodologies mentioned in Chapter Eleven. If this is not possible, summative evaluation efforts should take place later in program implementation.

In general, measurement of health communication programs relies on qualitative and quantitative methods. In the new media age, most of these methods can be implemented over various media platforms: in person or via telephone, texting, Skype, or online, just to cite a few examples. A detailed description of research and evaluation methods is beyond the scope of this book. Table 14.2 lists sample qualitative and quantitative methods.

Table 14.2   Sample Qualitative and Quantitative Methods for the Assessment of Health Communication Interventions

Qualitative Methods	Quantitative Methods
• In-depth interviews with members of intended audiences, program participants, or other key stakeholders before and after the program	• Pre- and postsurveys to be implemented in person, online, by telephone, or other methods (see Chapter Eleven)
• Focus groups	• Tracking surveys, which collect evaluation data at different time intervals
• Completion of evaluation forms after specific activities (for process evaluation only)	• Control and intervention groups in which groups are either randomized or selected in a way that one group will be exposed to the health communication intervention and the other will not
• Evidence of endorsement, such as letters of support or actual program participation from key influentials (for formative and process evaluation only)	• Online surveys and opinion polls to take the pulse of progress throughout program implementation and also to evaluate summative results
• Panel studies, that is, pre- and postintervention studies, which involve the same panel of key stakeholders or representatives of key groups and relevant communities	
• Community dialogue, public consultations, and other participatory research methods	

Most of these methods carry several limitations, such as in the case of control and intervention groups for which other differences may exist and have an impact on evaluation data (National Cancer Institute at the National Institutes of Health, 2002). As qualitative and quantitative methods can elucidate important aspects of program assessment, the use of mixed methods is increasingly supported by existing literature and applied in program assessment (Tucker-Brown, 2012; Schiavo, Gonzalez-Flores, Ramesh, and Estrada-Portales, 2011; Schiavo, Estrada-Portales, and Hoeppner, 2012) either by combining different methods or within the same method (for example, the inclusion of open-ended questions in surveys). In fact, "**mixed methodology** is a design for collecting, analyzing, and mixing both quantitative and qualitative data in a single study or series of studies to understand an evaluation problem" (Tucker-Brown, 2012). There are several reasons to conduct mixed method evaluations, of which some of the most important include the mutual validation of qualitative and quantitative findings and the richness of multiple perspectives that can be derived only from the strategic use of integrated research methods to explain the magnitude, percentages, context, and reasons for program results. Ultimately, the selection of specific evaluation methods depends on several factors, including budget, purpose of the evaluation, audience characteristics, needs, preferences, type of health organization, the extent to which the method enables input and participation of key groups and stakeholders, health issue–related factors, donor, partner, or client requirement and preferences, and many others.

mixed methodology
"Mixed methodology is a design for collecting, analyzing, and mixing both quantitative and qualitative data in a single study or series of studies to understand an evaluation problem" (Tucker-Brown, 2012)

Establishing Evaluation Parameters: A Consensus Process

Effective health communication programs include mutually agreed-on evaluation terms (Cole and others, 1995) and parameters, as decided via a consensus process that includes the health communication team, key partners, donors, and representatives of key groups. This is a common procedure in participatory evaluation as it is important to focus everyone's efforts on common goals as well as to minimize the possibility for misunderstanding and unrealistic expectations about the potential program's outcomes. As Sarriot (2002) describes, "There can be benefits, particularly improved collective learning in agreeing on shared and critical dimensions of evaluation." This includes "the contextual definition and selection of indicators of progress" (p. 91). This general principle applies to all forms of evaluation.

For process evaluation, the commercial sector as well as many health communication agencies have been using models that rely on mutually agreed-on parameters. Although this method may take various empirical formats, the overall premise is to set specific qualitative and quantitative parameters for each activity or material of a health communication program. Data collection methods are also included for each parameter. These criteria are discussed and agreed on by the program's funder, partners, health communication agencies, and all other key stakeholders involved in program planning. A written report is usually provided on the basis of the parameters previously agreed. (See Appendix A for a sample chart: "A7: Process and Progress Evaluation: Establishing Mutually Agreed Parameters.") This method is also suitable to provide a structured framework for all kinds of interactions on evaluation matters between the health communication team, key communities, and stakeholders.

Although this method is currently being used primarily for process evaluation, the overall principle of establishing mutually agreed-on parameters is important to all forms and phases of evaluation. Health communication is an integrated approach that frequently involves diverse stakeholders and uses multiple approaches. Potential evaluation parameters should reflect the diversity of approaches and stakeholders. Unifying these parameters under a mutually agreed-on principle helps meet the expectations that have been set with donors, communities, partners, team members, key groups, and stakeholders.

Integrating Evaluation Parameters That Are Inclusive of Vulnerable and Underserved Populations

As previously discussed throughout this book, public health and global health have been broadening their focus to go beyond traditional preventive or medical interventions. Today's emphasis is on improving the health of an entire population with the aim of reducing health disparities among populations' groups. This approach to public health is also referred to as *population health* and addresses a broad range of social determinants of health that affect health outcomes on a population level, such as environment, social structure, resource distribution, social support, access to services, information, socioeconomic opportunities, and many others.

Health communication has an important role within this agenda. As a reminder, the goal of *Healthy People 2020* for health communication interventions over one decade is to "use health communication strategies and health information technology (IT) to improve population health outcomes and health care quality, and to achieve health equity" (US Department of Health and Human Services, 2012b). Within this framework, evaluating outcomes of health communication interventions also needs to consider research questions and parameters that are specifically suited to assess results within vulnerable and underserved groups of a given population. Although such questions need to be specific to the health or social issue and key group, sample questions should attempt to assess the intervention's impact on health equity, as for example in the following:

- Were vulnerable or underserved populations included, and could they effectively access key components of the communication intervention? Did they have a chance to participate in the design of the overall intervention and data and issue analysis? If yes, how do results among these groups compare to results within the rest of the population vis-à-vis the program's outcome and communication objectives?

- If these groups were not included to a satisfactory extent (for example, in large percentages), are results relevant and which specific issues should be addressed to maximize inclusion of such groups as part of program refinement? What kinds of organizations or community leaders should be partnering on this intervention to maximize cultural competence, use, and access to communication activities, materials, channels, and media among vulnerable and underserved groups?

Because evaluation is an essential component of the health communication cycle, we may effectively create change only by making sure that our measurement strategies and key research questions also include parameters that are inclusive of vulnerable and underserved populations. The standardization of this practice will generate important lessons and evidence-based data that are sure to contribute toward the *Healthy People 2020* goal for health communication.

Evaluating New Media-Based Interventions: Emerging Trends and Models

A key question in approaching the evaluation of new media–based interventions is whether key assumptions should be the same or different from the assumptions we discussed in this chapter for the evaluation of comprehensive health communication interventions. New media have broken new ground and provided us with unlimited possibilities to connect with people across the globe. At the same time, we seek to use them strategically to influence health and social change, so we use or should use them in integration with other communication areas, activities, and channels because we want to make sure to reach people in all places where they discuss and engage with health and illness and their root causes.

With that said, the summative evaluation of new media–based interventions may rely on a different set of research tools and terminology but it is still grounded in the communication planning and evaluation principles used by other kinds of media. The scope of this book does not include providing specific information on the evaluation of specific new media. Our focus in this section is on general principles that should be considered throughout new media evaluation. To this aim, Figure 14.2 frames the contribution of different components of the health communication intervention as they may relate to results, and ultimately, improved public health outcomes at the general population level. The integration of a variety of media and health communication areas should be reflected also in the way we approach evaluation. See "A8: Evaluation of New Media–Based Interventions: A Proposed (and Evolving) Logic Model" in Appendix A.

Use of Mixed Methods (Online and Offline)

New media have provided health communication teams and researchers with opportunities to test communication interventions for the efficacy of messages, visual appeal, and other key elements. "The Internet, in

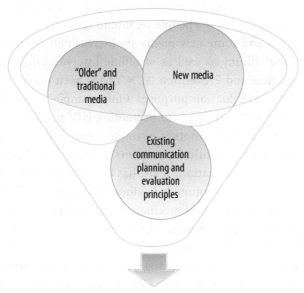

Behavioral, social, and organizational results that support improved public health outcomes

Figure 14.2 Integrating New Media and Other Communication Areas in Approaching Health Communication Planning and Evaluation

particular, provides tremendous opportunities to expose study participants to messages, assign them to experimental conditions, and test message effects" (Evans, Davis, and Zhang, 2008).

Other authors have also discussed the difference between **online efficacy** (the efficacy of a communication intervention as it relates to people's ability to understand and act on key communication messages and activities within an online or new media setting or virtual world) and **offline effectiveness** (the effectiveness of an online or new media–based intervention as it relates to people's ability to integrate recommendations from the same communication intervention in their everyday life vis-à-vis behavioral, social, and organizational objectives) as key principles in the evaluation of new media–based interventions. In fact, Evans, Davis, and Zhang (2008, p. 142) clarify that "an efficacy study is designed to evaluate the effects of an intervention under optimum conditions whereas an effectiveness study evaluates the effects of an intervention under real world conditions (Flay, 1996). But without first determining the efficacy of the campaign messages, results of effectiveness studies can be difficult to interpret." This principle applies to the importance of pretesting and formative research but also to the implications of process and progress evaluation vis-à-vis the assessment of behavioral, social, and organizational outcomes. Yet we should keep in mind that what works online may not work in real life given potential existing barriers within the living, working, and aging environment of the people we intend to reach.

The Internet and some new media are increasingly used for the evaluation of online efficacy as well as of offline interventions. The Centers for Disease Control and Prevention (CDC) have been on the forefront of new media use for evaluation purposes. One example is the CDC's *Take Charge. Take the Test* campaign for promoting HIV testing (Davis, Uhrig, Rupert, and Harris, 2008). Another example, again from the CDC, is the use of Whyville, a virtual world for preteens for both a health communication campaign and its evaluation. "CDC has been participating in Whyville for the past few years to promote behavioral health changes." "Using their avatars, students can get virtual vaccinations, wash their hands, cover their mouths when they cough, and more. But if they aren't vigilant, they can catch the 'WhyFlu' as well as spread it. The avatars can also earn badges that say 'I've been vaccinated in real life', giving CDC an idea of self-reported adoption among kids" (Chief Information Officer Council, 2009), which may be also an indication of real-life action and offline effectiveness among users. Figure 14.3 is an image of the 2009 flu vaccine campaign in Whyville. The use of Whyville or other virtual worlds may be helpful for online efficacy studies because it provides an opportunity to test messages and activities.

online efficacy
The efficacy of a communication intervention as it relates to people's ability to understand and act on key communication messages and activities within an online or new media setting or virtual world

offline effectiveness
The effectiveness of an online or new media–based intervention as it relates to people's ability to integrate recommendations from the same communication intervention in their everyday life vis-à-vis behavioral, social, and organizational objectives

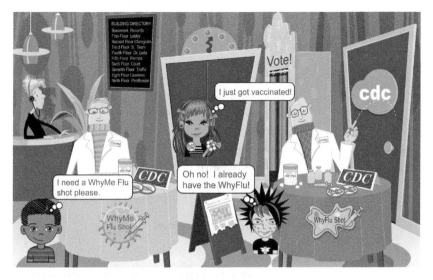

Figure 14.3   Flu Vaccine Campaign 2009 in Whyville

Source: Flu Vaccine Campaign 2009 in Whyville. www.whyville.net/smmk/nice?source=cdc. Copyright © 2009 Numedeon, Inc. Used by permission.

Yet new media–based evaluation is not likely to reach everyone, because it may leave out less-experienced new media users or nonusers as well as disadvantaged groups. Several factors point to the importance of continuing to use mixed methods (qualitative and quantitative and online and offline) to combine online efficacy and offline effectiveness assessments. Such reasons include the importance of (1) a participatory approach to evaluation in which vulnerable, underserved, and low health literacy populations are included; (2) assessing offline effectiveness in real-world settings where group dynamics, qualitative data, and multiple perspectives can shed light on important aspects of the communication intervention; and (3) considering that there is no real substitution to the human factor when we attempt to create ownership and commitment on health and social issues.

Other key factors for method selection may be specific to a given methodology, health topic, or group. For example, the moderator has a much more limited role in online focus groups and, therefore, it may be more difficult to make sure that everyone participates. Also, the cultural competence of specific methods (both offline and online) should be assessed because it relates to key groups. As for the evaluation of all kinds of health communication interventions, these and other factors should be considered in selecting the right combination of online and offline research tools. Table 14.3 includes examples of offline and online research tools and methods. Many of these methodologies can be implemented in both settings.

Table 14.3   Sample Tools for the Evaluation of New Media—Based Interventions

Online tools	Analytics (used to track process indicators such as number of visitors, page views)
	Web-based panels
	Survey tools
	Monitoring systems (used to monitor trends, opinions, news)
	Social media—specific analytical tools
	Virtual worlds
Offline and Online	*Quantitative methods*
	• Pre- and postsurveys
	• Tracking surveys
	• Satisfaction surveys
	• Control and intervention groups
	Qualitative Methods
	• Pre- and post-in-depth interviews of members of intended audience, program participants, key stakeholders
	• Panel studies
	• Focus groups
	• Monitoring systems
	• Evidence of endorsement from key influentials (formative and process evaluation only)

Monitoring: An Essential Element of Program Evaluation

Monitoring primarily addresses four areas:

- News and trends on the health or disease area, intended audiences, socially determined factors influencing a specific health issue or topic, and policies
- Ongoing feedback by key groups and stakeholders on program content or key elements (vehicles)
- Process and progress indicators throughout program implementation
- Collection of summative evaluation data

Information from these four areas contributes to the program's implementation, potential success, and refinement in various ways. For example, monitoring of news and trends on the health or disease area, as well as related policies, key groups, and contributing factors, may provide the health communication team with an opportunity to react promptly to emerging needs and audience preferences, new scientific data, health products, services, or media that need to be considered by or incorporated in the intervention. Monitoring news and trends can also help address and manage criticisms from other constituency groups or develop new alliances by being informed on current thinking and key players in a specific health or social field.

Evaluation data should be monitored and collected in relation to the process and progress indicators and the outcome parameters established by the evaluation plan. Because monitoring has a variety of purposes, some of the methods to collect, share, and use data may be different, and others may overlap. For example, monitoring news and trends relies primarily on the review of relevant media coverage and online and peer-reviewed publications and social media sites. Ongoing contacts and conversations with key opinion leaders and stakeholders in a specific health field can point to emerging trends and information, which are used to secure ongoing feedback and input from key groups and relevant communities on different aspects of program implementation, content, media, core messages, and materials.

In collecting data that will be used for process or summative evaluation, the health communication team should refer to the indicators and methods described in the original evaluation plan. Process and progress evaluation data can be collected at various times in program implementation and for each specific activity. They can also be used to adjust the content or the process of specific communication vehicles, media, and channels. For example, if the public relations component of a health communication program does not secure the expected media coverage (which should be quantified in terms of number of impressions or relevant articles on major publications; see Chapter Five), the team may need to consider different story angles or timing for the release of additional news about the communication intervention. Similarly, if a physician workshop does not attract the desired number of attendees, several factors (including the workshop's venue, the appeal of key speakers, the event's timing, or the extent of publicity efforts to announce the workshop) should be evaluated and reconsidered in preparation for the next event. Specific process indicators (for example, audience reach, level of satisfaction with the logistics and appeal of a specific activity, message retention) should be included as part of the evaluation plan. Progress indicators (for example, short-term changes in awareness, knowledge, or skills or the discussion of a new policy or plans to improve the transportation system or access to nutritious food in a given neighborhood) should be evaluated periodically at regular intervals (depending on the kind of indicator).

In-depth interviews, postevent questionnaires, surveys, focus groups, observation, and other methods described in Chapter Eleven as well as in this chapter are used to monitor and track summative evaluation data and process and progress indicators. Sometimes specific services can be used to track process indicators such as audience reach. For example, in the United States, the reach of mass media campaigns that aim to secure television coverage can be assessed using the Nielsen Station Index, a TV audience service that generates data on the number of people or households who are watching a specific program in a given television market (geographical area). Also, Google News provides a service for which users can select key words on the topic of their interest (for example, *global hand washing*) and receive daily or weekly reports on all kinds of print and online coverage on the topic. Such information can be helpful in analyzing the frequency and the tone with which the health communication intervention is covered by the media as well as new trends and facts on the specific health issue.

All monitoring data should be collected and discussed with key team members, partners, key groups, and stakeholders in the health communication program. This is usually accomplished through periodic reports and presentations that also provide a strategic analysis of the data being collected and their implications for the health communication intervention. The input and feedback of all recipients of these reports will contribute to the analysis of the data in relation to potential adjustments the program needs to make. For a while now, the overall tendency and recommended path in health communication has been to maximize participation of key stakeholders, team members, and audience representatives in the monitoring and analysis of all data collected during program implementation (Health Communication Partnership, 2003; Exchange, 2001). Table 14.4 gives examples of methods for the collection and reporting of various kinds of monitoring data.

Linking Outcomes to a Specific Health Communication Intervention

contribution analysis
The analysis of other plausible alternatives or concomitant interventions, if any, that may have contributed to the results of a health communication intervention

Different professionals often ask how they can link outcomes to a specific health communication intervention. As previously mentioned, communication takes place in a real-world environment, so it is always possible that other external factors also contributed to results. Yet several methods can be used to analyze and make a correlation between a program and its potential outcomes.

For example, **contribution analysis** (the analysis of other plausible alternatives or concomitant interventions, if any, that may have contributed

Table 14.4   Examples of Areas of Monitoring with Related Data Collection and Reporting Methods

Monitoring	Data-collection methods	Reporting
News and trends	Literature review (including peer-reviewed and trade publications, organizational newsletters, annual reports, and so on) Review and analysis of mass media coverage Internet searches and new media monitoring Online monitoring services Informal conversations and meetings with key stakeholders, key groups, health organizations, colleagues, community members, and others	Periodic media analysis reports (at least monthly) Presentation and discussion at team meetings E-mail summaries to all key program stakeholders and team members
Ongoing audience and stakeholder feedback	Informal conversations and meetings with key stakeholders and other relevant organizations and groups Activity-specific methods that are already part of process and progress monitoring	Presentation and discussion at team meetings E-mail summaries Can be incorporated in monthly media analysis reports
Process and progress indicators	Activity- or material-specific methods	
	Events	
	◦ Postevent questionnaires for audience feedback	Event evaluation summary for distribution to team members and program stakeholders*
	Mass media and new media campaigns	
	◦ Collection of media clips generated by the program to analyze message tone and frequency, audience reach, and so on	Monthly media coverage reports*
	◦ Use of specific services (Nielsen Index Rating) for audience reach of television coverage	
	◦ New media monitoring (including content of posts by users)	
	◦ Virtual worlds	
	Online activities and materials	
	◦ Number of hits on home page or specific content pages of a program-related website (to assess Internet traffic)	Monthly reports*
	All activities and materials	
	◦ Pre- and postactivity in-depth interviews with audience representatives, key stakeholders, and others	Can be incorporated as part of reports listed previously*
Summative evaluation data (in relation to the original evaluation plan and indicators)	Collection methods (offline and online) vary and should reflect the evaluation plans. They can include focus groups, in-depth interviews, panel studies, surveys, and others.	Final evaluation report to be developed, shared, and discussed with all team members, key program stakeholders, and key groups. It should include process and summative evaluation as well as data collected for other areas and phases of monitoring. Can be presented at professional conferences as well as distributed and publicized using different communication channels.

*These reports can be summarized in a preliminary process report and should be included as part of the final evaluation report.

to the results of a health communication intervention) can help isolate the actual impact of the communication intervention. The use of consistent models for program planning and evaluation—along with the development of specific outcomes and communication objectives to be expressed in measurable terms—also contributes to the accuracy of this kind of analysis by establishing a clear and logical path for the intervention and its potential results. Other key methods include the existence of sound monitoring systems, the collection and analysis of process and progress indicators, and the use of mixed research methods to validate findings via different perspectives and data sets. In general terms, monitoring and reporting on various process and progress indicators should make it easier to show a natural progression (or lack of) toward potential results as they relate to a specific communication intervention.

The following criteria to link outcomes to communication interventions were developed by Parks, Shresta, and Chitnis (2008, p. 28) as part of *Essentials for Excellence*, a research, monitoring, and evaluation methodology for UNICEF, and could be useful in assessing program linkages to actual outcomes:

- "Outcomes appeared at an appropriate time after your efforts began.
- Outcomes faded when your efforts stopped.
- Only those outcomes appeared that you should have affected.
- Outcomes appeared only where or when the program was active.
- The biggest outcomes appeared where or when you did the most.
- There are no plausible alternatives that could account for the outcomes, or if there are, you have recognized these other explanations and objectively accounted for them in your conclusion."

Evaluation Report

The evaluation report should include a detailed analysis of all data collected for process, progress, and summative evaluation in relation to the original evaluation plan, methods, and indicators. The evaluation framework and its theoretical basis should be consistent throughout the intervention. Interim progress and summative evaluation reports should be addressed in different sections of the final evaluation report.

Evaluating can be a "moving target" (Kennedy and Abbatangelo, 2005, p. 13), at least in reference to process and progress evaluations. Although potential revisions of the original evaluation plan always should be minimized, it is possible that certain aspects of the health communication intervention will be changed or refined in response to specific process evaluation data (Kennedy and Abbatangelo, 2005). Such revisions are justified primarily by emerging needs and preferences of key groups and stakeholders and specific observations and data collected during program implementation.

Take the example of a town hall meeting, which included the participation of breast cancer prevention organizations and patient groups as well as breast cancer survivors. At the end of the town hall meeting, all participants were asked to complete an evaluation questionnaire about the quality, duration, content, venue, and format of the event. If participants' responses suggest that additional topics should be included or that the duration or venue of the town hall meeting may limit attendance, these points should be addressed in preparation for the next event. If adequately designed, evaluation models can accommodate changes in process indicators or in core materials, media, and procedures (Kennedy and Abbatangelo, 2005).

Outcome indicators (for example, behavioral and social change) for summative evaluation should be consistent throughout the program. Changing outcome indicators suddenly or too soon in the lifespan of the communication intervention may complicate the overall evaluation process and compromise the accuracy of all analyses on the potential impact of the intervention on expected outcomes.

Evaluation reports should be customized to meet the intervention and audience needs. Special considerations should be given to the potential limitations of evaluation data (for example, sample size, limits of self-reported frequency of performing a recommended behavior, sequential implementation of new behaviors and social norms that may lead to social change, length of time dedicated to the evaluation process, organizational constraints), which should be described and considered as part of the report. In general, an evaluation report should do the following (National Cancer Institute at the National Institutes of Health, 2002; Office of Adolescent Pregnancy Programs, 2006):

- Refer to the key theoretical assumptions, models, and data from the situation and audience analysis that have influenced the design of the health communication program as well as the evaluation plan

- Provide an overview of the health communication intervention and its sociopolitical contexts (including an analysis of key obstacles to the adoption and sustainability of new behaviors, social norms, and policies)

- Restate expected program outcomes

- Highlight key research objectives in relation to expected outcomes

- Describe methods for data collection and analysis, as well as the composition of the evaluation and monitoring teams

- Provide a report on process indicators and each program activity or material, as well as progress indicators (intermediate steps and key milestones) as measured at regular intervals

- Report key evaluation findings and their implications for current or future interventions as they relate to expected outcomes and other evaluation indicators

- Highlight key lessons learned and future directions

- Discuss barriers to the achievement of expected outcomes (for example, as they relate to key social determinants of health or vulnerable and underserved populations) and highlight how they can be minimized or eliminated in the future

Program evaluation serves multiple purposes. In fact, not only do evaluation data provide information on the efficacy and impact of a program on expected outcomes but they also help define program refinement as well as future programs in the same health field (National Cancer Institute at the National Institutes of Health, 2002). An example of a multifaceted health communication program was developed and implemented by the Hamilton-Wentworth Drug and Alcohol Awareness Committee in collaboration with the Health Communication Unit of the University of Toronto (2004). The program aimed at "reducing the number of children born with Fetal Alcohol Spectrum Disorder" in Hamilton, Ontario, Canada. Summative evaluation showed that there was "still uncertainty among women of reproductive age regarding a safe level of alcohol consumption during pregnancy." These data and other postevaluation analyses contributed to the definition of many of the elements of the second phase of the campaign, and refocused the intervention on creating awareness of issues related to the fact that there is no safe level of alcohol during pregnancy.

Because of their relevance to program reassessment and refinement, evaluation reports should be shared with as many key stakeholders as possible. These include members of key groups, opinion leaders, partners, and professional organizations. Ideally, all of these stakeholders should participate in evaluation design, data collection and analysis, and the compilation of the final report. Although most of the time evaluation reports rely on the expertise of communication research consultants, agencies, or research centers, securing the involvement of key stakeholders and key groups may add to the accuracy and relevance of the evaluation analysis. As for other components of program planning, this is in line with the participatory model of communication planning (see Chapter Ten).

Incentives for participation should be identified for all key stakeholders (Exchange, 2001) and audiences and may include organizational visibility, the chance to be a part of a major health or social change at the community level, personal experiences about a specific health or disease area, peer pressure, and access to special services. These incentives also apply to other areas of program planning and implementation.

Finally, evaluation reports should be used to showcase the results of the communication intervention whenever possible, as well as the overall contribution of health communication to the solution of health issues. Evaluation reports should be presented at professional conferences and meetings, posted on relevant websites, distributed through direct mail and online summaries, and publicized through the mass media, new media, websites, and all appropriate channels. Most important, evaluation reports should be used to advocate for intervention refinement and scaling up so that relevant communities are not left without the tools and resources they need just when they had started to mobilize for action and to work on long-term solutions together with professionals from multiple sectors.

Key Concepts

Evaluation Plan

• The evaluation of health communication programs is a much debated and evolving topic.

• Evaluation starts with program planning and is an integral part of the overall health communication cycle. Outcome objectives should be set at the onset of program planning. The evaluation plan should be developed at the same time as the action plan and include evaluation parameters and methods.

• In health communication, behavioral, social, and organizational outcomes are key evaluation parameters. Behavioral outcomes at different levels of society are key parameters in the assessment of health communication programs, even in the context of social change interventions (see Figure 14.1).

• Evaluation of health communication programs presents several limitations and challenges but should not prevent program planners from considering it.

• Although evaluation should always be part of health communication, health organizations and programs may opt for different evaluation plans that represent diverse combinations of evaluation needs, costs, and other program-specific factors.

- Given the variety of evaluation parameters and models, establishing mutually agreed-on measurement parameters with key program stakeholders, team members, partners, and donors is the latest wisdom in the evaluation of health communication programs. This helps focus everyone's efforts on common goals and limits the possibility for misunderstandings and unrealistic expectations about potential program outcomes. Participatory evaluation is an important feature of the evaluation process.

- Another key trend in the evaluation of health communication programs is the use of consistent models. Maintaining the same theoretical assumptions and planning framework throughout the health communication cycle may be helpful in preserving the accuracy of program evaluation.

- Other key topics in this chapter include the importance of integrating evaluation parameters that are inclusive of vulnerable and underserved populations; new trends and strategies in the evaluation of new media–based intervention as well as methods and criteria to link outcomes to a specific communication intervention. Additional tools on some of these topics are included in Appendix A.

Monitoring

- Monitoring, an essential component of program implementation, refers to the collection and analysis of data and information relevant to the implementation, evaluation, and potential success of the health communication intervention:
  - News and trends on the health or disease area, intended audiences, socially determined factors influencing a specific health issue or topic, and policies
  - Ongoing feedback by key groups and stakeholders on program content or key elements (vehicles)
  - Process and progress indicators throughout program implementation
  - Collection of summative evaluation data
- Methods for data collection may vary and sometimes overlap across the different areas of monitoring.

Evaluation Report

- The evaluation report summarizes process and summative evaluation findings in relation to the original evaluation plan, methods, and indicators.

⋄ An evaluation report includes a summary description of these elements:

  • Key theoretical assumptions and models used in program and evaluation design

  • Expected program outcomes

  • Formal research objectives in relation to expected outcomes

  • Methods for data collection and analysis as well as the composition of the evaluation team

  • Progress report in relation to process indicators and specific activities and materials

  • Key evaluation findings and their implications for current or future programs

  • Key lessons learned and future directions

  • Existing barriers to expected outcomes and potential approaches to overcome them (for example, as they relate to key social determinants of health or vulnerable and underserved populations)

⋄ Evaluation reports (as well as the overall evaluation process) are used not only to assess the intervention's results but also to inform program refinement and future programs. For this reason, participation of all key stakeholders should be maximized in developing the evaluation report.

⋄ Evaluation reports should be shared with all team members, partners, key groups, and other key stakeholders. Publicity of the report's key findings should be used to showcase program results and to advocate for scaling up or additional funds, as well as to communicate the overall contribution of health communication to the public health, health care, and community development fields.

FOR DISCUSSION AND PRACTICE

1. Discuss the significance, pros and cons, and implications of current trends and core principles in the evaluation of health communication programs as described in this chapter (for example, participatory evaluation, mutually agreed-on parameters). Whenever possible, use practical examples or observations to support your discussion points.

2. Your communication team is establishing process indicators for a new website that focuses on increasing awareness of a vaccine-preventable childhood disease among parents and

health care providers. The website includes sections for health care providers and parents (in English and Spanish); a time line on the history of the disease; a section that highlights testimonials of parents whose children suffered or died from the disease; a contact e-mail to submit case studies, testimonials, questions, or suggestions for professionals and parents; a media section with recent news, facts, and statistics on the disease; a list of available speakers or experts to address media questions; links to social media sites that are part of this national communication intervention; and a resources section with links to other organizations that work in this disease area and relevant publications. Identify examples of process indicators that could be established to evaluate the success of this website, and discuss which methods you would use to monitor them.

3. After reviewing the evaluation report section of this chapter, draft the outline of a potential evaluation report that is related to a health communication case study or program of which you are aware. List the categories your report should include.

4. Design a model for a virtual world to be used for the online efficacy assessment of an intervention that aims to reduce chronic diseases within a population of your choice.

5. Research a recent communication evaluation case study. Highlight research questions and parameters the case study may feature to assess impact on key social determinants of health and among vulnerable and underserved populations. Develop and discuss what kinds of research questions and evaluation parameters you may include to assess impact on health equity and health disparities.

KEY TERMS

behavioral impact

contribution analysis

evaluation

evaluation plans

impact

metrics

mixed methodology

offline effectiveness

online efficacy

outcomes

process evaluation

program assessment

progress indicators

return on investment (ROI)

social change indicators and social impact

summative evaluation

CASE STUDIES AND LESSONS FROM THE FIELD

Part Four provides readers with additional case studies that can be used as a framework for discussion and practice on key lessons learned as well as to identify potential other communication approaches, strategies, and activities that may also be suitable in approaching similar health and social issues. This section complements other resources, materials, examples, and case studies that have been included throughout this book.

Part Four includes two chapters: Chapter Fifteen focuses on US-based case studies, and Chapter Sixteen focuses on global health communication and includes case studies from a variety of different country settings. Yet, as global health and social development issues transcend national boundaries and are interconnected, the division of the case studies in two different chapters should be considered only as instrumental to ease of use and chapter flow, a mere device to meet readers' preferences in case they want to focus solely on either the United States or international country settings. Lessons learned, key themes, and intervention models and methods discussed in this section may be relevant to different kinds of health and social areas and transcend specific country settings.

CHAPTER 15

HEALTH COMMUNICATION IN THE UNITED STATES:
Case Studies and Lessons from the Field

Health communication is a constantly evolving field, which is influenced by and influences different social determinants of health, and leads and adapts to new trends, group-specific preferences, and evolving media. One of the fundamental premises of this book is that health communication practice is shaped by and also shapes theory and planning models. Therefore, a case study analysis may reveal trends and approaches that are being used in the realm of practice and have relevant lessons or implications for other programs or future directions in health communication.

The case studies featured in this chapter as well as in Chapter Sixteen, which focuses on international case studies, were contributed by different organizations and colleagues to whom I am very grateful. For the most part, they follow specific guidelines and format that intend to provide information on the situation, health issue, and other needs that prompted the health communication intervention, as well as the intervention's specific goal and objectives, strategies, activities, lessons learned, and potential future directions (as it applies).

CHAPTER OBJECTIVES

The primary objective of including the case studies in this chapter is to review them and draw lessons that can be learned by others embarking in the complex process of designing, implementing, and evaluating a health communication intervention. Another objective is to provide readers with materials that can be used as a framework for discussion on how this applies to their professional experience as well as to identify other communication approaches, strategies, and activities that may also be suitable in similar cases.

From Theory to Practice: Select Case Studies from the United States

Because many topics in public health, health care, and community development are strictly interconnected, lessons learned from these case studies transcend the specific health areas for which the health communication intervention was designed, and have a broader application in a variety of settings. It is thus not an objective of this chapter to evaluate the outcomes of the programs featured in the case studies, but rather to extrapolate communication trends, strategies, and other lessons of general application as they relate to the theoretical and practical models discussed so far in this book. A discussion is included in the "Emerging Trends and Lessons" section of this chapter.

In this chapter, the individual case studies are categorized under the health or social field (for example, mental health) for which the health communication intervention was designed, and referred to by the name of the program they feature (for example, WhyWellness). Yet, this is done only for ease of reference, because the focus of the analysis is on extrapolating lessons learned that may apply to health communication interventions across different health and social areas and settings, and also to prompt discussion among readers on other potential approaches that may be suitable for implementation as they refer to a specific case study, health area, or their own professional endeavors.

Mental Health

WhyWellness

virtual world
"An online community that takes the form of a computer-based simulated environment through which users can interact with one another and use and create [both characters and] objects" (Bishop, 2009)

As youth throughout the United States "struggle daily with issues such as stress, anxiety, depression, bullying, and suicide" (Hannah, Reilly, and Sun, 2013), the WhyWellness case study features collaborative work between academia and the private sector that leverages the use of the Internet and cell phones to provide emotional health information, support, and role modeling to children and to help them address stress and other mental, emotional, and behavioral issues. The intervention uses an online **virtual world**—"an online community that takes the form of a computer-based simulated environment through which users can interact with one another and use and create [both characters and] objects" (Bishop, 2009)—and games to promote mental health and prevention of social and emotional issues and mental disorders among older children and teens, and seeks to incorporate in future programming other strategies and activities that would also engage significant adults, such as parents, teachers, and caretakers.

BOX 15.1. WHYWELLNESS: COMMUNICATING ABOUT MENTAL HEALTH WITHIN A GAMING COMMUNITY

Need

Innovative programming that addresses children's mental health needs are critical, as youth throughout the nation struggle daily with issues such as stress, anxiety, depression, bullying, and suicide. Mental, emotional, and behavioral (MEB) disorders occur commonly among children, and many start at young ages with the onset of major mental illness beginning as early as seven to eleven years of age (National Research Council and Institute of Medicine, 2009). In any given year, the percentage of young people with an MEB is estimated to be between 14 and 20 percent (National Research Council and Institute of Medicine, 2009). Over 50 percent of students with a mental disorder age fourteen and older drop out of high school—the highest dropout rate of any disability group (National Alliance on Mental Health, 2013). The annual quantifiable cost of such disorders among youth was estimated in 2007 to be $247 billion (McMorrow and Howell, 2010). The costs to society as a result of not addressing children's mental health needs are enormous, both economically and emotionally, because of tremendous suffering incurred and potential lost. Unfortunately, there is often a lag time (as long as ten years) between clinical innovation and its implementation into common practice. Although these statistics are alarming, research strongly supports mental health promotion, psycho-education, and skill building as effective ways to reduce risk of emotional disorders in youth. Helping children learn skills to address adversity is critical, because it allows them to identify risk factors and risky behaviors and develop skills for early action and prevention (National Research Council and Institute of Medicine, 2009).

Goals and Objectives

The Massachusetts School of Professional Psychology (MSPP) is partnering with Numedeon, Inc., to introduce emotional management skills to children through Whyville, an educational virtual world for children with 7.5 million registered users. Given that a large part of this generation's social and emotional development is occurring while on the Internet and on cell phones, leveraging this platform is critical. The goals of this project include creating a safe space where children can learn about and discuss topics related to emotional health, practice coping skills, self-regulation, and ultimately, for children to better cope with complex emotional issues.

Sample Communication Strategies and Activities

MSPP and Numedeon created a pilot project that focuses on stress, involving three typical situations that generate stress for children of this age group and skills for coping with these situations. In this activity, an automated avatar (see definition in Chapter Five) wanders into a virtual destination in Whyville where Whyville participants are chatting and playing (see Figure 15.1). The automated avatar looks sad and worried, and the Whyville participants respond by selecting question envelopes to figure out the problem collectively and offer advice envelopes accordingly. After receiving sufficient appropriate advice, the avatar expresses relief, and the participants are rewarded as virtual coins rain from the sky.

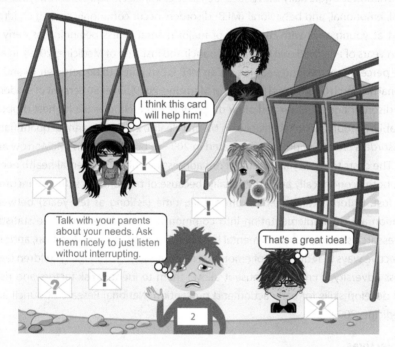

Figure 15.1   WhyWellness Virtual World

Source: © 2013 Numedeon, Inc. Used by permission.

Key Results

The efficacy using this site to provide children with information of emotional health and wellness has been astounding. When a prototype activity was launched on the site, within one month more than sixteen thousand games were played. In a poll involving 878 respondents, 82 percent of those who played the game liked it, 53 percent indicated an interest in learning more ways to deal with stress, and 34 percent indicated that the game helped them learn new ways to deal with stress.

Future Direction

As we extend this collaboration, MSPP and Numedeon will create WhyWellness Center in Whyville, offering youth content information and collaborative activities, including live coaching, that build wellness skills based on principles of neuroscience, prevention, and learning for youth. The collaboration will evaluate the efficacy of an online virtual world in addressing mental health promotion and prevention for youth. We will also incorporate additional programming that involves important adults in children's lives, including parents, caretakers, and teachers. By bringing together children and adults via this platform, we hope to foster a natural environment for continued support, mentoring, and eventually workforce development.

References

McMorrow, S., and Howell, E. M. "State Mental Health Systems for Children. A Review of the Literature and Available Data Sources." Urban Institute. August Aug. 2010. Report funded by the National Alliance for Mental Illness.

National Alliance on Mental Illness. "Mental Illness: Facts and Numbers." www.nami.org /Template.cfm?Section=About_Mental_Illness&Template=/ContentManagement /ContentDisplay.cfm&ContentID=53155. Retrieved Feb. 2013.

National Research Council and Institute of Medicine. (2009). *Preventing Mental, Emotional, and Behavioral Disorders Among Young People: Progress and Possibilities.* Committee on the Prevention of Mental Disorders and Substance Abuse Among Children, Youth, and Young Adults: Research Advances and Promising Interventions. (Mary Ellen O'Connell, Thomas Boat, and Kenneth E. Warner, eds.) Board on Children, Youth, and Families, Division of Behavioral and Social Sciences and Education. Washington, DC: The National Academies Press.

Source: Hannah, M., Reilly, N., and Sun, J. "WhyWellness: Communicating About Mental Health Within a Gaming Community." Unpublished Case Study, 2013. Used by permission.

• • •

WhyWellness Case Study Discussion: Read, Reflect, and Practice in Groups

1. Are you familiar with online virtual worlds? Reflect on what you know about them and how this compares to the definition provided in this chapter as well as the one emerging from the case study.

2. Think about other potential applications of online virtual worlds in health communication interventions. Discuss how you would integrate this kind of media with other program components and communication areas so that online interaction can translate into real-life action.

3. Because the intervention discussed in the WhyWellness case study is preparing to develop "additional programming that involves important adults in children's lives, including parents, caretakers, and teachers," discuss and develop with fellow group members a communication plan for each of these groups. Include all the different components of a communication plan as discussed in this book and use a PowerPoint format to present your plan.

4. Discuss key indicators you may use to evaluate the success of this multisectoral partnership between academia and the private sector. What other sectors or organizations (if any) do you think should be involved to further the impact of this effort and ensure its sustainability in the long term?

Obesity and Chronic Diseases

"BodyLove"

The first of the two case studies under this category discusses a communication intervention to address chronic disease disparities among low-literacy African Americans living in rural communities. "BodyLove" uses a radio serial drama format and on-air community leader engagement "to increase knowledge, positively change attitudes, improve self-efficacy, and connect listeners with local health services" (Chen, Kohler, Schoenberger, Suzuki-Crumly, Davis, and Powell, 2009). Future directions include program expansion in other regions and urban areas of the United States as well as the integration of elements of the current program with traditional and new media.

BOX 15.2. "BODYLOVE"—CASE STUDY SUMMARY

Need, Situation, Health Issues

Health disparities among African Americans are well documented, especially regarding chronic disease–related health outcomes. "BodyLove," a radio serial drama, was developed with the goal of addressing health disparities, reducing the risk for chronic health conditions, such as diabetes, hypertension, and cardiovascular disease, and improving health outcomes by promoting the adoption of healthy behaviors. "BodyLove" targeted low-income and low-literacy African Americans over the age of thirty-five, living in rural communities, who typically do not respond to conventional health promotion interventions.

Goals and Objectives

"BodyLove"'s communication objectives were to increase knowledge, positively change attitudes, improve self-efficacy, and connect listeners with local health services. "BodyLove" provided health information in an entertaining format, and used modeling to influence attitudes and increase self-efficacy, and connected the audience with local health services via radio program hosts and guests who answered callers' questions following the drama episode. The program aimed to address health disparities on three levels of prevention: (1) primary, by including technical information about diet and exercise; (2) secondary, by encouraging screening and regular medical care; and (3) tertiary, by encouraging patients to manage their chronic conditions.

Communication Strategies and Activities

From 2004 to 2007, eighty-three episodes of "BodyLove" were aired weekly on fifteen local radio stations in Alabama. These communities were chosen based on their high diabetes mortality rates and large African American populations. Each fifteen-minute episode was usually followed by a live question-and-answer call-in period, moderated by community leaders, including clergy and health professionals. "BodyLove"'s culturally appropriate storyline included positive, negative, and transitional models who modeled adherence, or the lack thereof, to behaviors such as screening, exercise, and healthy eating to shape listener outcome and efficacy expectations. Some of the healthy behaviors discussed in episodes included controlling chronic conditions such as elevated blood pressure and diabetes, modifying eating habits to reduce fat and sodium intake, and increasing exercise levels. The importance of social support in lowering stress associated with initiating and maintaining healthy behaviors in everyday life was a common theme.

The entertainment-education (E-E) format used had the benefit of engaging and affecting listener attitudes over an extended period of time, and allowed the audience to identify with character struggles and become emotionally invested in the drama. However, the impact of E-E can be difficult to evaluate, especially in media-saturated environments. Radio represents an important forum in the African American community, and tends to be low cost and widely accessible. "BodyLove" used positive, negative, and transitional role models as defined by the social cognitive theory to help listeners recognize the positive and negative consequences of their behavior.

Key Results and Future Directions

Preliminary evaluation based on a mailed longitudinal survey (a baseline survey followed by four waves of follow-up surveys) shows that frequent listeners were more likely than seldom listeners to report that "BodyLove" influenced them to discuss diabetes, get screened for diabetes and hypertension, start or increase physical activity, and start eating a healthier diet. The "BodyLove" team plans to expand into other regions and urban centers of the United States by tapping a blend of traditional and new media, and is considering rerecording the show in a more suitable, shorter, three-minute format. An updated "BodyLove" website went live in November 2008 in an effort to brand the program with the goal of using the power of social networks to promote "BodyLove" and increase the degree of social diffusion. Future evaluation could measure social diffusion or the indirect impact of health communication efforts within social networks.

Source: Chen, N., Kohler, C., Schoenberger, Y., Suzuki-Crumly, J., Davis, K., and Powell, J. "BodyLove: The Impact of Targeted Radio Educational Entertainment on Health Knowledge, Attitudes and Behavior Among African-Americans." *Cases in Public Health Communication & Marketing,* 2009, *3,* 92–113. Available from: www.casesjournal .org/volume3. Accessed Oct. 1, 2012. Copyright © 2009, *Cases in Public Health Communication & Marketing.* Used by permission. All rights reserved.

• • •

"BodyLove" Case Study Discussion: Read, Reflect, and Practice in Groups

1. Research and discuss key features of two to three community radio channels from your city as well as their health-related programs. Are these programs intended for a specific audience or the general public? How do they compare to "BodyLove"?

2. Within the context of "BodyLove" or similar programs, what other kinds of strategies and activities can you think of to increase community leader engagement and participation both on air and within community settings?

3. What other kinds of media and communication strategies (outside of radio and community leader engagement) can you think of to address chronic disease disparities among low-literacy African Americans living in rural areas?

4. Research and discuss the role of radio programs and community radio in health communication. Discuss key elements and success factors of potential radio programs that seek to address chronic diseases, and analyze synergies with other components of the health communication intervention.

5. Interview a radio host who specializes in or covers health issues, and discuss relevant facts and anecdotes from his or her experience. Discuss your findings, including key learnings on tools and resources, that may be helpful in pitching a story on health topics to community radios or the radio host you interviewed.

VERB Campaign

Coordinated by the Centers for Disease Control and Prevention (CDC), the VERB campaign (2002–2006), which is featured in this case study, sought to address the growing epidemic of childhood obesity by encouraging an active lifestyle and physical activities. The case study provides some interesting learnings on the integrated and strategic use of different mass media and new media in health communication (in integration with marketing models and theory), and has implications for peer-to-peer communication in the new media age.

BOX 15.3. CASE STUDY—NEW MEDIA AND THE VERB CAMPAIGN

Need, Situation, Health Issues

Sedentary lifestyles in children are associated with negative health outcomes, and linked to the growing epidemic of childhood obesity in the United States. "VERB It's What You Do" was a national social marketing campaign, coordinated by the Centers for Disease Control and Prevention (CDC), with the goal of increasing and maintaining physical activity among tweens (children aged nine to thirteen years). The campaign ran from 2002 to 2006.

Objective, Strategies, and Activities

The campaign's objectives were to improve tween attitudes and beliefs about participation in physical activity, increase parental and influencer support, and facilitate opportunities to participate in regular physical activity. The campaign used paid advertising on cable channels; marketing strategies, including school and community promotions, and Internet and other mass media; and partnerships with national organizations and local communities to reach tweens, and other key audiences, such as parents and other adult influencers (teachers, youth leaders, coaches, physical education and health professionals, etc.). An integrated marketing approach was employed so that all marketing and advertising had a single message that physical activity is fun, cool, and a social opportunity. The new media component of VERB consisted of three elements:

1. *A VERB website for tweens:* On VERBnow.com, tweens could engage with virtual "sidekicks," find places to be active in their area, record their physical activity, view tutorials from sports celebrities, and get ideas about making up games.

2. *Cell phone technology:* In a summer program called *8372* (spelling VERB on a cell keypad), cell phone messaging and a website were used to send prompting messages encouraging tweens to be physically active.

3. *VERB's Yellowball:* This multicomponent promotion that combined electronic interactivity and blogging encouraged tweens to play with one of the five hundred thousand

yellowballs distributed throughout the United States, pass the ball to another tween, and then blog about how they had played with the ball. Interactive projections of yellowballs also appeared on the floors of many shopping malls. For its innovative mix of marketing and social networking, Yellowball earned numerous public health and advertising industry awards.

Key Results

The VERB campaign was evaluated using the nationally representative Youth Media Campaign Longitudinal Survey (YMCLS). YMCLS used computer-assisted telephone interviewing to assess tweens' awareness of the campaign and understanding of its messages and the effects of the campaign on tweens' attitudes and physical activity behaviors. In the 2006 YMCLS, 75 percent of tweens reported being aware of the VERB campaign. The VERB campaign lasted for over four years, and during this period VERBnow site visitors climbed steadily, with site registration increasing by over 500 percent. At the end of the three-month text messaging program, more than 250,000 tweens had opted to receive online activity messages, and 25,000 tweens opted to receive text messages. The VERB Yellowball promotion generated 17,000 blogs and more than 170,000 videos.

Future Directions

Evaluation of the campaign showed that tweens who were aware of the campaign engaged in more physical activity in their free time than tweens who were unaware of the campaign, even one year after being exposed to the campaign. Contrary to assumptions that VERB awareness would diminish in the absence of mass media support after the campaign ended, website views and registrations continued for over a year and tweens kept VERB alive on networks such as YouTube for several years. This suggests the enormous potential of new media and electronic networking, essentially tween-to-tween marketing, that public health can tap as a communication tool. The number of tweens who interacted with VERB's new media indicates that digital technology is a promising public health communication tool, and that new media can be an important part of a marketing strategy that aims to surround an audience with messages in the places they frequent, including online.

Source: Huhman, M. "New Media and the VERB Campaign: Tools to Motivate Tweens to Be Physically Active." *Cases in Public Health Communication & Marketing,* 2008, *2,* 126–139. Available from: www.casesjournal.org/volume2. Accessed Oct. 1, 2012. Copyright © 2008, *Cases in Public Health Communication & Marketing.* Used by permission. All rights reserved.

• • •

VERB Campaign Case Study Discussion: Read, Reflect, and Practice in Groups

1. Discuss and reflect on any personal or professional experience that you may recall about peer-to-peer health communication interventions, whether online or offline. How does this compare to the approach and media used by the VERB campaign? What kinds of communication strategies did you or the program in which you participated use or plan to use?

2. What kinds of additional communication tools, resources, or training do you think may be helpful to include as part of a mass media and new media communication intervention to further expand its reach after the program ends?

3. Reflect on lessons learned from the VERB campaign and discuss how you would apply them to a program you are currently working on or another relevant case study focusing on adolescent health or chronic diseases that you may find in literature.

Social Determinants of Health

Health Equity Exchange

Because "health equity is a new and complex concept for most people" (Health Equity Initiative, 2012a), this case study features the Health Equity Exchange, an integrated multimedia communication program that seeks to engage US communities in discussing health equity and "to provide a proof-of-concept of the many different faces of health equity" (Health Equity Initiative, 2012a) as well as the need for community-specific solutions. The Exchange uses a blog platform, which acts as a virtual town hall, to solicit opinions and showcase different community-based or individual definitions of health equity as well as key priorities toward potential progress. Community, event, and social media outreach are also all integrated with the online forum. Several ideas for future directions for this or similar programs are also discussed.

BOX 15.4. HEALTH EQUITY EXCHANGE: USING AN INTEGRATED MULTIMEDIA
COMMUNICATION APPROACH TO ENGAGE U.S. COMMUNITIES ON
HEALTH EQUITY

Need

"Health equity is a new and complex idea for most people" (Health Equity Initiative, 2013a). Yet, health disparities compromise the ability of vulnerable and underserved communities to thrive. Improving the limited levels of awareness of these disparities and their root causes is "a necessary first step toward changing behavior and compelling action" (Benz, Espinosa, Welsh, and Fontes, 2011, p. 1860).

Disparities are linked to diverse factors, which are intrinsic to the living, working, and aging environment where people live. The influence and importance of each factor is likely to be community specific. Achieving health equity—"providing every person with the same opportunity to stay healthy, and/or effectively cope with disease or health-related emergencies" (Health Equity Initiative, 2012b)—therefore, must begin with an understanding that there are community-specific needs, and that communities must be involved in identifying their priorities and developing community-based indicators of progress toward health equity. Consequently, the advancement of health equity needs the support and engagement of communities across the United States, as well as a community-specific definition of health equity.

In 2011, Health Equity Initiative (HEI), a nonprofit organization working to encourage community action in support for health equity, launched Health Equity Exchange, which provides a space where people throughout the United States can speak specifically to two main issues: what health equity means to them, their families, peers, and community, and what they believe should be the top priorities in their community to make progress toward health equity.

Goals and Objectives

The project's goal is to actively engage different segments of the society to define their own road map to health equity. It also seeks to serve as a proof-of-concept of the many faces of health equity by collecting different community-based meanings, perspectives, and priorities, and inform future programs and policies through accurate reporting on emerging themes.

Sample Communication Strategies and Activities

Using an integrated multimedia communication and community engagement approach, including an online forum (functioning as a virtual town hall), community outreach, celebrity-sponsored messaging, and new media outreach, the Exchange seeks to engage individuals to be part of the discourse on health equity, and strengthens their capacity to be agents of change.

The Exchange's online forum uses a blog format innovatively to collect and document community voices in contrast to the more traditional path of using a blog to disseminate information and opinions. This methodology facilitates an open-ended and honest national dialogue that remains unmediated by HEI. The Exchange's online forum is complemented by (1) a free downloadable campus kit, including suggested activities and resources that are designed to enable college students and their groups to engage nearby communities to share their ideas on the Exchange and mobilize for a common cause, (2) a PowerPoint presentation with talking points to be used by students and others to introduce the Health Equity Exchange,

(3) social media promotion via HEI's media accounts, and (4) celebrity outreach and messaging via HEI's celebrity charity ambassador.

Emerging Themes

Several themes have emerged from the virtual town hall as supported by event and community outreach conducted using the campus kit and at HEI's events. For example, some of the participants in the online forum associate "health equity" and related progress to increased "cultural competence" in clinical settings in order to improve health outcomes among immigrant or underserved populations. Others refer to the importance of interventions that would improve living conditions in their communities or neighborhoods, such as access to affordable housing, nutrition, and health care services. Responses are quite diverse as they relate to health equity definitions, opinions, and progress-related priorities. Preliminary themes and other information on the Health Equity Exchange were presented at the 2012 Summit on the Science of Eliminating Health Disparities organized by the US National Institutes of Health (NIH) and the US Department of Health and Human Resources (DHHS) (Schiavo, Boahemaa, Watts, and Hoeppner, 2012b), as well as featured in August 2012 by the *Journal of Communication in Healthcare* (Schiavo, Boahemaa, Watts, and Hoeppner, 2012a).

Next Steps and Future Directions

HEI will develop and disseminate a report on key themes that emerge from the Health Equity Exchange to showcase community voices and priorities and to analyze them within the context of existing literature and other experiences. Preliminary results of the emerging themes from this project suggest the importance of a community-specific approach to health equity. Future directions to be considered for this or similar projects include the development of online tools to be used by visitors to share photos and videos within the online forum, which can help increase participation by low-health-literacy communities, and increased outreach, support, and training to college and graduate students and other community ambassadors for the program, who may engage in discussions on health equity and gather input in libraries, supermarkets, and community health and social centers. Event-based outreach has also emerged as a valuable approach to increase participation in online forums.

References

Benz, J. K., Espinosa, O., Welsh, V., and Fontes, A. "Awareness of Racial and Ethnic Health Disparities Has Improved Only Modestly over a Decade." *Health Affairs*, 2011, *30*(10), 1860–1867.

Health Equity Initiative. "Health Equity Exchange." www.healthequityinitiative.org/hei/what-we-do/community-engagement-and-mobilization/health-equity-exchange. Retrieved Jan. 2013a.

Schiavo, R., Boahemaa, O., Watts, B., and Hoeppner, E. "Raising the Influence of Community Voices on Health Equity: Introducing Health Equity Exchange." *Journal of Communication in Healthcare*, Aug. 2012a. http://maneypublishing.com/images/pdf_site/Health_Equity_Exchange_-_Renata_Schiavo.pdf.

Schiavo, R., Boahemaa, O., Watts, B., and Hoeppner, E. "Raising the Influence of Community Voices on Health Equity via an Integrated Communication and Community Engagement Approach." Poster presented at the 2012 Summit on the Science of Eliminating Health Disparities, National Harbor, MD, Dec. 18, 2012b.

Source: Health Equity Initiative (2012c). Used by permission.

. . .

Health Equity Exchange Case Study Discussion: Read, Reflect, and Practice in Groups

1.   Develop a blog to talk about your own definition of and interest in health equity or another complex topic of your choice, and encourage people to participate in the discussion via a variety of communication channels and activities.

2.   Identify communication strategies, activities, channels, and venues to secure input on a community-specific definition of health equity within your school, workplace, neighborhood, or other kind of community. Present a report on key definitions that emerge from this effort, as well as lessons learned related to the communication strategies and activities you used to engage relevant groups.

3.   Research and discuss a health communication case study or a specific example of media (interpersonal, traditional, community based, mass media, new media, etc.) that highlights and seeks to raise awareness and address the root causes (social determinants of health) of a health issue of your selection.

4.   Develop a policy brief (see Chapter Nine) to address the need for policy change in relation to a health disparity issue within a community or population of your choice.

Sustainable Food, Nutrition, and the Environment

Sustainable Table

The Sustainable Table case study highlights the interconnection among food, nutrition, health, and the environment as well as different communication areas (mass media, new media, and community mobilization). Sustainable Table, a program of GRACE Communications Foundation, aims to build community around sustainable food, and raise awareness of the implications of factory farming (corporation led, industrial-sized factory farms, also known as concentrated animal feeding operations [CAFOs]) on public health, socioeconomic conditions of local communities, and the environment. Since this case study was published, Sustainable Table's website moved to a new site, which also includes GRACE's water and energy programs and further demonstrates the interconnections among these apparently separate fields (GRACE Communications Foundation, 2013).

BOX 15.5. RAISING AWARENESS OF SUSTAINABLE FOOD ISSUES AND BUILDING COMMUNITY VIA THE INTEGRATED USE OF NEW MEDIA WITH OTHER COMMUNICATION APPROACHES

Over the past few decades, there has been an increasing shift from local family-owned farms, to corporation led, industrial-sized factory farms, also known as concentrated animal feeding operations (CAFOs). Factory farming practices are not only harmful to the animals they house, but also pose significant public health, environmental, and community-related risks because of:

- Overuse of antibiotics can create resistant forms of bacteria that can make treating human diseases more difficult;

- Improper storage and excess waste leads to air, water and soil pollution; and

- Negative impact on ecosystems, local communities and family-owned farms.

Sustainable farming is designed to minimize the use of antibiotics, minimally impact the environment, provide humane conditions for animals, and promote and enhance local farming communities. However, many Americans seem unable to fully support sustainable foods or lack the confidence to purchase them. There is a need for educators and mentors to promote and communicate about the sustainable food movement, continue to engage additional audiences, and limit the health, environmental and community impact of factory farming practices.

Goals and Objectives

A program of the GRACE Communications Foundation, Sustainable Table was started in 2003 to inform and educate consumers and relevant communities about the serious implications of factory farming on public health, socio-economic conditions of local communities, and the environment; to support sustainable farming methods; and to build community around food. The program aimed to raise awareness of key issues related to factory farming practices among the general public and other key stakeholders (for example local farms, community members, consumers, and relevant organizations) by: (1) providing information and resources, as well as (2) engaging them on issues related to sustainable food.

Communication Strategies and Activities

Sustainable Table has relied on an integrated approach in its communication interventions, employing new media and Internet-based communications, complemented by community outreach and mobilization as well as mass media communications. Communication efforts target consumers, who are the program's primary audience, while also reaching out to public health professionals, healthcare providers, educators, and other key stakeholders, who are all important secondary audiences because of their influence on attitudes and habits of the consumers. Key elements of the Sustainable Table outreach and communication program included:

- The program's main website, www.sustainabletable.org, supplied consumers and other key audiences with issue-specific information on sustainable food and factory farming, tools, and resources.

- *The Meatrix* series of award-winning short videos was developed to warn consumers about the dangers of factory farming (www.themeatrix.com). The videos use a cartoon format to encourage consumers to adopt healthier and sustainable food practices. The comprehensive promotion plan involved participation in film festivals, blast e-mails to organizations in relevant fields, merchandising, and promotion on social media networks. Some key features of this video series include: "the simplicity of its message; the animation format that removes viewers from thinking about grotesque scenes of animal cruelty, thus helping them focus on key issues and messages; and its use of graphic devices such as a bullet point banner that acts as a reminder of key messages on the bottom of the video screen" (Williams, Zraik, Schiavo, and Hatz, 2013).

- The Eat Well Guide (www.eatwellguide) was developed to offer an online directory of sustainable food stores, restaurants, small farms, and other outlets throughout the US and Canada. Consumers could go on-line, key in their state, city or zip code and retrieve a range of resources (e.g., farms, farmers markets, etc.) within a specific geographic area. By providing consumers a resources for buying locally produced, sustainable food, the guide aimed to lessen people's dependence on factory farms, as well as shift consumer eating and purchasing habits towards foods and products produced via sustainable agriculture and farming.

- A blog called *The Daily Table* and a monthly electronic newsletter called *The Pasture Post* were designed to keep consumers updated on various issues and to build the sustainable food community.

- As part of the national community outreach effort, Sustainable Table's key program staff traveled across the country for 40 days in 2007 on their Eat Well Guided Tour of America, which received coverage from national and local media, blogs, and magazines.

Key Results and Future Direction

The communications and outreach efforts were assessed in 2006–2008 primarily using website metrics. Data were collected by Sustainable Table via NetTracker, a web statistics service. Via its websites and Internet-based tools, Sustainable Table reached over 6.6 million unique visitors from February 2006 to April 2008. An analysis of the US zip codes that were most searched for on the Eat Well Guide, indicated that a large majority of the Guide's users were searching for sustainable food in large urban areas. Also, the *Pasture Post* Newsletter counted around 45,360 subscribers by March 2008.

Moreover, the Meatrix had been influencing older U.S. children. "In 2007, Pork Checkoff, an activist group led by the National Pork Board," conducted a study "assessing the impact and influence of food activist groups on children." "After viewing The Meatrix (either online or via its DVD format), nearly two-thirds of the children stated that their opinions and meat eating habits had been changed" (Williams, Zraik, Schiavo, and Hatz, 2013; National Pork Board, 2008a, 2008b).

Some of the key lessons learned included "the importance of a comprehensive new media promotion plan that includes both online and offline strategies and channels;" as well as of "taking risks with experimenting with new types of media" (Williams, Zraik, Schiavo, and Hatz, 2013).

Future directions at the time of this case study included expanding on Sustainable Table partnership-building efforts with other groups having similar goals and target audiences. Other plans and programs included a downloadable educational kit for teachers, students, and community members, and other online and offline tools to further its mission.

Post-case study note (2013): Sustainable Table, part of the GRACE food program, recently moved its website to a new site, www.gracelinks.org/food, which also integrates the GRACE water and energy programs to illustrate the interconnection among all of these issues, and to provide better resources and tools that promote a more holistic way of thinking—for consumers, advocates and educators alike. *The Daily Table* and the *Pasture Post* were also replaced by GRACE's new blog, *Ecocentric*, and a monthly newsletter (*GRACEnotes*) and weekly news briefs RSS feed (*EcoNews*). GRACE is also active throughout the social media landscape, including Facebook, Twitter and LinkedIn.

References

National Pork Board. "Activist Groups and Your Kids." *Pork Checkoff Report*, 2008a, *27*(1). www.pork.org/filelibrary/PorkCheckoffReport/2008SpringCheckoffReport.pdf.

National Pork Board. "Checkoff Tracks Activist Groups' Influence on Kids." 2008b. www.pork.org /News/645/Feature325.aspx#.USaKAB2–1Bk.

Williams, A., Zraik, D., Schiavo, R., and Hatz, D. "Raising Awareness of Sustainable Food Issues and Building Community via the Integrated Use of New Media with Other Communication

Approaches." *Cases in Public Health Communication and Marketing*, 2008, *2*, 159–177. Available from http://www.casesjournal.org/volume2. http://sphhs.gwu.edu/departments/pch/phcm/casesjournal/volume2/invited/cases_2_10.cfm.

• • •

Sustainable Table Case Study Discussion: Read, Reflect, and Practice in Groups

1. Go to the Eat Well Guide and identify sustainable food stores and restaurants in your zip code. Think about what other communication strategies and activities could be implemented in your neighborhood, community, or city to raise awareness of sustainable food issues and encourage people to buy sustainable foods. Discuss such strategies within your group or present recommendations via a PowerPoint presentation.

2. How does this case study relate to your food shopping and consumption habits? Reflect on the case study's content and discuss information and communication resources on the same topic you may have seen in your community, read about in the media (online of offline), or have researched for this discussion.

3. Select three different programs that aim to raise awareness of the connection between a specific health or nutrition issue and other fields. Research and compare communication strategies and program elements from these three programs. Highlight lessons learned and how these correlate to the results obtained by each program.

4. Develop and present a poster presentation on a case study that uses an integrated approach to health communication including the mass media, new media, and community mobilization and engagement.

Urban Health and Related Social Determinants

Mass in Motion

In addressing the high incidence of overweight and obesity among high school and middle school students living in an urban setting, Mass in Motion (MiM) makes the connection between health and the place where we live, go to school, work, and play, and the challenges this presents in urban health settings. This multifaceted initiative integrates community engagement and mobilization, new media and mass media communication, traditional media, public advocacy, constituency relations, and interpersonal communication to develop a sample intervention that is based on multisectoral partnerships and "could be potentially replicated . . . to address childhood obesity among the underserved" (Hamel, 2012).

BOX 15.6. WHAT DO SIDEWALKS HAVE TO DO WITH HEALTH?

Need, Situation, Health Issues

Although Massachusetts compares favorably to most other states, overweight and obesity remain major public health problems. More than one-half of the adults and almost one-third of high school and middle school students are overweight or obese and in recent years, the percentage of adults with diabetes has almost doubled. Unless the numbers decrease, overweight and obesity will soon pass smoking as the leading cause of preventable death across the nation.

The City of New Bedford, the "Whaling City," is proud of its history as a fishing and whaling port that is still a working seaport today. With a population of approximately ninety-five thousand (white, Portuguese, Hispanic, Latino, and black residents), 38 percent speak languages other than English at home and the median income is $36,000. Unfortunately, the childhood obesity rate is higher than the state average in this community (37.2 percent versus 33.4 percent). Social determinants research demonstrates that where we live, go to school, work, and play can seriously affect one's health. The urban health challenges of this multicultural city present a good example of this. So, how best to raise awareness of these issues in this community?

Goals and Objectives

In 2009, municipal health and wellness grants, supported by the Massachusetts Department of Public Health (MDPH; www.mass.gov/eohhs/gov/departments/dph) and private funders established a multifaceted initiative called Mass in Motion (MiM; www.mass.gov/massinmotion, an initiative of the Massachusetts Department of Public Health) to promote policy, systems, and environmental changes to address obesity in health care, schools, worksite sectors, community organizations, and the community at large (from fourteen cities in 2009 to fifty-three communities in 2012).

As one of the original MiM cities, New Bedford built a coalition of community partners to address childhood obesity in the city. One of many steps taken by the partnership was to raise awareness of safe routes to school (SRTS; www.saferoutesinfo.org) programs that bring parents, schools, community leaders, and local, state, and federal governments together to improve the health of children by encouraging them to walk and bicycle to school.

Sample Activities

To address the public health problems related to obesity, inactivity, and equity, MiM New Bedford (www.massinmotionnewbedford.org) teamed up with Greater New Bedford Allies for Health and Wellness (GNB Allies) to launch the GNB Health Equity Initiative (HEI), with a kick-off event that coincided with International Walk to School Day on October 5, 2011.

Linking the SRTS walk and a healthy living day at a local middle school with existing equity issues in the city allowed participants to hear leaders and community members outline successes and challenges through traditional speeches, PowerPoint and photovoice presentations, followed with a school rally and an energetic walk so all could see the need for improved infrastructure (sidewalks, crosswalks, lighting), safer pedestrian and bicycle-friendly routes, and community collaboration. Planning the HEI launch to coincide with an established SRTS event brought together leaders from federal (EOHHS), state (MDPH), and municipal levels (the mayor and his team, community development, parks and recreation, the regional health care system, community health center, school administrators, and human service organizations) to walk and talk with students, parents, and teachers. It also generated great attention from area homeowners and businesses as they watched a happy, interactive, intergenerational group of people march down city streets!

Sample Communication Strategies

The city's public information officers, local radio managers, and health beat reporters were contacted. The MiM coordinator provided additional information via meetings, interviews, websites, e-mail, and follow-up phone calls, which led to press releases, cable access, radio, and newspaper coverage. Numerous announcements, flyers, and programs were widely distributed as were "New Bedford is on the Move" pedometers.

Though social media is an excellent tool to generate interest during event planning, urban networking sometimes requires more basic interpersonal and word-of-mouth communications to get wheels turning, build trust, and gain momentum. Follow-up was critical, especially in days after the event. Video and photos of the event were shared on websites and in subsequent programs and presentations. (Never underestimate the reach of cable-access stations that some city residents watch daily; repeated programming reinforces the message!)

Key Results

Walking alongside decision makers empowered the community because people interacted and shared concerns for their neighborhoods. Some parents and grandparents didn't even know they were neighbors until they began this conversation! Participation led to better interpersonal, organizational, and community-level communication, and also increased ownership of the issues, trust, and development of future partnerships to ensure sustainability.

Low budgets and minimal staff necessitate creative solutions in health communication. Subsequent SRTS events have included mayoral participation (including a city proclamation), a greater number of spotlight schools, and continued support from the media that raises awareness of obesity and health equity issues as well as infrastructure needs in this community. A new interest in bicycling has emerged, and a committee was established to work with the city on safe bicycling, pathways, bike lanes, and helmet use. Walking and bicycling audits and a state infrastructure assessment are planned as a regional south coast bikeway continues to evolve. A health equity summit was recently held, and regular HEI meetings continue. New websites, Facebook pages, friends, and followers grow every day.

Future Directions

Mass in Motion Kids, a CDC childhood obesity research demonstration project, is underway. Multilevel strategies (including a comprehensive health communication campaign) that support change at the individual, institutional, and community levels will build on the coalition and infrastructure already in place in the city with a focus on two- to twelve-year-olds in multiple sectors (health care, schools and afterschool programs, childcare, and the community-at-large). MDPH, in partnership with the Harvard School of Public Health, and the National Initiative for Children's Healthcare Quality are collaborating to develop this integrated childhood obesity–prevention intervention that could be potentially replicated throughout the state and beyond in the future to address childhood obesity among the underserved.

References

Mass in Motion. www.mass.gov/eohhs/consumer/wellness/healthy-living/mass-in-motion-english.html. Retrieved Dec. 2012.

Mass in Motion New Bedford. http://massinmotionnewbedford.org. Retrieved Dec. 2012.

Massachusetts Department of Public Health. www.mass.gov/eohhs/gov/departments/dph. Retrieved Dec. 2012.

National Center for Safe Routes to School. http://www.saferoutesinfo.org. Retrieved Dec. 2012.

US Census Bureau. http://quickfacts.census.gov/qfd/states/25/2545000.html.

Source: Pauline C. Hamel, project coordinator, Mass in Motion New Bedford/Mass in Motion Kids, New Bedford, Massachusetts, October 2012. Used by permission

• • •

Mass in Motion (MiM) Case Study Discussion: Read, Reflect, and Practice in Groups

1. Analyze the case study in light of any element you may consider innovative or new to you. Describe how this relates to your personal and professional experience.

2. What additional strategies and activities would you recommend to further involve local business and homeowners in this initiative? Develop key strategies and elements of a partnership plan using as a framework the information discussed in Chapters Eight and Thirteen.

3. The case study refers to the importance of creativity in health communication planning in light of limited economic and human resources. What other kinds of cost- and time-effective strategies and activities can you think of to complement existing program components from this case study?

Emerging Trends and Lessons

Collectively, the five case studies included in this chapter address most of the different areas of health communication as described in this book and cover a variety of public health and social development challenges through different interventions. Several themes and trends emerged from these case studies. Although sample themes, lessons, or trends apply for the most part across all experiences discussed in this chapter, case studies more strongly related to a specific theme are included in parentheses within the specific bullet point. Many of these themes also resonate with the key concepts and existing literature we discuss in this book, and are presented here in the format of communication tips.

- *Reach people how and where they want to be reached or find themselves frequently*, whether online or via traditional media or in community settings (WhyWellness, "BodyLove," VERB, Mass in Motion) or, even better, via a combination of culturally competent and group-specific venues and media.

- *Use multisectoral partnership as a key approach* to bring to health communication programming different skills, perspectives, and competencies (WhyWellness, Mass in Motion) that may help enhance creativity, program design and implementation, and ultimately potential results.

- *Understand social support as an emerging theme associated with helping people adopt and maintain healthy behaviors* (WhyWellness, "BodyLove," VERB). Always strive to factor in program components that are inclusive of groups, strategies, media, and activities aiming to increase social support for health and social change.

- *Consider peer-to-peer communication as an important strategy in reaching out to older children, tweens, teens, and other vulnerable or at-risk groups.* Social networking and new media provides communicators with additional options to create peer-to-peer connections (WhyWellness, VERB) within groups that are frequent users and health literate of such media.

- *Engage communities, their leaders, and other community mobilization partners* to ensure sustainability and credibility of all efforts as well as potential community commitment and ownership of health and social issues and their solutions ("BodyLove," Health Equity Exchange, Mass in Motion).

- *Integrate different media and communication areas* at the outset of your communication program, or at least in the scale-up phase, to maximize program reach and potential or actual impact ("BodyLove," VERB, Mass in Motion, Health Equity Exchange, Sustainable Table).

- *Be aware that online and new media–based interventions have a longer lifespan that goes beyond program funding and duration*, because visitors continue to keep websites alive and share information on relevant social media and social networking sites (VERB). Plan accordingly to maximize long-term reach.

- *Recognize that many complex issues are community specific and should be addressed by community-driven solutions* (Health Equity Exchange, Mass in Motion).

- *Consider policymakers not only as key decision makers for policy change but also as key partners in community mobilization and public engagement* (Mass in Motion).

- *Look for links among different fields and issues* that may appear unrelated in addressing health and social issues to improve health outcomes and promote community development (Health Equity Exchange, Sustainable Table, Mass in Motion).

- *Increase the appeal of messages and materials via the strategic use of videos, animation, and other graphic or visual devices* that contribute to message simplicity (Sustainable Table, VERB, WhyWellness) both within online and offline settings.

Key Concepts

- Health communication is a constantly evolving field, which is influenced by and influences different social determinants of health as well as leads and adapts to new trends, group-specific preferences, and evolving media.

- Case study analysis may reveal trends and approaches that are being used in the realm of practice and have relevant lessons or implications for other programs or future directions in health communication.

- Case studies provide a framework to discuss themes, trends, and lessons that can be learned by others embarking in the complex process of designing, implementing, and evaluating a health communication intervention. Another objective is to provide readers with discussion materials on how this applies to their professional experience as well as what other communication approaches, strategies, and activities may be suitable in similar cases.

FOR DISCUSSION AND PRACTICE

1. Case study–specific discussion questions and exercises are included at the end of each case study, so please review them for discussion and practice.

2. Reflect on and discuss additional themes or lessons learned that you think may emerge from multiple case studies. Reflect on how they may be relevant to your current or future professional experience or similar programs you may be aware of.

3. Research additional information on the case studies featured in this chapter and analyze and present it in detail.

KEY TERM

virtual world

CHAPTER 16

GLOBAL HEALTH COMMUNICATION:
Case Studies and Lessons from the Field

Similar to Chapter Fifteen, this chapter features case studies and recent experiences, this time from global health communication. Yet, the distinction between US-based and global health communication case studies is included only for ease of use and chapter flow, and is used as a device to meet readers' preferences in case they want to focus solely on either the United States or international country settings.

In fact, different from **international health**, which "relates more to health practices, policies and systems in countries other than one's own and stresses more the differences between countries than their commonalities" (Global Health Education Consortium, 2013), **global health** refers to "health problems, issues and concerns that transcend national boundaries, and may be best addressed by cooperative actions" (Institute of Medicine, 1997, p. 1). This definition continues to shape and guide the role of professionals from multiple sectors in advancing global health.

More recently, "global health has become a rallying point for organizations, professionals, and individuals with a passion for social justice and for alleviating pain and suffering among human populations" (Ehiri, 2009, p. xix). Global health "stresses the commonality of health issues" (Global Health Education Consortium, 2013) and deals with partnership-based models and strategies that have the potential to address similar health issues across geographic boundaries—of course, always within a culturally competent and participatory framework for action so that the voices, preferences, and specific needs of local communities, partners, and stakeholders can be heard

international health
"Relates more to health practices, policies and systems in countries other than one's own and stresses more the differences between countries than their commonalities" (Global Health Education Consortium, 2013)

global health

Refers to "health problems, issues and concerns that transcend national boundaries, and may be best addressed by cooperative actions" (Institute of Medicine, 2007, p. 1)

and can inform local planning and implementation of all interventions. *Think globally, act locally* is now an established concept of great importance in many fields, including health, environment, urban planning, and education, and in most country settings and sectors. At the national level, the diversity of global health issues has brought governments, organizations, and professionals from the public health, health care, community development, and other sectors into a new kind of dialogue of which cultural competence, awareness of geopolitical issues, cross-cultural communication strategies and methods, and global coordination of most interventions are essential components. Within this framework, lessons learned, themes, and intervention models discussed in the US-based case studies in Chapter Fifteen may also be relevant for global health communication interventions and interventions in other specific country settings.

CHAPTER OBJECTIVES

As in Chapter Fifteen, key objectives of this chapter are to review and draw new trends, themes, and potential lessons from featured case studies so they may be considered for future programming and investigation; and most important, to provide readers with a framework for discussion on how this applies to their professional experience and what other communication approaches may be suitable in similar cases.

From Theory to Practice: Select Case Studies on Global Health Communication

This section is very similar to the one in Chapter Fifteen. It aims to provide an overview on how and why case studies are featured in this chapter. It is included again here to provide useful information to readers who may decide to approach this chapter first without having read Chapter Fifteen.

Because many topics in global health and social development are highly interconnected, lessons learned from these case studies transcend the specific health areas for which the health communication intervention was designed and have a broader application in a variety of settings. It was thus not an objective of this chapter to evaluate the outcomes of the programs featured in the case studies, but rather to extrapolate communication trends, themes, and other lessons that may be of general application as they relate to the theoretical and practical models discussed so far in this book.

This discussion is included in the "Emerging Trends and Lessons" section of this chapter.

In this chapter, the individual case studies are categorized under the health or social field (for example, epidemics and emerging diseases) for which the health communication intervention was designed, and referred to by the name of the country they feature (for example, Egypt). Yet, this is done only for ease of reference, because the focus of the analysis is on extrapolating lessons learned that may apply to health communication interventions across different health and social areas and settings, and also to prompt discussion among readers on other potential approaches that may be suitable for implementation as they refer to a specific case study, health area, or their own professional endeavors.

Epidemics and Emerging Diseases

This section includes three case studies that address risk and emergency communication in epidemics and disease outbreak settings as previously defined in this book. Some of the case studies in this section refer to interventions on similar topics in different countries, which may serve to highlight both commonalities and differences in addressing comparable health and community development issues in diverse settings.

Egypt

The first of the three case studies (Egypt) features a partnership-based communication intervention "led by UNICEF and concerned national partners" (Hegazi, 2012) to mitigate the impact of avian influenza (AI) in the general population, and more specifically among women and children, who have a high risk of contracting the virus. The intervention was designed to increase risk perception and promote "life-saving practices" (Hegazi, 2012) among different communities. It also used multiple strategies and media with community- and school-based communication as "cornerstones in the communication strategy" (Hegazi, 2012).

BOX 16.1. COMMUNICATION INTERVENTIONS: HELPING EGYPTIAN FAMILIES AND CHILDREN STAY SAFE FROM AVIAN INFLUENZA

Egypt is one of the world's countries most affected by the avian influenza (AI), caused by the virus H5N1. Since its first outbreak in February 2006 to June 2012, a total of 168 cases, 60 of which were fatal, were officially registered in the country. Women and children are most at risk to contract the virus, because they are those mainly involved in poultry breeding in or around the dwelling, which is found to be the main channel of spreading the virus in Egypt. Since its first outbreak, the Egyptian government recognized the serious social and economic threats represented by the spread of AI and the importance of undertaking massive efforts to step up control efforts, including early outbreak detection and reporting as well as community education efforts (see Figure 16.1).

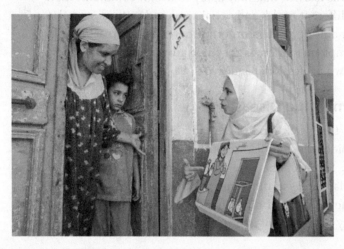

Figure 16.1   Egypt: Community Outreach Workers in Action
Source: UNICEF, Egypt. Used by permission.

A National Plan for Avian and Human Influenza (INPAHI) was developed and led by Ministries of Health, Agriculture, and Education as well as UNICEF and other UN concerned agencies in 2007. The main approach was "catch and contain" the AI H5N1 virus in the bird population before it spread to humans, and to provide citizens with the necessary information on safe breeding practices. Hence, communication for behavior change is a central strategy to achieve this objective. Led by UNICEF and concerned national partners, communication interventions were formulated based on several strategies including policy advocacy, capacity building of more than thirteen thousand community outreach workers and eleven thousand primary school teachers, national radio campaign and mobile information caravans, and finally community education program. The community component included house-to-house education and community outdoor campaign in twenty-four governorates (out of twenty-seven) over a period of four years (2006–2010). In addition, a school program was undertaken and was based on edutainment methods to promote protective messages of wash, stay away, separate, and notify. The community and school interventions were the cornerstones in the communication strategy to reach an estimated 4.8 million households and more than 3.8 million primary schoolchildren with the protective messages.

The interventions were designed according to the risk perception and behavioral analysis framework. The framework assumes that change of behavior is an outcome of the interaction between the perception of threat and efficacy to address this threat. The interventions were also based on a national baseline survey that was undertaken by UNICEF in 2006 and it highlighted the need to promote a number of minimum life-saving practices to increase the chances of protection from AI. These include washing hands with soap after dealing with poultry, covering nose and mouth when dealing with poultry, separating poultry from living areas, and reporting cases of sick or dead poultry.

An independent evaluation of the program conducted in 2009 by UNICEF based on a postintervention survey showed that families and children who were exposed to the community interventions had higher knowledge of the protective measures. When women were asked if they could protect themselves from AI, 98 percent reported they could, compared to 77.7 percent in the baseline. Eighty percent reported washing hands after dealing with poultry as a protection measure compared to 40 percent in the baseline. Meanwhile, breeding practices of households visited by community outreach workers significantly improved compared with the baseline. For covering nose and mouth the percentage reached 46 percent compared to 5 percent in the baseline and the same was achieved for wearing a special dress (47 percent versus 6 percent). When the breeding practices of intervention areas were compared with control areas, differences in shifted practices were also observed.

The community education program proved to be capable of accelerating change and in a cost effective way. $US1 will allow three children to acknowledge information on AI protective practices and with the same amount three rural households will be reached with valuable information about easy-to-apply protective practices from AI.

References

El Rabbat, M. *Avian Influenza Community Assessment: Focus on Backyard Poultry Breeding*. Post Intervention Qualitative Study. Egypt: UNICEF, 2007.

Hegazi, S. "*Successes and Challenges in Communicating Influenza in Egypt.*" Paper presented at the American Public Health Association, 2010.

Kasperson, R. E., and others. "The Social Amplification of Risk: A Conceptual Framework." *Risk Analysis*, 1988, *8*(2), 177–187.

SPAN Consultants. *Evaluation of Avian Influenza Community Education Interventions in Rural Egypt*. Summary Report. Egypt: UNICEF, 2010.

Source: Hegazi, S. *Communication Interventions: Helping Egyptian Families and Children Stay Safe from Avian Influenza*. Egypt: UNICEF, 2012a. Used by permission.

• • •

Egypt Case Study Discussion: Read, Reflect, and Practice in Groups

1. Research and compare other case studies on avian flu communication. Identify key elements of the communication strategy and discuss how they compare to key activities and strategies from the Egypt case study.

2. What other kinds of communication interventions and strategies can you think of to protect high-risk groups such as women and children from avian flu? Discuss pros and cons of each potential option and focus primarily on interventions that may effectively encourage community participation and mobilization.

3. Research and discuss the socioeconomic implications of avian flu in a country of your choice and related communication strategies and programs. Make sure to conduct a few in-depth interviews with organizations and stakeholders who work on this issue in the country you selected.

4. What can we learn from school-based health communication? Recall and discuss any personal or professional experience that included schools as a key communication setting for health-related topics. Analyze key success factors and other components of the intervention that appealed to you.

Canada

pandemic

A geographical widespread outbreak of an infectious disease in which many people are infected at the same time; occurring throughout a region or even throughout the world (Heymann and Rodier, 2001)

"With many experts at the time expecting a severe influenza **pandemic**" (Nacinovich and MacDonald, 2012), the second case study in this section features "regional planning efforts [that] were developed to anticipate and respond effectively" (Nacinovich and MacDonald, 2012) to pandemic flu in the Calgary Health Region of Canada. When several experts and organizations warned in 2005 about the potential imminence of a pandemic (see definition within the case study), "Canada was one of the first countries to have a pandemic influenza plan in place" (Nacinovich and MacDonald, 2012). The case study discusses the benefits of communication preparedness as well as key components of the plan and activities that were developed in the Calgary Health Region.

BOX 16.2. PREPARING FOR A NIGHTMARE IN THE CALGARY HEALTH REGION—PLANNING FOR PANDEMIC INFLUENZA

Need, Situation, Health Issues

Understanding the nature of a pandemic is an important step in the adequate preparation and crisis scenario planning regarding accurate and timely health care communications. A **pandemic** is a geographical widespread outbreak of an infectious disease in which many people are infected at the same time occurring throughout a region or even throughout the world (Heymann and Rodier, 2001). In 2005, the World Health Organization (WHO) and the Public Health Agency of Canada warned that "an influenza (flu) pandemic" is both "inevitable" and "imminent" (World Health Organization, 2005d) Canada was one of the first countries to have a pandemic influenza plan in place with the development of its Canadian Pandemic Influenza Plan at the national level (Public Health Agency of Canada, 2012). With many experts at the time expecting a severe influenza pandemic, regional planning efforts were developed to anticipate and respond effectively (Harper, Fukuda, Uyeki, Cox, & Bridges, 2005). These efforts were advanced to assist in the "proper understanding of the nature of the threat, its likely impact on Calgary, and to reassure people that Calgary Health Region is ready to respond" (Calgary Health Region, 2005).

Goal and Objectives

Goal

The Calgary Health Region needed to focus on communicating with its stakeholders by developing and implementing a detailed communication plan as part of its contingency plan.

Objectives

- Develop and implement an overall pandemic response communication plan.
- Provide employers, health professionals, and the community with a better understanding of pandemic influenza and its impact.

Approach

This case includes some of the planning highlights and communication activities developed in coordination at the health region level. With each region responsible for developing contingency plans to reduce the impact of an influenza pandemic, key stakeholders within Calgary Health Region, Alberta Health and Wellness, and local municipalities during this time frame in Canada came together to set out specific measures and actions.

Sample Communication Strategies and Activities

- Communication planning workshop for representatives of all the business units in the Calgary Health Region (i.e., HR, emergency services, operations, medical, etc.) to work through audiences, messages, and priorities
- Overall communications plan and development of the Calgary Health Region's main operational plan, *Pandemic Response Plan* (Volume 1 was 185+ pages, Volume 2 was 475 pages)
- First public document, *Explaining Pandemic Influenza*, in April 2005 and its revised second release in December 2005
- Quick facts booklets for three separate audiences—community, employees, and physicians
- Creative communication elements focused on promoting best practices in general hygiene included prevention posters and various educational tools
- Pandemic micro-site strategically integrated into Calgary Health Region's existing website
- Pandemic intranet site for employees
- Presentations at the Calgary Chamber of Commerce to reach the local business community and increase awareness with regard to pandemic preparedness and its importance to businesses

Key Results

During the initial phase of the pandemic influenza preparedness, Calgary Health Region was very successful in building awareness of the importance of pandemic influenza preparedness among all audience groups including the local community, businesses, and Calgary Health Region staff. The print and online materials were well received and helped Calgary Health Region become a recognized leader in the pandemic influenza preparedness process by engaging its staff and ensuring the local community had access to necessary and useful information.

Future Directions

During a pandemic, it is far too late to be thinking about refining crisis plans or putting a plan in place to protect your respective interests. The mere concept of a pandemic threat should immediately motivate government officials and business leaders to begin the complex preparations for how to maintain adequate continuity and how best to plan for the breadth and depth of needs and challenges associated with health care communications that will be critical to each stakeholder group. With the choices between "wait and see" and "plan for the worst and hope for the best," developing the pandemic planning and communication infrastructure now demonstrates innovative, forward thinking based on established best practices that will ultimately yield long-term benefits for all stakeholders. Ultimately, it is far easier to explain why you effectively planned ahead and invested in the development of a plan than to need to explain during or following a pandemic why a plan was not put in place.

References

Calgary Health Region. *Explaining Pandemic Influenza: A Guide from the Medical Officer of Health.* Calgary, AB: Calgary Health Region, 2005.

Harper, S. A., Fukuda, K., Uyeki, T., Cox, N. J., & Bridges, C. B. "Prevention and Control of Influenza—Recommendations of the Advisory Committee on Immunization Practices (ACIP)." *MMWR*, 2005, *54 (Early Release)*, 1–40. www.cdc.gov/mmwr/preview/mmwrhtml/rr54e713a1 .htm.

Heymann, D. L., and Rodier, G. R. "Hot Spots in a Wired World: WHO Surveillance of Emerging and Re-emerging Infectious Diseases." *Lancet*, 2001, *1*(5), 345–353.

Public Health Agency of Canada. "The Canadian Pandemic Influenza Plan for the Health Sector." www.phac-aspc.gc.ca/cpip-pclcpi/index-eng.php. Retrieved Nov. 2012.

World Health Organization. "Responding to the Avian Influenza Pandemic Threat— Recommended Strategic Actions." 2005d. www.who.int/csr/resources/publications/influenza /WHO_CDS_CSR_GIP_05_8-EN.pdf.

Source: Nacinovich Jr., M. R., and MacDonald, M. "Preparing for a Nightmare in the Calgary Health Region— Planning for Pandemic Influenza." Unpublished Case Study, 2012. Used by permission.

• • •

Canada Case Study Discussion: Read, Reflect, and Practice in Groups

1. Research and review lessons learned from past pandemic flu or other epidemics and disease outbreaks as they relate to communicating risk in an emergency setting as well as encouraging the adoption and sustainability of lifesaving behaviors and relevant social measures. Draw commonalities and differences among two or three case studies to identify key elements of effective communication in the preparedness, readiness, and response phases (see Chapter Six).

2. Identify and discuss potential community- and household-based communication interventions to integrate existing elements of the Calgary Health Region communication preparedness plan as highlighted by the Canada case study. Reflect on how you will build on existing strategies and activities discussed by the case study and how you can maximize community participation and citizen engagement in support of an effective response.

3. Research the role of local business and health care providers within a pandemic setting. What kind of information and training is it important for them to receive in order to respond

to a potential pandemic (or also during a disease outbreak) both effectively and safely? Draw your observations from published papers on this topic, personal experience, and available case studies or organizational resources.

4. Analyze media coverage during a recent pandemic or disease outbreak in your country or region and reflect on the roles and responsibilities of the mass media during a public health emergency. Focus on issues of accuracy, clarity of recommended emergency behaviors, responsible reporting, and other features that are particularly important at times of uncertainty and crisis such as during a pandemic, epidemic, or disease outbreak. Also, what are the main messages and do you think underserved, vulnerable, or low-literacy populations would be able to act on them? If not, what else would you do to make sure no one is left behind?

India

Because interpersonal communication is a key area of health communication, this case study (India) reflects on the lessons learned from two different interventions (addressing a polio upsurge and an avian flu outbreak, both in India) for which interpersonal communication was the most prominent element of communication programming. These experiences associate the effectiveness of interpersonal communication to "the personal credibility of community mobilizers and influencers" (Ateeq, 2012), and also identify sample issues that may undermine such credibility.

BOX 16.3. INTERPERSONAL COMMUNICATION: LESSONS LEARNED IN INDIA

Polio Eradication
On February 25, 2012, after more than sixteen years of polio immunization campaigns, WHO officially announced India as nonpolio endemic and removed it from the list of polio-endemic countries.

Background
There was an upsurge in wild polio virus (WPV) cases in 2002, with more than 1,600 reported WPV cases. This outbreak revealed that the impact of WPV was disproportionately high in children belonging to Muslim communities in most parts of India. However, a deeper analysis of the affected children's profiles revealed that poverty and not religion was the primary common factor among them.

Barriers and Challenges

Poor social and economic conditions; lack of access to basic services, including health, nutrition, and sanitation; unhealthy behaviors, such as open defecation and low usage of sanitary toilets; unsafe and contaminated water sources; and unhygienic food caused serious threats to the health of vulnerable sections and decreased their immunity. Therefore, despite taking multiple oral polio vaccine (OPV) doses, some children contracted WPV infection.

Preventive health practices, such as immunization, were hardly a priority for poor parents who were busy working hard to support their families. Other barriers included misconceptions, such as the belief that polio vaccine causes infertility, lack of trust in the government, fatigue due to repeated polio immunization rounds, sensationalized media stories, and so on.

Evidence-based BCC (Behavior Change Communication)

Many parents in various high-risk areas (HRAs) of polio with predominantly poor Muslims were not participating in immunization campaigns, and their children were not taking adequate numbers of OPV doses. This situation demanded more systematic and focused communication interventions in these HRAs, and these strategies led poor parents to accept immunization for their children. However, a sizable number of children who missed vaccination formed a cohort of susceptible children who constituted a wide enough immunity gap for the virus to circulate and infect others.

Interpersonal Communication and Social Mobilization

UNICEF India Country Office supported the deployment of more than six thousand local community mobilization coordinators (CMCs). Mostly local women, they were trained in interpersonal communication (IPC) skills and deployed in HRAs and in nonendemic states. Each CMC covered around three hundred families with children under the age of five, and pregnant and lactating mothers. This unique community mobilization deployment contacted over 1.5 million families for IPC at least four times during each polio immunization round and also during the routine immunization sessions between polio rounds.

Underserved Strategy

In 2003, an underserved strategy (USS) was developed to strengthen the ongoing social mobilization activities. The initiative was led by the government and supported by WHO, Rotary, UNICEF, and full-fledge universities founded to provide education to poor and underprivileged segments of society such as Aligarh Muslim University (AMU), Jamia Millia Islamia (JMI), and Jamia Hamdard. The strategic influence of these institutions was spread through other networks and forums including many local schools and madrasah. By 2006 more than 350 national-, state-, district-, and community-level social, religious, spiritual, and occupational institutions and forums were involved in various social mobilization activities including developing culture-specific local information, education, and communication materials, issuing appeals and endorsements for immunization programs at social and cultural events, sermons, masjid, and temple announcements.

These activities were helpful in establishing and strengthening interaction among local groups, parents, and immunization teams. Polio advocacy and immunization activities at various shrines helped immunize over 240,170 children across different priority districts of Uttar Pradesh in 2006.

Avian Influenza (AI)

Lessons learnt from the successful implementation of community mobilization for polio immunization were effectively used for avian flu (AI) prevention in the state of West Bengal. West Bengal experienced the worst AI outbreak in 2008 when all nineteen districts of the state were affected by the disease, killing about 115,710 birds. However, subsequent recurrences were less intensive, and the last couple of high seasons saw no cases of AI. IPC played a critical role in AI prevention.

The high density of poultry population in West Bengal, over 75 percent of which is backyard poultry in unorganized farming; movement of poultry across its porous border with Bangladesh where AI outbreaks are more common; water bodies that attract migratory birds, including ducks, that are H5N1 carriers and share living spaces with hens; and poor bio security for poultry made West Bengal particularly vulnerable to AI. AI can spread fast from birds to humans because farmers' families often share living space with their poultry.

The culling operations and communication activities during the very first outbreak also revealed the lack of information and unsafe behaviors prevalent in the poor sections of the population. In many rural areas and urban slums people were found buying and consuming cheap poultry transported from the AI-affected areas. Backyard poultry farmers often did not comply with culling operations and hid their sick poultry from the rapid response teams (RRTs) deployed by the government to swiftly complete the culling operations in the affected areas.

AI Communication

UNICEF had print- and broadcast-ready prototypes that were shared with the government for mass production and dissemination. This support was critical to deal with the crisis situation as the messages on dos and don'ts, particularly on safe poultry practices and culling operations, were helpful to inform public and create general awareness.

IPC for AI prevention

Later in 2008, UNICEF supported the training and deployment of 161 NGO and CBO volunteers across 125 gram panchayats (local self-governments at the village or small town level in India) in twenty-five blocks of five priority districts for social mobilization and IPC with backyard poultry farmers. The NGO-trained mobilizers conducted social mobilization activities, including focused IPC, dissemination of information, education, and communication material, and delivered messages on safe poultry practices. These included keeping poultry outside living areas and not mixing newly bought poultry with the old; preventing children from touching and playing with birds in case there is suspected poultry disease in the area; washing hands with soap after touching and handling poultry, cleaning their fences, and changing water at regular intervals; sharing information with farmers regarding vaccination; reporting to local animal health workers if birds show any symptoms of bird flu; refusing consumption of sick or dead birds; burying dead poultry and not dumping them in the open; and extending fullest cooperation with the RRTs by letting them cull poultry and complete disinfection operations following official notification of bird flu outbreak in the area.

Wave Effect Mobilization

About ten special teams, each with two to three community mobilizers, were formed to support culling and disinfection operations in resistant villages. The community influencers and mobilizers entered the villages first and counseled the poultry owners regarding serious risks involved in not parting with their poultry for culling and spoke about compensation to cover the loss. As soon as they obtained the families' cooperation they would ask the waiting RRTs to come in. The team would then swiftly move to the next resistant village.

This process formed a wave effect to deal with resistant backyard poultry owners and was highly effective in completing culling operations in the state. The first phase of social mobilization covered about 0.6 million in five districts and continue to expand.

IPC Contribution to AI Prevention

Qualitative and quantitative evaluations done by external agencies show that 70 percent of backyard poultry farmers could demonstrate knowledge of safe poultry practices across the five priority districts, and over 50 percent of them perform safe poultry practices. The most tangible effect attributed to communication interventions, especially to IPC, is that the behavior of hiding sick birds by the backyard poultry farmers is now almost nonexistent in the focused districts. The assessment reports show that farmers now report to local animal health workers if they observe any unhealthy or abnormal symptoms in their poultry, and demand vaccination for poultry from the government.

Challenges and Limitations of IPC

The effectiveness of interpersonal communication depends on the personal credibility of community mobilizers and influencers who are trained and deployed to conduct IPC. Issues that undermine the credibility of IPC can have a negative impact on the initiative.

- *IPC and routine immunization (RI):* It has been observed that RI sessions function erratically in underserved and hard-to-reach areas. Often vaccinators turn up late or not at all for RI sessions, keeping parents and children waiting; change the location of the session; or not have all the required antigens. This adversely affects the credibility of CMCs and influencers, who provide parents with IPC and urge them to attend the RI sessions.

- *IPC and latrine and water supply:* Despite the demand generated by IPC for toilet use to prevent open defecation, scarcity of water and supply issues with toilet hardware can undermine the efforts of IPC.

- *IPC and AI vaccination:* Poor government response to AI vaccination and delayed disbursement of postculling compensation in West Bengal also has serious implications for IPC.

Source: Ateeq, N. "Interpersonal Communication: Lessons Learned in India. Some Experiences from Communication for (i) Polio Eradication, (ii) Avian Influenza Prevention in India." UNICEF ICO. Unpublished Case Study, 2012. Used by permission.

● ● ●

India Case Study Discussion: Read, Reflect, and Practice in Groups

1. Think of policy communication and public advocacy interventions that may be helpful to address obstacles to community mobilizers' credibility, as described in the India case study, and to promote policy change and enforcement and advocate for further resource allocation for routine immunization and water and sanitation interventions. What kinds of constituency groups should be involved in these efforts? What kinds of communication strategies do you think may be effective in leading to policy change, monitoring, and adequate enforcement?

2. Research the issue of absent teachers and medical and community health workers in developing countries and present your findings as well as examples of communication programs that have attempted to address such issues (including relevant lessons learned). As an additional option, interview international or local organizations on this issue to gain their perspective. Use a PowerPoint format for your group presentation.

3. Identify and view existing videos on polio eradication in developing countries and use them as a framework to reflect on and discuss key communication messages, constituency groups, and spokespeople of polio eradication campaigns.

Infectious Diseases

United States–Mexico

Because "TB morbidity and mortality are higher along the United States–Mexico border region" (de Heer, Moya, and Lacson, 2008) than in other US regions, this initiative implemented in two cities aimed at increasing "TB awareness, cross-border collaboration, and treatment adherence" (de Heer, Moya, and Lacson, 2008). The intervention used a photovoice project as a tool for storytelling and communication with various groups and stakeholders for "empowering and mobilizing persons affected by TB to present their stories to decision makers, securing public commitments from decision makers to contribute to TB awareness and eradication, securing funding for existing prevention and control programs, disseminating important messages about TB, developing a support system by and for patients, and improving adherence to treatment" (de Heer, Moya, and Lacson, 2008). Future directions are also included in this case study.

BOX 16.4. CASE STUDY—VOICES AND IMAGES (TUBERCULOSIS)

Need, Situation, Health Issues

Despite available cost-effective treatment, every minute, tuberculosis (TB), an infectious disease caused by the *Mycobacterium tuberculosis*, kills four people and affects fifteen more worldwide. If left untreated, each person with active TB will infect an average of ten to fifteen people a year. Failure to treat persons with active TB results in high costs at the individual, community, and societal levels. In 2004, the TB rate in foreign-born persons living in the United States was 8.7 times that of native US citizens, with individuals of Hispanic (primarily Mexican) descent representing the largest percentage of all new TB cases (29 percent). TB morbidity and mortality are higher along the United States–Mexico border region, where geographical, social, and economic factors, including Mexico's higher TB rate, lower socioeconomic status, limited access to health care services, migration to the United States, lack of TB education, and language barriers, contribute to an elevated incidence of TB.

Goals and Objectives

In 2005, the Amaya-Lacson initiative initiated the TB Photovoice Project in the binational El Paso and Ciudad Juarez metropolitan community, with the aim of increasing TB awareness, crossborder collaboration, and treatment adherence. The site was chosen based on TB prevalence, socioeconomic and environmental conditions, and the community leadership's interest in the project.

The mission of the TB Photovoice Project was to facilitate the use of images, stories, and dialogue to elevate the voices of individuals directly impacted by tuberculosis so that they as well as their communities could improve their overall health. Program objectives included empowering and mobilizing persons affected by TB to present their stories to decision makers, securing public commitments from decision makers to contribute to TB awareness and eradication, securing funding for existing prevention and control programs, disseminating important messages about TB, developing a support system by and for patients, and improving adherence to treatment.

Communication Strategies and Activities

Photovoice or picture stories is a participatory action research (PAR) strategy developed by Caroline Wang and Mary Ann Burris (1994, 1997) that involves providing cameras to vulnerable groups to document their lives from their unique perspectives, and using photographs to encourage individuals to talk about everyday health and work realities. Since cameras are easy to use, people who do not read or write and who are socially isolated or stigmatized with a health condition such as TB are enabled to have a voice. Photovoice functions as a tool of empowerment and enables those with little money, power, or status to communicate to decision makers. It is based on the understanding that effective policies are derived from the integration of local knowledge from affected populations.

Participants recruited were receiving or had completed TB treatment, and included men, women, and children living in a binational area. They were asked to shoot one roll of film per week for five weeks, focusing on their community and the impact of TB on their lives.

Participants were asked to select two or three photos that captured their concerns and perspectives on TB. These photos were shared and discussed with the group and emerging themes were identified. Participants grouped the photographs and accompanying stories into four categories: personal history with TB, social norms and values, emotional aspects, and social aspects and ideas for advocacy and change. This process helped them identify themes such as allocation of financial and human resources for education and treatment, development of support services, clinically trained and culturally competent providers, and addressing the needs of patients beyond TB, including poverty, hunger, and housing. These themes served as a basis for an international call to action that was presented to global leaders and advocates during the Thirty-Eighth International Conference on Tuberculosis and Lung Diseases in South Africa.

Key Results

Photographs and stories selected by participants were utilized to create an exhibit that was presented on over twenty-five occasions, reaching an estimated 3,600 conference attendees.

At a forum at World TB day, the TB Photovoice Project participants presented their concerns and perspectives to influential decision makers. Twenty-five local and national decision makers made public commitments to address TB in the border area. Compared to 2006, newspaper coverage regarding TB doubled in the area in 2007. Participants in this project had 100 percent treatment adherence and were instrumental in establishing the first-ever support group for individuals with TB in Ciudad Juarez.

Future Directions

The TB Photovoice Project method (see www.tbphotovoice.org) is being implemented for TB in eleven additional sites in Mexico and other countries, and its feasibility is being explored for other health issues, such as HIV/AIDS and diabetes. The culture- and community-specific messages elicited by this method can be used to bridge the gap between patients and policymakers, and promote social change.

References

Wang, C., and Burris, M. "Empowerment Through Photo Novella: Portraits of Participation." *Health Education Quarterly*, 1994, *21*(2), 171–186.

Wang, C., and Burris, M. "Photovoice: Concept, Methodology, and Use for Participatory Needs Assessment." *Health Education & Behavior*, 1997, *25*(3), 369–387.

• • •

United States–Mexico Case Study Discussion: Read, Reflect, and Practice in Groups

1. Discuss other potential future directions as they relate to the design and implementation of the TB Photovoice Project in the United States–Mexico case study. What would you do to expand on the project's current reach and impact?

2. Have you used photovoice before? Are you familiar with this important communication tool to reach out to low-literacy and underserved populations? Describe any professional or personal experience you may have had with photovoice.

3. Develop a photovoice project in your community, school, workplace, or neighborhood. Share and discuss photos and stories or organize an exhibit to engage additional community members to participate in the project.

Maternal and Child Health

Cambodia

"In 2002 Cambodia's Ministry of Health identified behavior change communication as one among a set of key strategies to improve the health of women and children in the country" (Tan and others, 2012). This case study (Cambodia) focuses on a five-year communication intervention to increase antenatal care (ANC) (also referred to as *prenatal care*) among pregnant women and birth delivery by skilled birth attendants. The intervention relied on a strategic blend of mass media, interpersonal, and community engagement strategies and activities, integrates two different communication models and strategic planning frameworks (C4D and COMBI—see Chapter Two for additional information) and is being expanded to most regions in Cambodia.

BOX 16.5. APPLYING C4D TO CURB MATERNAL MORTALITY IN CAMBODIA

For the first time in decades, families in the Kingdom of Cambodia have adopted health-seeking behaviors that may finally curtail the nation's high maternal mortality, which is among the highest in the East Asia and Pacific region. Between 2005 and 2010 antenatal care (ANC) and delivery by skilled birth attendants has increased significantly. A key contributing factor behind this has been sustained support from UNICEF and the European Commission since 2005 to strengthen the national health promotion capacity.

In 2002 Cambodia's Ministry of Health identified behavior change communication as one among a set of key strategies to improve the health of women and children in the country. The European Commission and UNICEF therefore jointly established the Health Behavior Change Communication (BCC) Project to provide technical assistance and five million euros to strengthen the national health promotion capacity between 2005 and 2009. The implementing partner was Cambodia's National Center for Health Promotion (NCHP) with sixty staff based in the capital Phnom Penh, supported by provincial health promotion units (PHPUs) in each of the twenty-four provinces. While nationwide in scope, the BCC project was in particular focused on demonstrating good BCC practices in seven of the least-developed provinces. Activities were implemented in close collaboration with provincial maternal and child health managers and supervisors.

For the first three years the project provided intensive capacity-building support at the national and provincial levels and by 2008 Cambodia had reattained a robust and qualified national system to engage effectively with communities and families to improve health-seeking behaviors. To demonstrate its renewed capacity, the National Health Congress made an evidence-based decision to prioritize promotion of ANC. NCHP was awarded the responsibility for developing, implementing, and monitoring a campaign to increase the use of recommended ANC services in Cambodia.

NCHP successfully took on the challenge and with technical support from UNICEF developed a communication strategy using a C4D (communication for development) and COMBI (communication for behavioral impact) planning model. UNICEF and NCHP hired a professional advertising agency and jointly oversaw the development of innovative and engaging audio-visual and printed campaign materials targeting mothers, fathers, and other family members. This was guided by consultations and pretesting with representative community members, families, and health staff. Simultaneously, NCHP and PHPUs oversaw the training of around three hundred health workers from health centers and 4,400 village health volunteers in the seven demonstration provinces to provide and promote quality ANC services. Many of these were volunteers and mother support groups that UNICEF had also successfully nurtured and worked with in the past to promote exclusive breastfeeding.

In January 2009 Cambodia launched the ANC campaign on national television and radio (see Figure 16.2) supported by the trained interpersonal communicators in the seven demonstration provinces. Throughout the country, potentially pregnant women were encouraged by colorful, innovative, and captivating radio and TV spots, mobile phone ringtones, posters, banners, and leaflets, to come in for their first ANC visit within a month of missing their period. This core message was communicated massively and intensively in the media several times a day, and reinforced at community level by the trained interpersonal communicators. Everybody talked about it—some even whistled the catchy campaign tune.

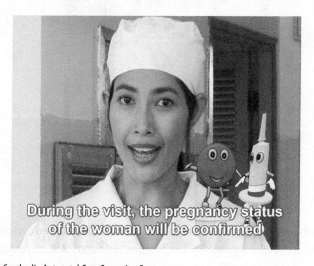

Figure 16.2 Cambodia Antenatal Care Campaign Spot

Source: UNICEF. Used by permission.

The twelve-month communication objective was to increase the percentage of women seeking ANC within the first eight weeks of pregnancy from 5 percent to 25 percent in the seven demonstration provinces. In turn this would enable them to receive a set of ANC services including confirmation of the pregnancy and related medical checkups, vaccination against tetanus, iron-folate tablets, and education on birth planning and proper health and nutrition during pregnancy. An external evaluation of the BCC project and the ANC campaign in 2011 documented that the communication objective was met well beyond expectations: already within the first twelve months of the ANC campaign, 36 percent of potentially pregnant women came in for their first ANC visit within the first eight weeks of pregnancy. This supported the achievement of key maternal health program objectives; the proportion of pregnant women completing all four recommended ANC visits and receiving the recommended two tetanus toxoid vaccinations almost doubled in the demonstration provinces. Key to the success of the campaign was the use of mass media and interpersonal communicators, which added credibility to the campaign and enabled genuine community engagement on the importance of ANC. Other key enabling factors were provision of financial incentives for midwives for delivering a live birth as well as improved road infrastructure (see Figure 16.3).

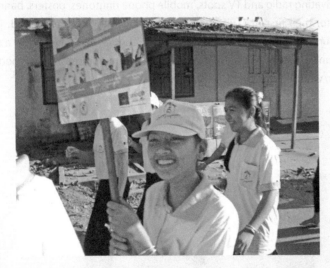

Figure 16.3 Volunteers Launch the ANC Campaign in Stung Treng, Cambodia, January 2009
Source: UNICEF. Used by permission.

The Cambodia Demographic and Health Survey (CDHS) in 2010 registered and documented the related and overall improved maternal health indicators. Since 2005, ANC coverage increased from 69 to 89 percent, delivery by skilled birth attendants increased from 44 to 71 percent, and delivery in health facilities increased from 22 to 53 percent. Furthermore, the proportion of women delivering with the support of traditional birth attendants at home decreased from

55 percent in 2005 to 28 percent in 2010. The ANC campaign has now been expanded to intensively provide and promote ANC in sixteen out of the twenty-four provinces in Cambodia.

Source: Written by Try Tan, C4D specialist, UNICEF Cambodia, and Tomas Jensen, communication specialist, UNICEF Pacific (Health Education Specialist, UNICEF Cambodia from 2005–2009)—in collaboration with Denise Shepherd-Johnson, chief of communication, UNICEF Cambodia; Penelope Campbell, chief, Health & Nutrition, UNICEF Cambodia; Malalay Ahmadzai, MCH specialist, UNICEF Cambodia; Vanny Ung, health education officer, UNICEF Cambodia; Viorica Berdaga, chief, Health & Nutrition, UNICEF Lao PDR (chief of Health & Nutrition, UNICEF Cambodia from 2008–2012); and Everold Hosein, founder of COMBI, 2012. Used by permission.

• • • •

Cambodia Case Study Discussion: Read, Reflect, and Practice in Groups

1. Research and discuss similar programs on maternal and child health in developing countries. Identify key components and success factors, and compare them with key learnings from the Cambodia case study.

2. Innovation is an important aspect of today's health communication. Think of potential innovations as they refer to communication programs on maternal and child health to be implemented in low-income country settings.

3. Develop two to three discussion questions as they refer to further exploration of the content of the Cambodia case study. Discuss them within your group or use them to facilitate a moderated discussion and ideas-sharing session on this case study.

Role of Health Sciences Librarians in Health Communication

International

Different from other experiences discussed in this chapter, we will refer to this case study as *international* because it does not cover information and activities that took place in a specific country. Yet, just to reiterate, these labels are used only for ease of reference because most of the themes and lessons that could be extrapolated from all case studies in this chapter transcend geographical boundaries and health areas and may find application for future global health communication programs. This case study discusses and provides examples of the role of health sciences librarians in health communication as well as in the education and training of future public health practitioners, and advocates for the need to build capacity among health sciences librarians so that they can further contribute to health communication interventions.

BOX 16.6. THE ROLE OF THE HEALTH SCIENCES LIBRARIAN IN HEALTH COMMUNICATION: CONTINUITY IN EVIDENCE-BASED PUBLIC HEALTH TRAINING FOR FUTURE PUBLIC HEALTH PRACTITIONERS

Health sciences librarians are professionally trained with a minimum of a master's degree and attend continuing education courses and professional workshops to ensure that we have the requisite information and skills to practice in the area of health communication. We use a variety of electronic tools such as listservs, blogs, and social media to assist one another in helping professionals, students, and lay people through instruction, literature searching, and a host of information-related tasks. One of these tools, LibGuides, is touted as "the most widely used system for creating research guides and sharing knowledge." It's an effective tool that helps us support those who must make day-to-day decisions in health care. As you read the following scenario, you will see how health sciences librarians can play an essential role in the field of health communication.

Think of polycystic ovarian syndrome (PCOS) treatment—search Google and more than 1,700,000 records are retrieved in a fraction of a second, 0.18 seconds. Search Google Scholar to filter these results and approximately 58,200 fair to high-quality results are retrieved in .08 seconds. There is an abundance of health-related, easy-to-use, and freely accessible databases and search engines via the Internet. Many students, health care practitioners, and general consumers looking for health information use general and health care databases and search engines with little or no skill to ensure optimal retrieval results and source credibility to answer health-related questions.

Evidence-based practice using the PICO (patient, problem, and/or population intervention comparison or control, and outcome) framework to generate clinical questions has enabled health sciences librarians to become key players in the field of health communication teaching different groups how to ask the properly framed question and filter the results for quality evidence. From PICO, a clinical question is generated that lends itself to searching the literature.

The PICO framework, however, does not lend itself to addressing the needs of public health practitioner. As a result, Brownson and others (2011) established an evidence-based public health (EBPH) framework using three types of evidence: type 1 recognizes a health care problem and states something should be done, type 2 states what should be done specifically to address the problem, and type 3 states specifically how to do it. By combining the PICO and EBPH frameworks, we now have an effective method in which to frame and address questions and find relevant information to be shared (see the EBP/EBPH framework in Figure 16.4).

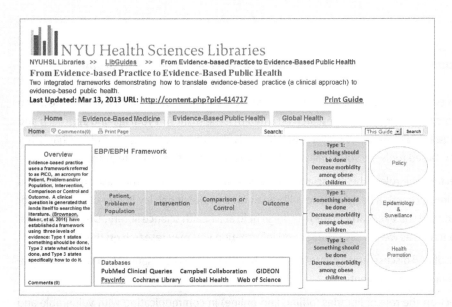

Figure 16.4 Sample Screenshot from LibGuides

Source: Springshare, LibGuide. Used by permission.

Using LibGuides, librarians share and adapt guides for effective health communication on a variety of topics. Figure 16.4 shows a page from LibGuides of how this can be used to frame a health issue and to find evidence-based information to communicate about it. The tabs allow easy navigation among topics. Comments can be submitted from both librarians and library patrons. The white space on the right is where the image of a librarian and contact information is typically displayed. Often, a chat box is available for librarians on duty to speak directly with their patrons. Polls can be added easily to address any kind of question.

LibGuides is an essential tool to build capacity among health sciences librarians so that they can have a significant role in health communication. Information can be easily shared and updated between librarians and their clientele. The next steps are to evaluate the effectiveness of resources such as LibGuides and continue to assess the information-seeking and critical-appraisal skills of library users.

Reference

Brownson, R. C., and others. *Evidence-Based Public Health.* (2nd ed.) New York: Oxford University Press, 2011.

Source: Vieira, D. L. "The Role of the Health Sciences Librarian in Health Communication: Continuity in Evidence-Based Public Health Training for Future Public Health Practitioners." Unpublished Case Study, 2013. Used by permission.

· · ·

International Case Study Discussion: Read, Reflect, and Practice in Groups

1. Because health communication is an evidence-based discipline, reflect on the tools you use to conduct preliminary research on a health issue to inform yourself and approach and engage others. Are you familiar with the tools described in this case study? What other library-based tools are you familiar with? What are some of their key features?

2. Reflect on the role of health sciences librarians in the context of this case study. Did you ever interact with a health sciences librarian (as a professional, lay library user, student, or other)? Did you ever participate in a course held at a health science library? Discuss personal experiences as well as case studies and information you may research on this topic.

3. Think of and discuss strategies to integrate health sciences librarians in health communication teams and interventions.

4. Reflect on the role of libraries (offline and online) in communicating with vulnerable and underserved groups.

Emerging Trends and Lessons

As in Chapter Fifteen, the six case studies included in this chapter address different areas of health communication, and in some cases also provide an opportunity to review similar interventions in different countries. Several themes, trends, and potential suggestions emerged from these case studies, and are discussed in the following. Although similar themes emerged for the most part across all experiences discussed in this chapter, case studies that are more strongly related to a specific topic and discuss it more explicitly are included in parentheses within the specific bullet point to which they refer. Most of these observations are also validated from other existing experiences, theories, and literature that are discussed in other chapters of this book, and reflect current practice in health communication as well as this author's own experience. They are presented here in the format of communication planning tips:

- *Provide opportunities for community ownership and participation* to expand program reach, "accelerating change" (Hegazi, 2012) and enabling inclusion of low-literacy, isolated, and other vulnerable populations, whether via community mobilization, school based, or door-to-door communication, interpersonal communication, photovoice, or other community-centered interventions (Egypt, India, Cambodia, United States–Mexico).

- *Focus on capacity building and training of community mobilization partners and national systems* on key communication areas including community outreach and mobilization, information dissemination, and interpersonal communication as an important step "to engage effectively with communities and families to improve health-seeking behaviors" (Tan and others, 2012) (Egypt, India, Cambodia).

- *Consider a strategic blend of communication areas, strategies, and channels* (mass media, print media, interpersonal, online, community based) to add credibility to the intervention, and enable community, partner, and staff engagement (Cambodia, Canada).

- *Establish clear behavioral objectives* on the basis of rigorous planning frameworks, evidence-based assumptions, and an in-depth understanding of perceived risk and potential obstacles to behavior change (Egypt, India, Cambodia).

- *Be aware that as in other communication areas, the "effectiveness of interpersonal communication depends on the personal credibility of community mobilizers"* (Ateeq, 2012), which in turn may be linked to social norms, policies, spotless execution of all program components, and resource allocation for related interventions (India).

- *Make sure to build capacity of groups that are either influential or provide essential services* (business community, health sciences librarians, and many others) so that they can either be an effective participant in the communication process or help educate and train future professionals (Canada, International).

- *Raise the influence of community voices and patients on policies and future programs* by developing culturally friendly tools that are inclusive of low health literacy, socially isolated, stigmatized, and other vulnerable populations (United States–Mexico).

- *Use research tools that allow you to frame and understand a health issue within the context of different communication interventions* (for example, policy, community, advocacy) (International).

Finally, some of the themes that emerged from the case studies in this chapter are more specifically related to risk and emergency communication in the context of pandemics, epidemics, and emerging diseases:

- *Recognize the importance of advance communication planning in preparation for a pandemic threat.* Despite all kinds of potential reasons and conflicting priorities for not acting quickly to preserve lives, "it is far easier to explain why you effectively planned ahead and invested in the development of a plan than to need to explain during or following a pandemic why a plan was not put in place" (Nacinovich and MacDonald, 2012) (Canada).

- *Community-based interventions are an integral and critical component of communication interventions in epidemics and emerging disease settings* (Egypt, India).

Key Concepts

- Health communication is a constantly evolving field, which is influenced by and influences different social determinants of health as well as leads and adapts to new trends, group-specific preferences, and evolving media.

- Case study analysis may reveal trends and approaches that are being used in the realm of practice and have relevant implications for other programs or future directions in health communication.

- Case studies provide a framework to analyze emerging themes, trends, and lessons that can be learned by others embarking in the complex process of designing, implementing, and evaluating a health communication intervention. Another objective is to provide readers with discussion materials on how this applies to their professional experience as well as what other communication approaches, strategies, and activities may be suitable in similar cases.

- Case studies in this chapter are related to global health communication. Yet, because global health refers to "health problems, issues and concerns that transcend national boundaries and may be best addressed by cooperative actions" (Institute of Medicine, 1997, p. 1), the distinction with US-based case studies is primarily related to the book's logic flow and ease of use.

- Think globally, act locally is now an established concept of great importance in many fields, including health, environment, urban planning, and education, and in most country settings and sectors. Within this framework, trends, lessons, themes, and intervention models, discussed by the US-based case studies in Chapter Fifteen, may also be relevant to global health communication interventions and country-specific interventions in other settings.

FOR DISCUSSION AND PRACTICE

1. Case study–specific discussion questions and exercises are included at the end of each case study and could be used to practice key concepts in this chapter within group settings.

2. Reflect and discuss about additional themes, trends, or lessons that you think emerge from multiple case studies. Reflect on how they may be relevant to your current or future professional experience, or similar programs you may be aware of.

KEY TERMS

global health   pandemic

international health

EXAMPLES OF WORKSHEETS AND RESOURCES ON HEALTH COMMUNICATION PLANNING

Topics in this appendix are organized within two main categories: (1) examples of planning worksheets and sample questions and (2) online resources. Many of these resources refer to multiple chapters in the text.

A1: Situation and Audience Analysis Worksheet: Sample Questions and Topics

This list of questions and topics is not all inclusive and may not apply to all health issues. Therefore, it should be used only as an example. As described in this book, the situation and audience analysis should be completed via a variety of participatory and traditional research methods. Questions within the categories in the following worksheet are often interconnected and are listed in a specific order only to simplify the use of this template.

Category	Key topics and questions
Condition or health issue	Description Prevalence or incidence Trends (for example, decreasing, staying the same, increasing) Degree of severity in different groups Risk factors (for example, socioeconomic conditions, age, gender, specific ethnic groups, geographical region, marital status, lifestyle) Overview of prevention and treatment methods Most common causes and symptoms Comorbidities (if relevant) Quality-of-life issues Other relevant issues
Key groups and stakeholders	Identify key groups and stakeholders (primary and secondary audiences) of the health communication program State reasons for prioritizing engagement of specific groups over others (for example, in the case of multiple key groups and limited program resources that set the need for prioritizing specific groups)
Social, political, and other determinants of health	Predominant health beliefs, attitudes, and behaviors within a given group Social norms Existing policies, laws, and regulations Trends and other factors that may influence the intervention's ability to address the health issue (for example, social, economic, demographic, political) Key characteristics of the living, working, and aging environment (social determinants of health) Access to services and information, such as primary care services, transportation, nutritious food, parks, recreational facilities, and other essential resources Other relevant issues or topics
Audience profile and segmentation	Key characteristics of primary and secondary audiences, including health beliefs, attitudes, behaviors, lifestyle issues, demographics, socioeconomic conditions, and geographical factors Audience segments (by behavioral and social stage and other common characteristics)

	Professional organizations, patient support groups, community groups, and other kinds of groups or associations that already work on the health issue or represent or attend key audiences
	Key opinion leaders (for example, community leaders, prominent health care providers, patient advocates, celebrities who may be frequently quoted on the health issue)
	Preferred communication channels
Existing programs, initiatives, and resources	Existing programs that seek to address the same health issue; existing coalitions or partnerships on the health or social issue
	Existing resources (for example, books, websites, social media sites, print materials, and community meetings dedicated to the topic)
	For all of these factors: lessons learned, trends, key success factors, program assumptions and theoretical foundations, key groups and stakeholders, key messages, activities and channels, key spokespeople, and other relevant information
	Potential opponents to the intervention's approach or key premises and existing initiatives and groups (for example, animal rights activists in the case of a program supporting animal research)
Unmet communication needs	An analytical description of potential messages, topics, or activities that have not been covered yet (or have been only partially or ineffectively covered) by existing programs and should be addressed by the health communication intervention
	This topic could be covered as a stand-alone section of the situation analysis or integrated in other sections
Barriers to program implementation or the adoption of the recommended change	Existing barriers that may complicate program implementation and should be addressed to achieve expected outcomes; examples are cost, time, socioeconomic factors, cost-cutting interventions, current beliefs and attitudes toward recommended health behavior, social norms, and lack of essential services (for example, transportation, primary care, nutritious food stores, and others)
Program goals and outcome objectives	To be included at the beginning of the analysis and restated at the end of it; if research findings do not reinforce preliminary program goals and outcome objectives, changes should be made to reflect research findings
References or bibliography	Primary and secondary sources of key data and findings

A2: Ranking and Selecting Communication Strategies: Sample Criteria

	Communication strategy option 1	Communication strategy option 2	Communication strategy option 3
Does the strategy support communication objectives? If yes, how?			
Key benefits			
Disadvantages			
Barriers to strategy implementation			
Is the strategy supported by key communities, groups, partners, and stakeholders? If yes, why?			
Are available resources (for example, funds, staff, and partners) sufficient for strategy implementation?			
Organizational capability in relation to strategy execution (include strengths and weaknesses)			
Strategy ranking (with final comments)			
Does the strategy address some of the key social and political factors, and other issues and obstacles that may contribute to the health issue within people's living, working, and aging environments?			
Is the strategy inclusive of the preferences and needs of vulnerable and underserved populations? If yes, does it effectively address issues of equity as they relate to projected outcomes of the health communication intervention?			

A3: Sample Communication Channels and Venues and Examples of Related Vehicles (Tactics)

	Channels	Vehicles (tactics)
Mass media	Print and broadcast media, the Internet, and select new media that may already act as mass media because of their reach as it relates to health topics	Editorials, feature articles, letters to the editor, online quizzes, online workshops and courses, television documentaries, public service announcements, illustrations, journal supplements, websites, blogs, webinars, podcasts, radio actualities, videos, radio programs, and virtual newsrooms
New media	Social media, social networking sites, mobile technology, and short message service (SMS)	Virtual town halls, mobile applications (apps), texting, videos, and Instagrams
Interpersonal media	Counseling, one-on-one meetings, peer education, provider-patient encounters, stakeholder-led communications, or other interactive channels	Presentations, courses, speeches, workshops, symposia, lectures, home visits, training, coaching, open discussions, questioning, and meet-the-expert sessions
Community-specific channels and venues (traditional channels)	Local or traditional media, poetry, traditional folk media, theater, exiting community meetings, churches, local markets, and towns' main squares	Theater workshops, comedies, dramas, rallies, presentations, lectures, workshops, sermons, poetry contests, poetry books, health information kiosks, comic books, and community dialogue
Professional media	Conferences, annual meetings, summits, office or department meetings, and other professional venues and settings	Panels, lectures, workshops, seminars, presentations, scientific briefings, and internal communication brochures

A4: Pretesting Messages, Materials, and Activities: Sample Questions

- What is the key point or message of these materials?
- What do you think people should do after reading them?
- Is any relevant information missing from them?
- What are the elements that you most dislike about this message or these materials, and why?
- What are some of the strengths and weaknesses of the illustrations and images in the materials?
- Will you use or distribute these materials? If yes, why, and in which kinds of situations or venues?
- What do you think of the role models that have been used in this public service announcement? What do you like or dislike about them?
- What do you think of the idea of appealing to people's hope for a cure? Will that work for you? If yes, why?
- Is there any social or political factor (for example, access to transportation, nutritious food, social norms, socioeconomic conditions, and many others) that contributes to this health issue, and the information and materials you reviewed have not addressed and should instead include?
- Is there anything you suggest to improve these materials or activities?

A5: Program Time Line: Sample Forms

Example 1

Activity	Estimated time for project completion	Notes or comments
Development of core communication materials for physician workshop	Three to five months	Time frame is contingent on a four-week time line for approval of first draft by all partners

Example 2

Use different colors for specific program phases—for example, yellow for project planning and development, red for project launch and implementation, and green for evaluation and reporting. Alternatively, use different patterns or shades of black and gray, as in the following example.

Activities	First quarter	Second quarter	Third quarter	Fourth quarter
Local media outreach	- - - - -	*******	******* ######	######

Notes:
- - - - - Project planning and development
******* Project launch and implementation
Evaluation and reporting

A6: Budget Sample Form

Activity description	Estimated cost
Disease awareness kit for local hospitals *Assumes the following materials:* cover sheet; fact sheet on disease symptoms, early signs, and diagnostic tools; camera-ready feature article for publication in hospital or organizational e-newsletters; list of online and peer-reviewed resources; includes print and online versions *Estimated costs:* research (database search, article fees), agency fee for materials development, printing and distribution costs (assumes ten thousand copies), graphic design and web development for online versions, kit development and design, assembly and shipment of print copies, cost of meetings with local hospitals or other relevant organizations (travel, refreshments, room rental), online and social media distribution, website update	

A7: Process and Progress Evaluation: Establishing Mutually Agreed-on Parameters

Preimplementation Sample Chart

Activity	Anticipated quantitative and qualitative results
Health care provider workshop series	• Reach audience of thirty to one hundred depending on venue • 80 percent positive response to evaluations • 70 to 80 percent speaker endorsement of key messages • Message retention assessed using pre- and posttest survey with health care providers in target practices and hospitals • Behavioral intention assessment reveals that participants have intention to implement 60 percent of new procedures or cross-cultural communication strategies covered by the workshop
Radio public service announcement	• Twenty to twenty-five million radio impressions during a one-year period • Ten to fifteen thousand requests for additional information using the program's website and other relevant contact information
School-based parental outreach	• Program endorsement by five to seven schools per city • Message retention assessed using pre- and posttest research with parents in target area • Increase by 15 to 30 percent parental awareness and suspicion of disease (assessed using a pre- or postsurvey with health care providers attending families in target regions) • Five to ten thousand requests for materials fulfilled in each city after initial distribution

Activity	Anticipated quantitative and qualitative results
Website	• Two million unique visitors within first year from launch
	• 20 percent of visitors look for additional information by accessing city-specific resources on the health topic
	• 10 percent of visitors share the site via their social media
	• 40 percent of visitors download printable resources
	• 60 percent of visitors are from key groups the intervention seeks to reach and engage (for example, teens)
	• 20 percent of unique visitors share feedback via the site's interactive features and opinion polls

A8: Evaluation of New Media–Based Interventions: A Proposed (and Evolving) Logic Model

Health issue	One or two sentences describing the health issue you are addressing and its relevance
Overall goal or impact	Defined in terms of changes in measurable parameters (incidence, prevalence, morbidity, mortality, quality of life, etc.) re: current health issue. This goal is supported by the achievement of measurable outcome objectives, which are defined early during the planning phase.

People and situations: contributing factors	List key factors and social determinants of health from formative participatory research and existing literature that contribute to current situation and health issue. Also include group-specific factors for each community, stakeholder or key group.
Resources	Economic, human, and time-related resources vis-à-vis potential conflicting priorities and activities; organizational capacity and existing competencies (internal or through partnerships), etc.
New media strategies and activities	List and describe key new media strategies and activities per each new media channel.
Integration with other program components	Discuss how new media–based strategies are integrated with each other as well as offline program elements and other communication areas (e.g., interpersonal communication, public advocacy, mass media communication, community outreach and mobilization, etc.).
Short-term results	Include process indicators, measurable communication objectives and other intermediate indicators (progress indicators) established during planning phase. Examples of *process indicators* include new media reach, tracking data (total and unique visitors, page views, number of followers), quality and numbers of posts, and so on. Examples of *progress indicators* include message retention, awareness, user feedback and participation, community building, new skills, behavioral intentions, and so on. These are all group-specific results for each community, stakeholder, or key group. Include vulnerable and underserved populations. Highlight connection with previous elements of this model.

Health issue	One or two sentences describing the health issue you are addressing and its relevance
Long-term outcomes	Correspond to and expand on measurable outcome objectives (behavioral, social, policy, organizational) established during planning phase in support of achieving the overall program goal. These are specific to each community, stakeholder, or key group. Include results related to individual, community, social, policy, and organizational levels. Include vulnerable and underserved groups.

Source: Copyright © Renata Schiavo. "Emerging Trends and Strategies on Evaluating New Media–Based Programs." Presented at the International Conference on Technology, Knowledge and Society, Bilbao, Spain, Mar. 25–27, 2011a.

Online Resources

Health Literacy Resources

- Centers for Disease Control and Prevention, www.cdc.gov /healthliteracy/pdf/simply_put.pdf

- Emory University—Rollins School of Public Health, www.sph.emory .edu/WELLNESS/reading.html

- Harvard School of Public Health, www.hsph.harvard.edu /healthliteracy/practice/innovative-actions

- MedlinePlus, www.nlm.nih.gov/medlineplus/etr.html

- Plain Language Action and Information Network, www.plainlanguage .gov

- US Department of Health and Human Services, Office of Disease Prevention and Health Promotion, www.health.gov/healthliteracyonline, www.health.gov/communication/literacy/quickguide/healthinfo.htm

Strategic Partnerships and Coalitions

- Alliance for the Prudent Use of Antibiotics—*Guidelines on Interaction with Commercial Enterprises*, pp. 14–15, www.tufts.edu/med/apua /intl_chapters/network_22_891897744.pdf

- American Marketing Association, www.marketingpower.com
- The Canadian Council for Public-Private Partnerships, www.pppcouncil.ca
- The Communication Initiative Network (case studies on successful partnerships), www.comminit.com
- Community-Academic Partnership Model—*Healthier Wisconsin Partnership Program*, www.mcw.edu/healthierwipartnerships/aboutus/partnershipmodel.htm
- The Community Toolbox—*Developing Multisector Collaborations*, http://sitefinity.myctb.org/en/tablecontents/sub_section_main_1385.aspx
- National Council for Public-Private Partnerships, www.ncppp.org
- United Nations Foundation, *Understanding Public-Private Partnerships*, http://business.un.org/en/documents/444
- World Health Organization—*WHO's Interaction with Civil Society and Nongovernmental Organizations*, www.who.int/civilsociety/documents/en/RevreportE.pdf

Logic Model Development: Resources and Templates

- Harvard Family Research Project, www.hfrp.org/publications-resources/browse-our-publications/learning-from-logic-models-in-out-of-school-time
- The Health Communication Unit, University of Toronto, guidebook: www.thcu.ca/infoandresources/publications/logicmodel.wkbk.v6.1.full.aug27.pdf; template: www.thcu.ca/infoandresources/publications/logic_model.pdf
- Office of Minority Health, US Department of Health and Human Services, http://minorityhealth.hhs.gov/templates/content.aspx?ID=7828&lvl=2&lvlID=6
- UNICEF—*Essentials for Excellence*, www.unicef.org/cbsc/files/Essentials_for_excellence.pdf
- University of Wisconsin Extension, www.uwex.edu/ces/pdande/evaluation/evallogicmodel.html
- W.K. Kellogg Foundation Logic Model Development Guide, www.wkkf.org/knowledge-center/resources/2006/02/wk-kellogg-foundation-logic-model-development-guide.aspx

Policy Briefs

- Food and Agricultural Organization, www.fao.org/docrep/014/i2195e /i2195e03.pdf

- International Development Research Centre (IDRC CRDI), Canada, www.idrc.ca/EN/Resources/Tools_and_Training/Documents/how -to-write-a-policy-brief.pdf

- Research to Action, www.researchtoaction.org/tasks/writing-policy -briefs

SAMPLE ONLINE RESOURCES ON HEALTH COMMUNICATION

Listings are in alphabetical order. For listings in the "Communication Centers" and "Graduate Programs" sections, alphabetical order is based on the organization's name and includes only programs that have a focus or concentration on health communication. This list is obviously not all-inclusive, and is only intended to provide sample resources and examples of the variety and breadth of offerings in the field of health communication. Moreover, because of its multidisciplinary nature, health communication is an integral component (as a required or elective course) of the curricula of many other excellent graduate and undergraduate programs in public health, communication studies, design, nursing, medicine, and health care administration, just to name a few relevant areas.

Websites

AudienceScapes, www.audiencescapes.org. Data and analysis on communication, media use, and information, communication, and technology (ICT) access trends. Includes country profiles, outlining information, communication, and the media environment in selected developing countries.

Coalition for Health Communication, www.healthcommunication.net. The website of the Coalition for Health Communication, formed by the American Public Health Association's PHEHP Health Communication Working Group, the Health Communication Division of the International Communication Association, and the Health Communication Division of the National Communication Association. It provides information on resources, job openings, conferences, and journals in the field.

The Communication Initiative Network, www.comminit.com. A multidisciplinary partnership between US and international organizations. Includes health communication–related articles, resources, planning models, programs, events, job openings, and links to other sources of information.

Gateway to Health Communication & Social Marketing Practice, www.cdc.gov/healthcommunication. Developed by CDC, this site contains resources to help build your health communication or social marketing campaigns and programs.

Health Communication, Health Literacy, and e-Health. www.health .gov/communication. Key tools, research and reports, and resources consolidated by the Office for Disease Prevention and Health Promotion.

Health Communication Partnership, www.hcpartnership.org. A multi-disciplinary partnership of educational institutions, national organizations, and international organizations to strengthen public health in the developing world through strategic communication programs. The content includes health communication theory and practice, case studies, news, and other resources and links.

Healthy People: Health Communication, http://healthypeople.gov/2020 /topicsobjectives2020/overview.aspx?topicid=18. Provides science-based, ten-year national objectives for improving the health of all Americans, which includes health communication–related goals. Current version is *Healthy People 2020.*

Healthy Roads Media, www.healthyroadsmedia.org/index.htm. A library of health information in multiple languages and formats.

Media/Materials Clearinghouse, www.m-mc.org. An international searchable resource on health communication materials: pamphlets, posters, audiotapes, videos, training materials, job aids, electronic media, and other media and materials designed to promote public health.

Partners in Information Access for the Public Health Workforce, http://phpartners.org/index.html. A collaboration of US government agencies, public health organizations, and health sciences libraries that provides access to selected public health resources on the Internet.

Journals

Cases in Public Health Communication and Marketing, www .casesjournal.org. Online annual journal featuring peer-reviewed case studies in public health communication and marketing.

Case studies can be written by graduate students, public health practitioners, or other health professionals.

Communication Research, http://crx.sagepub.com. Peer-reviewed bimonthly journal that explores the processes, antecedents, and consequences of communication in a variety of societal systems.

Communication Theory, http://onlinelibrary.wiley.com/journal/10 .1111/%28ISSN%291468–2885. A journal of the International Communication Association (ICA) publishing research into the theoretical development of communication from across a wide array of disciplines.

Health Communication, www.tandfonline.com/action/aboutThis Journal?show=readership&journalCode=hhth20. Peer-reviewed bimonthly journal on health communication. Articles focus on topics such as provider-patient or family interaction, communication and cooperation, health information, health promotion, interviewing, and health public relations.

Journal of Communication in Healthcare, www.maney.co.uk/index.php /journals/cih. Peer-reviewed quarterly journal on health communication's best practices and new thinking in communicating with patients, public, communities, media, and health care professionals.

Journal of Health Communication, www.tandfonline.com/loi/uhcm20# .UexakW0fo4c. Peer-reviewed bimonthly journal on health communication issues and news, including research studies in risk communication, health literacy, social marketing, interpersonal and mass media communication, psychology, government, policy-making, and health education around the world.

The Nation's Health, http://thenationshealth.aphapublications.org. Monthly newspaper of the American Public Health Association (APHA) that often includes news on communication programs from different parts of the United States and on health communication sessions of APHA annual meetings.

RECIIS—Electronic Journal of Communication Information and Health Innovation, www.reciis.cict.fiocruz.br/index.php/reciis/index. A peer-reviewed bilingual electronic journal, which publishes results of scientific research on the following areas: information, communication and technological advances, economics, institutional, social and public politics. All articles are published in English and Portuguese.

Organizations and Groups

American Academy of Health Behavior, www.aahb.org/index.php. A multidisciplinary society of health behavior scholars and researchers.

American Medical Writers Association, www.amwa.org. An association promoting excellence in medical communications.

American Public Health Association, PHEHP Health Communication Working Group, www.apha.org/membergroups/sections /aphasections/phehp/HCWG. The Health Communication Working Group (HCWG) is part of the APHA Public Health Education and Health Promotion (PHEHP) section. HCWG is dedicated to creating a forum for interaction and information exchange by building a network of health communication and public health professionals, researchers, students, and medical practitioners. The group's main forum and moderated listserv is found at http://health.groups.yahoo.com/group/HCWG-APHA.

Association for Education in Journalism and Mass Communication, www.aejmc.org/home. A nonprofit, educational association of journalism and mass communication educators, students, and media professionals, which includes a health communication interest group.

Centers for Disease Control and Prevention (CDC), www.cdc.gov. Resources and links to CDC communication models and activities such as training opportunities, fellowships in health communication, health communication programs in specific disease areas, entertainment, education, and health literacy.

Central States Communication Association, www.csca-net.org /aws/CSCA/pt/sp/home_page. Professional, academic organization of teachers, students, professors, and communication professionals; includes a health communication interest group.

Communication for Social Change Consortium, www.communication forsocialchange.org. Includes news, publications, resources, and case studies on communication for social change.

Eastern Communication Association, http://associationdatabase.com /aws/ECA/pt/sp/p_Home_Page. Professional organization of scholars, teachers, and students, and includes a health communication interest group.

Health and Science Communications Association, http://hesca.net. Information on association conferences, activities, media festivals, job opportunities, and other events and resources.

International Communication Association, www.icahdq.org. Information on association conferences, activities, publications, special events, and other areas. The International Communication Association has a health communication division.

National Communication Association, www.natcom.org. Information on association conferences, activities, publications, special events, and other areas. The National Communication Association has a health communication division.

National Public Health Information Coalition, www.nphic.org. Information on emergency and crisis communication, health promotion, and the organization's conferences and events.

Pan American Health Organization, www.paho.org/Project.asp?SEL= TP&LNG=ENG&ID=152#. Organization activities, publications, multimedia resources on social communication and several disease areas, and health statistics.

Rockefeller Foundation, www.rockfound.org. News, publications, and case studies related to communication for social change.

UNICEF, Communication for Development, www.unicef.org/cbsc/index .php. Resources and case studies on UNICEF's communication for development theory and practice.

Western States Communication Association, www.westcomm.org. Association of communication professionals with a health communication interest group.

World Health Organization, www.who.int. News and case studies on communication for behavioral impact programs, publications, resources, disease-related information and statistics, and activities in different fields and disciplines.

Communication Centers

The Centre for Health Communication Research and Excellence, Buckinghamshire New University, England, http://bucks.ac.uk/research /research_institutes/chcr. The center focuses on communication challenges and issues in the health sector, media coverage of the health services, lifestyle health campaigns, and other issues

Center for Public Health Readiness and Communication, Drexel University, http://publichealth.drexel.edu/cphrc. Center works to enhance community resilience and the ability of health professionals, emergency managers, and public safety officials to meet the needs of all communities in times of disaster and public health emergency.

The Center for Health & Risk Communication, George Mason University, http://chrc.gmu.edu. Provides a framework for stimulating health and risk communication research collaborations, health promotion intervention projects, and community interventions.

Center for Health Communication, Harvard University, www.hsph .harvard.edu/research/chc. Information about the center's health communication projects and key activities. The center focuses primarily on researching and analyzing the contribution of mass communications to behavior change and policy.

Native Health Communication Center, Healthy Native Communities Partnership, www.hncpartners.org/HNCP/Health_ Communications_Center.html. Center aims to develop Native American–specific health communication media.

Center for Health Media & Policy, Hunter College, http://centerfor healthmediapolicy.com. Center advances public conversations about health and health policy through media, research, education, and public forums.

Global Health Communication Center, Indiana University–Purdue University, http://liberalarts.iupui.edu/directory/role/IRSI-GHC. Center focuses on relational, organizational, and cultural transformation and change, and global health issues.

Indiana Center for Intercultural Communication (ICIC), Indiana University, http://liberalarts.iupui.edu/icic/health_communication. ICIC conducts research in many areas in intercultural health communication, including health literacy, prescription medication labeling, medication adherence, physician-patient interaction, the language and cultural training needs of international medical graduates, and the effect of health beliefs on the management of chronic diseases.

Center for Communications Programs, Johns Hopkins University, www.jhuccp.org. The center partners with other organizations to design and implement strategic communication programs. This site includes publications and resources on population, health communications, and development.

Centre for Health Communication and Participation, La Trobe University, Australia, www.latrobe.edu.au/chcp. The center aims to improve health communication with consumers and caregivers through evidence-based policy and decision making.

Ørecomm, Centre for Communication and Global Change, Malmo University, Sweden, and Roskilde University, Denmark, http://orecomm.net. A binational research group focusing on communication for development and the relation among media, communication, and social change processes at global and local levels.

Health and Risk Communication Center, Michigan State University, College of Communication Arts & Sciences, http://hrcc.cas.msu.edu. Center conducts communication-based education, outreach, and research related to risk education and health promotion.

The Health Communication Unit, Public Health Ontario, www.thcu.ca. The unit provides health promotion and knowledge exchange resources.

Center for Communication and Health Issues, Rutgers University, http://commandhealthissues.rutgers.edu/index.html.   Center works to explore communication in health decision making as it affects communities, especially college students and youth, and design, implement, and evaluate campus- and community-based education, intervention, and prevention programs and policies.

Center for Health, Intervention, and Prevention, University of Connecticut, www.chip.uconn.edu. The center itself studies the dynamics of health risk behavior and the processes of health behavior change, and one of the research areas of the center focuses on health communication and marketing.

Center for Health and Risk Communication, University of Georgia, http://chrc.uga.edu. The center advances knowledge about the role of communication processes in enhancing human health and safety, and houses the Southern Center for Communication, Health, and Poverty.

Southern Center for Communication, Health, and Poverty, University of Georgia, www.southerncenter.uga.edu. A health marketing and health communication center that focuses primarily on research and interventions aimed at reducing health disparities in the southern United States and underserved populations. This is a "center of excellence" funded by the US Centers for Disease Control and Prevention.

Center for Health and Risk Communication, University of Maryland, Department of Communication, www.healthriskcenter.umd.edu. Center studies communication processes and effects related to health and risk issues such as food safety and nutrition, health risks, environmental hazards, and disasters.

The Herschel S. Horowitz Center for Health Literacy, University of Maryland, www.healthliteracy.umd.edu/about. The center advances health literacy science, serves as a resource, and promotes community engagement to improve health literacy.

Center for Health Communications Research, University of Michigan, http://chcr.umich.edu. Designated a center of excellence in cancer communications research by the National Cancer Institute, the center conducts health-related research projects involving a broad range of topics, populations, settings, and communication channels.

Health Communication Research Center, University of Missouri, Missouri College of Journalism, http://hcrc.missouri.edu. The research center uses evidence-based communication tools to help strengthen public health; website includes case studies.

The Annenberg Public Policy Center, University of Pennsylvania, www.annenbergpublicpolicycenter.org/Default.aspx. The health communication area of the center addresses public awareness of health policy and health-related behaviors. The Center for Health Behavior and Communication Research at the Public Policy Center seeks to develop theory-based, culturally sensitive, and developmentally appropriate strategies to reduce health-risk behaviors.

Centre for Communication and Social Change, The University of Queensland, Australia, www.uq.edu.au/ccsc. The center conducts study, research, and practical application of communication processes in sustainable development.

Science and Health Communication Research Group, University of South Carolina, http://sc.edu/healthcomm/research/aboutus.html. Research group composed of scholars from various disciplines on USC's campus including journalism, public health, library and information science, and select institutes and centers, among others.

Centre for Health Communication, University of Technology Sydney, Australia, www.centreforhealthcom.org. The center's focus is on the communication processes of frontline staff.

Program on Effective Health Communication, Vanderbilt University, The Institute for Medicine and Public Health, http://medicineandpublichealth.vanderbilt.edu/center.php?userid=1815073&id=&displaypro=1. The center works to improve the communication of health-related information between and among patients, physicians, students, other health care professionals, and the general public through original investigation, education, and dissemination of effective strategies.

Center for Media and Health Promotion, The Edward R. Murrow College of Communication, Washington State University, http://communication.wsu.edu/mcmhp/mcmhp.htm. The center develops and evaluates health communication campaign strategies across a wide range of media platforms.

Health Communication Research Laboratory, Washington University in St. Louis, http://4c.wustl.edu. The research laboratory works to eliminate health disparities by increasing the reach and effectiveness of health information to disadvantaged populations.

Graduate Programs

Online Master of Science in Health Communication, Boston University, http://healthcommunication.bu.edu.

Master of Science in Health Risk and Crisis Communication, Brandman University, www.brandman.edu/academics/programDetails.asp?code=UC.MS.HRCC.

Master of Science in Health and Strategic Communication, Chapman University, www.chapman.edu/scst/crean-school-health/academic-programs/ms-health-communication/index.aspx.

Master of Public Health with a focus in health communication, Colorado State University, www.publichealth.colostate.edu/GPPH/HCfocus.asp.

Master of Arts in Health Communication, DePaul University, http://communication.depaul.edu/Programs/Graduate/HTHC.asp.

Master of Arts in Communication with an emphasis in health communication, East Carolina University, www.ecu.edu/cs-cfac/comm/graduate.

Master's Degree Program in Health Communication, Emerson College and Tufts University School of Medicine, www.emerson.edu /academics/departments/communication-sciences-disorders /graduate-degrees/health-communication, http://publichealth .tufts.edu/Academics/MS-Health-Communication-Microsite. A collaborative effort between Emerson College and Tufts University School of Medicine. Information can be found on the websites of both universities.

Master of Arts in Communication with an emphasis in health communication, George Mason University, http://communication.gmu.edu /programs.

Master of Public Health and Graduate Certificate in Public Health Communication and Marketing, George Washington University, http://sphhs.gwumc.edu/departments/preventioncommunity health/academicprograms/publichealthcommunicationmarketing, www.gwumc.edu/sphhs/academicprograms/programs/MPH_ Graduate_Certificate/PHCM.pdf.

Health Communication Concentration, Harvard University, www.hsph .harvard.edu/health-communication.

Master and Doctoral Degree in Public Health with a certificate in health communication, Johns Hopkins University, http://www.jhsph .edu/academics/certificate-programs/certificates-for-hopkins -students/health-communications.html.

Master of Science in Communication with a concentration in health communication, Lasell College, http://lasell.edu/Academics /Graduate-and-Professional-Studies/MS-in-Communication /Health-Communication.html.

Master's Degree Program in Health and Risk Communication, Michigan State University, www.cas.msu.edu/programs/masters-in-health- and-risk-communication.

Master of Arts in Communication with a focus on health communication and social influence, Ohio State University, www.comm.ohio -state.edu/graduate-soc/areas-of-study/49-graduate/areas-of -study/349-health-communication-and-social-influence.html.

Master of Arts in Communication and Development Studies, Ohio University, www.commdev.ohio.edu.

Master of Arts in Health Communication, Purdue University, www .cla.purdue.edu/communication/healthcommunication/pd.shtml.

Master of Arts in Communication with a focus in health communication, Texas A&M University, http://communication.tamu.edu/html /grad-degree-programs.html.

Master of Arts in Mass Communication in Science/Health Communication, University of Florida, www.jou.ufl.edu/grad/shcomm.

Health Communication Online Master of Science Program, University of Illinois at Urbana-Champaign, www.hcom.illinois.edu.

Master of Science in Community and Behavioral Health with a subtrack in health communication, University of Iowa, http://cph.uiowa .edu/cbh/programs/ms-hc.html.

Master of Arts in Health Communication, University of Miami, http://com.miami.edu/graduate-health-communication.

Master of Arts in Health Journalism and Communication, University of Minnesota, http://sjmc.umn.edu/grad/hjComm.html.

Master of Arts in Mass Communication (Interdisciplinary Health Communication), University of North Carolina at Chapel Hill, http://ihc.unc.edu/index.php?option=com_content&view=article &id=62&Itemid=73.

Master of Arts in Communication with a focus in health communication, University of North Carolina at Charlotte, http://gradcomm.uncc.edu.

Master of Arts in Communication with a focus in health communication, University of Oklahoma, http://cas.ou.edu/health-communication.

Master of Arts in Communication Management with a focus in health and social change communication, University of Southern California, http://annenberg.usc.edu/Prospective/Masters/CMGT.aspx.

Conferences and Meetings

American Public Health Association, www.apha.org/meetings. Annual meeting with several scientific sessions, presentations, and events on health communication organized by the APHA Health Communication Working Group (HCWG) of the Public Health Education and Health Promotion section (PHEHP).

American Public Health Association Film Festival, www.apha.org /meetings/highlights/Films.htm. Organized by the PHEHP Section's Health Communication Working Group (HCWG) and the International Health Section, the Public Health Film Festival showcases films, videos, and other media promoting public health.

Centers for Disease Control and Prevention, National Conference on Health Communication, Marketing, and Media, www.cdc.gov /NCHCMM. Brings together academia, public health researchers, and practitioners from government and private sectors.

Central States Communication Association, www.csca-net.org /aws/CSCA/pt/sp/convention_overview. Annual convention.

D.C. Health Communication Conference, http://chrc.gmu.edu /DCHC.html. Biennial conference.

Digital Health Communication Extravaganza, http://dhcx.hhp.ufl.edu. Annual conference.

Eastern Communication Association, http://associationdatabase.com /aws/ECA/pt/sp/p_convention_papers. Annual convention.

Health and Science Communications Association, http://hesca.net. Annual conference.

International Communication Association, www.icahdq.org/conf/index .asp. Annual conference with presentations and events on health communication.

Kentucky Conference on Health Communication, http://comm.uky.edu /kchc. Biannual conference.

National Communication Association, www.natcom.org/convention .aspx?id=3139#. Annual convention and other events with presentations and resources on health communication.

National Public Health Information Coalition, www.nphic.org. Annual symposium and other summits.

Society for Public Health Education, www.sophe.org/meetings.cfm. Annual meeting with several presentations on health communication.

Western Communication Association, www.westcomm.org /conventions/conventions.asp. Annual convention.

World Health Assembly, www.who.int/mediacentre/events /governance/wha/en. Sponsored by the World Health Organization.

Job Listings

American Public Health Association Public Health Career Mart, http://careers.apha.org/jobs. Lists positions in public health, including health communication.

CDC Health Communication Intern/Fellow Program, http://www.cdc
.gov/healthcommunication. Information on the Health Communication Intern/Fellow Program at the Centers for Disease Control and Prevention.

Coalition for Health Communication, www.healthcommunication.net
/CHC/jobs.htm.

Communication Initiative, www.comminit.com/job_vacancies.

Communication, Research, and Theory Network, http://lists1.cac.psu
.edu/cgi-bin/wa?SUBED1=crtnet&A=1. A listserv managed by the National Communication Association that lists research and academic positions in communication.

HHS Careers, www.hhs.gov/careers. Opportunities at the US Department of Health and Human Services (HHS).

Idealist, www.idealist.org. Information on jobs, organizations, volunteer opportunities, and internships in nonprofits, including those that work in health care, public health, health communication, and development.

International Jobs Center, www.internationaljobs.org. A comprehensive source of international jobs for professionals, including international health care positions and jobs in international understanding, education, communication, and exchange.

National Cancer Institute Internship in Health Communication,
https://hcip.nci.nih.gov. Information on internships offered in the area of health communication by the National Cancer Institute.

National Communication Association, www.natcom.org/findajob.

Nonprofit Career Network, www.nonprofitcareer.com.

Public Relations Society of America Job Center, www.prsa.org/jobcenter
/candidates/jobs.asp. Most positions advertised here are in the public relations area but sometimes include other communication areas.

Riley Guide, www.rileyguide.com/firms.html. A link to US and international executive search firms that specialize in different fields including health care, public health, health communication, and related areas.

US Department of Health and Human Services, www.hhs.gov/careers.
Federal employment opportunities at the HHS.

ACTION PLAN A detailed, actionable, and strategic description of all communication messages, materials, activities, media, and channels, as well as the methods that will be used to pretest them with key audiences. The plan is audience specific and relates to the different areas of health communication. It also includes a detailed time line for the program implementation, an itemized budget for each communication activity or material, and a partnership plan with roles and responsibilities that have been agreed to by all team partners, key groups, and stakeholders. Also called *tactical plan* or *implementation plan*.

ADVOCACY BRIEFS Policy briefs that "argue in favor of a specific course of action" (Food and Agricultural Organization, 2013, p.143).

ATTITUDES Positive or negative emotions or feelings toward a behavior, a person, or a concept or an idea that may affect health or social behavior (Health Communication Partnership, 2005e) and policies.

AUDIENCE ANALYSIS A comprehensive, research-based, participatory, and strategic analysis of all key groups' characteristics, demographics, needs, preferences, values, social norms, attitudes, and behavior. See *audience profile*.

AUDIENCE PROFILE An analytical report on key findings from audience-related research (also called *audience analysis*) and one of the key sections of the situation analysis. A comprehensive, research-based, and strategic description of all characteristics, demographics, needs, values, attitudes, and behaviors of key groups and stakeholders. It includes both primary and secondary audiences. See also *audience analysis, primary audiences, secondary audiences*, and *situation analysis*.

AUDIENCE SEGMENTATION The subdivision of key audiences into groups (segments) with similar characteristics and behavioral stages; one of the key steps of the situation and audience analysis and completes the audience profile. It is defined as the practice of understanding large groups and populations as part of smaller groups that have similar characteristics, preferences, and needs.

BEHAVIORAL BELIEFS   A term used within the theory of reasoned action (see Chapter Two), which refers to a person's own beliefs about the consequences of a given behavior.

BEHAVIORAL IMPACT   The specific behavioral results of a health communication program; measured in relation to specific behavioral indicators that have been established at the onset of planning.

BEHAVIORAL OBJECTIVES   Outcome objectives that explicitly highlight what key groups are expected to do as the result of the health communication program; can be synonymous with *behavioral indicators*. See also *outcome objectives*.

BLOG(s)   An abbreviation of the term *web log* and a discussion or an online informational site consisting of brief and conversational entries called *posts*.

BRAIN DRAIN   The large-scale emigration of health workers from developing countries.

CHANNELS   See *communication channels*.

CITIZEN ENGAGEMENT   The process of creating a better-informed citizenry so that people from different sectors and walks of life can effectively contribute to policy and economic decisions that ultimately affect their lives. Citizen engagement is community mobilization at scale, which more specifically aims to involve the general public in political processes and policy debates.

COLLABORATIVE AGREEMENTS   A special kind of partnership involving universities, health care professionals, and organizations.

COMMUNICATION CHANNELS   The path selected by program planners to reach the intended audience with health communication messages and materials. There are five broad categories of communication channels: mass media channels, new media channels, interpersonal channels, community-specific channels and venues (traditional channels), and professional channels and venues.

COMMUNICATION CONCEPTS   Concepts that describe "ways of presenting the information to intended audiences" (National Cancer Institute at the National Institutes of Health, 2002, p. 55) as well as the overall content-related and visual appeal (fear, hope, action, progress) key groups and stakeholders may connect with. Concepts are preliminary to message and materials development.

COMMUNICATION OBJECTIVES   The intermediate steps that need to be achieved in order to meet the overall program goals as complemented by specific behavioral, social, and organizational objectives. They usually highlight changes in knowledge, attitudes, skills, and other intermediate and necessary steps to behavioral or social change.

COMMUNICATION STRATEGY   A statement describing the overall approach (the "how") used to accomplish communication objectives.

COMMUNICATION VEHICLES   A category that includes materials, events, activities, or other tools for delivering a message using communication channels (Health Communication Unit, 2003b). For example, if the communication channel is a consumer magazine, potential vehicles are feature articles and advertorials.

COMMUNITIES OF PRACTICE   A group of people who share interests in an aspect of human endeavor and who participate in collective learning activities that both educate and create bonds among those involved" (Slotnick and Shershneva, 2002, p. 198). This definition may apply to groups of health care providers as well as to other community-based or professional groups.

COMMUNITY(IES)   Indicates a variety of social, ethnic, cultural, or geographical associations, for example, a school, workplace, city, neighborhood, organized patient or professional group, or association of peer leaders. Communities tend to share similar values, causes, needs, beliefs, overall objectives, and priorities.

COMMUNITY DEVELOPMENT   Refers to a field of research and practice that involves community members, average citizens, professionals, grantmakers, and others in improving various aspects of local communities.

COMMUNITY DIALOGUE   A process that seeks to create a favorable environment in which communities feel comfortable putting forward their ideas and interests and providing input and opinions on specific matters on which they are consulted.

COMMUNITY-DRIVEN ASSESSMENT   See *participatory-needs research.*

COMMUNITY MOBILIZATION   One of the key areas of health communication. A bottom-up and participatory process. Using multiple communication channels, it seeks to involve community leaders and the community at large in addressing a health issue, becoming part of the key steps to behavioral or social change or practicing a desired behavior. Closely related to *social mobilization.*

COMMUNITY-NEEDS ASSESSMENT   See *participatory-needs research.*

COMMUNITY-SPECIFIC CHANNELS   Local or traditional media, poetry, traditional folk media, theater, churches, local markets, and existing community meetings, for example. Also *traditional channels.*

CONSENSUS-BUILDING WORKSHOPS   These workshops facilitate the building of consensus as well as keep momentum on key priority issues and innovative ways to address them. These meetings should lead to a shared vision of the future that communities want to build for themselves and their children as it relates to a specific health or social issue. They may be embedded as part of community meetings.

CONSTITUENCY RELATIONS   The process of convening, exchanging information, and establishing and maintaining strategic relationships with key stakeholders, communities, and organizations with the intent of identifying common goals that can contribute to the outcomes of a specific communication program or health-related mission.

CONSTITUENTS   Individuals, communities, and groups that are influenced by or can influence a specific issue. In health care and global health, they include patients, physicians, and other health care providers, hospital employees, professional and advocacy groups, nonprofit organizations, academia, pharmaceutical companies, public health departments, the general public, and policymakers, as well as groups that have a stake in a health issue and can influence its solutions. See also *stakeholders.*

CONTRIBUTION ANALYSIS   The analysis of other plausible alternatives or concomitant interventions, if any, that may have contributed to the results of a health communication intervention.

COUNSELING   The help provided by a professional on personal, psychological, health, or professional matters, including via one-on-one interactions, personal selling, and other interpersonal communication approaches.

CRISIS AND EMERGENCY RISK COMMUNICATION   Integrates risk and crisis communication in preparing for, responding to, and recovering from epidemics, emerging disease outbreaks, and other hazards (CDC, 2011c). See *risk communication, emergency risk communication.*

CROSS-CULTURAL HEALTH COMMUNICATION   A systematic approach to health communication programming and interpersonal communication that emphasizes one key aspect of the health communication process: the ability to communicate across cultures, be culturally competent, be inclusive and mindful of diversity, as well as to bridge cultural differences so that community and patient voices are heard and properly addressed.

CULTURAL COMPETENCE   The ability to relate to other people's values, feelings, and beliefs across different cultures, and effectively address such differences as part of all interactions.

DELIVERED DIALOGUE   A method for public dialogue and consultation that usually relies on the use of specific discussion tools, including a discussion guide, sequence of questions, and briefing materials and instructions for dialogue facilitators.

EMERGENCY RISK COMMUNICATION   Risk communication as applied to public health and humanitarian emergency settings. See *risk communication.*

EVALUATION   The science and process of appraising the value or worth of a health communication intervention.

EVALUATION PLANS   Detailed descriptions of the behavioral, social, or organizational indicators as well as other parameters for assessing program outcomes. They should describe methods for data collection, analysis, and reporting, as well as related costs and time lines.

EXTERNAL OR ENVIRONMENTAL FACTORS   Political, social, market, and other social determinants of health or external influences that shape or contribute to a specific situation or health problem as well as influence key groups and stakeholders.

FOCUS GROUP   One of the most common marketing and communication research methodologies consisting of small-group discussions. Participants in focus groups are representatives of key program audiences.

FORMATIVE EVALUATION   An evaluation phase that informs, guides, and helps validate all elements of a health communication program. It occurs prior to program development and implementation and includes the analysis of all research data gathered as part of the situation and audience analysis, and pretesting studies.

GATEKEEPERS   All individuals, groups, or organizations that may provide access to intended audiences. Sometimes they control access to specific communication channels (for example, journalists who control access to the mass media).

GLOBAL HEALTH   Refers to "health problems, issues and concerns that transcend national boundaries, and may be best addressed by cooperative actions" (Institute of Medicine, 2007, p. 1). Global health "stresses the commonality of health issues" (Global Health Education Consortium, 2013) and deals with partnership-based models and strategies that have the potential to address similar health issues across geographic boundaries.

HEALTH COMMUNICATION   Health communication is a multifaceted and multidisciplinary field of research, theory, and practice. It is concerned with reaching different populations and groups to exchange health-related information, ideas, and methods in order to influence, engage, empower, and support individuals, communities, health care professionals, patients, policymakers, organizations, special groups, and the public so that they will champion, introduce, adopt, or sustain a health or social behavior, practice, or policy that will ultimately improve individual, community, and public health outcomes.

HEALTH DISPARITIES   Diseases or health conditions that discriminate and tend to be more common and more severe among vulnerable and under-served populations; or overall differences in health outcomes (Health Equity Initiative, 2012b).

HEALTH EQUITY   Providing every person with the same opportunity to stay healthy or to effectively cope with disease and crisis, regardless of race, gender, age, economic conditions, social status, environment, and other socially determined factors (Health Equity Initiative, 2012b).

HEALTH LITERACY   "The degree to which individuals have the capacity to obtain, process, and understand basic health information and services needed to make appropriate health decisions" (US Department of Health and Human Services, 2005, p. 11-20; Selden and others, 2000).

HEALTH LITERACY–HEALTH COMMUNICATION CONTINUUM   Health literacy improves communication and at the same time communication improves health literacy levels (Schiavo, 2009d).

HITS   Total number of downloads (photos, text, HTML, etc.) on all the pages, including all times users came in contact with any of the different elements and components on all pages of a given site.

IMPACT   An outcome in relation to a specific change or, alternatively, the long-term change influenced by a program in relation to the overall program goal. This term may also have other connotations in different models.

IMPLEMENTATION PLAN   See *action plan.*

IN-DEPTH INTERVIEWS   A research method that consists of one-on-one interviews (for example, telephone or in-person interviews) with internal and external stakeholders, members of key groups, or representatives of relevant health organizations.

INSTITUTIONAL REVIEW BOARD (IRB)   A group of research experts who are faculty members of an academic institution or research hospital or are part of an independent IRB. IRBs review research protocols and methods to ensure protection of human subjects.

INTENDED AUDIENCES All groups the health communication intervention is seeking to engage in the communication process. See also *key groups*.

INTERNATIONAL HEALTH "Relates more to health practices, policies and systems in countries other than one's own and stresses more the differences between countries than their commonalities" (Global Health Education Consortium, 2013).

INTERPERSONAL CHANNELS Counseling, one-on-one meetings, peer-to-peer trainings, provider-patient encounters, stakeholder-led meetings, or other interactive channels and venues that are used for interpersonal communication.

INTERPERSONAL COMMUNICATION A key health communication area that uses interpersonal channels. Includes personal selling and counseling, provider-patient communications, community dialogue, and other kinds of group or one-on-one interactions and communications.

KEY GROUPS All groups the health communication program is seeking to engage in the communication process. In this book, the terms *intended audience* and *key group* are used interchangeably. Yet, the term *key group* may be better suited to acknowledge the participatory nature of well-designed health communication interventions in which communities and other key groups are the lead architects of the change process communication can bring about. See *intended audiences*.

KEY INFLUENTIALS ROADMAP Identifying and mapping groups and stakeholders whose opinions, moral values, and expectations actually matter in the eyes of specific groups or populations.

KEY PROGRAM AUDIENCES See *intended audiences*.

KEYWORD MENTIONS Total count of mentions of the program's name or issue on the web (on websites, blogs, social media, and others).

LOGIC MODELING A flexible framework that has been used for program planning and evaluation in the fields of education (Harvard Family Research Project, 2002), public-private partnerships (Watson, 2000), health education (University of Wisconsin, Extension Program Development, 2005), and many other programmatic areas. In general, it is a one-page summary of key factors that contribute to a specific health or social issue; the program's key components; the rationale used in defining program strategies, objectives, and key activities; and expected program outcomes and measurement parameters that will be used in evaluating them.

LOW HEALTH LITERACY   "The inability to read, understand and act on health information" (Zagaria, 2004, p. 41).

MASS COMMUNICATION   A field of research and practice that is concerned with communication with large segments of the population and the general public, which is also a key action area in health communication.

MASS MEDIA   Means of communication to reach large audiences or percentages of a given population. What can act as mass media may vary in different countries or groups.

MASS MEDIA CHANNELS   Print and broadcast media, the Internet, and other new media.

MEDIA ADVOCACY   Consists of public advocacy strategies and activities that rely heavily on the use of the mass media and new media. See *public advocacy*.

MEDIA PITCH   A brief summary statement, letter, or e-mail message that explains why a piece of information is new, relevant to a journalist's intended audience, and worth covering.

METRICS   Another term for *evaluation parameters*. Metrics should be quantifiable and define a system of parameters to assess periodically specific program elements or outcomes (for example, process-related results or changes in attitude and behavior).

mHEALTH   The use of mobile and wireless technology devices for health-related interventions that seek to improve patient and public health outcomes.

MIXED METHODOLOGY   "Mixed methodology is a design for collecting, analyzing, and mixing both quantitative and qualitative data in a single study or series of studies to understand an evaluation problem" (Tucker-Brown, 2012).

MONITORING   Monitoring is an essential function in program implementation and evaluation and is related primarily to four areas: (1) program activities and related process; (2) ongoing feedback by key groups and stakeholders on the intervention's key elements, overall content, messages, and progress-related updates; (3) news and trends about the specific health areas, determinants of health, key policies, intended audiences, and other relevant facts and events; and (4) the collection and analysis of evaluation data.

MULTISECTORAL PARTNERSHIPS   Partnerships that result when governments, nonprofit, private, and public organizations, academia, community groups, individual community members, and others "come together to solve problems that affect the whole community or a specific population" (Community Tool Box, 2013).

NEW MEDIA   "Those media that are based on the use of digital technologies, such as the Internet, computer games, digital television, and mobile devices, as well as the remaking of more traditional media forms to adopt and adapt to new media technologies" (Williams, Zraik, Schiavo, and Hatz, 2008, p. 161; Flew, 2002, p. 11).

NEW MEDIA CHANNELS   Social media, social networking sites, mobile technology, and others.

NORMATIVE BELIEFS   A term used within the theory of reasoned action (see Chapter Two) that refers to whether a person may believe significant others will approve or not of his or her behavior.

OBJECTIVE BRIEFS   Policy briefs that only "give objective information for the policy maker to make up his or her mind" (Food and Agricultural Organization, 2013, p.143).

OFFLINE EFFECTIVENESS   The effectiveness of an online or new media–based intervention as it relates to people's ability to integrate recommendations from the same communication intervention in their everyday life vis-à-vis behavioral, social, and organizational objectives.

ONLINE EFFICACY   The efficacy of a communication intervention as it relates to people's ability to understand and act on key communication messages and activities within an online or new media setting or virtual world.

ORGANIZATIONAL OBJECTIVES   Refers to the change that should occur within an organization in terms of its focus, priorities, or structure in relation to the specific health issue addressed by a health communication intervention.

OUTCOME OBJECTIVES   The desired outcomes the health communication program is seeking to achieve through behavioral, social, and organizational objectives. These objectives are used as key indicators of change in the evaluation of health communication interventions and should be set at the onset of program planning.

OUTCOMES   A general term describing changes in knowledge, comprehension, attitudes, skills, behavior, policies, or social norms as established by the program's outcome and communication objectives (Coffman, 2002; Freimuth, Cole, and Kirby, 2000). Outcomes are measured in relation to the estimated influence the health communication program had on each change. *Short-term outcomes* are usually related to process indicators as well as intermediate steps and key milestones as those set by the communication objectives (for example, changes in awareness, knowledge, skills). *Long-term outcomes* are the ultimate results of health communication programs and relate to the achievement of behavioral, social, and organizational objectives (outcome objectives).

OVERALL PROGRAM GOAL   Describes the overall "health improvement" (National Cancer Institute at the National Institutes of Health, 2002, p. 22) or "overall change in a health or social problem" (Weinreich, 1999, p. 67; 2011) that the program is seeking to achieve.

PAGE VIEWS   Total number of times users viewed each unique page on a given site, meaning the total number of pages users viewed when they visited a specific site.

PANDEMIC   A geographical widespread outbreak of an infectious disease in which many people are infected at the same time; occurring throughout a region or even throughout the world (Heymann and Rodier, 2001).

PANEL STUDIES   A research method that consists of creating a panel of representatives of key groups or stakeholders, and then contacting them at various and regular times during the research and program evaluation phases (for example, every six months or every year).

PARTICIPATORY INFLUENTIAL ROAD MAPPING   A participatory and community-driven process to identify key stakeholders and other influentials who need to be engaged as part of the community mobilization and citizen engagement process.

PARTICIPATORY NEEDS ASSESSMENT   See *participatory research.*

PARTICIPATORY RESEARCH   A collaborative research effort that involves community members, researchers, community mobilizers, and interested agencies and organizations. It is a two-way dialogue that starts with the people, and through which the community understands and identifies key issues, priorities, and potential actions. Participatory research should inform and guide all phases of the community mobilization effort. Also referred to as *community-driven assessment, participatory needs assessment,* and *community-needs assessment.* Yet, these terms may have different meanings in different planning models.

PARTNERSHIP PLAN   A summary of the collective efforts that result in the creation of a strategic partnership on a given intervention, as well as roles and responsibilities and expectations of all partners and related time lines. It should be integrated in the action plan, and includes two different phases as described in Chapter Thirteen.

PERSONAL SELLING   Refers to (1) one-on-one engagement of different groups in their own homes, offices, or places of work and leisure (personal selling and counseling) and (2) the ability to sell one's image and expertise, an important skill in most counseling activities. It is an acquired communication skill that requires training but is also dependent on individual, social, and cultural factors. The two definitions are strongly connected and interdependent in their practical application.

PERSONAL VALUES   Emotions and feelings that derive from personal, group, or community past experiences.

PHOTOVOICE   Participatory photography.

PODCASTS   Multimedia digital files made available on the Internet for downloading to a portable media player or computer.

POLICY BRIEFS   A concise summary of an issue of public interest, potential policy solutions, and some recommendations on what may be the best policy option. They are important communication tools in both policy communication and public advocacy.

POLICY COMMUNICATION   Communicating about health or scientific data in support of policy change, or a new or existing policy and its implementation and evaluation.

POSITIONING   A core concept that communication borrows from marketing and social marketing. Positioning identifies the fit between what key groups are seeking and what the product (whether tangible or intangible such as a health behavior or social norm) could actually deliver or represent for them (Kotler and Roberto, 1989; Lefebvre, 2013).

PRETESTING   An essential phase of formative research that uses several research methods to assess whether communication concepts, messages, media, and materials meet the needs of intended audiences, are culturally appropriate, and are easily understood.

PRIMARY AUDIENCES   The people whom the program seeks to engage more directly and would most benefit from change—for example, people at risk for a certain medical condition or already suffering from it; parents or other caregivers responsible for pediatric care decisions for their children; or other groups in the case of programs of limited scope that seek to influence only one audience. Also referred to as *key primary groups*.

PROCESS EVALUATION   Used to compare key steps of the program's implementation with the original program plan and to measure expected results for specific activities, materials, media, and messages.

PROFESSIONAL CHANNELS AND VENUES   Professional conferences and summits, online forums dedicated to a specific profession, organizational communication channels (such as those of a professional association).

PROFESSIONAL CLINICAL COMMUNICATION   See *professional medical communication.*

PROFESSIONAL MEDICAL COMMUNICATION   A key health communication area that seeks to influence the behavior and the social contexts of these professionals directly responsible for administering health care. Professional medical communications aim to (1) promote the adoption of best medical and health practices; (2) establish new concepts and standards of care; (3) publicize recent medical discoveries, beliefs, parameters, and policies; (4) change or establish new medical priorities; and (5) advance health policy changes. Professional medical communication has evolved from the concept of scientific exchange as a peer-to-peer communication approach intended for physicians, nurses, physician assistants, and all other health care providers. This term is used interchangeably with *professional clinical communications.*

PROGRAM ASSESSMENT   A general term used to indicate program-specific evaluation.

PROGRAM OUTCOMES   Changes in knowledge, attitudes, skills, behavior, social norms, policies, and other parameters measured against those anticipated in the planning phase.

PROGRESS INDICATORS   Include intermediate steps and key milestones, which are assessed as part of progress evaluation. Sample progress indicators include short-term changes in awareness, knowledge, attitudes, skills, community participation levels, or other intermediate steps that may occur as a result of specific communication messages, activities, media, or materials.

PUBLIC ADVOCACY   The strategic use of communication to affect changes in public opinion and attitudes so that it influences policymakers or other decision makers and promotes changes in behaviors, social norms, policies, and resource allocation to benefit a community, group, population, or organization. It relies on multiple tools and activities, including community or town hall meetings and one-on-one encounters with policymakers and decision makers. A fundamental component of public advocacy efforts is the use of the mass media. Also called *media advocacy*, reflecting public advocacy that heavily relies on the strategic use of the mass media and new media.

PUBLIC CONSULTATION A process in which the general public is asked to provide input on policies or other matters that may affect them.

PUBLIC ENGAGEMENT See *citizen engagement*.

PUBLIC-PRIVATE PARTNERSHIPS "A collaboration between public bodies, such as central government or local authorities, and private companies" (*PPP Bulletin International*, 2012) or organizations. PPPs "involve at least one private for-profit organization and at least one not-for-profit or public organization" (Reich, 2002, p. 3).

PUBLIC RELATIONS (PR) Defined as "the art and science of establishing and promoting a favorable relationship with the public" (*American Heritage Dictionary of the English Language*, 2011). Functions of PR include public affairs, community relations, issues or crisis management, media relations, and marketing PR. PR relies on the skillful use of culturally competent and audience-appropriate mass media and new media as well as other communication channels to place a health issue on the public agenda, advocate for its solutions, and highlight the importance that the government and other key stakeholders take action.

QUALITATIVE RESEARCH Research methods and approaches that are used to collect data in relatively small groups. Qualitative data are not statistically significant and focus on opinions, trends, and insights.

QUANTITATIVE RESEARCH Research methods and data that are statistically significant and are usually collected from large samples. It aims to provide the health communication team with exact numbers about different kinds of external factors or audience-specific characteristics and behaviors.

REFERENDUM A vote on a ballot question in which the entire electorate is asked to accept or reject a policy change.

RESPONSES TO TEXT MESSAGES Total number of mobile users who reply to program texts or number of total responses per user received in reply to a text messaging program.

RETURN ON INVESTMENT (ROI) The economic benefits that may derive from having invested funds and other resources (for example, human resources, time) in a program or activity. This parameter is commonly used in the commercial sector to assess the impact of marketing and communication activities on product sales. In public health and community development, it may be useful in assessing the benefits of specific communication interventions. For example, the return could be calculated in terms of the percentage of people who changed knowledge, attitude, or behavior or benefited from a specific change in social norms, policies, and related practices or the cost-saving benefits of interventions that promote preventative measures. Includes a discussion and related actions about risk types and levels as well as methods, strategies, and activities for managing risks in a variety of settings.

RISK COMMUNICATION "An interactive process of exchange of information and opinion among individuals, groups, and institutions" (US Department of Health and Human Services, 2002). "The dissemination of individual and population health risk information" (US Department of Health and Human Services, 2005, p. 11-13).

SECONDARY AUDIENCES All individuals, groups, communities, and organizations that may influence the decisions and behaviors of the primary audiences. Also called *secondary key groups*. See also *primary audiences*.

SITUATION ANALYSIS The analysis of all individual, community, social, political, and behavior-related factors that can affect attitudes, behaviors, social norms, and policies about a health issue and its potential solutions.

SOCIAL CHANGE INDICATORS AND SOCIAL IMPACT Indicators—and their impact—that measure changes in social interactions, norms, policies, and practices, as well as changes in the issues of concern (for example, poverty reduction, HIV/AIDS rates) (Rockefeller Foundation Communication and Social Change Network, 2001) or any of the key social determinants of health (for example, the living, working, and aging environment of key groups, access to services or information).

SOCIAL DETERMINANTS OF HEALTH Different socially determined factors (e.g., socioeconomic conditions, race, ethnicity, culture, as well as having access to health care services, a built environment that supports physical activity, neighborhoods with accessible and affordable nutritious food, health information that's culturally appropriate and accurately reflects literacy levels, and caring and friendly clinical settings), which affect health outcomes as well as influence and are influenced by health communication.

SOCIAL MEDIA A subgroup of new media and social sites that aim primarily to create community and connect people. Social media (for example, YouTube) are tools for sharing and discussing information (Stelzner, 2009).

SOCIAL MOBILIZATION The "process of bringing together multisectoral community partners to raise awareness, demand, and progress for the initiative's goals, processes and outcomes" (Patel, 2005, p. 53). Closely related to *community mobilization.*

SOCIAL NETWORKING   A type of new media that uses "communities of interest to connect to others" (Stelzner, 2009). Some media (for example, Facebook and Twitter) combine both social media and social networking functions (Stelzner, 2009).

SOCIAL NORMS   Group-held beliefs on how people should behave in a social situation or group setting.

SOCIAL OBJECTIVES   Outcome objectives that highlight the policy, practice, or social change that the program is seeking to achieve or implement.

STAKEHOLDERS   All individuals and groups who have an interest or share responsibilities in a given issue, such as policymakers, community leaders, special groups, and community members. They may represent the primary audience or influence them. *See also* constituency groups and constituents.

SUMMATIVE EVALUATION   A phase of evaluation that measures the program's efficacy in relation to the outcome and communication objectives initially established by the program.

TABLETS   One-piece mobile computers, such as the iPad or the Kindle.

TACTICAL PLAN   See *action plan.*

TACTICS   Refer to different components of a plan of action (tactical plan) that includes communication messages, activities, media, materials, and channels and is developed to serve the program's strategies and objectives.

TEXT MESSAGING READERSHIP   Total number of mobile users who report reading messages from a text messaging program.

THIRD-PARTY GROUPS   Key constituency groups in constituency relations, and include nonprofit, special interest, and advocacy organizations.

UNDERSERVED POPULATIONS   Include geographical, ethnic, social, or community-specific groups who do not have adequate access to health or community services and infrastructure or adequate information.

UNIQUE VISITORS   The total count of how many different people accessed a specific website or media.

UNIVERSAL VALUES   Emotions and feelings that people may share across different groups within the same culture or in some cases across cultures.

USE OF MOBILE INTERACTIVE FEATURES   Total number of mobile users who use interactive features associated with the mHealth program (for example, apps, links to websites, and digital resources, etc.).

VEHICLES   See *communication vehicles*.

VIRTUAL NEWSROOMS   Dedicated webpages where the event announcements or other newsworthy items are linked to videos and other resources that can help reporters, online newsletter editors, and bloggers write the story or just link to it.

VIRTUAL WORLD   An online community that takes the form of a computer-based simulated environment through which users can interact with one another and use and create [both characters and] objects (Bishop, 2009).

VISITS   Total number of visits (including returning visitors and users who are no longer unique) on a given webpage or website.

VULNERABLE POPULATIONS   Include groups who have a higher risk for poor physical, psychological, or social health in the absence of adequate conditions that are supportive of positive outcomes (for example, children, the elderly, people living with disability, migrant populations, and special groups affected by stigma and social discrimination).

ABC News. "Poll: What Americans Eat for Breakfast." May 17, 2005. www.abcnews .com/GMA/PollVault/story?id=762685. Retrieved Nov. 2005.

Abroms, L. C., and others. "Text2Quit: Results from a Pilot Test of a Personalized, Interactive, Mobile Health Smoking Cessation Program." *Journal of Health Communication*, 2012, *17*(1), 44–53.

Abroms, L. C., and Lefebvre, R. C. "Obama's Wired Campaign: Lessons for Public Health Communication." *Journal of Health Communication*, 2009, *14*, 415–423.

Abroms, L. C., Padmanabhan, N., Thaweethai, L., and Phillips, T. "iPhone Apps for Smoking Cessation." *American Journal of Preventative Medicine*, 2011, *40*(3), 279–285.

Abroms, L. C., Schiavo, R., and Lefebvre, R. C. "New Media Cases in Cases in Public Health Communication & Marketing: The Promise and Potential." *Cases in Public Health Communication & Marketing*, 2008, *2*, 3–10. www.casesjournal .org/volume2.

Adams, J. "Successful Strategic Planning: Creating Clarity." *Journal of Healthcare Information Management*, 2005, *19*(3), 24–31.

Ad Council. "About Asthma." www.noattacks.org/about. Retrieved Feb. 2006a.

Ad Council. "Preventing Attacks." www.noattacks.org/preventing-attacks. Retrieved Feb. 2006b.

Ader, M., and others. "Quality Indicators for Health Promotion Programmes." *Health Promotion International*, 2001, *16*(2), 187–195.

Advertising Law Resource Center. "Children and Tobacco, Executive Summary, Final Rule: U.S. Food and Drug Administration." Aug. 2006. www.lawpublish .com/fdarule.html. Retrieved Mar. 2006.

Agriculture and Agri-Food Canada. "Community Dialogue Toolkit. Supporting Local Solutions to Local Challenges." 2013. www4.agr.gc.ca/AAFC-AAC /display-afficher.do?id=1239289563390&lang=eng. Retrieved Jan. 2013.

Agunga, R. A. *Developing the Third World: A Communication Approach.* Commack, NY: Nova Science, 1997.

Ahorlu, C., and others. "Malaria-Related Beliefs and Behaviour in Southern Ghana: Implications for Treatment, Prevention and Control." *Tropical Medicine and International Health*, 1997, *2*(5), 488–499.

Ajzen, I., and Fishbein, M. *Understanding Attitudes and Predicting Social Behavior.* Upper Saddle River, NJ: Prentice Hall, 1980.

Alcalay, R., and Bell, R. Promoting Nutrition and Physical Activity Through Social Marketing: Current Practices and Recommendations. For the Cancer Prevention and Nutrition Section of California Department of Health Services. Davis: Center for Advanced Studies in Nutrition and Social Marketing, University of California, Davis, June 2000. http://communication.ucdavis.edu/people /rabell/AlcalayBell.pdf.

Al-Khayat, M. H. *Health: An Islamic Perspective*. Alexandria, Egypt: World Health Organization, Regional Office for the Eastern Mediterranean, 1997. www.emro.who.int/Publications/HealthEdReligion/IslamicPerspective /Chapter1.htm. Retrieved Oct. 2006.

American Academy of Family Physicians. "Good Communication Is Sign of Good Medicine for FP of the Year." *FP Report*, Oct. 1999. www.aafp.org/fpr /991000fr/10.html. Retrieved June 2005.

American Academy of Pediatrics. "Periodic Survey of Fellows, Periodic Survey #43—Part 1, Characteristics of Pediatricians and Their Practices: The Socioeconomic Survey." www.aap.org/research/periodicsurvey/ps43aexs.htm. Retrieved Nov. 2005a.

American Academy of Pediatrics. "Periodic Survey of Fellows, Periodic Survey #54—Part 1, Characteristics of Pediatricians and Their Practices: The Socioeconomic Survey." www.aap.org/research/periodicsurvey/ps54aexs.htm. Retrieved Nov. 2005b.

American Association for the Advancement of Science. "Malaria and Development in Africa: A Cross-Sectoral Approach." www.aaas.org/international/africa /malaria91/rec6.html. Retrieved Feb. 2006.

American Diabetes Association, "Diabetes and Your Weight." www.diabetes .org/weightloss-and-exercise/weightloss/diabetes.jsp. Retrieved Oct. 2005.

American Folklife Preservation Act. Public Law 94–201, 94th Congress, H.R. 6673, Jan. 2, 1976.

American Heart Association. Office of Tobacco Control. "The American Heart Association Youth Fitness and Tobacco Prevention/Education Project." www.fsu.edu/~ctl/Tobacco2.htm. Retrieved Mar. 2006a.

American Heart Association, "Public Advocacy: What Is Public Advocacy?" www.americanheart.org/presenter.jhtml?identifier=4758. Retrieved Mar. 2006b.

American Heritage Dictionary of the English Language. "Search Term: Public Relations." http://ahdictionary.com/word/search.html?q=public+relations &submit.x=-1103&submit.y=-210. 2011. Retrieved June 2013.

American Heritage Dictionary of the English Language. Search Term: "Constituents." 2004a. Retrieved June 2005

American Heritage Dictionary of the English Language. Search Term: "Evaluate." 2004b. www.answers.com/topic/evaluate. .Retrieved Oct. 2005.

American Heritage Dictionary of the English Language. Search Term: "Tactics." 2004c. http://dictionary.reference.com/browse/tactics. Retrieved Oct. 2005.

American Lung Association. "Asthma & Children Fact Sheet." 2012. www.lung
.org/lung-disease/asthma/resources/facts-and-figures/asthma-children-fact
-sheet.html#4.

American Medical Association. "AMA to *New York Times*: Good Physician-
Patient Communication Helps All Doctors." Dec. 2005a. www.ama-assn.org
/ama/pub/category/15788.html. Retrieved Jan. 2006.

American Medical Association. "Partnership for Clear Health Communication."
www.ama-assn.org/ama/pub/category/11128.html. Retrieved June 2005b.

American Medical Association. "Partnership for Clear Health Communication—
What Can Providers Do?" www.askme3.org/PFCHC/what_can_provid.asp.
Retrieved June 2005c.

American Medical Association. "Partnership for Clear Health Communication—
What Is Ask Me 3?" www.askme3.org/PFCHC/what_is_ask.asp. Retrieved June
2005d.

American Medical Association. "An Ethical Force Program Consensus Report.
Improving Communication—Improving Care. How Health Care Organizations Can Ensure Effective, Patient-Centered Communication with People from Diverse Populations." 2006a. www.ama-assn.org/ama1/pub/upload
/mm/369/ef_imp_comm.pdf. Retrieved July 2012.

American Medical Association. "Eliminating Health Disparities." www.ama
-assn.org/ama/pub/physician-resources/public-health/eliminating-health
-disparities.page. Retrieved Jan. 2013.

American Medical Student Association. "Cultural Competency in Medicine: A
Project-in-a-Box." www.amsa.org/programs/gpit/cultural.cfm. Retrieved Oct.
2005.

American Public Health Association. "Media Advocacy Session." 133rd Annual
Meeting and Exposition, Philadelphia, Dec. 2005.

American Public Health Association. Health Communication Working Group.
"What Is Health Communication?" www.hehd.clemson.edu/Publichealth
/PHEHP/HealthComm/define.htm. Retrieved Feb. 2006.

American Public Health Association. "Public Health Is ROI. Save Lives, Save
Money." *American Public Health Association Meeting Blog*. Oct. 29, 2012.

Amoah, S. O. "Mobilizing Community Support for a Radio Serial on HIV." Paper
presented at the American Public Health Association's 129th Annual Meeting,
Atlanta, Oct. 2001.

Andersen, M. R., and Lobel, M. "Predictors of Health Self-Appraisal: What's
Involved in Feeling Healthy." *Basic and Applied Social Psychology Bulletin*,
1995, *16*(1–2), 121–136.

Andreasen, A. R. Marketing *Social Change: Changing Behavior to Promote Health,
Social Development and the Environment*. San Francisco: Jossey-Bass, 1995.

Annulis, H. M., and Gaudet, C. H. "Developing Powerful Program Objectives." In
P. P. Phillips (ed.), *ASTD Handbook of Measuring and Evaluating Training*.
Alexandria, VA: American Society for Training and Development, 2010.

Arias, J. R., Monteiro, P. S., and Zicker, F. "The Reemergence of Visceral Leishmaniasis in Brazil." *Emergency Infectious Diseases*, 1996, *2*(2), 145–146.

Association of American Medical Colleges. "AAMC Report Aims to Enhance Communications Skills Training at U.S. Medical Schools, AAMC Issues Doctor-Patient Communications Fact Sheet, Launches 'Doctoring 101.'" 1999. www.aamc.org/newsroom/pressrel/1999/991026.htm. Retrieved Nov. 2005.

Association of Cancer Online Resources. "Join the Pediatric Cancers Online Community." www.acor.org/listservs/join/111. Retrieved Mar. 2013.

Association of Schools of Public Health. ASPH Education Committee. "Master's Degree in Public Health Core Competency Development Project. Version 2.3." May 2007. www.asph.org/userfiles/WordFormat-DomainsandCompetenciesOnly.doc. Retrieved Feb. 2013.

Association of Schools of Public Health. ASPH Education Committee. "Doctor of Public Health (DrPH) Core Competency Model. Version 1.3." Nov. 2009. www.asph.org/publication/DrPH_Core_Competency_Model/index.html. Retrieved Jan. 2013.

Ateeq, N. "*Interpersonal Communication: Lessons Learned in India.*" Unpublished Case Study, 2012.

Atkin, C., and Schiller, L. "The Impact of Public Service Advertising." In Henry Kaiser Family Foundation, *Background Papers. Shouting to Be Heard: Public Service Advertising in a New Media Age*. Menlo Park, CA: Kaiser Family Foundation, Feb. 2002.

AudienceScapes. "Ghana Communication Profile." www.audiencescapes.org/country-profiles/ghana/ghana/communication-profile-317. Retrieved Mar. 2013.

Aylward, R. B., and Heymann, D. L. "Can We Capitalize on the Virtues of Vaccines? Insights from the Polio Eradication Initiative." *American Journal of Public Health*, 2005, *95*(5), 773–777.

Babalola, S., and others. "The Impact of a Community Mobilization Project—Knowledge and Practices in Cameroon." *Journal of Community Health*, 2001, *26*(6), 459.

Babrow, A. "Tensions Between Health Beliefs and Desires: Implications for a Health Communication Campaign to Promote a Smoking-Cessation Program." *Health Communication*, 1991, *3*(2), 93.

Babrow, A. S. "Communication and Problematic Integration: Understanding Diverging Probability and Value, Ambiguity, Ambivalence, and Impossibility." *Communication Theory*, 1992, *2*, 95–130.

Babrow, A. S. "Problematic Integration Theory." In B. B. Whaley and W. Samterm (eds.), *Explaining Communication: Contemporary Theories and Exemplars*. Hillsdale, NJ: Lawrence Erlbaum, 2007, pp. 181–200.

Balog, J. E. "*An Historical Review and Philosophical Analysis of Alternative Concepts of Health and Their Relationship to Human Education.*" Unpublished doctoral dissertation, University of Maryland, 1978.

Bandura, A. "Self-Efficacy: Toward a Unifying Theory of Behavioral Change." *Psychological Review*, 1977, *84*, 191–215.

Bandura, A. *Social Foundations of Thought and Action: A Social Cognitive Theory.* Upper Saddle River, NJ: Prentice Hall, 1986.

Bandura, A. *Self-Efficacy: The Exercise of Control.* New York: Freeman, 1997.

Baranick, E., and Ricca, J. "Community Mobilization Within a Multi-Channel Behavior Change C-IMCI Framework Has Rapid Impact in Diverse Settings." Paper presented at the American Public Health Association 133rd Annual Meeting, Philadelphia, Dec. 2005. http://apha.confex.com/apha/133am /techprogram/paper_110778.htm. Retrieved Oct. 2006.

Barbato, C. A., Graham, E. E., and Perse, E. M. "Communicating in the Family: An Examination of the Relationship of Family Communication Climate and Interpersonal Communication Motives." *Journal of Family Communication,* 2003, *3*(3), 123–148.

Barbato, C. A., and Perse, E. M. "Interpersonal Communication Motives and the Life Position of Elders." *Communication Research,* 1992, *19*(4), 516–531.

Barney, L. J., Griffiths, K. M., Jorm, A. F., and Christensen, H. "Stigma About Depression and Its Impact on Help-Seeking Intentions." *Australian and New Zealand Journal of Psychiatry,* 2006, *40*(1), 51–54.

Bauchner, H., Simpson, L., and Chessare, J. "Changing Physician Behavior." *Archives of Disease in Childhood,* 2001, *84*(6), 459–462.

BBC News. "Fake Professor in Wikipedia Storm." 2007. http://news.bbc.co.uk/2 /hi/americas/6423659.stm. Retrieved Mar. 2013.

Beal, G. M., and Rogers, E. M. *The Adoption of Two Farm Practices in a Central Iowa Community.* (Special Report No. 26) Ames: Iowa State University, 1960.

Becker, M. H., Haefner, D. P., and Maiman, L. A. "The Health Belief Model in the Prediction of Dietary Compliance: A Field Experiment." *Journal of Health and Social Behaviour,* 1977, *18,* 348–366.

Belch, G. E., and Belch, M. A. *Advertising and Promotion: An Integrated Marketing Communications Perspective.* (6th ed.) New York: McGraw-Hill, 2004.

Belzer, E. J. "Improving Patient Communication in No Time." *Family Practice Management,* 1999, *6*(5), 3–28.

Benz, J. K., Espinosa, O., Welsh, V., and Fontes, A. "Awareness of Racial and Ethnic Health Disparities Has Improved Only Modestly over A Decade." *Health Affairs,* 2011, *30*(10), 1860–1867.

Bernhardt, J. M. "Communication at the Core of Effective Public Health." *American Journal of Public Health,* 2004, *94*(12), 2051–2053.

Bernhardt, J. M., and others. "Perceived Barriers to Internet-Based Health Communication on Human Genetics." *Journal of Health Communication,* 2002, *7*(4), 325–340.

Berns, R. M. *Child, Family, School, Community: Socialization and Support.* (9th ed.) Belmont, CA: Wadsworth, Cengage Learning, 2013.

Bertrand, J. T. "Evaluating Health Communication Programmes." *The Drum Beat,* no. 302, Communication Initiative. 2005. www.comminit.com/global/content /evaluating-health-communication-programmes. Retrieved June 2013.

Besculides, M., and Laraque, F. "Racial and Ethnic Disparities in Perinatal Mortality: Applying the Perinatal Periods of Risk Model to Identify Areas for Intervention." *Journal of the National Medical Association*, 2005, *97*(8), 1128–1132.

Best, S., and Kellner, D. *The Postmodern Adventure*. New York and London: Guilford Press and Routledge, 2001.

Betancourt, J. "Impact of the *Sesame Street* Brand on Influencing Preschoolers' Healthy Food Choices." Presented at the American Public Health Association 136th Annual Meeting, San Diego, Oct. 29, 2008. https://apha.confex.com /apha/136am/webprogram/Paper188419.html. Retrieved Mar. 2013.

Bicchieri, C. *The Grammar of Society: The Nature and Dynamics of Social Norms*. New York: Cambridge University Press, 2006.

Biotechnology Journal. "Talking Biotech with the Public." *Biotechnology Podcast*. Sept. 2007. www.wiley-vch.de/publish/en/journals/alphabeticIndex/ 2446/?jURL=http://www.wiley-vch.de:80/vch/journals/2446/2446_pod.html. Retrieved Feb. 2013.

Bishop, J. "Enhancing the Understanding of Genres of Web-Based Communities: The Role of the Ecological Cognition Framework." *International Journal of Web Based Communities*, 2009, *5*(1), 4–17.

Blanchard, J., and others. "In Their Own Words: Lessons Learned from Those Exposed to Anthrax." *American Journal of Public Health*, 2005, *95*(3), 489–495.

Blot, W. J., and others. "Smoking and Drinking in Relation to Oral and Pharyngeal Cancer." *Cancer Research*, 1988, *48*(11), 3282–3287.

Blount, L. T. "Promoting Voices from the Field: African Scientists as Malaria Advocates." Presented at the American Public Health Association 135th Annual Meeting and Expo, Washington, DC, Nov. 6, 2007. https://apha.confex.com /apha/135am/techprogram/paper_165814.htm. Retrieved Mar. 2013.

Bogart, L. M., and others. "HIV Misconceptions Associated with Condom Use Among Black South Africans: An Exploratory Study." *African Journal of AIDS Research*, 2011, *10*(2), 181–187.

Bogen, K. "The Effect of Questionnaire Length on Response Rates—A Review of the Literature." Washington, DC: US Bureau of the Census. www.census.gov /srd/papers/pdf/kb9601.pdf. Retrieved Mar. 2006.

Bongaarts, J., and Watkins, S. C. "Social Interactions and Contemporary Fertility Transitions." *Population and Development Review*, 1996, *22*(4), 639–682.

Borg, E. "Smoking Ban Near Dorms Not Enforced: University Police Not Ticketing Smokers by Residency Halls." 2004. www.spectatornews.com/index .php?s=Smoking+Ban+Near+Dorms+Not+Enforced&x=0&y=0. Retrieved June 2013.

Boruchovitch, E., and Mednick, B. R. "Cross-Cultural Differences in Children's Concepts of Health and Illness." *Revista de Saude Publica*, 1997, *31*(5), 448–456.

Boruchovitch, E., and Mednick, B. R. "The Meaning of Health and Illness: Some Considerations for Health Psychology." *Psico-USF*, 2002, *7*(2), 175–183.

Boslaugh, S. E., Kreuter, M. W., Nicholson, R. A., and Naleid, K. "Comparing Demographic, Health Status and Psychosocial Strategies of Audience Segmentation to Promote Physical Activity." *Health Education Research*, 2005, *20*(4), 430–438.

Bradac, J. B. "Theory Comparison: Uncertainty Reduction, Problematic Integration, Uncertainty Management, and Other Curious Constructs." *Journal of Communication*, 2011, *51*(3), 456–476.

Braunstein, S., and Lavizzo-Mourey, R. "How the Health and Community Development Sectors Are Combining Forces to Improve Health and Well-Being." *Health Affairs*, 2011, *30*(11), 2042–2051.

Bray, G. "Medical Consequences of Obesity." *Journal of Clinical Endocrinology and Metabolism*, 2004, *89*(6), 2583–2589.

Brennan, S. E. *"Seeking and Providing Evidence for Mutual Understanding."* Unpublished doctoral dissertation, Stanford University, 1990.

Brennan, S. E. "How Conversation Is Shaped by Visual and Spoken Evidence." In J. Trueswell and M. Tanenhaus (eds.), *World Situated Language Use: Psycholinguistic, Linguistic, and Computational Perspectives on Bridging the Product and Action Traditions.* Cambridge, MA: MIT Press, 2004.

Brennan, S. E., and Lockridge, C. B. "Computer-Mediated Communication: A Cognitive Science Approach." In K. Brown (ed.), *ELL2, Encyclopedia of Language and Linguistics.* (2nd ed.) New York: Elsevier, 2006. www.psychology .stonybrook.edu/sbrennan-/papers/BL_ELL2.pdf. Retrieved Nov. 2005.

Broadstock, M., Borland, R., and Gason, R. "Effects of Suntan on Judgements of Healthiness and Attractiveness by Adolescents." *Journal of Applied Social Psychology*, 1992, *22*(2), 157–172.

Brown, R. *Social Psychology.* New York: Free Press, 1965.

Brownson, R. C., *and others.* Evidence-Based Public Health. (2nd ed.) New York: Oxford University Press, 2011.

Burns, P. G. "Reducing Infant Mortality Rates Using the Perinatal Periods of Risk Model." *Public Health Nursing*, 2005, *22*(1), 2–7.

Burson-Marsteller. "Constituency Relations." www.bm.com/pages/functional /relations. Retrieved Feb. 2006.

Bush, S., and Hopkins, A. D. "Public-Private Partnerships in Neglected Tropical Disease Control: The Role of Nongovernmental Organisations." *Acta Tropica*, 2011, *120* (Suppl. 1), S169–S172.

Burstall, M. L. "European Policies Influencing Pharmaceutical Innovations." In A. C. Gelijins and E. A. Halm (eds.), *The Changing Economics of Medical Technology.* Washington, DC: National Academies Press, 1991.

Calgary Health Region. *Explaining Pandemic Influenza: A Guide from the Medical Officer of Health.* Calgary, AB: Calgary Health Region, 2005.

California Newsreel. "Unnatural Causes . . . Is Inequality Making Us Sick?" Video recording. 2008.

Calmy, A. "MSF and HIV/AIDS: Expanding Treatment, Facing New Challenges." 2004. www.doctorswithoutborders.org/publications/ar/i2004/hivaids.cfm. Retrieved Jan. 2006.

Campaign for Tobacco-Free Kids. "Who We Are." www.tobaccofreekidsw.org /who_we_are. Retrieved Feb. 2013.

Campbell, C., and Scott, K. "Community Health and Social Mobilization." In R. Obregon and S. Waisbord (eds.), *The Handbook of Global Health Communication*. Oxford, UK: Wiley-Blackwell, 2012.

Campbell, J. D. "Illness Is a Point of View: The Development of Children's Concept of Illness." *Children's Development*, 1975, *46*, 92–100.

Canadian Public Health Association. "ParticipACTION: The Mouse That Roared a Marketing and Health Communications Success Story." 2004. www.cpha.ca/en /about/media/media2004/participaction.aspx. Retrieved June 2013.

CancerBACKUP, "Why Improve Access to Cancer Information?" www.cancer bacup.org.uk/Healthprofessionals/Reachingmorecommunities/Beyondthe Barriers/Whyimproveaccess#6623. Retrieved Jan. 2006.

Caribbean Epidemiology Center. "Report of Communication Advisory Committee Meeting, Sub-Committee of the Technical Advisory Group." 2003. www.carec.org/documents/cccpcp/communication_advisory_report.doc. Retrieved Feb. 2006.

Cargo, M., and Mercer, S. L. "The Value and Challenges of Participatory Research: Strengthening Its Practice." *Annual Review of Public Health*, 2008, *29*, 325–350.

Carter, K. E. "Building a Constituency Through Outreach." 1994. www.stc .org/confproceed/1994/PDFs/PG5152.PDF. Retrieved Mar. 2006.

Cassell, M. M., Jackson, C., and Cheuvront, B. "Health Communication on the Internet: An Effective Channel for Health Behavior Change?" *Journal of Health Communication*, 1998, *3*, 71–79.

Castrucci, B. C., Gerlach, K. K., Kaufman, N. J., and Orleans, C. T. "Tobacco Use and Cessation Behavior Among Adolescents Participating in Organized Sports." *American Journal of Health Behavior*, 2004, *28*(1), 63–71.

Cave, L. *NIMH Establishes Outreach, Education Program*. Bethesda, MD: National Institutes of Health. http://nihrecord.od.nih.gov/newsletters /08_08_2000/story04. Retrieved June 2013.

Cendron, M. "Primary Nocturnal Enuresis: Current Concepts." *American Family Physician*, 1999, *59*(5), 1205–1213.

Center, A. H., and Jackson, P. *Public Relations Practices: Management Case Studies and Problems*. (5th ed.) Upper Saddle River, NJ: Prentice Hall, 1995.

Center for Consumer Freedom. "Humane Society of the United States." www .activistcash.com/organizations/136-humane-society-of-the-united-states. Retrieved June 2013.

Center for Health Equity Research and Promotion. "Intro to Health Disparities." www.cherp.research.med.va.gov/introhd.php. Retrieved Oct. 2005.

Centers for Disease Control and Prevention. *Addressing Emerging Infectious Disease Threats: A Prevention Strategy for the United States*. Atlanta, GA: Public Health Service, 1994a.

Centers for Disease Control and Prevention. Office on Smoking and Health. National Center for Chronic Disease Prevention and Health Promotion. "State

Laws on Tobacco Control—United States, 1998." *MMWR*, June 25, 1999, *48* (SS-03), 21–62. www.cdc.gov/mmwr/preview/mmwrhtml/ss4803a2.htm. Retrieved Mar. 2006.

Centers for Disease Control and Prevention. "HealthComm Key: Unlocking the Power of Health Communication Research."www.cdc.gov/od/oc/hcomm. Retrieved May 2001.

Centers for Disease Control and Prevention. "From Data to Action: Infant Sleep Position." Centers for Disease Control and Prevention. 2002. www.cdc.gov /PRAMS/dataAct2002/infant_sleep.htm. Retrieved Feb. 2006.

Centers for Disease Control and Prevention. "Colorectal Cancer: About the CDC Program." 2004/2005. www.cdc.gov/colorectalcancer/pdf/about2004.pdf. Retrieved Mar. 2006.

Centers for Disease Control and Prevention. "CDC-Funded Asthma Activities by State and Type of Funding." www.cdc.gov/asthma/nacp.htm. Retrieved Feb. 2006a.

Centers for Disease Control and Prevention. "Colorectal Cancer." www.cdc.gov /colorectalcancer. Retrieved Mar. 2006b.

Centers for Disease Control and Prevention. "Got a Minute? Give It to Your Kid: Audience Profile." www.cdc.gov/tobacco/parenting/audience.htm. Retrieved Feb. 2006c.

Centers for Disease Control and Prevention. "Heads Up: Brain Injury in Your Practice Tool Kit." www.cdc.gov/ncipc/pub-res/tbi_toolkit/physicians /introduction.htm. Retrieved Jan. 2006d.

Centers for Disease Control and Prevention. "Malaria Control in Endemic Countries." www.cdc.gov/malaria/control_prevention/control.htm. Retrieved Feb. 2006e.

Centers for Disease Control and Prevention. "Parasites—Leishmaniasis." www.cdc.gov/parasites/leishmaniasis/index.html. Retrieved Mar. 2006f.

Centers for Disease Control and Prevention. "Physical Activity for Everyone: The Importance of Physical Activity." www.cdc.gov/nccdphp/dnpa /physical/importance/index.htm. Retrieved Mar. 2006g.

Centers for Disease Control and Prevention. "Preventing Tetanus, Diphtheria, and Pertussis Among Adolescents: Use of Tetanus Toxoid, Reduced Diphtheria Toxoid and Acellular Pertussis Vaccines." *MMWR*, Feb. 23, 2006h, *55*, 1–34. www.cdc.gov/mmwr/preview/mmwrhtml/rr55e223a1.htm. Retrieved Mar. 2006h.

Centers for Disease Control and Prevention. Foodborne and Diarrheal Diseases Branch. "Safe Water System Manual." http://hetv.org/India/mh/plan /safewater/manual/ch_7.htm. Retrieved Jan. 2006i.

Centers for Disease Control and Prevention. "Syphilis Elimination Effort (SEE) Toolkit." www.cdc.gov/stopsyphilis/toolkit/default.htm. Retrieved Jan. 2006j.

Centers for Disease Control and Prevention. *Promoting Cultural Sensitivity: A Practical Guide for Tuberculosis Programs That Provide Services to Persons from*

China. Atlanta, GA: US Department of Health and Human Services, 2008a. www.cdc.gov/tb/publications/guidestoolkits/EthnographicGuides/China/chapters/china.pdf. Retrieved Jan. 2013.

Centers for Disease Control and Prevention. *Promoting Cultural Sensitivity: A Practical Guide for Tuberculosis Programs That Provide Services to Persons from Somalia*. Atlanta, GA: US Department of Health and Human Services, 2008b. www.cdc.gov/tb/publications/guidestoolkits/EthnographicGuides/Somalia/chapters/SomaliTBBooklet.pdf. Retrieved Jan. 2013.

Centers for Disease Control and Prevention. "Gateway to Health Communication & Social Marketing Practice. Health Communication Basics." 2011a. www.cdc.gov/healthcommunication/HealthBasics/WhatIsHC.html. Retrieved Oct. 2012.

Centers for Disease Control and Prevention. "The Health Communicator's Social Media Toolkit." 2011b. www.cdc.gov/socialmedia/tools/guidelines/pdf/socialmediatoolkit_bm.pdf. Retrieved Feb. 2013.

Centers for Disease Control and Prevention. "Crisis and Risk Communication Course (CERC)." 2011c. http://emergency.cdc.gov/cerc/overview.asp. Retrieved Mar. 2013.

Centers for Disease Control and Prevention. "Concussion and Mild TBI." www.cdc.gov/concussion. Retrieved Feb. 2013a.

Centers for Disease Control and Prevention. "Glossary." *CDCynergy Web. Your Guide to Effective Health Communication*. www.orau.gov/cdcynergy/web/BA/Content/activeinformation/glossaryframeset.htm. Retrieved Mar. 2013b.

Centers for Disease Control and Prevention. "Injury Prevention & Control: Traumatic Brain Injury. How Many People Have TBI?" www.cdc.gov/TraumaticBrainInjury/statistics.html. Retrieved June 2013c.

Centers for Disease Control and Prevention. "Pertussis (Whooping Cough). Outbreaks." 2013d. www.cdc.gov/pertussis/outbreaks/about.html. Retrieved Mar. 2013.

Centers for Disease Control and Prevention. "What CDC Is Doing About Colorectal Cancer." 2013e. www.cdc.gov/cancer/colorectal/what_cdc_is_doing/index.htm. Retrieved Mar. 2013.

Chan, S. "Parents of Exceptional Asian Children." In M. K. Kitano and P. C. Chinn (eds.), *Exceptional Asian Children and Youth*. Reston, VA: Council for Exceptional Children, 1986.

Chen, N., Kohler, C., Schoenberger, Y., Suzuki-Crumly, J., Davis, K., and Powell, J. "The Impact of Targeted Radio Educational Entertainment on Health Knowledge, Attitudes and Behavior Among African-Americans." *Cases in Public Health Communication & Marketing*, 2009, 3, 92–113. www.casesjournal.org/volume3. Retrieved Oct. 2012.

Cherry, J. D., and others. "Defining Pertussis Epidemiology: Clinical, Microbiologic and Serologic Perspectives." *Pediatric Infectious Disease Journal*, 2005, 24(5 Suppl.), S25–S34.

Chief Information Officer Council. "Flu Prevention Goes Viral at CDC." Jan. 1, 2009. https://cio.gov/flu-prevention-goes-viral-at-cdc. Retrieved May 2010.

Chiu, C., Krauss, R. M., and Lau, I. Y. "Some Cognitive Consequences of Communication." In S. R. Fussell and R. J. Kreuz (eds.), *Social and Cognitive Approaches to Interpersonal Communication*. Mahwah, NJ: Erlbaum, 1998.

Christopher and Dana Reeve Foundation. "Action Network." www.christopherreeve.org/site/c.ddJFKRNoFiG/b.4426041. Retrieved Feb. 2013.

Clark, H. H., and Brennan, S. E. "Grounding in Communication." In L. B. Resnick, J. Levine, and S. D. Teasley (eds.), *Perspectives on Socially Shared Cognition*. Washington, DC: APA Press, 1991.

Clark, H. H., and Schaefer, E. F. "Contributing to Discourse." *Cognitive Science*, 1989, *13*, 259–294.

Clark, H. H., and Wilkes-Gibbs, D. "Referring as a Collaborative Process." *Cognition*, 1986, *22*, 1–39.

Cleland, J., and Wilson, C. "Demand Theories of the Fertility Transition: An Iconoclastic View." *Population Studies*, 1987, *41*(1), 5–30.

Clift, E., and Freimuth, V. "Health Communication: What Is It and What Can It Do for You?" *Journal of Health Education*, 1995, *26*(2), 68–74.

Cline, R.J.W., and Haynes, K. M. "Consumer Health Information Seeking on the Internet: The State of the Art." *Health Education Research*, 2001, *16*(6), 671–692.

Coalition for Health Communication. "Welcome to Coalition for Health Communication." www.healthcommunication.net. Retrieved Feb. 2013.

Coalition for Healthy Children. "About Us." www.healthychildrencoalition.org/about.html. Retrieved Feb. 2013.

Coffman, J. "Public Communication Campaign Evaluation: An Environmental Scan of Challenges, Criticisms, Practice, and Opportunities." 2002. www.hfrp.org/evaluation/publications-resources/public-communication-campaign-evaluation-an-environmental-scan-of-challenges-criticisms-practice-and-opportunities. Retrieved June 2013.

Cohen, L. K. "*Live.Learn.Laugh.*: A Unique Global Public-Private Partnership to Improve Oral Health." *International Dental Journal*, 2011, *61*(Suppl. 2), 1.

Cole, G. E., and others. "Addressing Problems in Evaluating Health Relevant Programs Through Systematic Planning and Evaluation." *Risk: Health, Safety and Environment*, 1995, *37*(1), 37–57.

Colle, R. D., and Roman, R. "A Handbook for Telecenter Staffs." 2003. http://ip.cals.cornell.edu/commdev/handbook.cfm. Retrieved Mar. 2006.

Colwill, J. M., and Cultice, J. M. "The Future Supply of Family Physicians: Implications for Rural America." *Health Affairs*, 2003, *22*, 190–198.

Communication Initiative. "Change Theories: Cultivation Theory of Mass Media." July 2003a. www.comminit.com/changetheories/ctheories/changetheories-24.html. Retrieved Sept. 2005.

Communication Initiative. "Change Theories Precede-Proceed." Nov. 2003b. www.comminit.com/changetheories/ctheories/changetheories-42.html. Retrieved Dec. 2005.

Communication Initiative. The Drum Beat Issue 427. "Emergency Communication." 2008. www.comminit.com/global/drum_beat_427.html. Retrieved Jan. 2013.

Communication Initiative. "Strategic Communication in Urban Health Settings: Taking the Pulse of Emerging Needs and Trends." May 2010. www.comminit.com/en/global/node/316562. Retrieved Jan. 2013.

Community Tool Box. "Developing Multisector Collaborations." http://sitefinity.myctb.org/en/tablecontents/sub_section_main_1385.aspx. Retrieved Feb. 2013.

Conrad, P., and Stults, C. "The Internet and the Experience of Illness." In C. E. Bird, P. Conrad, A. M. Fremont, and S. Timinermans (eds.), *Handbook of Medical Sociology* (6th ed.). Nashville: Vanderbilt University Press, 2010.

Constance, H. "Animal Wars." *Science*, 2005, *309*(5740), 1485.

Cooney Waters Group. "Virtual Connections." www.cooneywaters.com/services/virtual_connections. Retrieved Feb. 2013.

Corrigan, P. "How Stigma Interferes with Mental Health Care." *American Psychologist*, 2004, *59*(7), 614–625.

Costas-Bradstreet, C. "Spreading the Message Through Community Mobilization, Education and Leadership: A Magnanimous Task." *Canadian Journal of Public Health*, 2004, *95*, S25–S29.

Couldry, N., and Curran, J. (eds.). *Contesting Media Power: Alternative Media in a Networked world*. Boulder, CO: Rowman and Littlefield, 2003.

Coursaris, C. K., and Liu, M. "An Analysis of Social Support Exchanges in Online HIV/AIDS Self-Help Groups." *Computers in Human Behavior*, 2009, *25*(4), 911–918.

Coward, H., and Sidhu, T. "Bioethics for Clinicians: 19. Hinduism and Sikhism." *Canadian Medical Association Journal*, 2000, *163*(9), 1167–1170.

Crystalinks. "Hippocrates." www.crystalinks.com/hippocrates.html. Retrieved Jan. 2006.

Curtis, V. A., Garbrah-Aidoo, N., and Scott, B. "Ethics in Public Health Research." *American Journal of Public Health*, 2007, *97*(4), 634–641.

Cutlip, S. M., Center, A. H., and Broom, G. M. *Effective Public Relations*. Upper Saddle River, NJ: Prentice Hall, 1994.

Dalhousie University. "Evaluation of Health Information on the Web." 2011. http://dal.ca.libguides.com/content.php?pid=88898&sid=661725. Retrieved Mar. 2013.

Das, A. K., Olfson, M., McCurtis, H. L., and Weissman, M. M. "Depression in African Americans: Breaking Barriers to Detection and Treatment." *Journal of Family Practice*, 2006, *55*(1), 30–39.

Davidson, B. "New Media and Activism." Africa Is a Country. 2012. http://africasacountry.com/2012/06/08/new-media-and-activism. Retrieved Mar. 2013.

Davis, K., Schoen, C., and Stremikis, K. "Mirror, Mirror on the Wall: How the Performance of the U.S. Health Care System Compares Internationally. 2010 Update." The Commonwealth Fund. 2010. www.commonwealthfund.org/~/media/Files/Publications/Fund%20Report/2010/Jun/1400_Davis_Mirror_Mirror_on_the_wall_2010.pdf. Retrieved Feb. 2013.

Davis, K. C., Uhrig, J., Rupert, D., and Harris, S. "The Take Charge. Take the Test. HIV Testing Social Marketing Campaign for African American Women." Report submitted to the Centers for Disease Control and Prevention. Research Triangle Park, NC: RTI International, 2008.

Debus, M. *Methodological Review: A Handbook for Excellence in Focus Group Research.* Washington, DC: Academy for Educational Development, 1988.

de Heer, H., Moya, E. M., and Lacson, R. "Voices and Images: Tuberculosis Photovoice in a Binational Setting." *Cases in Public Health Communication & Marketing*, 2008, *2*, 55–86. www.casesjournal.org/volume2. Retrieved Oct. 2012.

Dein, S., Cook, C.C.H., Powell, A., and Eagger, S. "Religion, Spirituality and Mental Health." *The Psychiatrist*, 2010, *34*, 63–64.

De Nies, T., and others. "Bringing Newsworthiness into the 21st Century." Presented at the 11th International Semantic Web Conference, 2012, Proceedings, 106–117. http://ceur-ws.org/Vol-906/paper11.pdf. Retrieved Feb. 2013.

DES Action Canada and Working Group on Women and Health Protection. "Protecting Our Health: New Debates." www.whp-apsf.ca/pdf/dtca.pdf. Retrieved Jan. 2006.

Deutsch, M. "A Theory of Cooperation—Competition and Beyond." In P.A.M. Van Lange, A. W. Kruglanski, and E. T. Higgins (eds.), *The Handbook of Theories of Social Psychology.* (vol. 2) London: Sage, 2012.

Development Communication and Media Advocacy. "Project 'Know Yourself' and Project 'HEART'" 2009. http://aranya-rmt.blogspot.com/2009/03/project-know-yourself-and-project-heart.html. Retrieved Mar. 2013.

Dholakia, U. M., Bagozzi, R. P., and Pearo, L. K. "A Social Influence Model of Consumer Participation in Network- and Small-Group-Based Virtual Communities." *International Journal of Research in Marketing*, 2004, *21*(3), 241–263.

Dillman, D., Sinclair, M. D., and Clark, J. R. "Effects of Questionnaire Length, Respondent-Friendly Design, and a Difficult Question on Response Rates for Occupant-Addressed Census Mail Surveys." *Public Opinion Quarterly*, 1993, *57*(3), 289–304.

DiMatteo, M. R., and others. "Physicians' Characteristics Influence Patients' Adherence to Medical Treatment: Results from the Medical Outcomes Study." *Health Psychology*, 1993, *12*(2), 93–102.

Dingfelder, S. F. "Stigma: Alive and Well." *Monitor on Psychology*, 2009, *40*(6), 56. www.apa.org/monitor/2009/06/stigma.aspx. Retrieved Mar. 2013.

Doak, C. C., Doak, L. G., and Root, J. H. *Teaching Patients with Low Literacy Skills.* Philadelphia: Lippincott, 1995.

Dolan, P. L. "Physicians Tell How Much Time Tablets Save Them." American Medical Association. 2013. www.amednews.com/article/20130107 /business/130109995. Retrieved Feb. 2013.

Donovan, R. J. "Steps in Planning and Developing Health Communication Campaigns: A Comment on CDC's Framework for Health Communication." *Public Health Reports,* 1995, *110*(2), 215–217.

Dougall, A. L., and Baum, A. "Stress, Health, and Illness." In A. Baum, T. A. Revenson, and J. Singer (eds.), *Handbook of Health Psychology.* (2nd ed.) New York: Psychology Press, 2012.

Drum Beat. "Health Communication vs. Related Disciplines." Communication Initiative. 2005. www.comminit.com/governance-africa/drum_beat_324.html. Retrieved June 2013.

Druss, B. G., and others. "Mental Disorders and Use of Cardiovascular Procedures After Myocardial Infarction." *Journal of American Medical Association,* 2000, *283*(4), 506–511.

Duhe, S. C. "Editor's Note." In S. C. Duhe (ed.), *New Media and Public Relations.* New York: Peter Lang, 2007.

Duignan, P., and Parker, J. "From Monologue to Dialogue: An Overview of Consultation Methods." 2005. www.parkerduignan.com/documents/133pdf.PDF.

du Pré, A. *Communicating About Health: Current Issues and Perspectives.* Mountain View, CA: Mayfield, 2000.

Dutta, M. J. "Emerging Trends in the New Media Landscape." In J. C. Parker and E. Thorson (eds.), *Health Communication in the New Media Landscape.* New York: Springer, 2009.

Economic and Social Research Council. "Top Ten Tips." www.esrc.ac.uk/funding-and-guidance/tools-and-resources/impact-toolkit/developing-plan/top-tips.aspx. Retrieved Dec. 2005a.

Economic and Social Research Council. "Why Media Relations Is Important." www.esrc.ac.uk/funding-and-guidance/tools-and-resources/impact-toolkit /tools/media/important.aspx. Retrieved Dec. 2005b.

Ehiri, J. *Maternal and Child Health: Global Challenges, Programs, and Policies.* New York: Springer, 2009.

Eisenberg, J. M., and others. "Legislative Approaches to Tackling the Obesity Epidemic." *Canadian Medical Association Journal,* 2011, *183*(13), 1496–1500.

Eisenberg, J. M., Kitz, D. S., and Webber, R. A. "Development of Attitudes About Sharing Decision Making: A Comparison of Medical and Surgical Residents." *Journal of Health and Social Behavior,* 1983, *24*, 85–90.

Eiser, J. R., and Pancer, S. M. "Attitudinal Effects of the Use of Evaluatively Biased Language." *European Journal of Social Psychology,* 1979, *9*, 39–47.

El Rabbat, M. *Avian Influenza Community Assessment: Focus on Backyard Poultry Breeding.* Post Intervention Qualitative Study. Egypt: UNICEF, 2007.

Emanoil, P. "The Key to Public Health Is Community." *Human Ecology*, 2002, *28*(2), 16.

eMarketer Digital Intelligence. "Where to Reach Women Online." 2010. http://totalaccess.emarketer.com/Article.aspx?R=1007826. Retrieved July 2011.

Emblen, J. D. "Religion and Spirituality Defined According to Current Use in Nursing Literature." *Journal of Professional Nursing*, 1992, *8*(1), 41–47.

Emerson College. "Integrated Marketing Communication." www.emerson.edu /academics/departments/marketing-communication/graduate-degrees/integrated-marketing-communication. Retrieved Jan. 2013.

Encarta Dictionary (English, North America). "Search Term: Communication." http://encarta.msn.com/dictionary_/communication.html. Retrieved Dec. 2005.

Engel, G. E. "The Need for a New Medical Model: A Challenge for Biomedicine." *Science*, 1977, *196*, 129–136.

Erickson, J. G., Devlieger, P. J., and Sung, J. M. "Korean-American Female Perspectives on Disability." *American Journal of Speech-Language Pathology*, 1999, *8*, 99–108.

European Network for Smoking Prevention. "Implementation of the EU Directive on Advertising Ban—Status on 1 July 2005 Implementation Deadline: 31 July 2005." 2005. http://old.ensp.org/files/adv_ban_implementation _april_2009.pdf. Retrieved Mar. 2006.

Evans, D., Davis, K. C., and Zhang, Y. "Health Communication and Marketing Research with New Media. Case Study of the National Speak Up National Campaign Evaluation." *Cases in Public Health Communication and Marketing*, 2008, *11*, 140–158.

Evans, W. D., and others. "Mobile Health Evaluation Methods: The Text4baby Case Study." *Journal of Health Communication*, 2012, *17*(Suppl. 1), 22–29.

Exchange. "Issues in Evaluation for Health and Disability Communication." Aug. 2001. www.healthcomms.org/comms/eval/le05.html.

Exchange. "Health Communication." www.healthcomms.org/comms. Retrieved July 2005.

Exchange. "Integrated Communication." www.healthcomms.org/comms/integ/ict -integ.html. Retrieved Mar. 2006.

Eysenbach, G. "Consumer Health Informatics." *British Medical Journal*, 2000, *320*, 1713–1716.

Eysenbach, G. "What Is E-Health?" *Journal of Medical Internet Research*, 2001, *3*(2), e20.

Fadiman, A. *The Spirit Catches You and You Fall Down: A Hmong Child, Her American Doctors, and the Collision of Two Cultures.* New York: Farrar, Straus and Giroux, 1997.

Families USA. Global Health Initiative. "Why Global Health Matters—Here and Abroad." www.familiesusa.org/issues/global-health/matters. Retrieved Dec. 2012.

Families USA. "Making Radio Work for You: An Advocate's Guide on How to Use Radio Actualities and Talk Radio to Move Your Agenda Forward." www.familiesusa.org/resources/tools-for-advocates/guides/radio -guide.html. Retrieved April 2013.

FamilyDoctor.org. "Health Information on the Web: Finding Reliable Information." 2010. http://familydoctor.org/familydoctor/en/healthcare-management/ self-care/health-information-on-the-web-finding-reliable-information.printer view.all.html. Retrieved Mar. 2013.

Faulkner, G., and others. "ParticipACTION: Baseline Assessment of the Capacity Available to the 'New ParticipACTION': A Qualitative Study of Canadian Organization." *International Journal of Behavioral Nutrition and Physical Activity*, 2009, *6*, 87. www.ijbnpa.org/content/6/1/87. Retrieved Feb. 2013.

Federico, B., Mackenbach, J. P., Eikemo, T. A., and Kunst, A. E. "Impact of the 2005 Smoke-Free Policy in Italy on Prevalence, Cessation and Intensity of Smoking in the Overall Population and by Educational Group." *Addiction*, 2012, *107*(9), 1677–1686.

Fielding, J. E. "Foreword." In R. C. Brownson, E. A. Baker, T. L. Leet, K. N. Gillespie, and W. R. True (eds.), *Evidence-Based Public Health*. New York: Oxford University Press, 2011.

Figueroa, M. E., Kincaid, D. L., Rani, M., and Lewis, G. *Communication for Social Change: An Integrated Model for Measuring the Process and Its Outcomes*. New York: Rockefeller Foundation and Johns Hopkins University Center for Communication Programs, 2002.

Finerman, R. "The Burden of Responsibility: Duty, Depression, and Nervios in Andean Ecuador." *Health Care for Women International*, 1989, *10*(2–3), 141–157.

Fischer, J. E. "Current Status of Medicine in the USA: A Personal Perspective." *Journal of the Royal College of Surgeons of Edinburgh*, 2001, *46*, 71–75.

Fishbein, M., Goldberg, M., and Middlestadt, S. *Social Marketing: Theoretical and Practical Perspectives*. Mahwah, NJ: Erlbaum, 1997.

Fisher, S. "Case Study—Viim Kuunga Radio Project—Burkina Faso." Communication Initiative. 2003. www.comminit.com/la/node/120105. Retrieved June 2013.

Flanagin, A. J., and Metzger, M. J. "Internet Use in the Contemporary Media Environment." *Human Communication Research*, 2001, *27*(1), 153–181.

Flay, B. R. "Efficacy and Effectiveness Trials (and Other Phases of Research) in the Development of Health Promotion Programs." *Preventive Medicine*, 1986, *15*(5), 451–474.

Flew, T. *New Media: An Introduction*. South Melbourne: Oxford University Press, 2002.

Fog, A. *Cultural Selection*. Norwell, MA: Kluwer, 1999.

Food and Agriculture Organization of the United Nations, International Labour Organization, Joint United Nations Programme on HIV/AIDS, United Nations

Children's Fund, United Nations Development Programme, United Nations Educational, Scientific and Cultural Organization, and World Health Organization. "Communication for Development: Strengthening the effectiveness of the United Nations." 2011. www.unicef.org/cbsc/files/Inter-agency_C4D_Book _2011.pdf. Retrieved Dec. 2012.

Food and Agricultural Organization. "Writing Effective Reports: Preparing Policy Briefs." www.fao.org/docrep/014/i2195e/i2195e03.pdf. Retrieved Mar. 2013.

FoodNavigatorUSA.com. "Innova Taps Trans Fat-Free Vegetable Oil Demand." 2005a. www.foodnavigator-usa.com/R-D/Innova-taps-trans-fat-free-vegetable -oil-demand. Retrieved June 2013.

FoodNavigatorUSA.com. "Seafood Producer Goes Trans Fat Free." 2005b. www .foodnavigator-usa.com/Suppliers2/Seafood-producer-goes-trans-fat-free. Retrieved June 2013.

Fox, S. "Participatory Medicine: Text of My Speech at the Connected Health Symposium—Susannah Fox." 2008. http://susannahfox.com/2008/11/03 /participatory-medicine-text-of-my-speech-at-the-connected-health -symposium. Retrieved Feb. 2013.

Frable, P. J., Wallace, D. C., and Ellison, K. J. "Using Clinical Guidelines in Home Care: For Patients with Diabetes." *Home Healthcare Nurse*, 2004, *22*(7), 462–468.

Freeman, R. E. *Strategic Management: A Stakeholder Approach*. Boston: Pitman, 1984.

Freimuth, V., Cole, G., and Kirby, S. *Issues in Evaluating Mass Mediated Health Communication Campaigns*. Copenhagen: WHO Regional Office for Europe, 2000.

Freimuth, V., Linnan, H. W., and Potter, P. "Communicating the Threat of Emerging Infections to the Public." *Emerging Infectious Diseases*, 2000, *6*(4), 337–347.

Freimuth, V. S., and Quinn, S. C. "The Contributions of Health Communication to Eliminating Health Disparities." *American Journal of Public Health*, 2004, *94*(12), 2053–2055.

Frey, K. A., Navarro, S. M., Kotelchuck, M., and Lu, M. C. The Clinical Content of Preconception Care: Preconception Care for Men. *American Journal of Obstetric Gynecology*, 2008, *199*(6 Suppl. B), S389–S395.

Friedman, H. S., and DiMatteo, M. R. "Health Care as an Interpersonal Process." *Journal of Social Issues*, 1979, *35*, 1–11.

Frisby, B. N., and Martin, M. M. "Interpersonal Motives and Supportive Communication." *Communication Research Reports*, 2010, *27*(4), 320–329.

Fritch, J. W., and Cromwell, R. L. "Evaluating Internet Resources: Identity, Affiliation, and Cognitive Authority in a Networked World." *Journal of the American Society for Information Science and Technology*, 2001, *52*, 499–507.

Futerra Sustainability Communications. "Heidelberg PR Campaign Analysis & Recommendation." Aug. 2010. www.citiesengage.eu/en/IMG/pdf/Heidelberg _campaign_analysis.pdf. Retrieved Feb. 2013.

Gaebel, W., Baumann, A. E., and Phil, M. A. "Interventions to Reduce the Stigma Associated with Severe Mental Illness: Experiences from the Open the Doors Program in Germany." *Canadian Journal of Psychiatry*, 2003, *48*(10), 657–662.

Gallup, J. L., and Sachs, J. D. "The Economic Burden of Malaria." *The American Journal of Tropical Medicine and Hygiene*, 2001, *64*(Suppl. 1), 85–96.

Gallus, S., and others. "Effects of New Smoking Regulations in Italy." *Annals of Oncology*, 2006, *17*, 346–347.

Gantenbein, R. E. *"E-Health: Using Information and Communication Technology to Improve Health Care."* Presentation at the IRI Conference, Las Vegas, Nov. 2001.

Gardenswartz, L., and Rowe, A. *Managing Diversity: A Complete Desk Reference and Planning Guide*. New York: McGraw-Hill, 1993.

Garrity, T. F., Haynes, R. B., Mattson, M. E., and Engebretson, J. T. (eds.). *Medical Compliance and the Clinical-Patient Relationship: A Review*. Washington, DC: US Government Printing Office, 1998.

Gay Men's Health Crisis. *The Gay Men's Health Crisis HIV/AIDS Timeline*. New York: Gay Men's Health Crisis, 2006.

Gay Men's Health Crisis. *Gay Men's Health Crisis HIV/AIDS Timeline*. New York: Gay Men's Health Crisis (GMHC), 2013.

George Mason University. "Review of Literature: Impact of Interactive Health Communications." F. Alemi (ed.). 1999. http://gunston.gmu.edu/healthscience/722/Review.htm. Retrieved Feb. 2013.

Gerbner, G. "Toward Cultural Indicators—Analysis of Mass Mediated Public Message Systems." *AV Communication Review*, 1969, *17*(2), 137–148.

Gerbner, G., Gross, L., Morgan, M., and Signorielle, N. "The Mainstreaming of America: Violence Profile No. 11." *Journal of Communication*, 1980, *30*, 10–29.

GETHealth Global Education and Technology Health Summit. www.gethealthsummit.org/about-the-summit.php. Retrieved Feb. 2013.

Gillis, D. "Beyond Words: The Health-Literacy Connection." 2005. www.nald.ca/library/research/cahealth/cover.htm. Retrieved June 2013.

Global Heath Education Consortium. "Global Health vs. International Health: What Is the Difference?" http://globalhealtheducation.org/Pages/GlobalvsInt.aspx. Retrieved Mar. 2013.

Glucksberg, S., and Weisberg, R. W. "Verbal Behavior and Problem Solving: Some Effects of Labeling in a Functional Fixedness Problem." *Journal of Experimental Psychology*, 1963, *71*, 659–664.

Godbout, J. P., and Glaser, R. "Stress-Induced Immune Dysregulation: Implications for Wound Healing, Infectious Disease and Cancer." *Journal of Neuroimmune Pharmacology*, 2006, *1*, 421–427.

Godfrey, F. "The Right Time for Europe to Stop Smoking." *Breathe*, 2005, *2*(1), 12–14.

GoGulf. "How People Spend Their Time Online [Infographic]." 2012. www.go-gulf.com/blog/online-time. Retrieved Feb. 2013.

Goodwin, J. S., Black, S. A., and Satish, S. "Aging Versus Disease: The Opinions of Older Black, Hispanic, and Non-Hispanic White Americans About the Causes and Treatment of Common Medical Conditions." *Journal of the American Geriatrics Society*, 1999, *47*(8), 973–979.

Gouin, J. P., and Kiecolt-Glaser, J. K. "The Impact of Psychological Stress on Wound Healing: Methods and Mechanisms." *Immunology and Allergy Clinics of North America*, 2011, *31*(1), 81–93.

GRACE Communications Foundation. www.gracelinks.org. Retrieved Mar. 2013.

Gray-Felder, D., and Dean, J. *Communication for Social Change: A Position Paper and Conference Report*. New York: Rockefeller Foundation Report, 1999.

Green, L. W., and Kreuter, M. W. *Health Promotion Planning: An Educational and Environmental Approach*. (2nd ed.) Mountain View, CA: Mayfield, 1991.

Green, L. W., and Kreuter, M. W. *Health Promotion Planning: An Educational and Environmental Approach*. (3rd ed.) Mountain View, CA: Mayfield, 1999.

Green, L. W., and Ottoson, J. M. *Community and Population Health*. (8th ed.) New York: McGraw-Hill, 1999.

Greenberg, D. P., von Konig, C. H., and Heininger, U. "Health Burden of Pertussis in Infants and Children." *Pediatric Infectious Disease Journal*, 2005, *24*(5 Suppl.), S39–S43.

Greenes, R. A., and Shortliffe, E. H. "Medical Informatics: An Emerging Academic Discipline and Institutional Priority." *Journal of the American Medical Association*, 1990, *263*(8), 1114–1120.

Grimley, D., Gabrielle, R., Bellis, J., and Prochaska, J. "Assessing the Stages of Change and Decision-Making for Contraceptive Use for the Prevention of Pregnancy, Sexually Transmitted Diseases, and Acquired Immunodeficiency Syndrome." *Health Education Quarterly*, 1993, *20*, 455–470.

Grimshaw, J. M., Eccles, M. P., Walker, A. E., and Thomas, R. E. "Changing Physicians' Behavior: What Works and Thoughts on Getting More Things to Work." *Journal of Continuing Education in the Health Professions*, 2002, *22*, 237–243.

Grol, R. "Beliefs and Evidence in Changing Clinical Care." *British Medical Journal*, 1997, *315*(7105), 418–421.

Grol, R. "Changing Physicians' Competence and Performance: Finding the Balance Between the Individual and the Organization." *Journal of Continuing Education in the Health Professions*, 2002, *22*, 244–251.

Gross, A. "Overview of Asia, Healthcare Markets and Regulatory Issues in the Region." Aug. 2001. www.pacificbridgemedical.com/publications/html/AsiaAugust01.htm. Retrieved Oct. 2005.

Grusec, J. E. "Socialization Processes in the Family: Social and Emotional Development." *Annual Review of Psychology*, 2011, *62*, 243–269.

GSMA. "African Mobile Observatory 2011. Driving Economic and Social Development Through Mobile Services." 2011. www.gsma.com/publicpolicy/wp-content/uploads/2012/04/africamobileobservatory2011–1.pdf. Retrieved June 2013.

Gudykunst, W. B. "Toward a Theory of Effective Interpersonal and Intergroup Communication: An Anxiety/Uncertainty Management (AUM) Perspective." In Richard L. Wiseman and Jolene Koester (eds.), *Intercultural Communication Competence: International and Intercultural Communication Annual.* Thousand Oaks, CA: Sage Publications, 1993, Vol. XVII, pp. 33–71.

Haider, M. (ed.). *Global Public Health Communication: Challenges, Perspectives, and Strategies.* Sudbury, MA: Jones and Bartlett, 2005.

Halpin, H. A., Morales-Suárez-Varela, M. M., and Martin-Moreno, J. M. "Chronic Disease Prevention and the New Public Health." *Public Health Reviews*, 2010, *32*, 120–154.

Halterman, J. S., Montes, G., Shone, L. P., and Szilagyi, P. G. "The Impact of Health Insurance Gaps on Access to Care Among Children with Asthma in the United States." *Ambulatory Pediatrics*, 2008, *8*(1), 43–49.

Hamel, P. C. *"What Do Sidewalks Have to Do with Health?"* Unpublished Case Study, 2012.

Hammond, D. "Tobacco Packaging and Labeling Policies Under the US Tobacco Control Act: Research Needs and Priorities." *Nicotine & Tobacco Research*, 2012, *14*(1), 62–74.

Hannah, M., Reilly, N., and Sun, J. *"WhyWellness: Communicating About Mental Health Within a Gaming Community."* Unpublished Case Study, 2013.

Haque, N., and Eng, B. "Tackling Inequity Through a Photovoice Project on the Social Determinants of Health: Translating Photovoice Evidence to Community Action." *Global Health Promotion*, 2011, *18*(1), 16–19.

Harper, S.A., and others. "Prevention and Control of Influenza—Recommendations of the Advisory Committee on Immunization Practices (ACIP)." *MMWR*, 2005, *54 (Early Release)*, 1–40. www.cdc.gov/mmwr/preview/mmwrhtml/rr54e713a1.htm. Retrieved Nov. 2012.

Harris, G. "Five Cases of Polio in Amish Group Raise New Fears." *New York Times*, Nov. 8, 2005.

Harvard Family Research Project. "Learning from Logic Models in Out-of-School Time." 2002. www.gse.harvard.edu/hfrp/projects/afterschool/resources/learning_logic_models.html. Retrieved Dec. 2005.

Hatcher, M. T., and Nicola, R. M. "Building Constituencies for Public Health." In L. F. Novick, C. B. Morrow, and G. P. Mays (eds.), *Public Health Administration: Principles for Population-Based Management.* (2nd ed.) Sudbury, MA: Jones and Bartlett, 2008.

Hayes, R. B., and others. "Tobacco and Alcohol Use and Oral Cancer in Puerto Rico." *Cancer Causes Control*, 1999, *10*(1), 27–33.

Health Canada, "What Do Canadians Think About Nutrition?" 2002. www.weightlosschat.net/what-do-canadians-think-about-nutrition-2002. Retrieved Oct. 2005.

Health Canada and Schizophrenia Society of Canada. "Schizophrenia: A Handbook for Families." 1991. www2.fiu.edu/~otweb/schhbk.htm. Retrieved June 2013.

Health Communication Partnership. "The New P-Process: Steps in Strategic Communication." Dec. 2003. www.jhuccp.org/resource_center/publications /field_guides_tools/new-p-process-steps-strategic-communication-2003. Retrieved Mar. 2006.

Health Communication Partnership. "HEART Program Offers Zambian Youth Hope for an HIV/AIDS-Free Future." Dec. 2004. www.jhuccp.org/sites/all /files/17.pdf. Retrieved Dec. 2012.

Health Communication Partnership. "About the Health Communication Partnership (HCP)." www.hcpartnership.org/About/about.php. Retrieved Sept. 2005a.

Health Communication Partnership. "CCP Graduate Seminar Series Convergence and Bounded Normative Influence Theory." www.k4health.org/sites /default/files/6%20CBNormTheory.ppt Retrieved Sept. 2005b.

Health Communication Partnership. "Introduction to Theories of Communication Effects: Diffusion Theory." www.hcpartnership.org/Topics /Communication/theory/2004–04–02.ppt. Retrieved Sept. 2005c.

Health Communication Partnership. "Introduction to Theories of Communication Effects: Social Learning Theory." www.hcpartnership.org/Topics /Communication/theory/256,1,Slide1. Retrieved Sept. 2005d.

Health Communication Partnership. "Introduction to Theories of Communication Effects: The Theory of Reasoned Action." www.hcpartnership.org/Topics /Communication/theory/2004–03–19.ppt. Retrieved Sept. 2005e.

Health Communication Partnership. "About the Health Communication Partnership (HCP): Using Strategic Communication, Engaging Communities for Change." www.hcpartnership.org/About/about.php. Retrieved Jan. 2006a.

Health Communication Partnership. "Africa, Namibia, Community Mobilization/ Participation." www.hcpartnership.org/Programs/Africa/Namibia/community _mobilization.php. Retrieved Jan. 2006b.

Health Communication Partnership. "How to Mobilize Communities for Health and Social Change." www.jhuccp.org/hcp/countries/usa/trusa1464.pdf. Retrieved Jan. 2006c.

Health Communication Unit. Center for Health Promotion. University of Toronto. "Overview of Health Communication Campaigns: Step 5 Set Communication Objectives." 1999. www.thcu.ca/infoandresources/publications/OHC _Master_Workbook_v3.1.format.July.30.03_content.apr30.99.pdf. Retrieved Feb. 2006.

Health Communication Unit. Center for Health Promotion. University of Toronto. "Lecturette on Health Communication Evaluation, Effectiveness and Why Campaigns Fail." Oct. 2003a. www.thcu.ca/infoandresources/publications/ StepTwelveEvaluationEffectivenessWhyCampaignsFailForWebOct9–03.pdf. Retrieved Mar. 2006.

Health Communication Unit. Center for Health Promotion. University of Toronto. "Selecting Channels and Vehicles Lecturette." Oct. 2003b. www.thcu.ca /infoandresources/publications/StepSixSelectChannelsVehiclesForWebOct9 –03.pdf. Retrieved Mar. 2006.

Health Communication Unit. Center for Health Promotion. University of Toronto. "Setting Communication Objectives Lecturette." Oct. 2003c. www.thcu.ca/infoandresources/publications/StepFiveSettingObjectivesForWebOct9–03.pdf. Retrieved Mar. 2006.

Health Communication Unit. Center for Health Promotion. University of Toronto. "Implementing THCU's Twelve Steps. PACE: A Campaign Preventing and Addressing FASD from the Hamilton-Wentworth Drug and Alcohol Awareness Committee." Nov. 2004. www.thcu.ca/infoandresources/publications/CaseStudy2.pace.v1.02.pdf. Retrieved Mar. 2006.

Health Communication Unit. Center for Health Promotion. University of Toronto. "Health Communication Resources." www.thcu.ca/infoandresources/health_communication.htm. Retrieved Mar. 2006.

Health Education Advocate. www.healtheducationadvocate.org. Retrieved Mar. 2013.

Health Equity Initiative. Health Equity Exchange. "What Does Health Equity Mean to You?" 2011. www.healthequityinitiative.org/hei/health-equity-exchange/what-does-health-equity-mean-to-you. Retrieved Jan. 2013.

Health Equity Initiative. *Health Equity Exchange: Using an Integrated Multimedia Communication Approach to Engage U.S. Communities on Health Equity.* Unpublished Case Study, 2012a.

Health Equity Initiative. "Why Health Equity Matters." 2012b. www.healthequityinitiative.org/hei/about/meeting-a-critical-need/why-health-equity-matters. Retrieved Jan. 2013.

Health Equity Initiative. "Health Equity Exchange." www.healthequityinitiative.org/hei/what-we-do/community-engagement-and-mobilization/health-equity-exchange. Retrieved Jan. 2013a.

Health Equity Initiative. *Sports for Health Equity: A Multi-faceted National Program.* Unpublished Case Study, 2013b.

Health Equity Initiative. "Workshop Descriptions." www.healthequityinitiative.org/hei/what-we-do/counseling-partnership-and-capacity-building/professional-development-workshops-summer/workshop-description. Retrieved Feb. 2013c.

Health Leads. "Our Impact." https://healthleadsusa.org/what-we-do/strategy-impact. Retrieved Feb. 2013.

Hegazi, S. *"Successes and Challenges in Communicating Influenza in Egypt."* Paper presented at the American Public Health Association, 2010.

Hegazi, S. *Communication Interventions: Helping Egyptian Families and Children Stay Safe from Avian Influenza.* Egypt: UNICEF, 2012a.

Hegazi, S. *Maintaining Egypt Polio Free: How Communication Made it Happen.* Egypt: UNICEF, 2012b.

Heimann, D. "Reaching Youth Worldwide: Part III—JHU/CCP Programmes—Latin America." The Communication Initiative Network, www.comminit.com/node/1772. Retrieved Sept. 2002.

Hester, E. L. *Successful Marketing Research.* Hoboken, NJ: Wiley, 1996.

Heurtin-Roberts, S. "High-pertension: The Uses of a Chronic Folk Illness for Personal Adaptation." *Social Science Medicine,* 1993, *37,* 285–294.

Heurtin-Roberts, S., and Reisin, E. "The Relation of Culturally Influenced Lay Models of Hypertension to Compliance with Treatment." *American Journal of Hypertension,* 1992, *5,* 787–792.

Heymann, D. L., and Rodier, G. R. "Hot Spots in a Wired World: WHO Surveillance of Emerging and Re-emerging Infectious Diseases." *Lancet,* 2001, *1*(5), 345–353.

Hill, P. C., and Pargament, K. I. "Advances in Conceptualization and Measurement of Religion and Spirituality: Implications for Physical and Mental Health Research." *American Psychologist,* 2003, *58*(1), 64–74.

hiv/aidstribe. www.hivaidstribe.com. Retrieved Mar. 2013.

Ho, G.Y.F., and others. "Cancer Disparities Between Mainland and Island Puerto Ricans." *Revista Panamericana de Salud Pública,* 2009, *25*(5), 394–400.

Hodge-Gray, E., and Caldamone, A. A. "Primary Nocturnal Enuresis: A Review." *Journal of School Nursing,* 1998, *14*(3), 38–42.

Hoffman, K. S. *Popular Leadership in the Presidency.* Lanham, MD: Lexington Books, 2010.

Hofstede, G. *Culture's Consequences: International Differences in Work-Related Values.* Thousand Oaks, CA: Sage, 1984.

Hofstede, G. *Culture's Consequences: Comparing Values, Behaviors, and Organizations Across Nations.* (2nd ed.) Thousand Oaks, CA: Sage, 2001.

Holtzman, D., and Rubinson, R. "Parent and Peer Communication Effects on AIDS-Related Behavior Among U.S. High School Students." *Family Planning Perspectives,* 1995, *27*(6), 235–240, 268.

Hoover, S. A. "Environmental Prevention. Community Prevention Institute (CPI) & Center for Applied Research Solutions (CARS)." 2005. www.ca-cpi.org/tarp/EP-Final.pdf. Retrieved Nov. 2008.

Hornik, R. C. "Evaluation Designs for Public Health Communication Programs." In R. C. Hornik (ed.), *Public Health Communication: Evidence for Behavior Change.* Mahwah, NJ: Erlbaum, 2002, 385–405.

Hornik, R. "Speaking of Health: Assessing Health Communication Strategies for Diverse Populations." 2003. http://foundation.acponline.org/healthcom/hcc2/hornik.ppt. Retrieved Feb. 2006.

Hornik, R. C. "Preface." In R. C. Hornik (ed.), *Public Health Communication: Evidence for Behavior Change.* Mahwah, NJ: Erlbaum, 2008a.

Hornik, R. C. "Public Health Communication: Making Sense of Contradictory Evidence." In R. C. Hornik (ed.), *Public Health Communication: Evidence for Behavior Change.* Mahwah, NJ: Erlbaum, 2008b.

Hosein, E. "Communication for Behavioral Impact (COMBI): An Overview of WHO's Model for Strategic Social Mobilization and Communication." Presented at the American Public Health Association 136th Annual Meeting, San Diego, Oct. 28, 2008. https://apha.confex.com/apha/136am/webprogram/Paper188764.html. Retrieved Jan. 2013.

Hosein, E., Parks, W., and Schiavo, R. "Communication-for-Behavioral-Impact: An Integrated Model for Health and Social Change." In R. J. DiClemente, R. A. Crosby, and M. C. Kegler (eds.), *Emerging Theories in Health Promotion Practice and Research: Strategies for Improving Public Health.* (2nd ed.) San Francisco: Jossey-Bass, 2009.

Hospitals and Health Networks. "Clinical Communication and Patient Safety." www.hhnmag.com/hhnmag_app/jsp/articledisplay.jsp?dcrpath=HHNMAG/ PubsNewsArticle/data/2006August/0608HHN_gatefold&domain=HHNMAG. Retrieved July 2012.

Houston, S. D. "The Archaeology of Communication Technologies." *Annual Review of Anthropology*, 2004, *33*, 223–250.

Hsu, M. H., Ju, T. L., Yen, C. H., and Chang, C. M. "Knowledge Sharing Behavior in Virtual Communities: The Relationship Between Trust, Self-Efficacy, and Outcome Expectations." *International Journal of Human-Computer Studies*, 2007, *65*(2), 153–169.

Hufford, M. "American Folklife: A Commonwealth of Cultures." 1991. www.loc .gov/folklife/cwc. Retrieved Oct. 2005.

Huhman, M. "New Media and the VERB Campaign: Tools to Motivate Tweens to Be Physically Active." *Cases in Public Health Communication & Marketing*, 2008, *2*, 126–139. www.casesjournal.org/volume2. Retrieved Oct. 2012.

Hustig, H. H., and Norrie, P. "Managing Schizophrenia in the Community." *Medical Journal of Australia*; 1998, *168*(4), 186–191.

Hwa-Froelich, D. A., and Vigil, D. "Three Aspects of Cultural Influence on Communication: A Literature Review." *Communication Disorders Quarterly*, 2004, *25*(3), 107.

Institute of Medicine. *Crossing the Quality Chasm.* Washington, DC: National Academies Press, 2001.

Institute of Medicine. *Speaking of Health Assessing Health Communication Strategies for Diverse Populations.* Washington, DC: The National Academies Press, 2002.

Institute of Medicine. Committee on Understanding and Eliminating Racial and Ethnic Disparities in Health Care. *Unequal Treatment: Confronting Racial and Ethnic Disparities in Health Care.* (full printed version) Washington, DC: The National Academies Press, 2003a.

Institute of Medicine. *Who Will Keep the Public Healthy?* Washington, DC: The National Academies Press, 2003b.

Institute of Medicine. "Report Brief. Apr. 2004. Health Literacy: A Prescription to End Confusion." Washington, DC: National Academies Press. www.iom.edu /~/media/Files/Report%20Files/2004/Health-Literacy-A-Prescription-to-End -Confusion/healthliteracyfinal.pdf. Retrieved June 2013.

Institute of Medicine. Board on International Health. *America's Vital Interest in Global Health: Protecting Our People, Enhancing Our Economy, and Advancing Our International Interests.* Washington, DC: The National Academies Press, 2007.

Institute of Medicine. "SMART Objectives." www.iom.edu/About-IOM/Making-a-Difference/Community-Outreach/~/media/Files/About%20the%20IOM/SmartBites/Planning/P1%20SMART%20Objectives.ashx. Retrieved Mar. 2013.

Institute for Public Relations. "Guidelines for Measuring the Effectiveness of PR Programs and Activities." 1997, 2003. www.instituteforpr.org/iprwp/wp-content/uploads/2002_MeasuringPrograms.pdf. Retrieved June 2013.

Institute for Public Relations. "Dictionary for Public Relations Measurement and Research." 2006. www.instituteforpr.org/iprwp/wp-content/uploads/PRMR_Dictionary.pdf. Retrieved June 2013.

International Center for Research on Women. "Disentangling HIV and AIDS Stigma in Ethiopia, Tanzania and Zambia." 2003. www.icrw.org/docs/stigmareport 093003.pdf. Retrieved Feb. 2006.

International Telecommunication Union. "Key Global Telecom Indicators for the World Telecommunication Service Sector." June 2012. www.itu.int/ITU-D/ict/statistics/at_glance/KeyTelecom.html. Retrieved Feb. 2013.

Internet World Stats. "Internet World Stats. Usage and Population Statistics." 2012. www.internetworldstats.com/stats.htm. Retrieved Feb. 2013.

ISeek Education. "Field of Study: Mass Communication Studies." www.iseek.org /education/fieldOfStudy?id=300103. Retrieved Feb. 2013.

Issue Management Council. "What Is Issue Management?" www.issuemanagement .org/documents/im_details.html#clarification%20of%20terms. Retrieved Dec. 2005.

Jack, B. W., and Culpepper, L. "Preconception Care: Risk Reduction and Health Promotion in Preparation for Pregnancy." *JAMA*, 1990, *264*(9), 1147–1149.

Janz, N. K., and Becker, M. H. "The Health Belief Model: A Decade Later." *Health Education Quarterly*, 1984, *11*(1), 1–47.

Javidi, M., Long, L. W., Long, P. N., and Javidi, A. *"An Examination of Interpersonal Communication Motives Across Age Groups."* Paper presented at the meeting of the Speech Communication Association, Chicago, Nov. 1990.

Jernigan, D. B., and others. "Investigation of Bioterrorism-Related Anthrax, United States, 2001: Epidemiologic Findings." *Emergency Infectious Diseases*, 2002, *8*(10), 1019–1028.

Jette, A. M., and others. "The Structure and Reliability of Health Belief Indices." *Health Services Research*, 1981, *16*(1), 81–98.

Jitaru, E., Moisil, I., and Jitaru, M. C. "Criteria for Evaluating the Quality of Health Related Sites on Internet." Paper presented at the Twenty-Second Romanian Conference on Medical Informatics Towards the Millennium, Nov. 1999. http://atlas.ici.ro/ehto/medinf99/papers/criteria_for_evaluating_the_qual.htm. Retrieved Feb. 2006.

Johns Hopkins University. Center for Communication Programs. "Avian Flu." 2005. www.jhuccp.org/topics/avian_flu.shtml. Retrieved May 2008.

Johnson & Johnson. *"Campaign for Nursing's Future Initiative."* Unpublished case study, 2005.

Jones, N., and Walsh, C. "Policy Briefs as a Communication Tool for Development Research." Overseas Development Institute Background Note. May 2008. www.odi.org.uk/sites/odi.org.uk/files/odi-assets/publications-opinion-files /594.pdf. Retrieved Mar. 2013.

Joppe, M. "The Research Process." www.ryerson.ca/~mjoppe/ResearchProcess. Retrieved Feb. 2006.

Joyner, A. M. "Eradication of a Disease: Keys to Success." July–Sept. 2001. www.popline.org/node/186790. Retrieved Mar. 2006.

Kahn, R., and Kellner, D. "New Media and Internet Activism: From the 'Battle of Seattle' to Blogging." *New Media and Society*, 2004, *6*(1), 87–95.

Kamateh, L. "Seven Must Haves to Launch an Effective Social Media Health Campaign." HealthCetera—Blog of Center for Health Media & Policy at Hunter College (CHMP), 2013. http://centerforhealthmediapolicy.com/2013/01/25 /seven-must-haves-to-launch-an-effective-social-media-health-campaign. Retrieved Feb. 2013.

Kapoor, S. C. "DOTS, NTP AND HIV." *Indian Journal of Pediatrics*, 1996, *43*(4), 177–222.

Kasperson, R. E., and others. "The Social Amplification of Risk: A Conceptual Framework." *Risk Analysis*, 1988, *8*(2), 177–187.

Katz, R., Mesfin, T., and Barr, K. "Lessons From a Community-Based m-Health Diabetes Self-Management Program: 'It's Not Just About the Cell Phone.'" *Journal of Health Communication*, 2012, *17*(1), 67–72.

Kaur, H., Hyder, M. L., and Poston, W. S. "Childhood Overweight: An Expanding Problem." *Treatments in Endocrinology*, 2003, *2*(6), 375–388.

Kellermann, K., and Reynolds, R. "When Ignorance Is Bliss: The Role of Motivation to Reduce Uncertainty in Uncertainty Reduction Theory." *Human Communication Research*, 1990, *17*, 5–75.

Kelman, I. "Linked Cultures: Breaking Out of the 'Disaster Management Rut.'" *UN Chronicle Online Edition*, 2004, *41*(3).

Kelmanson, I. A. "Risk Factors for Sudden Infant Death Syndrome and Risk Factors for Sleep Disturbances." *Early Child Development and Care*, 2011, *181*(5), 681–690.

Kennedy, M. G., and Abbatangelo, J. "Guidance for Evaluating Mass Communication Health Initiatives: Summary of an Expert Panel Discussion." 2005. www.cdc.gov/communication/practice/epreport.pdf. Retrieved Mar. 2006.

Kim, P., Eng, T., Deering, M. J., and Maxfield, A. "Published Criteria for Evaluating Health Related Web Sites: Review." *British Medical Journal*, 1999, *318*(7184), 647–649.

Kimbrell, J. D. "Coalition, Partnership, and Constituency Building by a State Public Health Agency: A Retrospective." *Journal of Public Health Management and Practice*, 2000, *6*(2), 55–61.

Kincaid, D. L. *The Convergence Model of Communication*. Honolulu: East-West Communication Institute, 1979.

Kincaid, D. L., and Figueroa, M. E. "Ideation and Communication for Social Change." Health Communication Partnership Seminar. Apr. 23, 2004. www .hcpartnership.org/Topics/Communication/theory/2004–04–23.ppt. Retrieved Oct. 2006.

Kincaid, D. L., Figueroa, M. E., Storey, D., and Underwood, C. *Communication and Behavior Change: The Role of Ideation.* Baltimore: Johns Hopkins University, Bloomberg School of Public Health, Center for Communication Programs, 2001.

Knowledge Networks and MediaPost Communications. "The Faces of Social Media—Wave 2." June 2011.

Korioth, T. "Podcasts a Convenient CME Option." *AAP News*, 2007, *28*(5), 18.

Kotler, P., and Roberto, E. L. *Social Marketing: Strategies for Changing Public Behavior.* New York: Free Press, 1989.

Krauss, R. M., and Fussell, S. R. "Social Psychological Models of Interpersonal Communication." In E. T. Higgins and A. W. Kruglanski (eds.), *Social Psychology: Handbook of Basic Principles.* New York: Guilford Press, 1996.

Kraut, R. E. "Social and Emotional Messages of Smiling: An Ethological Approach." *Journal of Personality and Social Psychology*, 1979, *37*, 1539–1553.

Krenn, S., and Limaye, R. "The Role of Social and Behavior Change Communication in Combating HIV/AIDS." In R. G. Marlink and S. T. Teitelman (eds.), *From the Ground Up: Building Comprehensive HIV/AIDS Care Programs in Resource-Limited Settings.* Washington, DC: Elizabeth Glaser Pediatric AIDS Foundation, 2009. http://ftguonline.org/ftgu-232/index.php/ftgu/article/view/2037/4070.

Kreps, G. L. "Engaging Health Communication." In T. J. Socha and M. J. Pitts (eds.), *The Positive Side of Interpersonal Communication.* New York: Routledge, 2012a.

Kreps, G. L. "The Maturation of Health Communication Inquiry: Directions for Future Development and Growth." *Journal of Health Communication*, 2012b, *17*(5), 495–497.

Kreps, G. L., Query, J. L., and Bonaguro, E. W. "The Interdisciplinary Study of Health Communication and Its Relationship to Communication Science." In L. Lederman (ed.), *Beyond These Walls: Readings in Health Communication.* Los Angeles: Roxbury, 2007.

Kreuter, M. W., and McClure, M. S. "The Role of Culture in Health Communication." *Annual Review of Public Health*, 2004, *25*, 439–455.

Kreuter, M. W., and Skinner, C. "Tailoring: What's in a Name?" *Health Education Research*, 2000, *15*, 1–4.

Krugman, D. M., Fox, R. J., and Fischer, P. M. "Do Cigarette Warnings Warn? Understanding What It Will Take to Develop More Effective Warnings." *Journal of Health Communication*, 1999, *4*, 95–104.

Kunst, H., Groot, D., Latthe, P. M., Latthe, M., and Khan, K. S. "Accuracy of Information on Apparently Credible Websites: Survey of Five Common Health Topics." *BMJ*, 2002, *324*, 581–582.

Laine, C., and Davidoff, F. "Patient Centered Medicine: A Professional Evaluation." *JAMA*, 1996, *275*(2), 152–156.

Lara, M., Allen, F., and Lange, L. "Physician Perceptions of Barriers to Care for Inner-City Latino Children with Asthma." *Journal of Healthcare for the Poor and Underserved*, 1999, *10*(1), 27–44.

Laulajainen, T. *"Tackling Oral Polio Vaccine Refusals Through Volunteer Community Mobilizer Network in Northern Nigeria."* Unpublished case study, 2012.

Lavery, S. H., and others. "The Community Action Model: A Community-Driven Model Designed to Address Disparities in Health." *American Journal of Public Health*, 2005, *95*(4), 611–616.

Lay, J. "Household Survey Data Basics." Kiel Institute for the World Economy. www.gtap.agecon.purdue.edu/events/conferences/2006/documents/HH SurveyBasics_GTAP_POSTCW06.pdf. Retrieved Mar. 2013.

Le, M. H., and Nguyen, T. U. "Social and Cultural Influences on the Health of the Vietnamese American Population." In G. J. Yoo, M. N. Le, and A. Y. Oda (eds.), *Handbook of Asian American Health*. New York: Springer, 2013.

Lea, M., Spears, R., and de Groot, D. "Knowing Me, Knowing You: Anonymity Effects on Social Identity Processes Within Groups." *Personality and Social Psychology Bulletin*, 2001, *27*(5), 526–537. http://personalpages.manchester.ac.uk/staff /martin.lea/papers/2001-EJ%20Lea%20Spears%20DeGroot%20Knowing%20 PSPB.pdf. Retrieved Jan. 2013.

Ledingham, J. A. "Explicating Relationship Management as a General Theory of Public Relations." *Journal of Public Relations Research*, 2003, *15*(2), 181–198.

Lee, K. K. "Healthy and Green Design." www.nyc.gov/html/hpd/downloads/pdf /Karen-Lee-presentation.pdf. Retrieved Dec. 2012.

Lefebvre, R. C. "The New Technology: The Consumer as Participant Rather than Target Audience." *Social Marketing Quarterly*, 2007, *13*(3), 31–42.

Lefebvre, R. C. Social *Marketing and Social Change: Strategies and Tools for Improving Health, Well-Being, and the Environment*. San Francisco: Jossey-Bass, 2013.

Lewin, F., and others. "Smoking Tobacco, Oral Snuff, and Alcohol in the Etiology of Squamous Cell Carcinoma of the Head and Neck." *Cancer*, 2000, *82*(7), 1367–1375.

Lewis, A. "Health as a Social Concept." *British Journal Society*, 1953, *4*, 110–115.

LexisNexis. "Search Terms: Baby and Sleep." www.lexisnexis.com. Retrieved Mar. 27, 2006.

Li, K. "African Immunization Campaign Strikes Back Against Global Polio Epidemic." 2005. UNICEF www.unicef.org/immunization/index_26945.html. Retrieved May 2005.

Lim, E.H.Y., Liu, J.N.K., and Lee, R.S.T. *Knowledge Seeker—Ontology Modelling for Information Search and Management: A Compendium*. Intelligence Systems Reference Library. (vol. *8*) Berlin: Springer-Verlag, 2011.

Lind, P., and Finley, D. "County Commissioners as a Key Constituency for Public Health." *Journal of Public Health Management and Practice*, 2000, *6*(2), 30–38.

Lipkin, M. J. "Patient Education and Counseling in the Context of Modern Patient-Physician-Family Communication." *Patient Education and Counseling*, 1996, *27*(1), 5–11.

Littlejohn, S. W., and Foss, K. A. "Anxiety/Uncertainty Management Theory" In *Encyclopedia of Communication Theory*. September 17, 2009a. http://knowledge.sagepub.com/view/communicationtheory/n15.xml.

Littlejohn, S. W., and Foss, K. A. "Problematic Integration Theory" In *Encyclopedia of Communication Theory*. September 17, 2009b. http://knowledge.sagepub.com/view/communicationtheory/n304.xml.

Liu, S., and Chen, G. M. "Communicating Health: People, Culture and Context." *China Media Research*, 2010, *6*(4), 1–2. www.chinamediaresearch.net/readmore/vol6no4/CMR100400%20Editor%20Introduction%20Liu%20and%20Chen%20Communication%20Health.pdf. Retrieved Jan. 2013.

Lu, M. C., and Lu, J. S. "Maternal Nutrition and Infant Mortality in the Context of Relationality." Joint Center for Political and Economic Studies, Health Policy Institute, 2007. www.jointcenter.org/sites/default/files/upload/research/files/MATERNAL%20FINAL%20-%2087%20pages.pdf. Retrieved Jan. 2013.

Lukoschek, P., Fazzari, M., and Marantz, P. "Patient and Physician Factors Predict Patients' Comprehension of Health Information." *Patient Education and Counseling*, 2003, *50*, 201–210.

Lund, S., and others. "Mobile Phones as a Health Communication Tool to Improve Skilled Attendance at Delivery in Zanzibar: A Cluster-Randomized Controlled Trial." *BJOG: An International Journal of Obstetrics & Gynaecology*, 2012, *119*, 1256–1264.

Lunn, M. R., and Sanchez, J. P. "Prioritizing Health Disparities in Medical Education to Improve Care." *Academic Medicine*, 2011, *86*(11), 1343.

Macartney, K. K., and Durrheim, D. N. "NSW Immunisation Performance: Continuing Progress but No Room for Complacency." *New South Wales Public Health Bulletin*, 2011, *22*(10), 169–170.

Macnamara, J. "PR Metrics: Research for Planning & Evaluation of PR & Corporate Communication." *Media Monitors*. Research Paper. 2006. http://195.130.87.21:8080/dspace/bitstream/123456789/231/1/Macnamara-PR%20metrics.pdf. Retrieved Feb. 2013.

Maibach, E. "Pan-Canadian Healthy Living Strategy: The Roles of Communication and Social Marketing." *Presentation at the Pan-Canadian Healthy Living Strategy, Public Information Strategic Direction: Social Marketing Roundtable*, Sept. 23–24, 2003. Ottawa, Canada. www.phac-aspc.gc.ca/hl-vs-strat/ppt/ed_maibach/index-fra.php. Retrieved June 2013.

Maibach, E., and Holtgrave, D. R. "Advances in Public Health Communication." *Annual Review of Public Health*, 1995, *16*, 219–238.

Malmo University. "Communication for Development Portal." http://wpmu.mah.se/comdev. Retrieved Jan. 2013.

Marcus, J. *Mesoamerican Writing Systems: Propaganda, Myth, and History in Four Ancient Civilizations.* Princeton, NJ: Princeton University Press, 1992.

Mashberg, A., and Samit, A. "Early Diagnosis of Asymptomatic Oral and Pharyngeal Squamous Cancers." *CA: A Cancer Journal for Clinicians*, 1995, *45*(6), 328–351.

Mashberg, A., and others. "Tobacco Smoking, Alcohol Drinking, and Cancer of the Oral Cavity and Oropharynx Among US Veterans." *Cancer*, 2006, *72*(4), 1369–1375.

Mass in Motion. www.mass.gov/eohhs/consumer/wellness/healthy-living/mass-in-motion-english.html. Retrieved Dec. 2012.

Mass in Motion New Bedford. http://massinmotionnewbedford.org. Retrieved Dec. 2012.

Massachusetts Department of Public Health. www.mass.gov/eohhs/gov/departments/dph. Retrieved Dec. 2012.

Mast, R. C., and Smith, A. B. "Elimination Disorders: Enuresis and Encopresis." In W. M. Klykylo and J. Kay (eds.), *Clinical Child Psychiatry.* (3rd ed.) Chichester, UK: Wiley, 2012.

Matiella, A. C., Middleton, K., and Thaker, N. *Guidebook to Effective Materials Development for Health Education.* Scotts Valley, CA: Tobacco Education Clearinghouse of California, California Department of Health Services, Tobacco Control Section, 1991.

Matsunaga, D. S., Yamada, S., and Macabeo, A. "Cross-Cultural Tuberculosis Manual." Kalihi-Palama Health Center, Association of Asian and Pacific Community Health Organizations, US Centers for Disease Control, Oct. 1998. www.hawaii.edu/hivandaids/Cross%20Cultural%20TB%20Manual.pdf. Retrieved June 2013.

Mayfield, Z. "Fear Appeal Messages and their Effectiveness in Advertising." Yahoo! Contributor Network, 2006. http://voices.yahoo.com/fear-appeal-messages-their-effectiveness-advertising-31626.html?cat=70. Retrieved Mar. 2013.

McDivitt, J. A., Zimicki, S., and Hornik, R. C. "Explaining the Impact of a Communication Campaign to Change Vaccination Knowledge and Coverage in the Philippines." *Health Communication*, 1997, *9*, 95–118.

McEwen, E., and Anton-Culver, H. "The Medical Communication of Deaf Patients." *Journal of Family Practice*, 1988, *13*, 51–57.

McGuire, W. J. "Public Communication as a Strategy for Inducing Health-Promoting Behavioral Change." *Preventive Medicine*, 1984, *13*(3), 299–313.

McMorrow, S., and Howell, E. M. "State Mental Health Systems for Children. A Review of the Literature and Available Data Sources." Urban Institute. Aug. 2010. www.urban.org/uploadedpdf/412207-state-mental.pdf. Retrieved Feb. 2013.

McQuail, D. *Mass Communication Theory.* (3rd ed.) Thousand Oaks, CA: Sage, 1994.

Medscape. "How Stigma Interferes with Mental Healthcare: An Expert Interview with Patrick W. Corrigan, PsyD." *Medscape Psychiatry and Mental Health*, 2004, *9*(2). www.medscape.com/viewarticle/494548. Retrieved Jan. 2006.

Meetoo, D., and Meetoo, L. "Explanatory Models of Diabetes Among Asian and Caucasian Participants." *British Journal of Nursing*, 2005, *14*(3), 154–159.

Mercer, S. L., Potter, M. A., and Green, L. W. *"Participatory Research: Guidelines and Lessons from the CDC's Extramural Prevention Research Program."* Paper presented at the American Public Health Association 130th Annual Meeting, Philadelphia, Nov. 2002.

Mercuri, M., and Gafni, A. "Medical Practice Variations: What the Literature Tells Us (or Does Not) About What Are Warranted and Unwarranted Variations." *Journal of Evaluation in Clinical Practice*, 2011, *17*(4), 671–677.

Mercy Corps. "Guide to Community Mobilization Programming." www.mercy corps.org/sites/default/files/CoMobProgrammingGd.pdf. Retrieved Feb. 2013.

Mermelstein, R., and others. "Social Support and Smoking Cessation and Maintenance." *Journal of Consulting and Clinical Psychology*, 1986, *54*(4), 447–453.

Metzger, M. J., Flanagin, A. J., and Medders, R. B. "Social and Heuristic Approaches to Credibility Evaluation Online." *Journal of Communication*, 2010, *60*(3), 413–439.

Michau, L. "Community Mobilization: Preventing Partner Violence by Changing Social Norms." *Expert paper prepared for Expert Group Meeting Prevention of Violence against Women and Girls*, Bangkok, Thailand, Sept. 17–20, 2012. www.unwomen.org/wp-content/uploads/2012/09/EGM-paper-Lori-Michau.pdf. Retrieved Feb. 2013.

Mintzes, B., and Baraldi, R. "Direct-to-Consumer Prescription Drug Advertising: When Public Health Is No Longer a Priority." www.whp-apsf.ca/en/documents/dtca_priority.html. Retrieved Jan. 2006.

Mo, P.K.H., and Coulson, N. S. "Developing a Model for Online Support Group Use, Empowering Processes and Psychosocial Outcomes for Individuals Living with HIV/AIDS." *Psychology & Health*, 2012, *27*(4), 445–459.

Mokhtar, N., and others. "Diet, Culture and Obesity in Northern Africa." *Journal of Nutrition*, 2001, *131*, 887S–892S.

Moment, D., and Zaleznik, A. *The Dynamics of Interpersonal Behavior.* Hoboken, NJ: Wiley, 1964.

Monfrecola, G., Fabbrocini, G., Posteraro, G., and Pini, D. "What Do Young People Think About the Dangers of Sunbathing, Skin Cancer, and Sunbeds? A Questionnaire Survey Among Italians." *Photodermatology, Photoimmunology and Photomedicine*, 2000, *16*, 15–18.

Montecino, V. "Criteria to Evaluate the Credibility of WWW Resources." Aug. 1998. http://mason.gmu.edu/~montecin/web-eval-sites.htm. Retrieved Feb. 2006.

Moon, R. Y., Oden, R. P., Joyner, B. L., and Ajao, T. I. "Qualitative Analysis of Beliefs and Perceptions About Sudden Infant Death Syndrome in African-American Mothers: Implications for Safe Sleep Recommendations." *The Journal of Pediatrics*, 2010, *157*(1), 92–97.

Morris, J. N. (ed.). *The Socio-Ecological Model: Uses of Epidemiology.* New York: Churchill Livingstone, 1975.

Morzinski, J. A., and Montagnini, M. L. "Logic Modeling: A Tool for Improving Educational Programs." *Journal of Palliative Medicine*, 2002, *5*(4), 566–570.

Moss, H. B., Kirby, S. D., and Donodeo, F. "Characterizing and Reaching High-Risk Drinkers Using Audience Segmentation." *Alcoholism: Clinical and Experimental Research*, 2009, *33*(8), 1336–1345.

Mshana, G., Dotchin, C. L., and Walker, R. W. "'We Call It the Shaking Illness': Perceptions and Experiences of Parkinson's Disease in Rural Northern Tanzania." *BMC Public Health*, 2011, *11*, 219. www.biomedcentral.com/content/pdf/1471-2458-11-219.pdf. Retrieved Jan. 2013.

MSNBC. "Trans Fat Free—The Next Food Fad? Companies Rush to Get Rid of Artery-Clogging Ingredient." www.msnbc.msn.com/id/6840122. Retrieved Jan. 2006.

Mueller, P. S., Plevak, D. J., and Rummans, T. A. "Religious Involvement, Spirituality and Medicine: Implications for Clinical Practice." *Mayo Clinic Proceedings*, 2001, *76*, 1225–1235.

Museum of Public Relations. "1992: The Case for PR Licensing." www.prmuseum.com/bernays/bernays_1990.html. Retrieved Nov. 2005.

Muturi, N. "Communication for HIV/AIDS Prevention in Kenya: Socio-Cultural Considerations." *Journal of Health Communication*, 2005, *10*, 77–98.

Nacinovich Jr., M. R., and MacDonald, M. *"Preparing for a Nightmare in the Calgary Health Region—Planning for Pandemic Influenza."* Unpublished case study, 2012.

National Alliance on Mental Illness. "Mental Illness: Facts and Numbers." www.nami.org/Template.cfm?Section=About_Mental_Illness&Template=/ContentManagement/ContentDisplay.cfm&ContentID=53155. Retrieved Feb. 2013.

National Association of Chain Drug Stores. "How to Effectively Communicate with Policymakers." http://meetings.nacds.org/rxImpact/pdfs/FS11_HowToCommunicate.pdf. Retrieved Feb. 2013.

National Association of Community Health Centers. "Press Kit." www.nachc.com/press-kit.cfm. Retrieved Feb. 2013.

National Association of Pediatric Nurse Practitioners. "HIB Disease." www.hibdisease.com. Retrieved Nov. 2005.

National Board of Public Health Examiners. www.nbphe.org/index.cfm. Retrieved Dec. 2011.

National Cancer Institute at the National Institutes of Health. *Making Health Communication Programs Work*. Bethesda, MD: National Institutes of Health, 2002.

National Cancer Institute. "Theory at a Glance: A Guide for Health Promotion Practice." www.cancer.gov/cancertopics/cancerlibrary/theory.pdf. Retrieved Oct. 2005a.

National Cancer Institute. "What You Need to Know About Skin Cancer: Cause and Prevention." www.cancer.gov/cancertopics/wyntk/skin/page5. Retrieved Oct. 2005b.

National Cancer Institute. "Pink Book—Making Health Communication Programs Work." www.cancer.gov/cancertopics/cancerlibrary/pinkbook/page1/AllPages. Retrieved Mar. 2013.

National Center for Safe Routes to School. www.saferoutesinfo.org. Retrieved Dec. 2012.

National CNS Competency Task Force. "Clinical Nurse Specialist Core Competencies. Executive Summary 2006–2008." 2010. www.nacns.org/docs/CNSCoreCompetenciesBroch.pdf. Retrieved Feb. 2013.

National Council for Public-Private Partnerships. "How Partnerships Work." http://ncppp.org/howpart/index.html. Retrieved Mar. 2006.

National Foundation for Infectious Diseases. "NFID Urges Use of New Childhood Vaccine Schedule." *Double Helix*, 1997, *22*(2).

National Foundation for Infectious Diseases. *"Flu Fight for Kids."* Unpublished case study, 2005.

National Institute of Child Health and Human Development. "Safe Sleep for Your Baby: Reduce the Risk of Sudden Infant Death Syndrome (SIDS) (African American Outreach)." Oct. 2005. www.nichd.nih.gov/publications/pubs/Documents/safe_sleep_general_brochure_2012.pdf. Retrieved Feb. 2006.

National Institute of Mental Health. "NIMH Outreach Partnership Program." www.nimh.nih.gov/outreach/partnership-program/index.shtml. Retrieved Feb. 2013a.

National Institute of Mental Health. "Office of Constituency Relations and Public Liaison (OCRPL)." www.nimh.nih.gov/about/organization/od/office-of-constituency-relations-and-public-liaison-ocrpl.shtml. Retrieved Feb. 2013b.

National Institutes of Health. "NIH News Release, February 28, 2003." 2003. www.nichd.nih.gov/new/releases/infant_sids_risk.cfm. Retrieved June 2005.

National Institutes of Health. "Improving Health Literacy." www.health.gov/communication/literacy. Retrieved Oct. 2005.

National Institutes of Health. "Human Subjects Research and IRBs." http://bioethics.od.nih.gov/IRB.html. Retrieved Mar. 2006.

National League for Nursing. "Core Competencies of Nurse Educators with Task Statements." 2005. www.nln.org/profdev/corecompetencies.pdf. Retrieved June 2013.

National Network for Election Reform. "Removing Voting Barriers for Citizens with Mental Disabilities." www.lawv.net/system/files/Removing%20Barriers%20Voters%20Mental%20Disabilities.pdf. Retrieved Mar. 2013.

National Opinion Research Center. University of Chicago. "Understanding the Impact of Health IT in Underserved Communities and those with Health Disparities." *Briefing Paper*. 2010. www.healthit.gov/sites/default/files/pdf/hit-underserved-communities-health-disparities.pdf. Retrieved Feb. 2013.

National Patient Safety Foundation. "Partnership for Clear Health Communication Joins Forces with the National Patient Safety Foundation." 2007. www.npsf.org/updates-news-press/press/partnership-for-clear-health-communication-joins-forces-with-the-national-patient-safety-foundation. Retrieved Jan. 2013.

National Planning Council, Colombia. "Traditional vs. Participatory Planning." Communication Initiative. 2003. www.comminit.com/polio/content/traditional-vs-participatory-planning. Retrieved June 2013.

National Pork Board. "Activist Groups and Your Kids." *Pork Checkoff Report,* 2008a, *27*(1). www.pork.org/filelibrary/PorkCheckoffReport/2008SpringCheckoffReport.pdf. Retrieved Feb. 2013.

National Pork Board. "Checkoff Tracks Activist Groups' Influence on Kids." 2008b. www.pork.org/News/645/Feature325.aspx#.USaKAB2–1Bk. Retrieved Feb. 2013.

National Research Council and Institute of Medicine. (2009). *Preventing Mental, Emotional, and Behavioral Disorders Among Young People: Progress and Possibilities.* Committee on the Prevention of Mental Disorders and Substance Abuse Among Children, Youth, and Young Adults: Research Advances and Promising Interventions. (Mary Ellen O'Connell, Thomas Boat, and Kenneth E. Warner, eds.) Board on Children, Youth, and Families, Division of Behavioral and Social Sciences and Education. Washington, DC: The National Academies Press.

National Public Radio. "Profile: How Sigmund Freud's Ideas Helped to Create the New Field of Public Relations." *Morning Edition,* Apr. 22, 2005.

National SIDS/Infant Death Resource Center. "SIDS Deaths by Race and Ethnicity 1995–2001." www.californiasids.com/UploadedFiles/Forms/SIDS%20Race%20and%20Ethnicity.pdf. Retrieved June 2013.

New School for Public Engagement. www.newschool.edu/public-engagement. Retrieved Feb. 2013.

New South Wales Department of Health, Australia. "Health Promotion Glossary." www.health.nsw.gov.au/public-health/health-promotion/abouthp/glossary.html. Retrieved Feb. 2006.

New York Academy of Sciences. "Prioritizing Health Disparities in Medical Education to Improve Care." www.nyas.org/Events/Detail.aspx?cid=cb76f217–8ed4–4e0b-8c9f-29b25483b181. Retrieved Dec. 2012.

New York City Department of Health and Mental Hygiene. "Health Department Launches New Smoking Cessation Campaign, Suffering Every Minute, Which Depicts the Health Consequences of Smoking." Sept. 2012. www.nyc.gov/html/doh/html/pr2012/pr023–12.shtml.

New York Times Company. "The New York Times Circulation Data." www.nytco.com/investors/financials/nyt-circulation.html. Retrieved Feb. 2013.

New York University. "Integrated Marketing Communication for Behavioral Impact in Health and Social Development 2006." http://steinhardt.nyu.edu/imc. Retrieved Jan. 2013.

Ngo-Metzger, Q., and others. "Surveying Minorities with Limited-English Proficiency: Does Data Collection Method Affect Data Quality Among Asian Americans?" *Medical Care,* 2004, *42*(9), 893–900.

Nielsen. "Three Screen Report." (vol. *8*) 1st Quarter 2010. 2010. www.nielsen.com/content/dam/corporate/us/en/reports-downloads/3%20Screen/2010/Three%20Screen%20Report%20(Q1%202010).pdf. Retrieved Feb. 2013.

Nielsen Norman Group. "Participation Inequality: Encouraging More Users to Contribute." Oct. 2006. www.nngroup.com/articles/participation-inequality. Retrieved Feb. 2013.

Nilsen, W., and others. "Advancing the Science of mHealth." *Journal of Health Communication*, 2012, *17*(Supp. 1), 5–10.

Nivet, M. "Commentary: Diversity and Inclusion in the 21st Century: Bridging the Moral and Excellence Imperatives." *Academic Medicine*, 2012, *87*(11), 1458–1460.

Nowak, G., and others. "The Application of 'Integrated Marketing Communications' to Social Marketing and Health Communication: Organizational Challenges and Implications." *Social Marketing Quarterly*, 1998, *4*(4), 12–16.

Nuzum, E. "On-Air Program Promotions Insight Study—Final Report." May 2004. www.aranet.com/library/pdf/doc-0111.pdf. Retrieved Jan. 2013.

Obayelu, A., and Ogunlade, I. "Analysis of the Uses of Information Communication Technology (ICT) for Gender Empowerment and Sustainable Poverty Alleviation in Nigeria." *International Journal of Education and Development using ICT*, 2006, *2*(3). http://ijedict.dec.uwi.edu/viewarticle.php?id=172.

Obregon, R., and Waisbord, S. "The Complexity of Social Mobilization in Health Communication: Top-Down and Bottom-Up Experiences in Polio Eradication." *Journal of Health Communication: International Perspectives*, 2010, *15*(Suppl. 1), 25–47.

O'Connell, M. E., Boat, T., and Warner, K. E. (eds.). *Preventing Mental, Emotional, and Behavioral Disorders Among Young People.* Committee on the Prevention of Mental Disorders and Substance Abuse Among Children, Youth, and Young Adults: Research Advances and Promising Interventions. (Mary Ellen O'Connell, Thomas Boat, and Kenneth E. Warner, eds.) Board on Children, Youth, and Families, Division of Behavioral and Social Sciences and Education. Washington, DC: The National Academies Press.

Office for Human Research Protections. "Office for Human Research Protections." www.hhs.gov/ohrp/about/facts/index.html. Retrieved Mar. 2006.

Office of Adolescent Pregnancy Programs. "Instructions for Completing the Adolescent Family Life Prevention Demonstration Project End of Year Report Template." www.hhs.gov/ocio/infocollect/pending/EOYInstructionsPrev.doc. Retrieved Mar. 2006.

Office of Behavioral and Social Sciences Research. National Institutes of Health. "Mobile Health (mHealth) Training Institutes." http://obssr.od.nih.gov/training_and_education/mhealth/. Retrieved Feb. 2013.

101PublicRelations.com. "Public Relations: How to Make Your Story Pitch Stand Out in the Email Jungle." http://101publicrelations.com/blog/cat_marketing_and_sales.html. Retrieved Dec. 2005.

101PublicRelations. "The Good, The Bad, and the Atrocious." http://101publicrelations.com/blog/the_good_the_bad_and_the_atrocious_000099.html. Retrieved Feb. 2013.

Ohio University. "Communication & Development Studies." www.commdev.ohio
.edu. Retrieved Jan. 2013.

O'Sullivan, G. A., Yonkler, J. A., Morgan, W., and Merritt, A. P. *A Field Guide
to Designing a Health Communication Strategy.* Baltimore: Johns Hopkins
Bloomberg School of Public Health, Center for Communication Programs,
2003.

Paek, H. J., and others. "Applying Theories of Behavior Change to Public Emergency
Preparedness: Implications for Effective Health and Risk Communication."
Paper presented at the Annual Meeting of the NCA 94th Annual Convention,
San Diego, Nov. 2008. www.allacademic.com/meta/p259806_index.html.

Painter, A. F., and Lemkau, J. P. "Turning Roadblocks into Stepping Stones: Teaching Psychology to Physicians." *Teaching of Psychology,* 1992, *19*(3), 183–184.

Paletz, D. L. *The Media in American Politics: Contents and Consequences.* New
York: Longman, 1999.

Paletz, D. L., Owen, D., and Cook, T. E. "Saylor.org's Comparative Politics/
Understanding Diverse Populations and Public Opinion. Public Opinion." 2012. http://en.wikibooks.org/wiki/Saylor.org's_Comparative_Politics
/Understanding_Diverse_Populations_and_Public_Opinion. Retrieved June
2013.

Pang, C. "The Koreans." In N. Palafox and A. Warren (eds.), *Cross Cultural Caring:
A Handbook for Health Care Professions in Hawaii.* Honolulu: Transcultural
Healthcare Forum, 1980.

Park, H. S., and Raile, A.N.W. "Perspective Taking and Communication Satisfaction
in Coworker Dyads." *Journal of Business and Psychology,* 2010, *25*(4), 569–581.

Parkin, D. M., and others (eds.). *Cancer Incidence in Five Continents.* Lyon: IARC,
1997.

Parks, W., and Lloyd, L. *Planning Social Mobilization and Communication for
Dengue Fever: A Step-By-Step Guide.* Geneva: World Health Organization,
2004. www.who.int/tdr/publications/documents/planning_dengue.pdf.

Parks, W., Shrestha, S., and Chitnis, K. Essentials for Excellence: Research, Mon-
itoring and Evaluating Strategic Communication for Behaviour and Social
Change with Special Reference to the Prevention and Control of Avian
Influenza/Pandemic Influenza. UNICEF Pacific Office, Fiji, 2008.

Partnering for Patient Empowerment Through Community Awareness (PPECA).
"PPECA Home Page." www.galter.northwestern.edu/ppeca. Retrieved June
2005.

Partnership at Drugfree.org. "Germans Defy Smoking Ban, and Enforcement Is
Lax." Jan. 16, 2008. www.drugfree.org/uncategorized/germans-defy-smoking-
ban-and. Retrieved Mar. 2013.

Partnership for Health in Aging. "Multidisciplinary Competencies in the Care of
Older Adults at the Completion of the Entry-Level Health Professional Degree."
www.americangeriatrics.org/files/documents/health_care_pros/PHA_Multi
disc_Competencies.pdf. Retrieved Feb. 2013.

Patel, D. "Social Mobilization as a Tool for Outreach Programs in the HIV/AIDS Crisis." In M. Haider (ed.), *Global Public Health Communication: Challenges, Perspectives, and Strategies.* Sudbury, MA: Jones and Bartlett, 2005.

Paunio, M., and others. "Increase of Vaccination Coverage by Mass Media and Individual Approach: Intensified Measles, Mumps, and Rubella Prevention Program in Finland." *American Journal of Epidemiology*, 1991, *133*(11), 1152–1160.

Peace Corps. "Culture Matters. The Peace Corps Cross-Cultural Workbook." 2011. wws.peacecorps.gov/wws/publications/culture/pdf/workbook.pdf. Retrieved Jan. 2013.

Pearson, J. C., and Nelson, P. E. *Understanding and Sharing.* (5th ed.) Dubuque, IA: Wm. C. Brown, 1991.

Pechmann, C. "A Comparison of Health Communication Models: Risk Learning Versus Stereotype Priming." *Media Psychology*, 2001, *3*(2), 189–210.

Perlotto, M. "The Invisible Partner: How the Marketing Department Supports Your Sales Efforts." 2005. www.spectroscopyonline.com/spectroscopy /article/articleDetail.jsp?id=160030. Retrieved June 2013.

Pernice, D., and others. "Italian Validation of the Royal Free Interview for Religious and Spiritual Beliefs." *Functional Neurology*, 2005, *20*(2), 77–84.

Pew Internet & American Life Project. "Bloggers: A Portrait of the Internet's New Storytellers." July 2006. http://pewinternet.org/~/media/Files/Reports /2006/PIP%20Bloggers%20Report%20July%2019%202006.pdf.pdf. Retrieved Feb. 2013.

Pew Internet & American Life Project. "E-patients with a Disability or Chronic Disease." Oct. 2007. www.pewinternet.org/~/media/Files/Reports/2007 /EPatients_Chronic_Conditions_2007.pdf.pdf. Retrieved Feb. 2013.

Pew Internet & American Life Project. "Demographics of Teen Internet Users." 2011a. http://pewinternet.org/Static-Pages/Trend-Data-(Teens) /Whos-Online.aspx.

Pew Internet & American Life Project. "Health Topics." 2011b. http://pewinternet .org/~/media//Files/Reports/2011/PIP_Health_Topics.pdf.

Pew Internet & American Life Project. "71% of Online Adults Now Use Video-Sharing Sites." 2011c. http://pewinternet.org/Reports/2011/Video-sharing -sites/Report.aspx.

Pew Internet & American Life Project. "Smartphone Adoption and Usage: Key Findings." 2011d. http://pewinternet.org/Reports/2011/Smartphones /Summary.aspx.

Pew Internet & American Life Project. "The Social Life of Health Information, 2011." 2011e. www.pewinternet.org/~/media//Files/Reports/2011 /PIP_Social_Life_of_Health_Info.pdf.

Pew Internet & American Life Project. "Demographics of Internet Users." 2012a. http://pewinternet.org/Trend-Data-(Adults)/Whos-Online.aspx. Retrieved Feb. 2013.

Pew Internet & American Life Project. "Older Adults and Internet Use." 2012b. www.pewinternet.org/Reports/2012/Older-adults-and-internet-use.aspx. Retrieved Feb. 2013.

Pew Internet & American Life Project. "Teens, Smartphones & Texting: Summary of Findings." 2012c. http://pewinternet.org/Reports/2012/Teens-and-smartphones/Summary-of-findings.aspx. Retrieved Feb. 2013.

Pew Internet & American Life Project. "Blogs." http://pewinternet.org/Topics/Activities-and-Pursuits/Blogs.aspx?typeFilter=5. Retrieved Feb. 2013a.

Pew Internet & American Life Project. "Pew Internet: Health." 2013b. http://pewinternet.org/Commentary/2011/November/Pew-Internet-Health.aspx. Retrieved Feb. 2013.

Pew Internet & American Life Project. "Pew Internet: Mobile." 2013c. http://pewinternet.org/Commentary/2012/February/Pew-Internet-Mobile.aspx. Retrieved Feb. 2013.

Pew Internet & American Life Project. "Pew Internet: Social Networking (Full Detail)." 2013d. http://pewinternet.org/Commentary/2012/March/Pew-Internet-Social-Networking-full-detail.aspx. Retrieved Feb. 2013.

Pew Research Center. "Are We Happy Yet?" Feb. 2006. http://pewsocialtrends.org/files/2010/10/AreWeHappyYet.pdf. Retrieved Jan. 2013.

Phillips, B. "5 Factors That Determine Whether a Journalist Will Cover Your Story." Dec. 2012. www.prdaily.com/Main/Articles/5_factors_that_determine_whether_a_journalist_will_10531.aspx#. Retrieved June 2013.

Photovoice. www.photovoice.org. Retrieved Mar. 2013.

Physicians for Human Rights. "An Action Plan to Prevent Brain Drain: Building Equitable Health Systems in Africa." *Health Action AIDS*. June 2004. http://allafrica.com/download/resource/main/main/idatcs/00010242:21e6b22 646882263f8b7aa73a71c810c.pdf. Retrieved June 2013.

Pikoulis, E., Waasdorp, B. S., Leppaniemi, A., and Burris, D. "Hippocrates: The True Father of Medicine." *American Surgeon*, 1998, *64*(3), 274–275.

Pinto E. "KAP Study: Common Practices and Attitudes Toward Malaria, 1998." Unpublished report. UNICEF, Luanda, Angola.

Piotrow, P. T., Kincaid, D. L., Rimon, J. G., and Rinehart, W. *Health Communication: Lessons from Family Planning and Reproductive Health.* Westport, CT: Praeger, 1997.

Piotrow, P. T., Rimon, J. G. II, Payne Merritt, A., and Saffitz, G. *Advancing Health Communication: The PCS Experience in the Field.* Baltimore: Johns Hopkins Bloomberg School of Public Health, Center for Communication Programs, 2003.

Population Reference Bureau. "Policy Communication Fellows." www.prb.org/EventsTraining/InternationalTraining/PolicyFellows.aspx. Retrieved Feb. 2013.

Porter, R. W., and others. "Role of Health Communications in Russia's Diphtheria Immunization Program." *Journal of Infectious Diseases*, 2000, *181*(Supp. 1), S220–S227.

Porter, S., and ten Brinke, L. "Reading Between the Lies: Identifying Concealed and Falsified Emotions in Universal Facial Expressions." *Psychological Science*, 2008, *19*(5), 508–514.

Powell, H. L., and Segrin, C. "The Effect of Family and Peer Communication on College Students' Communication with Dating Partners about HIV and AIDS." *Health Communication*, 2004, *16*(4), 427–449.

PPP Bulletin International. "What Is a Public Private Partnership?" 2012. www.pppbulletin.com/pages/whatisappp. Retrieved Feb. 2013.

Prochaska, J., and DiClemente, C. C. "Stages and Process of Self-Change of Smoking: Toward an Integrative Model of Change." *Journal of Consulting and Clinical Psychology*, 1983, *51*, 390–395.

Prochaska, J. O., and Vleicer, W. F. "The Transtheoretical Model of Health Behavior Change." *American Journal of Health Promotion*, 1997, *12*(1), 38–48.

Program for Appropriate Technology in Health. "Community Theater in Benin: Taking the Show on the Road." Unpublished case study, 2005a.

Program for Appropriate Technology in Health. *"How Bingwa Changed His Ways."* Unpublished case study, 2005b.

ProQuest. Search term: "Babies and Sleep." Retrieved April 2013. www.proquest.com/en-US.

Public Health Agency of Canada. "The Canadian Pandemic Influenza Plan for the Health Sector." www.phac-aspc.gc.ca/cpip-pclcpi/index-eng.php. Retrieved Nov. 2012.

Public-Private Partnership for Handwashing. "Mission." www.globalhandwashing.org/mission. Retrieved June 2013.

Public Relations Society of America. "PRSA Member Code of Ethics 2000." www.prssa.org/downloads/codeofethics.pdf. Retrieved Nov. 2005a.

Public Relations Society of America. "The Public Relations Profession: About Public Relations." www.prsa.org/_Resources/Profession/index.asp?ident=prof1. Retrieved Nov. 2005b.

Quebral, N. C. "Development Communication in the Agricultural Context." Paper presented at the symposium *In Search of Breakthroughs in Agricultural Development*. Laguna: University of the Philippines, College of Agriculture, 1971.

Quebral, N. "What Do We Mean by Development Communication?" *International Development Review*, 1972, *15*(2), 25–28.

Quebral, N. "Development Communication in a Borderless World." Paper presented at the national conference-workshop on the undergraduate development communication curriculum, *New Dimensions, Bold Decisions*. Los Baños: University of the Philippines, College of Development Communication, 2001, 15–28.

QuickMBA. "Marketing Research." www.quickmba.com/marketing/research. Retrieved Feb. 2006.

Ramirez, A. G., and others. "Advancing the Role of Participatory Communication in the Diffusion of Cancer Screening Among Hispanics." *Journal of Health Communication*, 1999, *4*(1), 31–36.

Randall, V. R. "Racial Discrimination in Health Care and CERD." Dayton, OH: Institute on Race, Health Care and the Law, University of Dayton School of Law. 2002. http://academic.udayton.edu/health/07HumanRights/racial01.htm. Retrieved Mar. 2006.

Ratzan, C., and others. "Education for the Health Communication Professional." *American Behavioral Scientist*, 1994, *38*(2), 361–380.

Raven, J. H., Chen, Q., Tolhurst, R. J., and Garner, P. "Traditional Beliefs and Practices in the Postpartum Period in Fujian Province, China: A Qualitative Study." *BMC Pregnancy & Childbirth*, 2007, *7*, 8.

Reeves, P. M. "Coping in Cyberspace: The Impact of Internet Use on the Ability of HIV-Positive Individuals to Deal with Their Illness." *Journal of Health Communication*, 2000, *5*(Suppl.), 47–59.

Reich, M. R. "Public-Private Partnerships for Public Health." In M. R. Reich (ed.), *Public-Private Partnerships for Public Health*. Cambridge, MA: Harvard Center for Population and Development Studies, 2002.

Reid, E. "Understanding the Word 'Advocacy' Context and Use." Online article. Urban Institute. Advocacy Research Seminars. www.urban.org/advocacy research/seminar1/Reid.pdf. Retrieved June 2013.

Renganathan, E., and others. "Communication-for–Behavioral-Impact (COMBI): A Review of WHO's Experiences with Strategic Social Mobilization and Communication in the Prevention and Control of Communicable Diseases." In M. Haider (ed.), *Global Public Health Communication: Challenges, Perspectives, and Strategies*. Sudbury, MA: Jones and Bartlett, 2005.

Reynolds, B. "Crisis and Emergency Risk Communication." *Applied Biosafety*, 2005, *10*(1), 47-56. www.absa.org/abj/abj/051001reynolds.pdf. Retrieved Feb. 2013.

Reynolds, B., and Seeger, M. W. "Crisis and Emergency Risk Communication as an Integrative Model." *Journal of Health Communication*, 2005, *10*, 43–55.

Rhode Island Department of Health. "Office of Minority Health African-American/Black Culture and Health." www.health.ri.gov/chic/minority/afr _cul.php. Retrieved Oct. 2005a.

Rhode Island Department of Health. "Office of Minority Health Latino/Hispanic Culture and Health." www.health.ri.gov/chic/minority/lat_cul.php. Retrieved Oct. 2005b.

Rhode Island Department of Health. "Office of Minority Health Native American Culture and Health." www.health.ri.gov/chic/minority/natcul.php. Retrieved Oct. 2005c.

Rhode Island Department of Health. "Office of Minority Health Southeast Asian Culture and Health." www.health.ri.gov/chic/minority/asi_cul.php. Retrieved Oct. 2005d.

Richardson, A. "New Media: A Potential Mechanism to Exacerbate Health-Related Disparities." *Journal of Mass Communication and Journalism*, 2012, *2*(1), e107. www.omicsgroup.org/journals/2165–7912/2165–7912-2-e107.php?aid= 3755. Retrieved June 2013.

Rienks, J., and others. "Evidence That Social Marketing Campaigns Can Effectively Increase Awareness of Infant Mortality Disparities." Paper presented at the Annual Meeting of the American Public Health Association, Philadelphia, Dec. 13, 2005.

Rimal, R. N., and Lapinski, M. K. "Why Health Communication Is Important in Public Health." *Bulletin of the World Health Organization*, 2009, *87*(4), 247. www.who.int/bulletin/volumes/87/4/08–056713/en. Retrieved June 2013.

Rimon, J. G. "Behaviour Change Communication in Public Health. Beyond Dialogue: Moving Toward Convergence." The Communication Initiative. 2002. www.comminit.com/strategicthinking/stnicroundtable/sld-1744.html. Retrieved Nov. 2005.

Robberson, M. R., and Rogers, R. W. "Beyond Fear Appeals: Negative and Positive Persuasive Appeals to Health and Self-Esteem." *Journal of Applied Social Psychology*, July 2006, 277–287.

Robert Graham Center. Policy Studies in Family Practice and Primary Care. "Patterns of Visits to Physicians' Offices, 1980 to 2003." *American Academy of Family Physicians*, 2005, *72*(5), 762.

Robert Wood Johnson Foundation. "Using ECHO (Extension for Community Healthcare Outcomes) to Train Primary Care Providers in Best Practices for Complex Health Conditions." www.rwjf.org/en/grants/grant-records/2009/02/using-echo—extension-for-community-healthcare-outcomes-to-trai.html. Retrieved June 2013.

Robinson, T. N., Patrick, K., Eng, T. R., and Gustafson, D. "An Evidence-Based Approach to Interactive Health Communication: A Challenge to Medicine in the Information Age." *Journal of the American Medical Association*, 1998, *280*, 1264–1269.

Rockefeller Foundation Communication and Social Change Network. "Measuring and Evaluating Communication for Social Change." Communication Initiative. June 2001. www.comminit.com/node/1849. Retrieved June 2013.

Rogers, E. M. *Diffusion of Innovations.* New York: Free Press, 1962.

Rogers, E. M. "Communication and Development: The Passing of the Dominant Paradigm." *Communication Research*, 1976, *3*(2), 213–240.

Rogers, E. M. *Diffusion of Innovations.* (3rd ed.) New York: Free Press, 1983.

Rogers, E. M. *Diffusion of Innovations.* (4th ed.) New York: Free Press, 1995.

Rogers, E. M., and Kincaid, D. L. *Communication Networks: Towards a New Paradigm for Research.* New York: Free Press, 1981.

Rogers, R. W. "A Protection Motivation Theory of Fear Appeals and Attitude Change." *Journal of Psychology*, *91*, 1975, 93–114.

Rogers, R. W. "Cognitive and Physiological Processes in Fear Appeals and Attitude Change: A Revised Theory of Protection Motivation." In J. Cacioppo and R. Petty (eds.), *Social Psychophysiology.* New York: Guilford Press, 1983.

Roll Call. "Senate Yet to Limit Smoking." June 12, 2012. www.rollcall.com/issues/57_149/Senate-Yet-to-Limit-Smoking-215259–1.html. Retrieved June 2013.

Roloff, M. E. *Interpersonal Communication: The Social Exchange Approach.* Thousand Oaks, CA: Sage, 1987.

Rosen, D., Stefanone, M. A., and Lackaff, D. "Online and Offline Social Networks: Investigating Culturally Specific Behavior and Satisfaction." In *Proceedings of the 43rd Hawai'i International Conference on System Sciences.* New Brunswick: Institute of Electrical and Electronics Engineers, Inc. (IEEE), 2010.

Rosenstock, I. M., and Kirscht, J. P. "The Health Belief Model and Personal Health Behavior." *Health Education Monographs,* 1974, *2,* 470–473.

Royce, R. "Health Care Reform in England—Commercial Opportunity or Another False Dawn?" *Managed Care,* 2012, *21*(8), 32. http://ftp.managedcaremag .com/archives/1208/1208.UK_Royce.html. Retrieved Jan. 2013.

Rubin, R. B., Perse, E. M., and Barbato, C. A. "Conceptualization and Measurement of Interpersonal Communication Motives." *Human Communication Research,* 1988, *14,* 602–628.

Ruxin, J., and others. "Emerging Consensus in HIV/AIDS, Malaria, Tuberculosis, and Access to Essential Medicines." *Lancet,* 2005, *356*(9459), 618–621.

Saba, W. "Why Invest in Health Communication?" The Communication Initiative. Feb. 21, 2006. http://forums.comminit.com/viewtopic.php?t=60061 andpostdays=0andpostorder=ascandandstart=45andsid=e3887d65f69451e3 949aae2a487b9601andstyle=1. Retrieved Mar. 2006.

Saba, W. "The Added-Value of Theoretical Models in Evaluating Mass Media Campaigns." Unpublished case study, 2012a.

Saba, W. "Using Process Evaluation Data to Refine an Entertainment-Education Program in Bolivia." Unpublished case study, 2012b.

Saba, W., and others. "The Mass Media and Health Beliefs: Using Media Campaigns to Promote Preventive Behavior." Unpublished case study, 1992, 1–25.

Sarriot, E. "Sustaining Child Survival: Many Roads to Choose, but Do We Have a Map. Background Document for the Child Survival Sustainability Assessment (CSSA)." Sept. 2002. http://projectlaunch.promoteprevent.org /resources/sustaining-child-survival-many-roads-choose-do-we-have-map. Retrieved June 2013.

Saunders, M.N.K., Lewis, P., and Thornhill, A. *Research Methods for Business Students.* (3rd ed.) Upper Saddle River, NJ: Prentice Hall, 2003.

Sawyer, R. "The Impact of New Social Media on Intercultural Adaptation." 2011. Senior Honor Projects, Paper 242. http://digitalcommons.uri.edu /srhonorsprog/242.

Schepens Eye Research Institute. "Media and Public Relations." 2003. www.schepens.harvard.edu/news-room/newsroom/newsroom.html. Retrieved Nov. 2005.

Schiavo, R. "UNICEF Marketing and Production Study Preliminary Analysis/Research Protocol: The Marketing and Distribution of Insecticide-Treated Mosquito Nets in Angola—A National Program." Unpublished report. Luanda, Angola: UNICEF, National Malaria Control Program, Dec. 18, 1998.

Schiavo, R. "Marketing and Production Study Final Report/Research Results: The Marketing and Distribution of Insecticide-Treated Mosquito Nets in Angola—A National Program." Unpublished report. Luanda, Angola: UNICEF, National Malaria Control Program, May 4, 2000.

Schiavo, R. "Strategies to Build Successful Multi-Sectoral Partnerships." Presented at Support Center for Nonprofit Management, 2006; Strategic Communication Resources, 2007; and Health Equity Initiative, 2012.

Schiavo, R. "Why Invest in Health Communication?" The Communication Initiative. http://forums.comminit.com/viewtopic.php?t=60061andpostdays=0and postorder=ascandandstart=60andstyle=1. Retrieved Mar. 2006.

Schiavo, R. "Communication Strategies to Influence Policy Makers: The Role of Media Advocacy in Policy and Social Change." Presented at the American Public Health Association 135th Annual Meeting and Expo, Washington, DC, Nov. 6, 2007a.

Schiavo, R. *Health Communication: From Theory to Practice*. San Francisco: Jossey-Bass, 2007b.

Schiavo, R. "The Rise of E-Health: Current Topics and Trends on Online Health Communications." *Journal of Medical Marketing*, 2008, *8*, 9–18.

Schiavo, R. "E-Health: Current Trends, Strategies, and Tools for Online Health Communications." Presented at the Office of Minority Health Resource Center, Rockville, MD, Mar. 24–25, 2009a.

Schiavo, R. Mapping & Review of Existing Guidance and Plans for Community- and Household-Based Communication to Prepare and Respond to Pandemic Flu. Research Report. New York: UNICEF, 2009b. www.unicef.org /influenzaresources/index_1072.html. Retrieved Jan. 2013.

Schiavo, R. *"Public Health Communications: Conceptual Frameworks and Models Relevant to Public Health Emergencies."* Presented at a WHO consultation, Geneva, Switzerland, Dec. 2009c.

Schiavo, R. *"Thinking Globally About Health Literacy: Looking at Key Issues and Multiple Communication Settings."* Presented at New York University, New York, Oct. 2009d.

Schiavo, R. "Public Health Communications: Conceptual Frameworks and Models Relevant to Public Health Emergencies." In World Health Organization *Social Mobilization in Public Health Emergencies: Preparedness, Readiness and Response*. Report of an Informal Consultation. Geneva: WHO, 2010a. http://whqlibdoc.who.int/hq/2010/WHO_HSE_GAR_BDP_2010.1_eng .pdf. Retrieved Jan. 2013.

Schiavo, R. "Training Paradigms for Health Communication in Urban Health Setting." Presented at the Ninth International Conference on Urban Health, New York, Oct. 2010b.

Schiavo, R. "Emerging Trends and Strategies on Evaluating New Media-Based Programs." Presented at the International Conference on Technology, Knowledge and Society, Bilbao, Spain, Mar. 25–27, 2011a. www.youtube.com/watch?v= DoKiGkuln1g. Retrieved Feb. 2013.

Schiavo, R. "Health Equity and Health Communication: A New Dawn?" *Journal of Communication in Healthcare*, 2011b, *4*(2), 67–69.

Schiavo, R. "Implementing a Social Determinants of Health Agenda: New Trends, Strategies and Case Studies." *Health Equity Initiative*. 2012a.

Schiavo, R. "Health Communication in the New Media Age: What Has Changed and What Should Not Change." Workshop presented at Health Equity Initiative, 2012b.

Schiavo, R. "Strategies to Build Successful Multi-Sectoral Partnerships." *Health Equity Initiative*. 2012c.

Schiavo, R., Boahemaa, O., Watts, B., and Hoeppner, E. "Raising the Influence of Community Voices on Health Equity: Introducing Health Equity Exchange." *Journal of Communication in Healthcare*, Aug. 2012a. http://maneypublishing .com/images/pdf_site/Health_Equity_Exchange_-_Renata_Schiavo.pdf. Retrieved Jan. 2013.

Schiavo, R., Boahemaa, O., Watts, B., and Hoeppner, E. "Raising the Influence of Community Voices on Health Equity via an Integrated Communication and Community Engagement Approach." Poster presented at the 2012 Summit on the Science of Eliminating Health Disparities, National Harbor, MD, *Dec. 18*, 2012b.

Schiavo, R., Estrada-Portales, I., and Hoeppner, E. "Preconception Health and Peer-to-Peer Communication: Assessing Results of a National Program for Infant Mortality Prevention." Presentation at the 2012 NIH Summit on the Science of Eliminating Health Disparities, National Harbor, MD, Dec. 17, 2012.

Schiavo, R., Estrada-Portales, I., Hoeppner, E., and Ormaza, D. "Building Community-Campus Partnerships to Prevent Infant Mortality: Lessons Learned from Building Capacity in Four U.S. Cities." Presented at the American Public Health Association 140th Annual Meeting and Expo, San Francisco, Oct. 29, 2012. https://apha.confex.com/apha/140am/webprogram /Paper268579.html. Retrieved Feb. 2013.

Schiavo, R., Gonzalez-Flores, M., Ramesh, R., and Estrada-Portales, I. "Taking the Pulse of Progress Toward Preconception Health: Preliminary Assessment of a National OMH Program for Infant Mortality Prevention." *Journal of Communication in Healthcare*, 2011, *4*(2), 106–117.

Schiavo, R., and Kapil, N. "Mapping and Review of Existing Guidance and Plans for Community and Household-Based Communication to Prepare and Respond to Pandemic Influenza." Poster presented at American Public Health Association 137th Annual Meeting and Expo, Philadelphia, Nov. 2009.

Schiavo, R., and Ramesh, R. "Strategic Communication in Urban Health Settings: Taking the Pulse of Emerging Needs and Trends." Online Report. New York: Strategic Communication Resources, May 2010. www.renataschiavo.com /surveyresultsnew.html. Retrieved Jan. 2013.

Schiavo, R., and Robson, P. *Workshop Sobre Éstrategias de Proteção Contra a Maláría em Angola* [Workshop on malaria protection strategies in Angola]. Unpublished report. Luanda, Angola: UNICEF, National Malaria Control Program, 1999.

Schober, M. F., and Clark, H. H. "Understanding by Addressees and Observers." *Cognitive Psychology*, 1989, *21*, 211–232.

Schoch-Spana, M., and others. "Disease, Disaster, and Democracy: The Public's Stake in Health Emergency Planning." *Biosecurity and Bioterrorism: Biodefense Strategy, Practice, and Science*, 2006, *4*(3), 313–319.

Scholl, H. J. "Applying Stakeholder Theory to E-Government: Benefits and Limits." Paper presented at the First IFIP Conference on E-commerce, E-business, E-government, Zurich, Switzerland, Oct. 2001. www.albany.edu/~hjscholl /Scholl_IFIP_2001.pdf. Retrieved July 2006.

Schultz, D., and Schultz, H. *IMC: The Next Generation*. New York: McGraw-Hill, 2003.

Schultz, D., Tannerbaum, S. I., and Lauterborn, R. F. *The New Marketing Paradigm: Integrated Marketing Communications*. Chicago: NTC Business Books, 1994.

Schuster, M., McGlynn, E., and Brook, R. "How Good Is the Quality of Care in the United States?" *Milbank Quarterly*, 1998, *76*, 517–563.

Schutz, W. C. *The Interpersonal Underworld*. Palo Alto, CA: Science and Behavioral Books, 1966.

Search Engine Land. "Infographic: The Top Three US Search Engines." 2011. http://searchengineland.com/infographic-the-top-three-us-search-engines -99036. Retrieved Mar. 2013.

Sebeok. T. A. *Signs: An Introduction to Semiotics*. Toronto: University of Toronto Press, 2001.

Sekhri, N., Feachem, R., and Ni, A. "Public-Private Integrated Partnerships Demonstrate the Potential to Improve Health Care Access, Quality, and Efficiency." *Health Affairs*, 2011, *30*(8), 1498–1507.

Selden, C. R., and others (eds.). *Health Literacy, January 1990 Through 1999*. Bethesda, MD: National Library of Medicine, Feb. 2000.

Sellors, J. W., and others. "Incidence, Clearance and Predictors of Human Papillomavirus Infection in Women." *Canadian Medical Association Journal*, 2003, *168*(4), 421–425.

Sengupta, S., and others. "HIV Interventions to Reduce HIV/AIDS Stigma: A Systematic Review." *AIDS and Behavior*, 2011, *15*(6), 1075–1087.

Sesame Workshop. "Healthy Teeth, Healthy Me." www.sesameworkshop.org /news/pressroom/oralhealth.html. Retrieved Mar. 2013.

Sheikh, A. "Book of the Month: Religion, Health and Suffering." *Journal of the Royal Society of Medicine*, 1999, *92*, 600–601.

Sindel, D. "Text Messaging Simplifies Communication for Nurses and Hospitals." *AMN Healthcare 2009*. 2009. www.nursezone.com/nursing-news -events/devices-and-technology/Text-Messaging-Simplifies-Communication -for-Nurses-and-Hospitals_24668.aspx. Retrieved Feb. 2013.

Skevington, S. M., Lotfy, M., and O'Connell, K. A. "The World Health Organization's WHOQOL-BREF Quality of Life Assessment: Psychometric Properties and Results of the International Field Trial. A Report from the WHOQOL Group." *Quality of Life Research*, 2004, *13*, 299–310.

Slater, M. D. "Theory and Method in Health Audience Segmentation." *Journal of Health Communication*, 1996, *1*, 267–283.

Slotnick, H. B., and Shershneva, M. B. "Use of Theory to Interpret Elements of Change." *Journal of Continuing Education in the Health Professions*, 2002, *22*, 197–204.

Smith, A. "Technology Trends Among People of Color." Pew Internet & American Life Project. Sept. 2010. www.pewinternet.org/Commentary/2010/September/Technology-Trends-Among-People-of-Color.aspx. Retrieved Feb. 2013.

Smith, R. D. "Psychological Type and Public Relations: Theory, Research, and Applications." *Journal of Public Relations Research*, 1993, *5*(3), 177–199.

Smith, W. A., and Hornik, R. "Marketing, Communication, and Advocacy for Large-Scale STD/HIV Prevention and Control." In K. K. Holmes and others (eds.), *Sexually Transmitted Diseases*. New York: McGraw-Hill, 1999.

Society for Neuroscience. "Programs." http://web.sfn.org/Template.cfm?Section= Programs. Retrieved Mar. 2006.

Solomon, M. Z. "The Enormity of Task: Support and Changing Practice." *Hastings Center Report*, 1995, *25*(6), S28–S32.

Solomon, M. Z., and others. "Toward an Expanded Vision of Clinical Ethics Education: From the Individual to the Institution." *Kennedy Institute of Ethics Journal*, 1991, *1*(3), 225–245.

Solomon, M. Z., and others. "Learning That Leads to Action: Impact and Characteristics of a Professional Education Approach to Improve the Care of Critically Ill Children and Their Families." *Archives of Pediatrics and Adolescent Medicine*, 2010, *164*(4), 315–322.

Solving Kids' Cancer. "Podcasts: This Week in Pediatric Oncology." http://solvingkidscancer.org/podcasts. Retrieved Dec. 2012.

Soul Beat Africa. "Situation Analysis Report on STD/HIV/AIDS in Nigeria." Communication Initiative. www.comminit.com/red-salud/node/214288. Retrieved Feb. 2006.

Southwest Center for the Application of Prevention Technologies. "Community Based Social Marketing." 2001. http://captus.samhsa.gov/southwest/resources/documents/307,12,Slide12. Retrieved Feb. 2006.

SPAN Consultants. Evaluation of Avian Influenza Community Education Interventions in Rural Egypt. Summary Report. Egypt: UNICEF, 2010.

Spickard Jr., A., and others. "Changes Made by Physicians Who Misprescribed Controlled Substances." Nashville: Vanderbilt University Medical Center. 2001. www.mc.vanderbilt.edu/root/vumc.php?site=cph&doc=1094. Retrieved Feb. 2006.

Spiegel, A. "Freud's Nephew and the Origins of Public Relations." www.npr.org/templates/story/story.php?storyId=4612464. Retrieved Nov. 2005.

Springston, J. K., Keyton, J., Leichty, G., and Metzger, J. "Field Dynamics and Public Relations Theory: Toward the Management of Multiple Publics." *Journal of Public Relations Research*, 1992, *4*(2), 81–100.

Springston, J. K., and Lariscy, R. A. "Health as Profit: Public Relations in Health Communication." Paper presented at the American Public Health Association 129th Annual Meeting, Atlanta, Oct. 2001. http://apha.confex .com/apha/129am/techprogram/paper_26391.htm. Retrieved Jan. 2006.

Standing Committee of European Doctors. "On Information to Patients and Patient Empowerment." July 2004. http://cpme.dyndns.org:591/adopted/CPME_AD _Brd_110904_080_EN.pdf. Retrieved Nov. 2005.

Steenholdt, D. "Enhancing Patient Outcomes Through the Utilization of Evidenced Based Best Practices." www.sdfmc.org/ClassLibrary/Page/Information/Data Instances/235/Files/1235/Enhancing_Patient_Outcomes_through_Utilization _of_Evidenced_Based_Best_Practices.pdf. Retrieved Jan. 2006.

Stelzner, M. "Social Media vs. Social Networking: What's the Difference?" May 2009. www.examiner.com/article/social-media-vs-social-networking-what-s -the-difference.

Step, M. M., and Finucane, M. O. "Interpersonal Communication Motives in Everyday Interactions." *Communication Quarterly*, 2002, *50*(1), 93–109.

Stock-Iwamoto, C., and Korte, R. "Primary Health Workers in North East Brazil." *Social Science and Medicine*, 1993, *36*(6), 775–782.

Strecher, V. J., and Rosenstock, I. M. *The Health Belief Model.* San Francisco: Jossey-Bass, 1997.

Suárez, E., and others. "Age-Standardized Incidence and Mortality Rates of Oral and Pharyngeal Cancer in Puerto Rico and Among Non-Hispanics Whites, Non-Hispanic Blacks, and Hispanics in the USA." *BMC Cancer*, 2009, 9, 129.

Sundar, S. "The MAIN Model: A Heuristic Approach to Understanding Technology Effects on Credibility." In M. Metzger and A. Flanagin (eds.), *Digital Media, Youth, and Credibility.* Cambridge, MA: MIT Press, 2008.

Sussman, M. State of the Blogosphere 2009. "Day 1: Who are the Bloggers? SOTB 2009." Oct. 2009. http://technorati.com/social-media/article/day-1-who-are- the-bloggers1. Retrieved Feb. 2013.

Swallow, E. "The Future of Public Relations and Social Media." Aug. 2010. http:// mashable.com/2010/08/16/pr-social-media-future. Retrieved Feb. 2013.

Tan, T. "Summary: Epidemiology of Pertussis." *Pediatric Infectious Disease Journal*, 2005, *24*(5 Suppl.), S35–S38.

Tan, T., and others. "*Applying C4D to Curb Maternal Mortality in Cambodia.*" Unpublished case study, 2012.

Tannebaum, R. D. "Emergency Medicine in Brazil." *Emedicine.* www.emedicine .com/emerg/topic930.htm. Retrieved Feb. 2006.

Tucker-Brown, A. "CDC Coffee Break: Using Mixed Methods in Program Evalua- tion." *Presentation by the Division for Heart Disease and Stroke Prevention at the Centers for Disease Control and Prevention. July 10, 2012.*

Tufts University Student Services. "Exploring the Health Professions Handbook." http://studentservices.tufts.edu/hpa/handbook.shtm. Retrieved Feb. 2006.

Twaddle, A. G., and Hessler, R. M. *A Sociology of Health*. New York: Auburn House, 1987.

Twitter. "Barack Obama @BarackObama." https://twitter.com/BarackObama. Retrieved Mar. 2013a.

Twitter. Search for "#gunviolence." https://twitter.com/search. Feb 27. 2013b.

UCLA Department of Epidemiology. School of Public Health and CNN. "Six Months Later: Anthrax Lessons Learned." www.ph.ucla.edu/epi/bioter/sixmoanthraxlessons.html. Retrieved Mar. 2002.

Ukrainian Catholic Church in Australia, New Zealand, and Oceania. "What Is the Meaning of Illness?" http://catholicukes.org.au/tiki/tiki-print_article.php?articleId=160. Retrieved Jan. 2006.

UMass Medical School. "Macy Initiative in Health Communication." www.umassmed.edu/macy. Retrieved Mar. 2006.

UNAIDS. "Community Mobilization." www.unaids.org/en/Issues/Prevention_treatment/community_mobilization.asp. Retrieved Sept. 2005.

UNAIDS. Promising Practices in Community Engagement for Elimination of New HIV Infections Among Children by 2015 and Keeping Their Mothers Alive. Geneva: UNAIDS, 2012.

Underhill, C., and Mckeown, L. "Getting a Second Opinion: Health Information and the Internet." *Health Reports*, 2008, *19*(1), 65–69.

UNFPA. "Linking Population, Poverty and Development." www.unfpa.org/pds/urbanization.htm. Retrieved Dec. 2012.

UNICEF. Division of Communication, Health Communication Materials. "Communication Programme Planning Work Sheet." Communication Initiative. 2001. www.stoptb.org/assets/documents/getinvolved/resmob/Communication%20Programme%20Planning%20Work%20Sheet.pdf. Retrieved June 2013.

UNICEF. National Immunization Day for the Eradication of Polio in Egypt: Post Assessment. Final Report. Egypt: UNICEF, 2006a.

UNICEF. "Right to Know Initiative: Communication Strategy Development Handbook." www.actforyouth.net/documents/comstrat_toolkit.pdf. Retrieved Mar. 2006b.

UNICEF. Strategic Communication for Behavior and Social Change in South Asia. Kathmandu, Nepal: Regional Office of South Asia, 2006c.

UNICEF. "Communication for Development. The Big Picture" www.unicef.org/cbsc/index.html. Retrieved Dec. 2012.

UNICEF. "Communication for Development. C4D Approaches." www.unicef.org/cbsc/index_42148.html. Retrieved Feb. 2013a.

UNICEF. "Negative and Positive Clichés." www3.extranet.unicef.org/myFolder/c-rights/neg-pos-imagery.html. Retrieved Mar. 2013b.

Unilever. "Unilever to Make Country Crock Soft Spreads Trans-Fat-Free." www.unileverusa.com/media-center/pressreleases/2005/Country_Crock_TFF.aspx. Retrieved Jan. 2006.

United Nations Development Programme. "The Legislature and Constituency Relations." http://mirror.undp.org/magnet/Docs/parliaments/notes/Constituency%20Relations%205%20.htm. Retrieved Feb. 2006.

United Nations Foundation. "Understanding Public-Private Partnerships." 2003. www.globalproblems-globalsolutions-files.org/unf_website/PDF/understand_public_private_partner.pdf.

United Nations Foundation. "mHealth Alliance." www.unfoundation.org/what-we-do/campaigns-and-initiatives/mhealth-alliance. Retrieved Feb. 2013.

United States Census Bureau. "New Bedford (city), Massachusetts". http://quickfacts.census.gov/qfd/states/25/2545000.html. Retrieved Dec. 2012.

University of British Columbia. "Evaluating Information Sources." 2012. http://help.library.ubc.ca/evaluating-and-citing-sources/evaluating-information-sources. Retrieved Mar. 2013.

University of Michigan Health System. Program for Multicultural Health. www.med.umich.edu/multicultural. Retrieved Oct. 2005.

University of Utah. "IMC: Integrated Marketing Communication Certificate Program." Communication Institute. University of Utah. http://communication.utah.edu/programs/integrated-marketing/index.php. Retrieved Jan. 2013.

University of Wisconsin, Extension Program Development. "Program Development and Evaluation." www.uwex.edu/ces/pdande/evaluation/evallogicmodel.html. Retrieved Dec. 2005.

US Agency for International Development. "Behavior Change Interventions." 1999. www.jhpiego.org/files/bcireport.pdf. Retrieved Feb. 2006.

US Department of Health and Human Services. *The Health Consequences of Using Smokeless Tobacco. A Report of the Advisory Committee to the Surgeon General.* Washington, DC: US Department of Health and Human Services, 1986.

US Department of Health and Human Services. *Preventing Tobacco Use Among Young People: A Report of the Surgeon General.* Washington, DC: US Department of Health and Human Services, 1994.

US Department of Health and Human Services. "Communicating in a Crisis: Risk Communication Guidelines for Public Officials." Washington, DC: US Department of Health and Human Services, 2002. www.hhs.gov/od/documents/RiskCommunication.pdf. Retrieved Apr. 2010.

US Department of Health and Human Services. Office of Disease Prevention and Health Promotion. *Healthy People 2010.* (vols. 1 and 2). 2005. www.healthypeople.gov/2010/Document/tableofcontents.htm#parta. Retrieved Oct. 2012.

US Department of Health and Human Services. Office of Disease Prevention and Health Promotion. "Making Better Health Communication a Reality: A Midcourse Check on *Healthy People 2010* Objectives." *Prevention Report,* 2006a, *20*(3, 4). http://odphp.osophs.dhhs.gov/pubs/prevrpt/Volume20/Issue3pr.htm. Retrieved July 2006.

US Department of Health and Human Services. Office of Minority Health. "What Is Cultural Competency?" 2006b. http://minorityhealth.hhs.gov/templates/browse.aspx?lvl=2&lvlID=11. Retrieved June 2013.

US Department of Health and Human Services. Office of Minority Health. "Evaluation Planning Guidelines for Grant Applicants." 2010. http://minorityhealth.hhs.gov/Assets/pdf/Checked/1/Evaluation%20Planning%20Guidelines%20for%20Grant%20Applicants.pdf. Retrieved Mar. 2013.

US Department of Health and Human Services. "Health Communication." www.health.gov/communication/resources/Default.asp. Retrieved July 2012a.

US Department of Health and Human Services. *Healthy People 2020*. "Health Communication and Health Information Technology." http://healthypeople.gov/2020/topicsobjectives2020/overview.aspx?topicid=18. Retrieved July 2012b.

US Department of Health and Human Services. Office of Minority Health. "Preconception Peer Educators (PPE) Program." http://minorityhealth.hhs.gov/templates/content.aspx?ID=8394. Retrieved Feb. 2013.

US Food and Drug Administration. "FDA Licenses New Vaccine for Prevention of Cervical Cancer and Other Diseases in Females Caused by Human Papillomavirus." *FDA News*, June 8, 2006. www.fda.gov/NewsEvents/Newsroom/PressAnnouncements/2006/ucm108666.htm. Retrieved June 2013.

US Food and Drug Administration. "FDA Approves New Indication for Gardasil to Prevent Genital Warts in Men and Boys." *FDA News Release*, Oct. 16, 2009. www.fda.gov/NewsEvents/Newsroom/PressAnnouncements/ucm187003.htm. Retrieved Mar. 2013.

Vancouver/Richmond Early Psychosis Intervention. "Early Intervention: Why Is It Needed?" www.hopevancouver.com/Early_Intervention-Why_is_it_Needed.html. Retrieved Mar. 2013.

Vanderford, M. L. "Communication Lessons Learned in the Emergency Operations Center During CDC's Anthrax Response: A Commentary." *Journal of Health Communication*, 2003, *8*(Suppl. 1), 11–12.

VanLeeuwen, J. A., Waltner-Toews, D., Abernathy, T., and Smit, B. "Evolving Models of Human Health Toward an Ecosystem Context." *Ecosystem Health*, 1999, *5*(3), 204–219.

Vartanian, T. P. *Secondary Data Analysis*. New York: Oxford University Press, 2011.

Veenhoven, R. "Healthy Happiness: Effects of Happiness on Physical Health and the Consequences for Preventive Health Care." *Journal of Happiness Studies*, 2008, *9*(3), 449–469. www.instituteofcoaching.org/images/pdfs/VeenhovenHealthHappiness2006.pdf. Retrieved June 2013.

Ventola, C. L. "Direct-to-Consumer Pharmaceutical Advertising." *Pharmacy and Therapeutics*, 2011, *36*(10), 669–674, 681–684.

Vernon, J. G. "Immunisation Policy: From Compliance to Concordance?" *British Journal of General Practice*, 2003, *53*, 399–404.

Vieira, D. L. "*The Role of the Health Sciences Librarian in Health Communication: Continuity in Evidence-Based Public Health Training for Future Public Health Practitioners*." Unpublished Case Study, 2013.

Virginia Public Health Association. "Events." http://vapha.org/events. Retrieved Mar. 2013.

Viswanathan, M., *and others.* Community-Based Participatory Research: Assessing the Evidence. Rockville, MD: Agency for Healthcare Research and Quality, Aug. 2004.

Vlahov, D., and others. "Urban as a Determinant of Health." *Journal of Urban Health*, 2007, *84*(Suppl. 1), 16–26.

Vlassoff, C., and Manderson, L. "Incorporating Gender in the Anthropology of Infectious Diseases." *Tropical Medicine and International Health*, 1998, *3*(12), 1011–1019.

Vovici. "Response Rates Driven by 16 Major Factors." 2010. http://blog.vovici.com /blog/bid/26604/Response-Rates-Driven-by-16-Major-Factors. Retrieved Mar. 2013.

Waelkens, M-P., and Greindl, I. *Urban Health: Particularities, Challenges, Experiences and Lessons Learnt.* Eschborn, Germany: Deutsche Gesellschaft für Technische Zusammenarbeit, 2001.

Waisbord, S. "Family Tree of Theories, Methodologies and Strategies in Development Communication." May 2001. Prepared for the Rockefeller Foundation. The Communication Initiative. www.comminit.com/?q=global/node/1547. Retrieved June 2013.

Waisbord, S., and Larson, H. *Why Invest in Communication for Immunization: Evidence and Lessons Learned.* Baltimore: Johns Hopkins Bloomberg School of Public Health, Center for Communication Programs, and New York: United Nations Children's Fund, June 2005.

The Waiting Room: 24 Hours, 241 Patients, One Stretched ER. Waiting Room. 2012. www.whatruwaitingfor.com. Retrieved Feb. 2013.

Wakefield, M. A., Loken, B., and Hornik, R. C. "Use of Mass Media Campaigns to Change Health Behavior." *Lancet*, 2010, *376*(9748), 1261–1271.

Wall Street Journal. "The Growing Clout of Online Patient Groups." June 2007. http://online.wsj.com/article/SB118168968368633094.html. Retrieved Feb. 2013.

Wallace Foundation. "Workbook H: Self-Administered Surveys: Conducting Surveys via Mail and Email." www.wallacefoundation.org/knowledge-center /after-school/collecting-and-using-data/Documents/Workbook-H-Self -Administered.pdf. Retrieved Mar. 2013.

Wang, C. C. "Photovoice: A Participatory Action Research Strategy Applied to Women's Health." *Journal of Women's Health*, 1999, *8*(2), 185–192.

Wang, C., and Burris, M. "Empowerment Through Photo Novella: Portraits of Participation." *Health Education Quarterly*, 1994, *21*(2), 171–186.

Wang, C., and Burris, M. "Photovoice: Concept, Methodology, and Use for Participatory Needs Assessment." *Health Education & Behavior*, 1997, *25*(3), 369–387.

Wang, S. S., Brownell, K. D., and Wadden, T. A. "The Influence of the Stigma of Obesity on Overweight Individuals." *International Journal of Obesity*, 2004, *28*(10), 1333–1337.

Washington State Department of Health. "Guidelines for Developing Easy-to-Read Health Education Materials." June 2000. www3.doh.wa.gov/here/howto/images/easy2.html. Retrieved Mar. 2006.

Watson, S. "Using Results to Improve the Lives of Children and Families: A Guide for Public-Private Child Care Partnerships." Fairfax, VA: National Child Care Information Center, 2000. www.eric.ed.gov/ERICWebPortal/search/detailmini.jsp?_nfpb=true&_&ERICExtSearch_SearchValue_0=ED449892&ERICExtSearch_SearchType_0=no&accno=ED449892. Retrieved June 2013.

Weinreich, N. K. *Hands-on Social Marketing: A Step-by-Step Guide*. Newbury Park, CA: Sage, 1999.

Weinreich, N. K. *Hands-on Social Marketing: A Step-by-Step Guide to Designing Change for Good*. (2nd ed.) Thousand Oaks, CA: Sage, 2011.

Weinstock, H., Berman, S., and Cates, W., Jr. "Sexually Transmitted Diseases Among American Youth: Incidence and Prevalence Estimates, 2000." *Perspectives on Sexual and Reproductive Health*, 2004, *36*(1), 6–10.

Weir, S. J., DeGennaro, L. J., and Austin, C. P. "Repurposing Approved and Abandoned Drugs for the Treatment and Prevention of Cancer Through Public-Private Partnership." *Cancer Research*, 2012, *72*(5), 1055–1058.

White House. "Engage and Connect." www.whitehouse.gov/engage/office. Retrieved Feb. 2013.

Wiggins, B. B., and Deeb-Sossa, N. "Conducting Telephone Surveys." 2000. www.irss.unc.edu/irss/bwiggins/shortcourses/telephonehandout.pdf. Retrieved Mar. 2006.

Wikipedia. "Blog." http://en.wikipedia.org/wiki/Blog. Retrieved Feb. 2013.

Williams, A., Zraik, D., Schiavo, R., and Hatz, D. "Raising Awareness of Sustainable Food Issues and Building Community via the Integrated Use of New Media with Other Communication Approaches." *Cases in Public Health Communication and Marketing*, 2008, *2*, 159–177. http://sphhs.gwu.edu/departments/pch/phcm/casesjournal/volume2/invited/cases_2_10.cfm. Retrieved Feb. 2013.

Winau, R. "The Hippocratic Oath and Ethics in Medicine." *Forensic Science International*, 1994, *9*(3), 285–289.

Witte, K., and Allen, M. "A Meta-Analysis of Fear Appeals: Implications for Effective Public Health Campaigns." *Health Education and Behavior*, 2000, *27*(5), 591–615.

Wood. J. T. *Gendered Lives: Communication, Gender, and Culture*. Boston: Wadsworth Cengage Learning, 2009.

Woods, J. E., and Kiely, J. M. "Short-Term International Medical Services." *Mayo Clinic's Proceedings*, 2000, *75*, 311–313.

World Bank, "Development Communication." http://web.worldbank.org/WBSITE/EXTERNAL/TOPICS/EXTDEVCOMMENG/0,,menuPK:34000201~pagePK:34000189~piPK:34000199~theSitePK:423815,00.html. Retrieved Feb. 2013.

World Health Organization. "Constitution of the World Health Organization." New York, July 22, 1946. www.who.int/governance/eb/who_constitution_en.pdf. Retrieved Oct. 2005.

World Health Organization. Mediterranean Centre for Vulnerability Reduction. "Mobilizing for Action, Communication-for-Behavioural-Impact (COMBI)." 2003. The Communication Initiative. www.comminit.com/combi/content /mobilizing-action-communication-behavioural-impact-combi.   Retrieved June 2013.

World Health Organization. Mediterranean Center for Vulnerability Reduction. "COMBI in Action: Country Highlights." 2004a. http://wmc.who.int/pdf /COMBI_in_Action_04.pdf. Retrieved Apr. 2006.

World Health Organization and Global Polio Eradication Initiative. "Polio Eradication in India." www.sciencedirect.com/science/article/pii/S0264410 X12018476. Retrieved Nov. 2004.

World Health Organization. "Social Mobilization to Fight Ebola in Yambio, Southern Sudan." Action Against Infection, 2004c. http://wmc.who.int/pdf /Action_Against_Infection.pdf. Retrieved Jan. 2006.

World Health Organization and Joint United Nations Programme on HIV/AIDS. "Access to HIV Treatment Continues to Accelerate in Developing Countries, but Bottlenecks Persist, Says WHO/UNAIDS Report." 2005a. www.who.int /3by5/progressreportJune2005/en. Retrieved Jan. 2006.

World Health Organization. Social Mobilization and Training Team. "Guidelines for Social Mobilization, Planning Communication-for-Behavioural-Impact (COMBI) in TB Control." www.stoptb.org/assets/documents/countries /acsm/TB-COMBI%20Guide%202.pdf. Retrieved Nov. 2005b.

World Health Organization. *Preventing Chronic Disease: A Vital Investment. WHO Global Report.* Geneva: WHO, 2005c. www.who.int/chp/chronic _disease_report/contents/part1.pdf. Retrieved Jan. 2013.

World Health Organization. "Responding to the Avian Influenza Pandemic Threat—Recommended   Strategic   Actions."   2005d.   www.who.int/csr /resources/publications/influenza/WHO_CDS_CSR_GIP_05_8-EN.pdf. Retrieved Nov. 2012.

World Health Organization. "Malaria and Travelers." www.who.int/malaria /preventionmethods.html. Retrieved Feb. 2006.

World Health Organization. "Appropriate Information-Communications Technologies for Developing Countries." *Bulletin of the World Health Organization,* 2007, 85(4). www.who.int/bulletin/volumes/85/4/07−041475/en. Retrieved Feb. 2013.

World Health Organization. "Defining Objectives and Preparing an Action Plan. 6.1 Defining Objectives." *Managing WHO Humanitarian Response in the Field.* 2008. www.who.int/hac/techguidance/tools/manuals/who_field _handbook/6/en/index1.html.

World Health Organization. *Social Mobilization in Public Health Emergencies: Preparedness, Readiness, and Response.* Geneva: WHO, 2010.

World Health Organization. "Communication for Behavioural Impact (COMBI). A Toolkit for Behavioural and Social Communication in Outbreak Response." 2012a. www.who.int/ihr/publications/combi_toolkit_outbreaks/en.

World Health Organization. "Global Polio Emergency Action Plan 2012–2013. Web Annex 1: List of Innovations in the India Polio Eradication Program." 2012b. www.polioeradication.org/Portals/0/Document/Resources/StrategyWork/EAP/EAP_annex1.pdf. Retrieved Jan. 2013a.

World Health Organization. "Polio Eradication Initiative. 3.2 Million Children Vaccinated in South Sudan." www.emro.who.int/polio/polio-news/3-million-children-vaccinated-south-sudan.html. Retrieved Jan. 2013b.

Wu, S. "Department of Health Targets Asians with Anti-Smoking Ads." *NYU-LOCAL.* March 6, 2012. http://nyulocal.com/city/2012/03/06/department-of-health-targets-asians-with-anti-smoking-ads. Retrieved Mar. 2013.

Yaxley, H. "Monitoring and Evaluation." In A. Theaker and H. Yaxley, *The Public Relations Strategic Toolkit: An Essential Guide to Successful Public Relations Practice.* New York: Routledge, 2013.

Zagaria, M.A.E. "Low Health Literacy: Raising Awareness for Optimal Health Communication." *U.S. Pharmacist*, 2004, *10*, 41–48.

Zaman, F., and Underwood, C. *The Gender Guide for Health Communication Programs.* Baltimore: Johns Hopkins Bloomberg School of Public Health, Center for Communication Programs, Mar. 2003.

Zarcadoolas, C. "The Simplicity Complex: Exploring Simplified Health Messages in a Complex World." *Health Promotion International*, 2011, *26*(3), 338–350.

Zarcadoolas, C., Pleasant, A. and Greer, D. S. *Advancing Health Literacy: A Framework for Understanding and Action.* San Francisco: Jossey-Bass, 2006.

Zolnierek, K.B.H., and DiMatteo, M. R. "Physician Communication and Patient Adherence to Treatment: A Meta-Analysis." *Medical Care*, 2009, *47*(8), 826–834.

Zorn, M., Allen, M. P., and Horowitz, A. M. "Understanding Health Literacy and Its Barriers: Bibliography on the Internet." Bethesda, MD: National Library of Medicine, May 2004. www.nlm.nih.gov/archive/20040830/pubs/cbm/healthliteracybarriers.htmle. Retrieved June 2013.

Zuger, A. "Doctors Learn How to Say What No One Wants to Hear." *New York Times*, Jan. 10, 2006.

Zunker, C., Rutt, C., and Meza, G. "Perceived Health Needs of Elderly Mexicans Living on the U.S.–Mexico Border." *Journal of Transcultural Nursing*, 2005, *16*(1), 50–56.

NAME INDEX